SYSTEMIC PATHOLOGY / THIRD EDITION

Volume 13 **The Breast**

SYSTEMIC PATHOLOGY / THIRD EDITION

Emeritus Editor W. St C. Symmers

Volume Editors

M. C. Anderson **Female Reproductive System**

I. D. Ansell **Male Reproductive System**

M. E. Catto and A. J. Malcolm **Bone, Joints and Soft Tissues**

B. Corrin **The Lungs**

M. J. Davies and J. Mann **The Cardiovascular System: Part B**

C. W. Elston and I. O. Ellis **The Breast**

I. Friedmann **Nose, Throat and Ears**

K. Henry and W. St C. Symmers **Thymus, Lymph Nodes, Spleen and Lymphatics**

P. D. Lewis **Endocrine System**

B. C. Morson **Alimentary Tract**

K. A. Porter, R. C. B. Pugh and I. D. Ansell **The Kidneys/The Urinary Tract**

W. B. Robertson **The Cardiovascular System: Part A**

D. Weedon **The Skin**

R. O. Weller **Nervous System, Muscle and Eyes**

S. N. Wickramasinghe **Blood and Bone Marrow**

D. G. D. Wight **Liver, Biliary Tract and Exocrine Pancreas**

For Churchill Livingstone

Commissioning Editor: Gavin Smith
Copy Editor: Carolyn Holleyman
Indexer: Liza Weinkove
Design Direction: Sarah Cape
Marketing: Susan Jerdan-Taylor

SYSTEMIC PATHOLOGY / THIRD EDITION

Emeritus Editor W. St C. Symmers

Volume 13

The Breast

EDITED BY

C. W. Elston
MD MBBS FRCPath

Professor of Tumour Pathology, Nottingham University Medical School;
Consultant Histopathologist, City Hospital, Nottingham, UK

AND

I. O. Ellis
MBBS MRCPath

Reader in Pathology, Nottingham University Medical School;
Consultant Histopathologist, City Hospital, Nottingham, UK

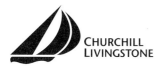

CHURCHILL LIVINGSTONE

EDINBURGH LONDON NEW YORK PHILADELPHIA SAN FRANCISCO SYDNEY TORONTO 1998

CHURCHILL LIVINGSTONE
A Division of Harcourt Publishers Limited

© Harcourt Brace and Company Limited 1998
© Harcourt Publishers Limited 2000

D is a registered trademark of Harcourt Publishers
Limited.

First published 1998
Reprinted 1999
Reprinted 2000

ISBN 0 443 03723X

British Library Cataloguing in Publication Data
A catalogue record for this book is available from the British
Library.

Library of Congress Cataloging in Publication Data
A catalog record for this book is available from the Library of
Congress.

Note
Medical knowledge is constantly changing. As new
information becomes available, changes in treatment,
procedures, equipment and the use of drugs become
necessary. The editors, authors, contributors and the
publishers have, as far as it is possible, taken care to ensure
that the information given in this text is accurate and up to
date. However, readers are strongly advised to confirm that
the information, especially with regard to drug usage,
complies with latest legislation and standards of practice.

The
publisher's
policy is to use
paper manufactured
from sustainable forests

Printed in Great Britain by Redwood Books Limited

Preface

In the previous edition of *Systemic Pathology* the breast was covered by a single chapter of 100 pages placed in Volume 4 as a somewhat uneasy bedfellow amongst the urinary, reproductive and endocrine systems. The elevation to an independent volume in this edition is a reflection of the enormous expansion of interest in breast disease in the ensuing 20 years, resulting in the establishment of breast pathology as a sub-specialty in its own right. There are, of course, a number of reasons for this, including the development of accurate pre-operative diagnostic techniques, expansion of the therapeutic options for the management of patients with breast cancer and the introduction of mammographic screening programmes. The role of the histopathologist has therefore changed dramatically, from a rather isolated and basic diagnostic arbitration of 'benign' or 'malignant' to full participation in multidisciplinary team decision-making on all aspects of diagnosis and management. At the same time there have been remarkable developments in molecular biology and genetics which have helped to improve our understanding of underlying disease processes, although it remains a paradox that in this technological era no consistent substitute has yet been found for careful evaluation of the morphological characteristics of breast lesions as far as patient management is concerned.

For the foreseeable future then, diagnostic histopathology will remain as an integral part of the clinical breast service, and in producing this book we have tried to give an appropriate emphasis to this multidisciplinary philosophy. In this respect we have been particularly fortunate in our close collaboration with colleagues in the Nottingham Breast Service, especially Professor Roger Blamey and Mr John Robertson, our surgeons, Drs Robin Wilson and Andrew Evans, our radiologists, and Drs David Morgan and Steven Chan, our clinical oncologists. We have drawn heavily on our own experience in treating over 4000 patients with breast cancer over the last 24 years, and many more with benign disease, but have also attempted to provide extensive reference to the published literature. For certain specific topics we felt the need to call on expertise from other centres and we are extremely grateful to our colleagues Vincenzo Eusebi and Maria Foschini for their chapter on rare carcinomas (Ch. 16); David Page, Roy Jensen and Jean Simpson for their chapters on epithelial hyperplasia (Ch. 5) and lobular neoplasia (Ch. 6) and John Sloane for his chapter on quality assurance in breast pathology (Ch. 24).

Our aim has been to provide a comprehensive account of the pathological aspects of breast disease of relevance to the diagnostic histopathologist and in keeping with the general philosophy of the *Systemic Pathology* series. Although we have concentrated on traditional histopathological characteristics, the role of newer techniques such as immunocytochemistry is emphasised where appropriate. We have already referred to the enhanced clinical role played by histopathologists in the modern management of patients with breast disease. There is perhaps no better evocation of our duty to the patient than the following quotation from Sir Robert Hutchinson (1871–1960):

From inability to leave well alone;
From too much zeal for the new and
contempt for what is old;
From putting knowledge before wisdom,
science before art and cleverness before
common sense;
From treating patients as cases and from

making the cure of the disease more grievous
than the endurance of the same,
Good Lord deliver us.

Christopher W. Elston

Nottingham 1998   Ian O. Ellis

Acknowledgements

In the Preface we indicated the close collaboration which we enjoy with our colleagues in the Nottingham Breast Service and we thank them all for their continued help and support. We are particularly grateful to Roger Blamey, Robin Wilson and Andrew Evans for their contributions to this book. Our sincere thanks are also due to Sarah Pinder, Clinical Research Fellow (now Senior Lecturer/Consultant Histopathologist, City Hospital, Nottingham), Helen Goulding, Lecturer in Pathology (now Consultant Histopathologist, Jersey Pathological Service) and David Poller, Senior Registrar (now Consultant Pathologist, Portsmouth) for their considerable help in the preparation of many of the chapters. We have received invaluable assistance from our laboratory and secretarial staff, but we must make special mention of members of the 'B' team: Jane Bell, Tracey Clarke, Glynn Donovan, Patrick Kumah, Heather Mounteney, Helen Naylor, John Ronan, Peter Wencyk and Jayne Whilding (who was responsible for most of the manuscript production). We are very grateful to Heather Mounteney for help with photomicrography, Lyndon Cochrane and Sandra Huskinson for line drawings and Geoffrey Gilbert and Sue Hirst for other photographic material. We are indebted to the editorial staff at Churchill Livingstone for their patience and helpful advice: initially, Lowri Daniels and Geoff Nuttall, and, latterly, Gavin Smith. Although William Symmers was no longer taking an active editorial role when this book was being produced, we should like to record our gratitude to him for inviting us to participate in the *Systemic Pathology* series. Finally, we must acknowledge the debt to our families for the sacrifices of time spent away from them and for their support in this venture.

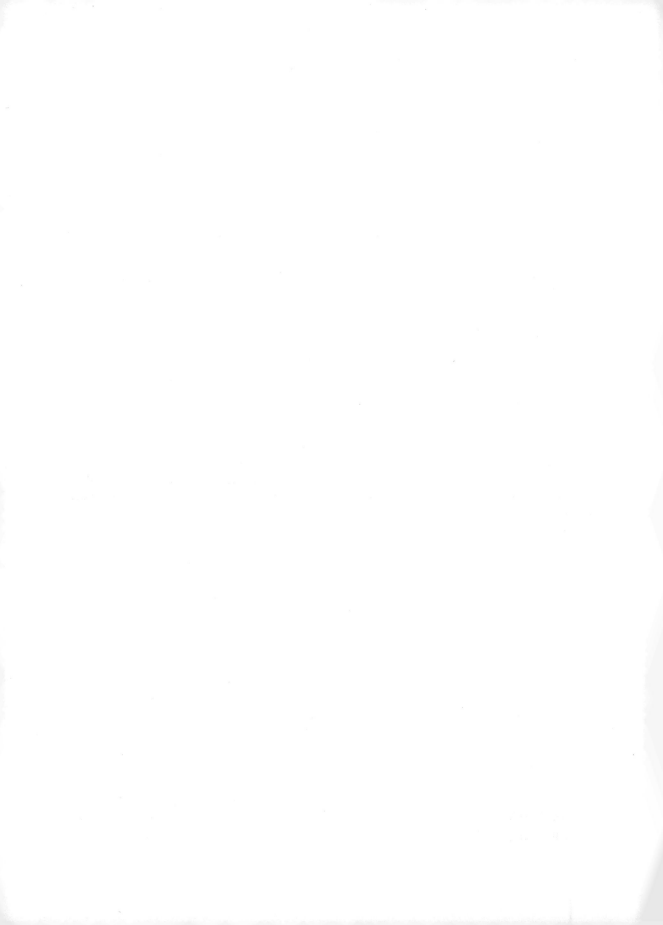

Contributors

R. W. Blamey
MD MA FRCS FRACS(Hon) FRCSG(Hon)
Professor of Surgical Science, University of Nottingham; Consultant Surgeon, Nottingham City Hospital, Nottingham, UK

I. O. Ellis
MBBS MRCPath
Reader in Pathology, Nottingham University Medical School; Consultant Histopathologist, City Hospital, Nottingham, UK

C. W. Elston
MD MBBS FRCPath
Professor of Tumour Pathology, Nottingham University Medical School; Consultant Histopathologist, City Hospital, Nottingham, UK

V. Eusebi
MD FRCPath
Professor of Pathology, Bellaria Hospital, University of Bologna, Bologna, Italy

A. J. Evans
MRCP FRCR
Consultant Radiologist, City Hospital, Nottingham, UK

M. P. Foschini
MD
Consultant Histopathologist, Bellaria Hospital, University of Bologna, Bologna, Italy

H. Goulding
BA MBBS MRCPath
Consultant Histopathologist, States of Jersey

Laboratory, The General Hospital, St Helier, Jersey

Roy A. Jensen
MD
Associate Professor of Pathology and Cell Biology, Department of Pathology, Vanderbilt University Medical Center, Nashville, USA

David L. Page
MD
Professor of Pathology and Director of Anatomic Pathology, Department of Pathology, Vanderbilt University Medical Center, Nashville, USA

S. E. Pinder
MBChB MRCPath
Senior Lecturer in Pathology, Nottingham University Medical School; Consultant Histopathologist, City Hospital, Nottingham, UK

D. N. Poller
MBChB MRCPath
Consultant Pathologist, Department of Pathology, Queen Alexandra Hospital, Cosham, Portsmouth, UK

Jean F. Simpson
MD
Associate Professor, Department of Pathology, Vanderbilt University Medical Center, Nashville, USA

J. P. Sloane
MB FRCPath

Professor of Pathology, University of Liverpool;
Honorary Consultant Pathologist, Royal
Liverpool University Hospitals, Liverpool, UK

A. R. M. Wilson
MBChB FRCR FRCP(E)

Consultant Radiologist, City Hospital,
Nottingham, UK

Contents

Normal structure and developmental abnormalities

EMBRYOLOGICAL DEVELOPMENT

The breasts are often described as modified sweat glands. This view oversimplifies their developmental history and helps little towards understanding either the complex physiological changes to which they are subject during reproductive life or the pathological changes to which their highly specialized structural and functional responses make them liable. The phylogenetic relationship of the mammary glands to sweat glands is, in fact, fully established;[1] their specialization, however, dates from a stage so far distant in evolution (more than 150 million years ago) that it is already apparent when the first evidence of their development is recognizable in the human embryo.

The mammary line (primitive milk streak, galactic streak), which is the initial stage in development of the breast tissue, appears at about the 7 mm stage of embryonic growth (fifth or sixth week) and extends on each side of the body from the axilla to the groin.[1] The caudal two thirds of each line disappears by the 20 mm stage (seventh or eighth week) and eventually only the mid portion of the cephalic third remains. It is from this residuum of the milk line that the mammary primordium develops. By the 60–90 mm stage (12–16 weeks) mesenchymal cells differentiate into the smooth muscle of the nipple and areola. Epithelial buds then develop and branch to form between 15 and 25 sprouts which represent the future secretory apparatus; adipose tissue forms around these sprouts. The secondary mammary anlage follows with hair follicle, sebaceous gland and sweat gland differentiation. It appears that the

1

developments which occur up to this stage are independent of hormonal influences.

From about the 20th–32nd week of pregnancy placental sex hormones enter the fetal circulation and induce canalization of the epithelial sprouts to form a branching system composed of 15–25 major ducts. Distinction into the two layers of epithelium, secretory and myoepithelial, can be recognized ultrastructurally at about 20 weeks,[2] but the biochemical phenotype is not yet established.[3] Between 32 and 40 weeks secretory activity begins, with the production of colostrum. The nipple-areolar complex develops further and becomes pigmented. Apart from minor growth and branching of the duct system, no significant changes occur in the mammary tissue from then until the onset of puberty.

ANATOMY AND MICROSCOPICAL STRUCTURE

The adult female breasts lie on the upper chest wall, the upper edges at the level of the second or third rib and the lower edge at the level of the sixth rib. Medially they extend to the edge of the sternum and laterally to the anterior axillary line, although the tail may extend further into the axilla. The breasts vary greatly in size from individual to individual, in general having a correlation with overall body mass. It is not unusual for one breast to be slightly larger than the other. The contour of the breasts is also variable. In the early post pubertal period it is usually domelike, but with increasing age, especially in parous women, the breasts become pendulous.

The detailed anatomy and microanatomy of the breast has been covered in greater depth elsewhere;[4–5] only a brief summary is provided here. The breasts consist of three major components, the skin, the subcutaneous adipose tissue and the functional glandular tissue which comprises both parenchyma and stroma (Fig. 1.1). The nipple-areolar complex which is centrally placed contains abundant sensory nerves and sebaceous and apocrine glands, but no follicles except at the very periphery. Morgagni's tubercles, located in the areola, are elevations formed by the openings of the ducts of Montgomery's glands. These are of sebaceous type. At the tip of the nipple are the

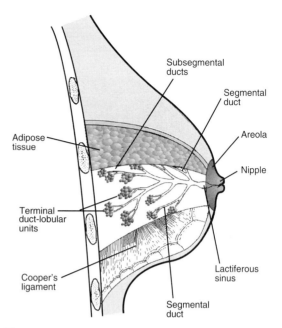

Fig. 1.1   Schematic cross-section of mature female breast to show the main anatomical structures.

openings of the collecting ducts through which the infant obtains milk at suckling. Immediately beneath the nipple the collecting ducts dilate to form the lactiferous sinuses which are surrounded by intertwining fascicles of smooth muscle continuous with the musculature of the nipple. Deep to this the breast is divided into 15–25 lobes, each based on a branching duct system leading from the collecting ducts via segmental and subsegmental ducts to the terminal duct-lobular units (TDLU) which are the functional site of milk production (Fig. 1.2). Each duct drains a lobe made up of 20–40 lobules. The main bulk of each lobe is made up of adipose tissue and fibrous stroma, the so-called inter- or peri-lobular connective tissue. The superficial pectoral fascia envelops the breast, which lies on the deep pectoral fascia; fibrous bands connect these two layers (Coopers suspensory ligaments), providing a degree of support to the breast. It is probable that increasing laxity of these ligaments with age and parity is responsible for the pendulous shape of the breast in older women.

In the nipple the stratified squamous epithelium of the surface extends for a variable but short distance into the collecting ducts. There is then a relatively abrupt change to the glandular epithe-

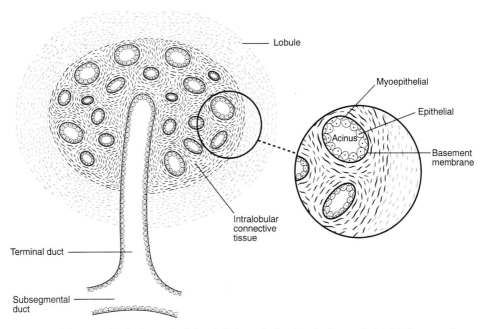

Fig. 1.2 Diagram of a single terminal duct-lobular unit showing the inter-relationship between the epithelial and stromal components.

lium which is present throughout the duct and lobular system. In keeping with its phylogenetic origin this epithelium is composed of two distinct types of cell, the secretory or luminal cell and the myoepithelial cell (Figs 1.3 and 1.4). In the collecting ducts the luminal cells are generally columnar whilst in the lobular acini they are more usually cuboidal. Detailed microanatomical studies have shown that there are two types of luminal secretory cell.[5] Basal cells have relatively clear cytoplasm and form microvilli where they are in contact with the lumen; the nucleus is oval and

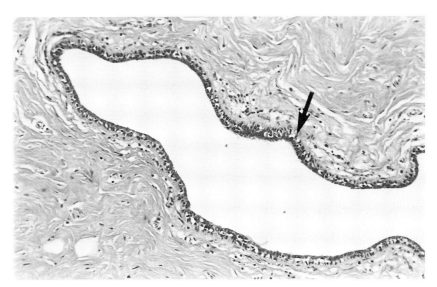

Fig. 1.3 Segmental breast duct. Even at this magnification the epithelial and myoepithelial cells (arrowhead) can be identified separately. Hematoxylin–eosin × 125.

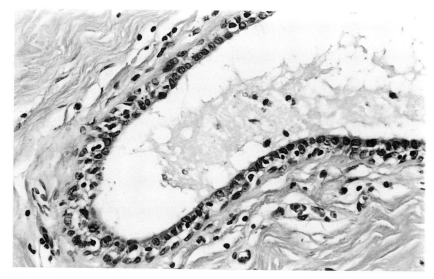

Fig. 1.4 Higher magnification of another breast duct showing the bilaminar structure of epithelial and myoepithelial cells, with some luminal secretion. Hematoxylin–eosin × 400.

lacks a nucleolus. Superficial cells are darker with basophilic cytoplasm rich in ribosomes. They undergo intercellular dehiscence, with swelling of mitochondria, forming buds within the lumen. The myoepithelial cells form a layer between the luminal secretory cells and the basement membrane. This is often discontinuous, the cells appearing small and flattened with dark nuclei and clear cytoplasm (Fig. 1.4), although they may be more numerous and form a complete layer. The myoepithelial cytoplasm contain myofibrils 50–80 nm in diameter which are inserted by hemidesmosomes into the basement membrane. These cells may be readily identified by immunostaining with anti-smooth muscle actin (Figs 1.5, 1.10 and 1.11).[3,6]

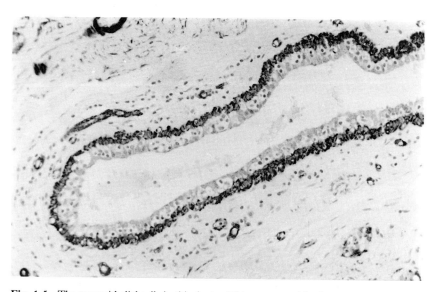

Fig. 1.5 The myoepithelial cells in this duct exhibit strong positive immunoreactivity for actin whilst the secretory epithelial cells are negative. Immunostaining for anti-smooth muscle actin × 185.

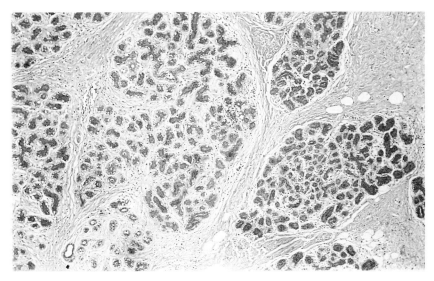

Fig. 1.6 Low power view of lobules from normal mature female breast tissue. Hematoxylin–eosin × 57.

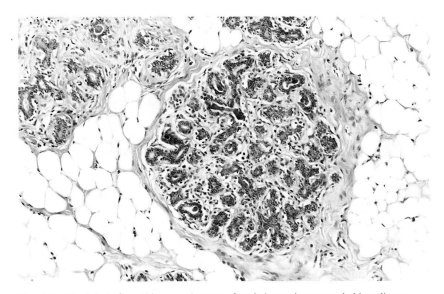

Fig. 1.7 The lobule from this normal mature female breast is surrounded by adipose tissue rather than interlobular connective tissue. Hematoxylin–eosin × 125.

The terminal duct-lobular units are set within an interlobular stroma which is composed of variable proportions of collagenous connective tissue and adipose tissue (Figs 1.6 and 1.7). It is not always appreciated by pathologists that both normal ducts and lobules may be entirely surrounded by adipose tissue; this is especially important in the understanding of the morphological features of entities such as microglandular adenosis (see

Ch. 7) and assessment of microinvasion in association with ductal carcinoma in situ (see Ch. 14).

The lobules are formed by multiple blind ending branches of the terminal duct which appear as acini in two dimensional cross-section (Figs 1.8–1.11). As noted above the same bilayer of secretory epithelial cells and myoepithelial cells seen in segmental and subsegmental ducts extends into the lobule. In addition to the epithe-

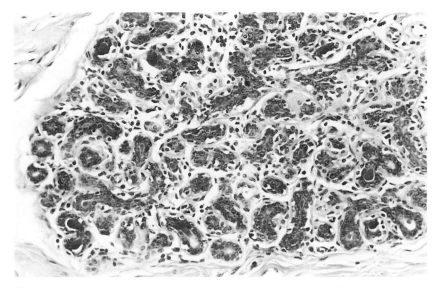

Fig. 1.8 Normal breast lobule, composed of acini in which both epithelial and myoepithelial cells are evident, together with cellular intralobular stroma. Hematoxylin–eosin × 185.

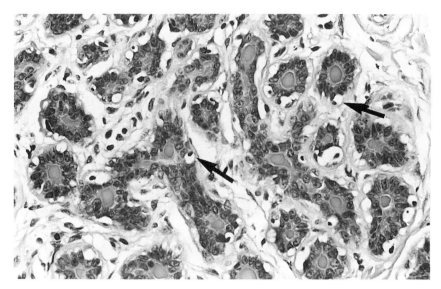

Fig. 1.9 Higher magnification of another lobule. The inter-relationship of epithelial, myoepithelial (arrowheads) and stromal cells is clearly seen. Hematoxylin–eosin × 400.

lial acini there is also a connective tissue component, the intralobular stroma (Fig. 1.9). This loose connective tissue is more cellular than the interlobular stroma, and mucopolysaccharide ground substance is also more abundant. A delicate meshwork of fine elastic fibers can be identified using special stains. Small numbers of lymphocytes, plasma cells, mast cells and macrophages are present in this intralobular stroma.

The breasts are supplied with a rich and complex network of lymphatic channels, and the major pathways to the loco-regional lymph nodes have been well documented.[5,7] The great majority of the lymphatic flow, over 95%, is directed

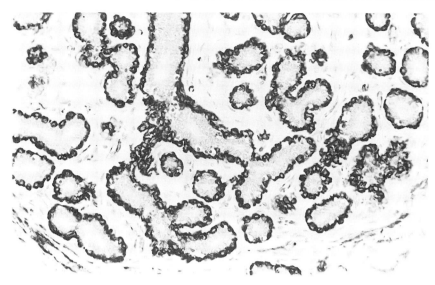

Fig. 1.10 The myoepithelial cells in this lobule show strong positive immunoreactivity for actin. Immunostaining for anti-smooth muscle actin × 185.

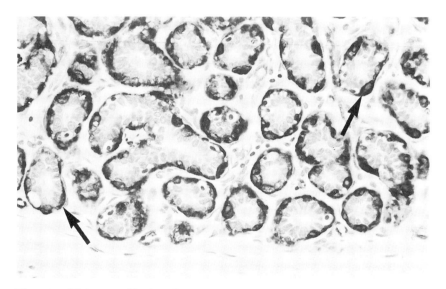

Fig. 1.11 Higher magnification of another lobule. Myoepithelial cells exhibit positive immunoreactivity for actin (arrowheads) whilst epithelial cells are negative. Immunostaining for anti-smooth muscle actin × 400.

towards the axillary lymph nodes, although drainage to the internal mammary chain can occur from any quadrant of the breast.[8] However, until recently the microanatomy of the fine lymphatic channels within the breast stroma was poorly understood. The elegant ultrastructural studies carried out by Hartveit[9] have shown that the breast, in common with other organs, possesses a lymphatic labyrinth,[10] an irrigation system in which the lumen of these fine lymphatic structures is 'open ended' and in continuity with the tissue spaces, allowing a free flow of lymph, including its cellular content, to the drainage system. It should also be noted that small intramammary lymph nodes may be present within the interlobular connective tissue in any quadrant of the breast.[11]

They are occasionally palpable and are also visible on mammography; in these situations diagnostic difficulty may be caused in their distinction from carcinoma, especially with fine needle aspiration cytology (see Ch. 2).

STRUCTURE AND FUNCTION IN RELATION TO PHYSIOLOGICAL CHANGES

The human female is distinguished from related mammalian species in the fact that breast development takes place without the stimulus of copulation or pregnancy. During childhood both male and female breasts are relatively insignificant structures composed only of a small nipple-areolar complex and underlying rudimentary duct system. At puberty the female breast develops its characteristic adult structure described above, and can then be regarded as being in its 'resting' state. Minor variations occur during the menstrual cycle, but major physiological changes are seen during pregnancy and lactation. Thereafter the appearances alternate between these two states until the menopause when there is a major regression which subsequently merges with the atrophy associated with aging. It is important to appreciate that unlike every other organ in the body these physiological changes result in radically different histological appearances which still fall within the range of normality. This is especially important when such appearances are compared with the pathological processes which occur in the breast; for this reason they are described in more detail below. A more comprehensive account is provided by Salazar[2] and a detailed description of the role of the myoepithelial cell is given by Gusterson.[3]

PUBERTY

The onset of puberty in Western European and North American girls occurs at an appreciably younger age in the latter part of the 20th century than in the 19th century (approximately 12 years compared with 16 years).[12] In the breasts elongation and branching of the ducts occurs, principally under the influence of estrogenic stimulation from the ovaries. Progesterone, growth hormone, adrenal cortical steroids, thyroxine and insulin are also thought to have a role in pubertal breast development,[13] but this is not as yet well understood. The end results of the epithelial proliferation is the formation of lobules which bud out from terminal ducts (Figs 1.2, 1.8) to form the normal adult resting breast structure. An increase in connective tissue stroma and interstitial matrix also occurs around the developing epithelial structures, but the characteristic outward growth of the breasts at this time is mainly the result of adipose tissue being laid down. The nipple-areolar complex also undergoes changes, with an increase in pigmentation and enlargement of the nipple itself.

It should be emphasized that the first sign of pubertal development of mammary tissue is a disc-like thickening in the tissues deep to the nipple. This does not always occur simultaneously on the two sides and in exceptional circumstances several months may pass before growth is detectable in the breast which develops later. Some girls have discomfort and even pain in the growing breasts, and the tissues may be tender; such findings, if unilateral, can be misinterpreted as pathological and clinicians must be aware that surgical intervention in cases of apparent anomalies of the breast in adolescence is potentially disastrous, and very rarely required.[7,14–15] If, through inexperience, a surgeon excises the 'lump', the outcome may be failure of that breast to develop or at best a notable disparity.

ADULT RESTING STATE

The majority of women experience cyclical changes in the breasts during the menstrual cycle. These usually take the form of an increase in size and nodularity during the latter part of the cycle, often with increased sensitivity. A distinct feeling of engorgement occurs in the 3 or 4 days before menstruation and the breasts then return to the resting state at the end of menstruation. It is tacitly assumed that these changes are related to the cyclical variation in the levels of ovarian hormonal secretion, but there has been considerable debate as to how far the responses are manifested in morphologically recognized parenchymal changes. The controversy has now been largely resolved,[16-18] and detailed accounts have been provided elsewhere.[5,19] In summary, during the follicular phase of the menstrual cycle proliferation of the breast epithelium occurs with an increase in mitotic index. In the luteal phase breast ducts and acini dilate and secretory changes occur in the acinar cells, with lipid material in the lumina. The premenstrual engorgement has been attributed to increased intralobular oedema and the epithelial proliferation. At the onset of menstruation secretory activity ceases and the breast epithelium returns to the resting state. It appears that apoptosis occurs approximately 3 days after the peak of mitotic activity in order to restore the balance between cell proliferation and cell death. Changes in the stromal cells during the menstrual cycle have not as yet been satisfactorily documented.

PREGNANCY AND LACTATION

Striking and well defined changes occur in the breast during pregnancy and lactation under the influence of estrogen, progesterone, placental lactogen and prolactin. These hormones stimulate the proliferation of ductular and lobular epithelium to form new lobular units. Microscopically little morphological change is seen in early pregnancy, but by the fifth or sixth month a great increase in the amount of lobular tissue has taken place (Fig. 1.12). Secretory activity becomes prominent within the luminal secretory cells, and lipid droplets appear in acinar lumina. Myoepithelial cells become flattened and relatively less prominent, as does the intralobular stroma (Fig. 1.13). Expansion of the lobules is so great that interlobular connective and adipose tissue also appear relatively insignificant. Little further change occurs until parturition when the uninhibited action of prolactin and the stimulus of suckling quickly lead to the establishment of lactation. Once lactation starts the acini become dilated and the appearance of the secretory cells reflects their activity (Fig. 1.14). The cells may be tall or columnar and their cytoplasm granular or vacuolated. As milk production seems, at least in part, to be an apocrine type of secretion, the free margin of the acinar cells has a frayed appearance. It should be noted that, in common with other endocrine target organs, not all groups of lobules, even within the same lobe, are at the same stage

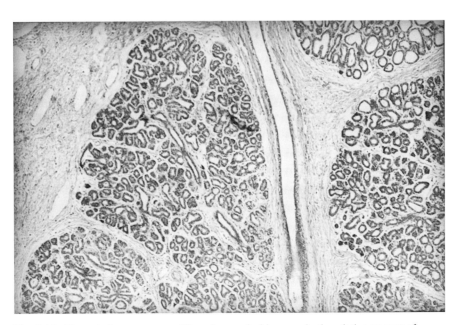

Fig. 1.12 Breast in late pregnancy. There is a marked increase in the relative amount of lobular tissue. Hematoxylin–eosin × 25.

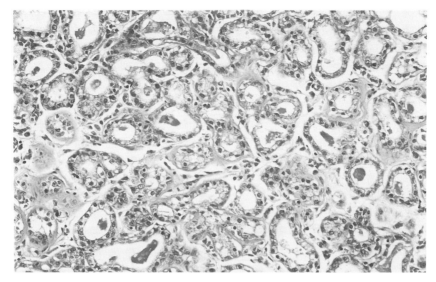

Fig. 1.13   Breast lobule in late pregnancy. Acini are dilated and myoepithelial cells relatively inconspicuous. Vacuolation of the cytoplasm of the epithelial cells is evident and luminal secretion is present. Hematoxylin–eosin × 185.

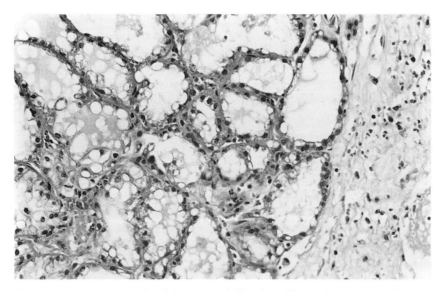

Fig. 1.14   Lactating breast. Acini show marked dilatation with cytoplasmic vacuolation and luminal secretion. The appearances are an exaggeration of those seen in Figure 1.13. Hematoxylin–eosin × 185.

of secretory activity at any one time. Secretory activity is cyclical within the breast, but the local controlling mechanism is not known. Milk is expressed at the nipple following sensory nerve stimulation by the infant which results in release of oxytocin by impulses travelling along the neurosecretory fibers of the hypothalamoneurohypophyseal tract. Oxytocin causes the myoepithelial cells of the breast acini to contract and eject milk into the duct system and then the lactiferous sinuses.

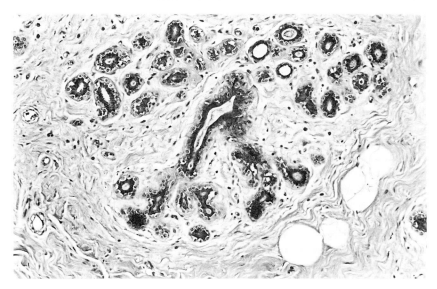

Fig. 1.15   Postlactational involution. Breast tissue from a 35-year-old woman 3 months after cessation of breast feeding in her third pregnancy. Note the focal loss of acini within the lobule. Hematoxylin–eosin × 125.

INVOLUTION

When lactation comes to an end there is a gradual return to the 'resting' state; it has been estimated that this takes, on average, 3 months.[19] It is not known whether the factors which control these changes are vascular, mechanical or hormonal, although it is assumed that the reduction in prolactin levels is a major influence. Involution of the epithelial tissue occurs, with regression towards the resting ratio of connective tissue to lobules. The breasts never return completely to their former state and there is undoubtedly a variation in the degree of involution from one area to another (Fig. 1.15). Disturbances in the process of normal involution may account for some apparent pathological changes seen when subsequent breast biopsies are carried out, particularly the minor degrees of cyst formation. This issue is discussed more widely in Chapter 4.

POSTMENOPAUSAL ATROPHY

At the end of reproductive life the profound reduction in ovarian hormonal activity is accompanied by progressive atrophy of the epithelial components of the breast.[20–21] There is a relative increase in the amount of adipose tissue, with hyalinization of connective tissue stroma. Much of the main duct system is preserved but there is considerable loss of lobular units. Those lobules which remain eventually show a marked reduction in size which appears to be due to loss of acini; hyalinization of intralobular stroma is also seen (Fig. 1.16). Some ducts may appear ectatic and focal microcyst formation is common in residual lobules (Fig. 1.17); such changes must not be mistaken for pathological processes (see Ch. 4). In the elderly any residual lobules become very small and indistinct (Fig. 1.18A) and ductal structures predominate within a dense hypocellular stroma (Fig. 1.18B). Not infrequently an apparent myoepithelial hyperplasia is seen in the atrophic lobules (Fig. 1.19A, B and C). Curiously this was called myoepithelial atrophy by Foote and Stewart[22] but we agree with Tavassoli[23] that such a term is inappropriate, given the predominance of the myoepithelial cells. These appearances must not be mistaken for the lobular proliferation of lobular neoplasia and the myoepithelial nature of the cells can readily be checked by immuno-staining for actin (Fig. 1.19D). Occasionally isolated apparently normal resting type lobules may be found in postmenopausal breast tissue, including those which exhibit secretory features,

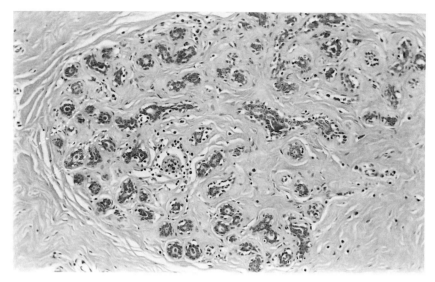

Fig. 1.16   Early postmenopausal atrophy. In this lobule there is a general loss of acini with focal hyalinization of intralobular stroma. Hematoxylin–eosin × 125.

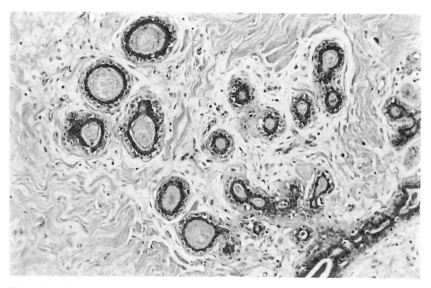

Fig. 1.17   Microcyst formation in postmenopausal atrophy. Note the relative lack of acini, many of which are dilated, with luminal secretion. Hematoxylin–eosin × 125.

the so-called 'lactational lobules' (Fig. 1.20). It is of interest that the latter have now been observed in nulliparous women.[24]

DEVELOPMENTAL ABNORMALITIES

INTRODUCTION

In general, abnormalities associated with the development of the breasts are uncommon, but affect females more frequently than males. They are considered under the following headings:

FAILURE OF NORMAL DEVELOPMENT

Congenital underdevelopment of the breasts is referred to as *hypoplasia*, complete absence of one

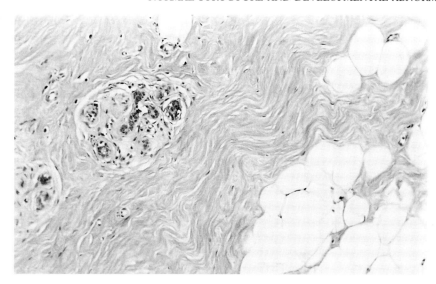

Fig. 1.18A   Atrophic lobule from an elderly female. Note the marked reduction in size of the lobule with scanty acini. Compare with Figure 1.7. Hematoxylin–eosin × 125.

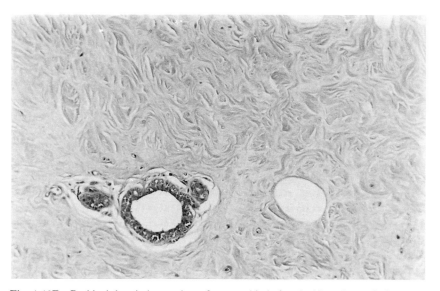

Fig. 1.18B   Residual duct in breast tissue from an elderly female. Note the marked hyalinization of the interlobular connective tissue. Same case as Figure 1.18A. Hematoxylin–eosin × 125.

or both breasts as *amastia* and if a nipple is present but there is no underlying breast disc the condition is termed *amazia*. The frequency of these congenital abnormalities has never been recorded accurately, but they are extremely rare and fewer than 100 cases have been reported in the literature.[7,15] In the majority of cases there appears to be no predisposing genetic factor, although rare familial inheritance has been noted.[25–26] Amastia and severe hypoplasia are associated with pectoral muscle hypoplasia in 90% of cases.[27] The abnormalities are more common in females than males and are more often unilateral than bilateral.

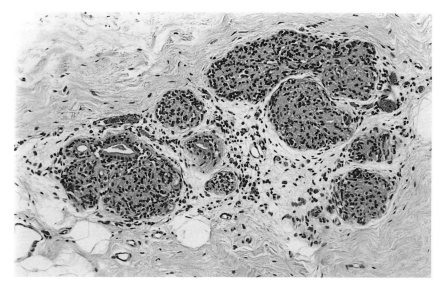

Fig. 1.19A Myoepithelial hyperplasia. The acini in this lobule have almost disappeared; they are replaced by a proliferation of myoepithelial cells. Hematoxylin–eosin × 125.

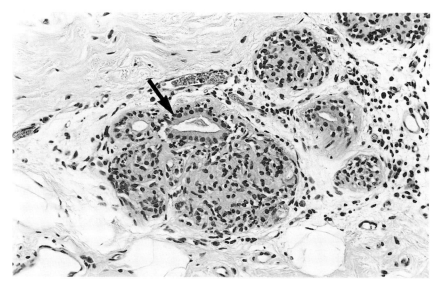

Fig. 1.19B Higher magnification of lobule in Figure 1.19A showing scanty residual acini (arrowhead) with adjacent myoepithelial hyperplasia. Hematoxylin–eosin × 185.

PREMATURE DEVELOPMENT

In normal females breast development is unusual before the age of 10 years. Patients with premature breast development (before the age of 8 and as early as 2 to 3 years) fall into three categories, true precocious puberty, precocious pseudopuberty and premature thelarche.

In *true precocious puberty* (constitutional or central precocious puberty) there is complete sexual maturation with full development of secondary sex characteristics. Free estradiol levels and estrone levels are elevated for the age,[28] but in most cases no etiological or predisposing factor has been identified.[15] Extremely rare cases such as optic glioma, pineal tumours, neurohypophyseal

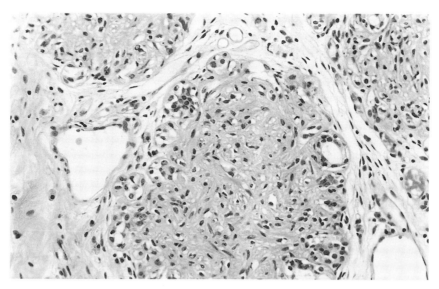

Fig. 1.19C Myoepithelial hyperplasia. In this example the myoepithelial proliferative process is undergoing sclerosis. Hematoxylin–eosin × 125.

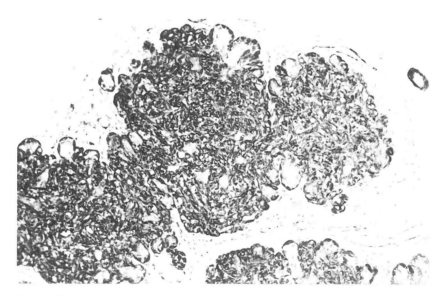

Fig. 1.19D Myoepithelial hyperplasia. Strong positive immunoreactivity for actin is seen in the proliferating myoepithelial cells. Immunostaining for anti-smooth muscle actin × 185.

infundibular glioma or hamartoma and hydrocephalus have been reported.[29–30]

In *precocious pseudopuberty* secondary sex characteristics are usually incompletely developed. The size of the breasts may fluctuate and large ovarian cysts or follicles may be present; these can be visualized on pelvic ultrasonography.[31] Rapid regression of the breast hypertrophy has been reported after limited resection of the functional ovarian cysts.[32] In a proportion of cases there is an underlying ovarian tumor, usually of granulosa cell or, more rarely, mixed germ cell type.[7,15]

Premature thelarche is the term used to describe patients in which early breast growth occurs without any other manifestations of sexual development. It is believed that premature thelarche

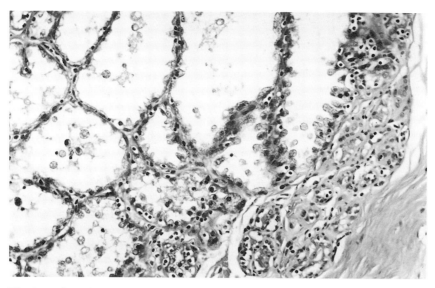

Fig. 1.20   Lactational lobule in an elderly patient. Part of an atrophic residual lobule is seen at the bottom right with 'lactational' features in the adjacent lobule. Hematoxylin–eosin × 185.

represents increased end-organ sensitivity to estrogen produced by luteinized or cystic graafian follicles in prepubertal girls.[14] No therapy is required, biopsy is contraindicated and in about 50% of patients the breasts will regress spontaneously.

No morphological abnormality is present in the breasts in patients with any of the types of precocious puberty described above.

ABNORMAL DEVELOPMENT AT PUBERTY

Failure of the breasts to develop normally at puberty is usually associated with ovarian dysfunction. This phenomenon is rare, and is usually seen as part of Turner's syndrome of sexual infantilism, short stature and webbed neck. These patients, who have the genotype 45X, develop only streak gonads. A degree of breast development may be induced by estrogen therapy.[15] Failure of breast development may also occurs in congenital adrenal hyperplasia.[33]

JUVENILE HYPERTROPHY

The more frequent but still uncommon abnor-

mality of growth related to puberty is hypertrophy, usually termed *adolescent* or *juvenile hypertrophy*. Instead of developing to within the normal limits for the size of the virgin breast in girlhood the breasts continue to enlarge, often rapidly, until they may constitute a serious physical handicap by reason of their size and weight, as well as being a social and psychological embarrassment. In general the cause is unknown, but it may on occasion be associated with hypothyroidism[34] and rare familial cases have been recorded.[35] Microscopical examination shows that the increased bulk of the breasts is due to an excess of apparently normal fibrous and adipose tissue, and, in the majority of cases, no significant abnormality is seen in the epithelial component. However, Eliasen et al[36] have reported the presence of atypical ductal hyperplasia as an incidental finding in five patients undergoing reduction mammoplasty for juvenile hypertrophy. On relatively short-term follow-up (5–68 months) none had developed breast carcinoma, but further surveillance will be required to determine the actual long-term risk.

Eventually, although it may not be for several years, the breasts cease to enlarge; the condition, however, does not regress spontaneously and surgical treatment is the only means of relief.

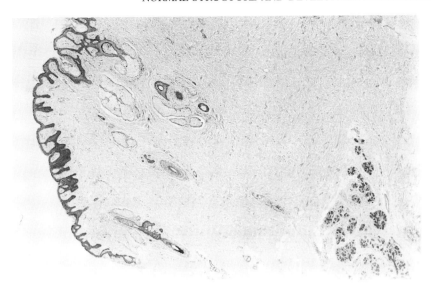

Fig. 1.21A Accessory nipple and breast. The nipple is seen at the upper left, with associated sebaceous glands, and the breast tissue is at the lower right. Hematoxylin–eosin × 25.

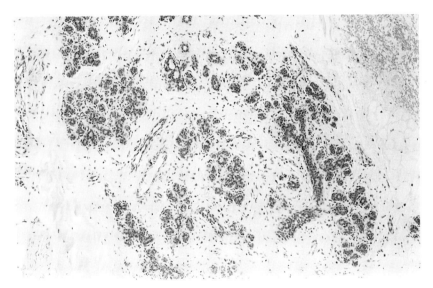

Fig. 1.21B Higher magnification of the field in Figure 1.21A. The typical lobular structure of the breast tissue is shown. Hematoxylin–eosin × 100.

Adolescent hypertrophy sometimes affects one breast much more than the other, and Haagensen[15] describes a case in which the condition was entirely unilateral, the other breast being completely normal. Such cases need to be distinguished from the so-called juvenile fibroadenoma (see Ch. 9).

ACCESSORY BREAST TISSUE

Polymastia, or multiplicity of mammary glands, and *polythelia*, the presence of accessory nipples, occur when primordial breast tissue survives and develops in sites along the milk line in which complete regression of the mammary anlage is usual. The presence of accessory breast tissue is uncommon and the incidence has been estimated at 1–2% in Caucasian subjects, although the anomaly is apparently more frequent in Orientals.[15]

Accessory breasts are usually situated just below the lower edge of the normal breast; the next most frequent site is the axilla.[15] They are occasionally bilateral. Radner[37] has reported the unusual occurrence of accessory breast tissue in the dorsal interscapular region. Accessory breasts are considerably smaller than normal breasts, but respond in the same way to physiological influences. They usually have a nipple and areola; when the nipple is absent the presence of the accessory tissue is likely to be overlooked, or it is taken for the axillary tail of the normal breast. The absence of a duct system may cause acute symptoms of obstruction, especially with the onset of lactation. The presence of such an indurated mass may be mistaken clinically for a carcinoma. Microscopically the structure is closely similar to that of normal breast tissue (Fig. 1.21A and B), and susceptible to the same pathological processes; fibrocystic change, fibroadenoma and carcinoma have all been recorded.[15,38]

Accessory nipples may be located anywhere along the line corresponding to the primitive milk streak, but are found most commonly immediately below the normal breast. Clinically they may be mistaken for nevi or other benign skin tumours. Microscopical sections may also be misinterpreted, especially if the associated rudimentary duct structures are sparse.

REFERENCES

1. Hamilton WJ, Boyd JD, Mossman HW. Human embryology. 4th ed. Cambridge: Heffer, 1972.
2. Salazar H, Tobon H, Josimovich HB. Developmental, gestational and postgestational modifications of the human breast. Clin Obstet Gynecol 1975; 18: 113–137.
3. Gusterson B, Laurence D, Anbazhagan R et al. The breast myoepithelial cell and its significance in physiology and pathology. Curr Diag Pathol 1994; 1: 203–211.
4. Parks AG. The micro-anatomy of the breast. Ann Roy Coll Surg, Engl 1959; 25: 235–251.
5. Osborne MP. Breast development and anatomy. In: Harris JR, Hellman S, Henderson IC, Kinne DW, eds. Breast diseases. 2nd ed. Philadelphia: Lippincott, 1991; 1–13.
6. Böcker W, Bier B, Freytag G et al. An immuno-histochemical study of the breast using antibodies to basal and luminal keratins, alpha-smooth muscle actin, vimentin, collagen IV and luminin. Part 1: normal breast and benign epithelial proliferative lesions. Virchow Arch A Pathol Anat 1992; 421: 315–322.
7. Haagensen CD. Anatomy of the mammary glands. In: Haagensen CD, ed. Diseases of the breast. 3rd ed. Philadelphia: Saunders, 1986a; 1–46.
8. Hultborn KA, Larsson L-G, Ragnhult I. The lymph drainage from the breast to the axillary and parasternal lymph nodes studied with the aid of colloidal AU 198. Acta Radiol 1955; 43: 52–64.
9. Hartveit F. Attenuated cells in breast stroma: the missing lymphatic system of the breast. Histopathol 1990; 16: 533–543.
10. Leak LV. The fine structure and function of the lymphatic vascular system. In: Handbook der Allgemeinen Pathologie, Berlin: Springer Verlag, 1972; 1149–1196.
11. Jadusingh IH. Intramammary lymph nodes. J Clin Pathol 1992; 45: 1023–1026.
12. Bodian C, Haagensen CD. Reproductive factors in breast carcinoma. In: Haagensen CD, ed. Diseases of the breast. 3rd ed. Philadelphia: Saunders, 1986; 424–439.
13. Frantz AG, Wilson JD. Endocrine disorders of the breast. In: Wilson JD, Foster DW, eds. Williams' Textbook of Endocrinology. 8th ed. Philadelphia: Saunders, 1992; 953–975.
14. Capraro VJ, Dewhurst CJ. Breast disorders in childhood and adolescence. Clin Obstet Gynaecol 1975; 18: 25–50.
15. Haagensen CD. Abnormalities of breast growth, secretion and lactation of physiological origin. In: Haagensen CD, ed. Diseases of the breast. 3rd ed. Philadelphia: Saunders, 1986b; 56–74.
16. Vogel PM, Georgiade NG, Fetter BF, Vogel FS, McCarty KS. The correlation of histologic changes in the human breast with the menstrual cycle. Am J Pathol 1981; 104: 23–34.
17. Potten CS, Watson RJ, Williams GT et al. The effect of age and menstrual cycle upon proliferative activity of the normal human breast. Brit J Cancer 1988; 58: 163–168.
18. Anderson TJ, Ferguson DJP, Raab GM. Cell turnover in the 'resting' human breast. Influence of parity, contraceptive pill, age and laterality. Brit J Cancer 1982; 46: 376–382.
19. Page DL, Anderson TJ. Stages of breast development. In: Page DL, Anderson TJ, eds. Diagnostic histopathology of the breast. Edinburgh: Churchill Livingstone, 1987; 11–29.
20. Hutson SW, Cowen PN, Bird CC. Morphometric studies of age related changes in normal human breast and their significance for evolution of mammary cancer. J Clin Pathol 1985; 38: 281–287.
21. Wellings SR, Jensen HM, Marcum RG. An atlas of subgross pathology of the human breast with special reference to possible precancerous lesions. J Natl Cancer Inst 1975; 55: 231–273.

22. Foote FW, Stewart FW. Comparative studies of cancerous versus non-cancerous breasts. Ann Surg 1945; 121: 574–585.

23. Tavassoli FA. Pathology of the breast. Norwalk: Appleton and Lange, 1992.

24. Tavassoli FA, Yeh IT. Lactational and clear cell changes of the breast in non lactating, non pregnant women. Am J Clin Pathol 1987; 87: 23–29.

25. Wilson MG, Hall EB, Ebbin AJ. Dominant inheritance of absence of the breast. Humangenetik 1972; 15: 268–270.

26. Burck Y, Held KR. Athelia in a female infant — heterozygous for anhidrotic ectodermal dysplasia. Clin Genet 1981; 19: 117–121.

27. Trier WC. Complete breast absence. Plast Reconstr Surg 1965; 36: 430–439.

28. Rosenthal IM, Weiss E. Precocious puberty and sexual immaturity. In: Gold JJ, Josimovich JB, eds. Gynecologic endocrinology. Hagerstown: Harper and Row, 1980; 625–641.

29. Kovacs K, Horvath E. Tumors of the neurohypophysis. In: Atlas of tumor pathology, 2nd Series, Fascicle 21, Tumors of the pituitary gland. Washington, DC: Armed Forces Institute of Pathology, 1986; 233–235.

30. Bridges NA, Brook CGD. Premature sexual development. In: Grossman A, ed. Clinical endocrinology. London: Blackwell Scientific Publications, 1992; 837–846.

31. Lyon AJ, de Bruyn R, Grant DB. Transient sexual precocity and ovarian cysts. Arch Dis Child 1985; 60: 819–822.

32. Kosloske AM, Goldthorne JF, Kaufman E, Hayek A. Treatment of precocious pseudo-puberty associated with follicular cysts of the ovary. Am J Dis Childh 1984; 138: 147–149.

33. Jones HW, Klingensmith GJ. Congenital adrenal hyperplasia. In: Shearman RP, ed. Clinical reproductive endocrinology. Edinburgh: Churchill Livingstone, 1985; 362–397.

34. Hollingworth DR, Archer R. Massive virginal breast hypertrophy at puberty. Am J Dis Childh 1973; 125: 293–295.

35. Kupfer D, Dingman D, Broadbent R. Juvenile breast hypertrophy: report of a familial pattern and review of the literature. Plast Reconstr Surg 1992; 90: 303–309.

36. Eliasen CA, Cranor ML, Rosen PP. Atypical ductal hyperplasia of the breast in young females. Am J Surg Pathol 1992; 16: 246–251.

37. Radner H, Berger A, Schmid KD. Mamma supernumeraria dorsalis interscapularis (paravertebralis). Ein klinisch-pathologischer Fallbericht mit Literaturübersicht. Pathologe 1987; 8: 310–315.

38. Badejo OA. Fungating accessory breast carcinoma in Nigerian women. Trop Geogr Med 1984; 36: 45–49.

2

I. O. Ellis, C. W. Elston, A. J. Evans, A. R. M. Wilson and S. E. Pinder

Diagnostic techniques and examination of pathological specimens

PREOPERATIVE DIAGNOSIS

INTRODUCTION

The use of preoperative techniques allows better use of resources, including operating time, and reduces patient anxiety; the psychological trauma of utilizing frozen section to determine the nature of a lesion and thus not knowing the extent of operation at the time of anesthesia is avoided in the vast majority of cases. In addition patients with benign lesions can elect to leave these in situ; in this way the number of benign biopsies is reduced.[1] In the 1970s preoperative diagnosis was largely confined to core biopsy of palpable mass lesions. With the use of mammographic screening in the 1980s, fine needle aspiration cytology (FNAC) became more popular and this technique is now widely used in the United Kingdom as well as the rest of Europe and Scandinavia. The development of automated 'guns' for core biopsy of breast lesions, which can be used on impalpable abnormalities has, however, led to increasing interest in this technique once again. Thus the debate has recommenced regarding the technique of choice for achieving an accurate preoperative diagnosis of a breast lesion. It is almost impossible to compare the two techniques reliably — series differ in patterns of disease, the nature and experience of the aspirators and interpretation of cytological and histological material; both methods of preoperative diagnosis however give a high sensitivity and specificity.[2]

It must be stressed that these pathological techniques should be used in combination with independent clinical examination and imaging techniques. FNAC is not the gold standard but must be used in conjunction with the 'triple approach'. When all three specialities concur a high predictive value and sensitivity of up to 100% is achieved.[3,4]

TRIPLE ASSESSMENT

Breast problems are best managed using an approach where clinician, radiologist and pathologist work closely together as a team following protocols based on the principles of triple assessment: clinical evaluation with imaging and needle cytology/histology. Triple assessment was first developed to manage abnormalities detected at mammographic screening, but its success soon led to its use in the diagnosis and management of all breast problems. Breast teams normally include specialist surgeons, radiologists, pathologists, clinical and medical oncologists, radiographers and breast care nurses with support from psychologists, medical geneticists and plastic surgeons.

The fundamental principle of the triple approach is that the clinician, radiologist and pathologist come to an independent opinion concerning a case which is discussed at a multidisciplinary meeting where the clinical, radiological and pathological findings are given equal weighting and a consensus on the best course of action agreed. Management is based on the most suspicious of the three opinions. For example, if a surgeon finds a clinically benign mass which appears radiologically malignant and yields a benign FNAC, diagnostic biopsy is required because of the radiological suspicion. Lesions are only to be left in the breast when there is a concordant benign opinion from all the team. Wide local excision may be agreed upon when at least two of the opinions point towards a malignant diagnosis, but mastectomy should not be performed on the basis of a malignant FNAC when the clinical and radiological opinion is of a benign process.

Added benefits of triple assessment are that it fosters greater understanding between the members of the team, facilitates multidisciplinary audit and education and encourages research and the development and evolution of detailed management protocols.

IMAGE GUIDED PROCEDURES

Many lesions detected by mammography and ultrasound are impalpable, increasingly so with the more widespread use of imaging as part of breast assessment and increasing participation in mammographic breast cancer screening. Many of these lesions require image guided procedures for FNAC, core biopsy or excision to achieve a definitive diagnosis.

Ultrasound is the imaging modality of choice for such procedures. The patient lies supine and the procedure of FNAC, core biopsy or marker wire localization is performed while real-time ultrasound images confirm the lesion is being accurately sampled/localized. Ultrasound procedures are easy to perform and are also significantly more comfortable for the patient as breast compression is not required. They are also quicker than X-ray-guided procedures taking only about 5 minutes to carry out. Most mass lesions and architectural distortions can be sampled under ultrasound control.

Calcifications are not usually visible on ultrasound. These, and other impalpable lesions not seen on ultrasound, require X-ray-guided biopsy which is best performed using stereotaxis. This can be done using either an add-on device to a normal mammogram machine or a dedicated stereotactic prone table. Both methods use stereoscopic images to calculate the position of a lesion to an accuracy of 0.1 mm. The procedure does, however, require the breast to be compressed in the device for 15 to 30 minutes and may thus be uncomfortable for the patient. X-ray stereotaxis is equally effective for FNAC, core biopsy and wire localization.

Core biopsy is the sampling method of choice for indeterminate and suspicious calcifications. Five to ten cores are obtained under local anesthesia. The core specimens are X-rayed to confirm that representative calcifications have been sampled and to indicate the reliance which can be placed on the histological report.

IMAGING OF BREAST DISEASE

INTRODUCTION

Imaging has an established and important role in

the diagnosis and management of breast problems. Of the techniques available for imaging the breast X-ray mammography is the preferred, having the highest sensitivity and specificity for breast carcinoma. Mammography is particularly sensitive for malignant disease and is the primary technique for breast cancer screening. It is less useful for the assessment of diffuse benign breast processes.

The sensitivity of mammography for disease is dependent on the radiological background pattern. Young women tend to have dense breasts where the sensitivity of mammography for malignancy may be as low as 50–75%. Older women more commonly have fatty breasts where the sensitivity of mammography is usually greater than 95%.[5]

Because mammography uses ionizing radiation to produce an image there is a theoretical risk that the procedure can induce breast cancer; in young women mammography should be confined to situations where there is a significant risk of malignant disease. In younger patients and in the further assessment of clinically benign abnormalities, ultrasound is the imaging technique of choice. In this situation ultrasound is highly sensitive in the detection of invasive malignancy (>90%).[6] However, this technique is poor at detecting DCIS (7%).[7] Ultrasound, unlike mammography, also provides differentiation of cystic from solid breast lesions. It is the imaging technique of first choice for image guided procedures.

Magnetic resonance imaging (MRI) is a highly sensitive technique for imaging the breast but is expensive, time-consuming and difficult. Its use is limited to particular situations where standard imaging techniques are less helpful. Indications include assessing the extent of malignant disease when determination of the size of the lesion is difficult using routine techniques, the detection of recurrent disease in the conserved breast when there are equivocal clinical or mammographic findings and in the assessment of silicone implant integrity.

Isotope scanning of the breast itself using specific labeling agents is under evaluation and may prove to be a useful tool in the future, particularly in the assessment of multi-focal malignancy and recurrence of breast cancer following treatment.

No imaging technique is completely reliable in the assessment of metastatic involvement of axillary lymph nodes, although good results can be obtained using Doppler ultrasound and MRI.

IMAGING FEATURES OF BREAST DISEASE

Imaging of the breast should not be carried out in isolation; it should be used as part of a multidisciplinary approach to the assessment of screen detected and symptomatic breast problems. Symptomatic and screen detected abnormalities should be managed on the basis of triple assessment where the clinical, imaging and cytological/histological findings are all taken into account before management decisions are made.

THE NORMAL BREAST

There is a wide variety of normal appearances on mammography, varying from a homogeneously dense pattern (Fig. 2.1) through a mixed fatty/dense pattern to a predominately fatty pattern (Fig. 2.2). There is, however, poor correlation between the mammographic pattern and the histology of the breast, but there is a tendency for the denser breast to show more fibrous and glandular tissue. There is also poor correlation between the background pattern and subsequent development of breast cancer, although dense breasts are slightly more likely to develop breast

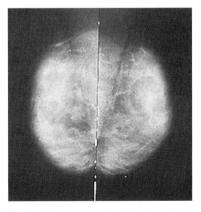

Fig. 2.1 Bilateral mammography showing a homogeneously dense background density which is associated with a reduced sensitivity for carcinoma.

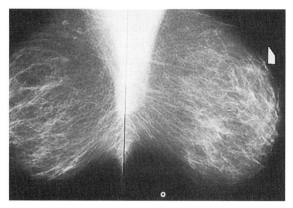

Fig. 2.2   Bilateral mammography showing a homogeneously fatty background density which is associated with a high sensitivity for carcinoma.

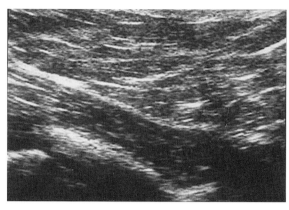

Fig. 2.4   Normal breast ultrasound demonstrating Cooper's ligaments as hyperechoic lines with intervening fat and the pectoralis major muscle posteriorly.

cancer. Normal structures seen using ultrasound include fat, breast parenchyma, Cooper's ligaments and retroareolar ducts (Figs 2.3, 2.4). The use of Doppler ultrasound enables the demonstration of blood vessels and the characterization of blood flow within abnormalities.

FEATURES OF BENIGN BREAST DISEASE

Fibrocystic change

Mammography will demonstrate areas of asymmetric density which often correspond to palpable thickenings. This is, however, a very non-specific feature and similar asymmetric densities are seen often on the mammograms of asymptomatic patients (Fig. 2.5).

Cystic change is most commonly demonstrated on mammography as single or multiple well-defined round or lobulated masses of varying size and low density (Fig. 2.6). Cysts, unlike fibroadenomas, can often be very large. Ultrasound is extremely useful in confirming the cystic nature of lesions, cysts demonstrated as well-defined anechoic masses with distal acoustic enhancement (Fig. 2.7).

Calcification is also a common feature of fibrocystic change/sclerosing adenosis. Typically this

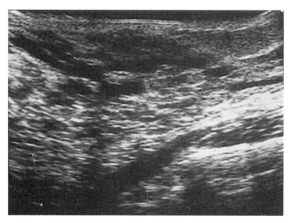

Fig. 2.3   Normal ultrasound of the retroareolar area showing normal ducts as anechoic tubular structures.

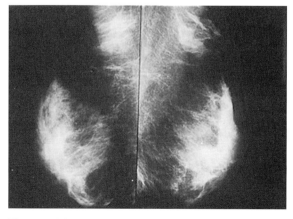

Fig. 2.5   Bilateral mammography showing separate islands of normal breast tissue in upper outer quadrants of both breasts. Such findings are often present unilaterally.

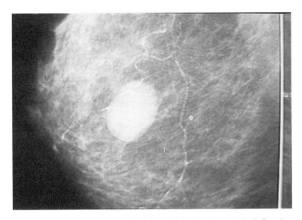

Fig. 2.6 Mammogram showing a low density well-defined mass due to a cyst.

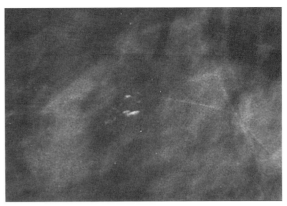

Fig. 2.8 Lateral magnification view of calcifications showing a 'tea cup' configuration due to layering of calcific fluid in small cysts.

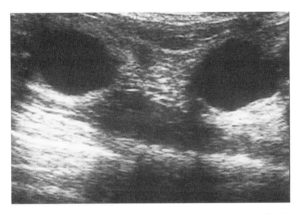

Fig. 2.7 Breast ultrasound image showing two well-defined anechoic masses with distal acoustic enhancement due to simple cysts.

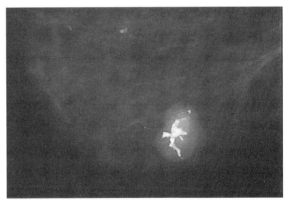

Fig. 2.9 Mammogram showing a fibroadenoma as a well-defined mass containing coarse popcorn calcification.

calcification is seen diffusely in both breasts although it may be asymmetric. The calcifications are seen within round clusters and are themselves round or punctate in shape. When calcification occurs in larger cysts (>2 mm), sedimentation of milk of calcium occurs within the cysts appearing as 'tea cup' shaped calcifications on lateral and occasionally oblique mammograms (Fig. 2.8).

Fibroadenoma

Fibroadenomas, like cysts, appear as well-defined round or lobulated masses on mammography. They may be solitary or multiple. Fibroadenomas commonly calcify in older women; this is often coarse and popcorn-like in character and is obviously benign (Fig. 2.9) but occasionally ductal calcification can occur which can mimic malignancy. Fibroadenomatoid hyperplasia can produce irregular calcification in a ductal distribution with no mass present and this is often indistinguishable radiologically from DCIS.

The ultrasound features of a fibroadenoma are of a well-defined, oval, homogeneous mass which may have distal bright up or distal attenuation depending on the fibrous content of the lesion (Fig. 2.10). Calcification within the mass can cause irregular attenuation at ultrasound which can mislead the radiologist unless the image is correlated with the mammographic findings.

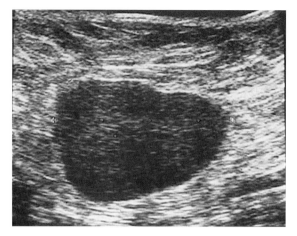

Fig. 2.10 A breast ultrasound image showing a well-defined, oval mass with a homogeneous internal echo pattern due to fibroadenoma.

Phyllodes tumor

These appear mammographically as well-defined masses which are often large and may contain calcification. The ultrasound appearances are similar to those of fibroadenomas except that many contain hyperechoic flecks and some show hyperechoic leaf-like septations, an appearance virtually pathognomic of phyllodes tumor (Fig. 2.11).

Hamartoma

Hamartomas appear mammographically as large well-defined masses that are often impalpable.

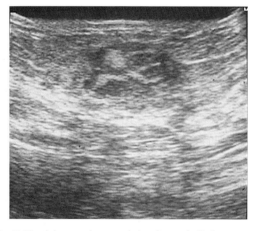

Fig. 2.11 A breast ultrasound showing a phyllodes tumor as a well-defined hypoechoic mass with echogenic septae.

About 50% contain radiographically visible fat, a feature which confirms the diagnosis. The ultrasound features of hamartomas are of well-defined masses of mixed soft tissue and fat echogenicity.

Hematoma

Hematomas appear mammographically as ill-defined masses or asymmetric densities often associated with focal trabecular thickening. At ultrasound examination hematomas commonly appear as poorly-defined masses with mixed cystic and solid components and thus may mimic malignancy. Distal bright up is however often present, a feature rarely seen in malignant disease.

Duct ectasia

The typical mammographic features of duct ectasia are prominent tubular structures of soft tissue density behind the nipple, representing dilated ducts. Calcification is also a common finding and it occurs in two forms: (a) coarse linear and branching intraductal calcification of uniform density ('broken needle' pattern) and (b) periductal calcifications giving a 'pipe stem' appearance. The latter is due to calcification secondary to fat necrosis, resulting from the periductal leakage of intraductal debris.

The dilated ducts of duct ectasia may be well demonstrated on ultrasound and this technique is also useful in demonstrating the periareolar abscesses that may complicate the disease (Fig. 2.12).

Fat necrosis

The typical features of fat necrosis of the breast are small round calcifications with lucent centers (liponecrosis microcystica calcificans) and are seen scattered throughout the breast of many normal middle aged and elderly women with pendulous breasts. Focal areas of fat necrosis can also occur following surgery, radiotherapy or trauma and this can give rise to a variety of radiological appearances: calcifications that, at first, are fine and linear but which eventually coarsen, ill-defined masses (both these appearances may mimic malignancy) and post-traumatic oil cysts which appear as well-defined masses of fat density.

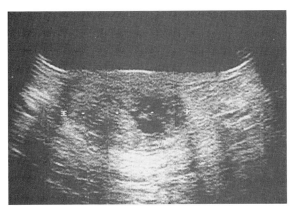

Fig. 2.12 A breast ultrasound image of a breast abscess. There is a hypoechoic mass with an anechoic, irregular center.

Radial scar and complex sclerosing lesion

Radial scars usually appear as architectural distortions without any central opacity (Fig. 2.13).[9] Punctate calcification is also commonly seen. Radial scars are visualized less frequently on ultrasound than carcinoma but when seen may be indistinguishable.[10]

Lobular carcinoma in situ (LCIS) and atypical lobular hyperplasia (ALH)

In the past it was thought that these conditions were the cause of some mammographic abnormalities. It has, however, recently been shown that there are no mammographic correlates of these two conditions and the existence of these lesions in marker biopsy specimens is fortuitous and is due to the coexistence of LCIS or ALH with other conditions capable of producing a mammographic abnormality.[11]

Atypical ductal hyperplasia (ADH)

Opinion is divided as to whether ADH produces radiological features. Some claim that it can produce fine microcalcification similar to that seen in low grade DCIS while others say that any calcification present mammographically is due to associated benign conditions.[12]

FEATURES OF MALIGNANT BREAST DISEASE

DCIS

Calcification is the commonest mammographic feature of DCIS, being found in 90% of cases.[13] Such calcification occurs unilaterally in irregularly shaped clusters (compared with fibrocystic change) and adopts a ductal distribution varying in size, shape and density (Figs 2.14, 2.15). The calcifications are often associated with an asymmetric density representing a lymphocytic infiltrate and may occasionally be associated with a mass.

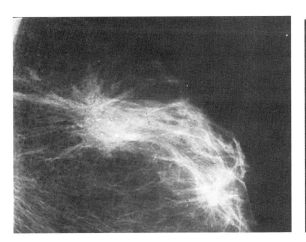

Fig. 2.13 Mammogram of a complex sclerosing lesion demonstrating an area of architectural distortion associated with punctate calcification.

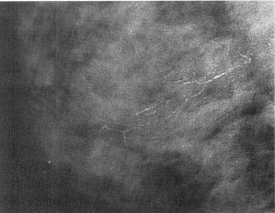

Fig. 2.14 Mammogram showing linear calcification with a striking ductal distribution due to high grade DCIS.

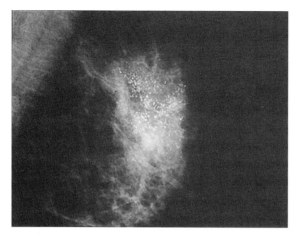

Fig. 2.15 Mammogram showing calcification which shows variation in shape, size and density in an irregularly shaped cluster due to high grade DCIS.

High grade DCIS nearly always calcifies; the calcifications tend to be linear and branching[14] and are due to the dystrophic calcification of intraductal necrotic debris. The extent of calcification in high grade DCIS correlates well with the extent of the lesion histologically.[15] Low grade DCIS, however, calcifies in only about 50% of cases; the calcifications often appear granular or oval and are due to calcification of mucin present in intercellular spaces. In low grade DCIS, however, the extent of calcification tends to underestimate the histological size of the lesion.[15]

Ultrasound has a very low sensitivity in the detection of DCIS due to its inability to consistently identify microcalcification. DCIS may nevertheless present as a mass and may then be identified as such on ultrasound imaging, often with indeterminate features.

Paget's disease

Mammography is only abnormal in about 50% of cases of Paget's disease of the nipple. However, as the treatment of Paget's disease is always mastectomy and the diagnosis is established by nipple biopsy not radiology there seems little to be gained from ipsilateral mammographic examination. When mammography is abnormal in Paget's disease, calcification due underlying DCIS is the commonest finding.[16]

Invasive carcinoma

The commonest mammographic features of invasive carcinoma are a spiculate mass (Fig. 2.16) or an ill-defined mass (Figs 2.17, 2.18). The positive predictive value (PPV) for malignancy of these features is 94% and 54% respectively.[17] Other radiological features of invasive carcinoma which are commonly seen are architectural distortion, suspicious calcification, developing and asymmetric density. The PPV for malignancy of these features varies from 45% for architectural distortion and suspicious microcalcification to 1% for asymmetric density.

Secondary mammographic features of breast carcinoma are occasionally seen and include

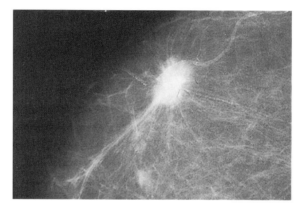

Fig. 2.16 Mammogram of an invasive carcinoma manifesting as a spiculate mass. The long spicules represent inpulling of normal breast structures and not tumor infiltration.

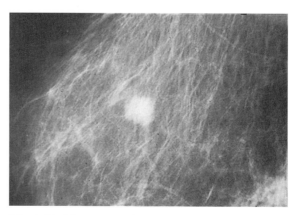

Fig. 2.17 Mammogram showing an ill-defined mass due to grade 3 invasive carcinoma.

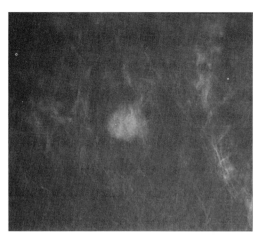

Fig. 2.18 Mammogram showing a similar ill-defined mass to that shown in Figure 2.17, but on this occasion the lesion was a fibroadenoma.

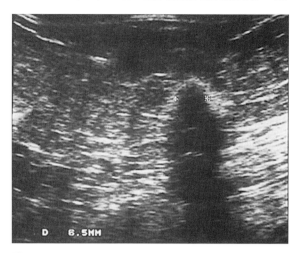

Fig. 2.19 Ultrasound image of an invasive carcinoma showing a hypoechoic ill-defined mass with an echogenic halo. There is marked distal acoustic attenuation. The mass is taller than it is wide.

nipple retraction, focal or generalized trabecular and skin thickening and tenting of the breast disc. Enlarged blood vessels and single dilated ducts are described in older text books as signs of breast cancer, but are very rarely seen.

Mammography is accurate in predicting the extent of invasive carcinoma and associated DCIS. It is more accurate than clinical examination in identifying multifocal disease. Mammography may also demonstrate a clinically occult carcinoma in the other breast. Enlarged axillary lymph nodes are frequently seen on mammograms, but they are a very poor predictor of metastatic involvement; mammographically normal sized nodes may contain metastases.

On ultrasound invasive carcinomas appear as ill-defined, irregularly shaped, hypoechoic masses. They often have an inhomogeneous internal echo-pattern, distal shadowing, an echogenic halo and appear taller than wide (benign masses are always wider than tall) (Fig. 2.19). Ultrasound is accurate in the prediction of the invasive size of breast carcinoma. Color Doppler may show areas of neovascularity within the tumor.

Variations in the radiological appearance of invasive breast cancer according to grade and type

Spiculation of carcinomas at mammography is due to a desmoplastic reaction which is more commonly seen in low grade carcinomas. Spiculate masses are therefore most frequently low grade carcinomas. The absence of a desmoplastic reaction seen in many high grade carcinomas means that the appearance of an ill-defined mass correlates with high histological grade. Suspicious calcification is also seen more commonly in high grade invasive carcinomas. The grade of invasive carcinoma correlates well with the grade of DCIS from which it arose and as high grade DCIS calcifies more commonly than low grade DCIS the correlation between high grade invasive cancer and suspicious calcification is to be expected.[18]

Ductal carcinomas of no special type tend to appear as large, ill-defined or spiculate masses often associated with calcification. Lobular carcinomas are more frequently radiologically occult and often appear as ill-defined masses or asymmetric densities. Calcification in lobular cancer is unusual.[19] Tubular cancers usually appear as small spiculate masses or architectural distortions[20] and calcification is an uncommon feature. Invasive cribriform carcinoma commonly appears as large spiculate masses.[21] Papillary carcinomas are often seen mammographically as partially well-defined masses which on ultrasound may be partly cystic (Fig. 2.20); spiculation is unusual in these lesions. Pure mucinous cancers also appear as partially well-defined lobulated masses which

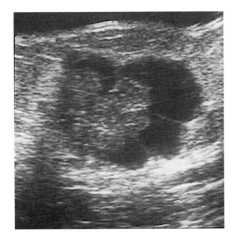

Fig. 2.20 Ultrasound image of a an encysted papillary carcinoma with invasive features manifesting as a mixed cystic/solid mass.

rarely spiculate.[22] In addition mucinous cancer is the only type of breast carcinoma which commonly causes distal bright up on ultrasound. Angiosarcomas appear mammographically as non-calcifying, ill-defined masses.[23]

FINE NEEDLE ASPIRATION CYTOLOGY

INTRODUCTION

It is now widely accepted that fine needle aspiration cytology (FNAC) can reliably be used to provide accurate preoperative diagnosis of both palpable and screen-detected breast lesions, using freehand, ultrasound or stereotactic techniques. Indeed in almost all published series, FNAC meets the minimum requirements suggested by the Cytology Sub-Group of the National Co-ordinating Committee for Breast Screening Pathology[24] who recommend as a minimum an absolute and complete sensitivity of more than 60% and 80% respectively with a specificity of more than 60%. In addition, a positive predictive value of more than 95%, a false negative rate of less than 5%, a false positive rate of less than 1% and an inadequate rate of less than 25% should be obtained. Nevertheless, despite the success of FNAC, some centers still regard the technique with suspicion; in a large series of 7495 FNAC specimens, a sensitivity of 83.9% and a specificity

of 99.5% was obtained with a predictive value for a negative result of 93.2% and for a positive result of 98.6%. The overall accuracy was 94.6%, but the authors nevertheless believe that 'frozen-section diagnosis could be bypassed only in selected cases'.[25] However other studies have shown that the diagnostic accuracy of FNAC is as high as that of frozen section.[26,27]

Some authors believe that FNAC should not be used to diagnose benign lesions due to an unacceptable high false negative rate[28] and feel that symptomatic lesions which are reported as benign cytologically should be excised.[29,30] We do not take this view at this time and are satisfied that lesions may be left 'in situ' if all specialities of the triple approach concur with a benign assessment.

FNAC is easy to perform with little equipment needed. Diagnosis can be made on a single sample taken in an outpatient setting without the need for an inpatient stay; thus both cost and patient anxiety are reduced. Complications are uncommon and generally minor, including hematoma formation and fainting. Very rarely pneumothoraces may develop in women with small breasts or in the aspiration of axillary lymph nodes.

The most important drawback of the technique of FNAC is the need for trained and experienced staff both to obtain and to examine the sample.[31] The proportion of technically inadequate specimens, for example, ranges from 9.8% for single experienced aspirators to 45.9% when inexperienced groups of clinicians are performing the aspiration.[32] Some cytopathologists, for this reason, perform the aspiration procedure themselves on symptomatic breast lesions and achieve very good yields compared with those of inexperienced clinicians or where the techniques of preparation are poor. In addition to instruction of aspirators, considerable training is required for reliable diagnosis of cytological preparations from breast lesions.

FNAC TECHNIQUE

Palpable masses

Palpable breast lesions are best aspirated by a freehand technique. Minimal equipment is required: a syringe of either 10 or 20 ml volume and needle of appropriate size. As a rule of thumb the smaller the needle, the less bleeding will be produced and a 23 gauge (blue) needle is appropriate if the length is adequate to reach the lesion within the breast. For deeper sampling a 21 gauge (green) needle may be needed. Some aspirators use a syringe holder, although this is a matter of personal choice. Although local anesthetic can be applied superficially, care must be taken not to inject deep to the dermis into the mass or area to be aspirated. Local anesthetic is used more frequently when sampling impalpable lesions as multiple punctures may be necessary.

The procedure for obtaining a breast aspirate from a palpable lesion is simple; the skin is cleansed and the lesion immobilized between thumb and forefinger. After introducing the needle into the skin and up to the anterior edge of the mass, negative pressure is applied to the syringe and several passes made through the lesion without removing the needle through the skin. Each pass is made at a different angle and the syringe is rotated simultaneously.

After releasing the negative pressure, the needle is then withdrawn from the skin. If the fluid which is seen in the hub of the needle is heavily blood-stained repeat aspiration may be helpful.

Impalpable lesions

Screen-detected abnormalities are aspirated by image-guided techniques. The most frequently used are ultrasound and stereotaxis; both are performed by specialist radiologists. Ultrasound guided FNAC is easier to perform, less uncomfortable for the patient and can be used to sample mass lesions. Stereotactic methods are required to obtain specimens from areas of microcalcification and are also often used to sample parenchymal deformities. By this latter technique the coordinates of the area to be aspirated are determined by calculation from stereo images and considerable experience on the part of the radiologist is required.

The cellularity of samples from impalpable lesions may be poorer than those from symptomatic masses due to the relatively smaller size of the former. In addition it is not possible to alter the angle of sampling through the lesion with a stereotactic device. Multiple passes with associ-ated punctures should therefore be made to ensure good yields from mammographically detected lesions. It is often recommended that the initial pass should be made through the center of the lesion and that subsequently the periphery be sampled.[24]

The aspirator can be certain of the location of the lesion with an ultrasound technique by direct visualization whilst obtaining the sample and less passes are thus required. Ultrasound jelly which is used to obtain 'coupling' between the probe and skin should not, however, be used during ultrasound FNAC sampling as it may mimic necrotic or mucinous material microscopically.

SMEAR PREPARATION, FIXATION AND STAINING

Many methods can be used to achieve a good spread of cells from the sample obtained. In principle the aim is to obtain a thin layer of cells to enable optimum assessment by microscopy. If the samples are subsequently to be processed through an air-dried Giemsa-stained technique they must be dried rapidly and a thin smear is necessary for this to occur. Although a pipette or a needle may be used to spread the aspirate manually, more commonly a drop of material is placed at the frosted end of one glass slide and the sample is spread by gliding a second slide over the first. Whichever technique is used, care must be taken not to spread the sample with excess force resulting in distortion of the cells and making interpretation impossible. If an aspirator continually or frequently produces slides spoiled by poor spreading, feedback with visual demonstration of the artefacts is helpful.

Once spread, the slides can be processed in several ways. In the United Kingdom breast FNAC samples are more commonly air-dried (75% of departments) than wet fixed (73% of laboratories).[33] Smears to be air-dried should be waved in air to ensure rapid drying or an electric fan or hair-dryer on the cold setting may be used. Conversely wet-fixed smears should be flooded with, or placed immediately into, fixative (most commonly alcohol[33]) before drying can commence.

Although the direct smear is assessed in up to

84% of laboratories and is the most common method of assessment of breast cytology samples, in 43% of units the cytospin technique is used.[33] This technique is especially helpful if problems are found with poor preparation of samples. This may particularly be the case if many and inexperienced aspirators are taking specimens.[34] In this technique a transport medium is utilized to transfer the aspirate to the laboratory where it is cytocentrifuged and a 'cytospin' or a 'cytoblock' preparation made.

Many cytopathologists use more than one method of preparation, fixation and staining.[33] The method used to stain the smear reflects the technique used to prepare the sample; in the United Kingdom, Giemsa is the first choice of preparation and is utilized by 54% of laboratories,[33] but Papanicolaou staining is used on wet-fixed smears. More rarely hematoxylin and eosin or Diff-Quick, PAS/Alcian blue and immunocytochemical stains can be used.

BREAST FNAC DIAGNOSIS

Introduction

It is vital that adequate clinical information is supplied with the smears before diagnosis is reached. Many false positive diagnoses and pitfalls can be avoided if full patient details are obtained; lactational change, for example, may result in cellular specimens composed of discohesive cells with prominent nucleoli which may mimic malignancy.

The NHS BSP Guidelines for reporting breast cytology recommend five categories of breast FNAC diagnosis and these have been widely accepted.[24,35] It must be stressed that definitive diagnosis is not possible on all breast FNAC specimens and, although the proportion decreases with experience, a number of cases must be classified into 'non-diagnostic' categories.

C1/Inadequate/unsatisfactory smears

The smears may have insufficient epithelial cells for assessment or the cells present may show preparation damage such that diagnosis is impossible. The former samples may be expected from some lesions such as lipomas and thus an 'inadequate' report may be clinically valuable. Other smears in this category may, however, contain sufficient epithelial cells for diagnosis but show air drying or crush artefacts. These may mimic cytological changes seen in malignancy and over-interpretation of a poorly prepared specimen is a well recognized pitfall resulting in false positive diagnoses. Alternatively the smear may be too thick for full examination with the epithelial cells present obscured by blood, fluid or other cells. It is recommended that further details on inadequate reports are provided to aspirators; explanation with visual feedback is helpful in improving quality of poor smears.

C2/Benign smears

The classification of a smear as benign implies a sufficient yield of cells. Benign specimens are often poorly to moderately cellular but are composed of cohesive, regular epithelial cells (Fig. 2.21). These may be seen in sheets with well-defined edges. Apocrine change may be identified. A background population of 'bare' or 'naked' nuclei is present and fatty tissue is also often seen. In some cases a more precise diagnosis such a fibroadenoma can be suggested.

C3/Atypia probably benign/equivocal smears

Although the smear in these cases has an overall benign appearance, as described above, additional features such as mild pleomorphism or loss of cohesion may be present such that a definite diagnosis of benignity cannot be made. Other features such as increased cellularity or nuclear changes may be identified which may be due to treatment or hormonal effects.[24] Nevertheless the majority of equivocal FNAC diagnoses will be derived from benign lesions (68% of excised lesions with a C3 diagnosis were benign in a recent audit in our unit[36]).

C4/Suspicious of malignancy

Suspicious smears show features which are suggestive of a malignant lesion but which are not

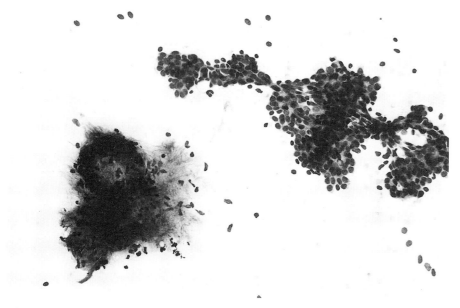

Fig. 2.21   An example of a benign cytology yield containing a large cohesive sheet of regular epithelial cells surrounded by scattered single nuclei and a fragment of stroma. Maygrunwald Giemsa ×185.

diagnostic. This may be because of poor preparation, poor preservation or low cellularity of the sample or because, whilst atypical, the cells do not show sufficient abnormalities for definitive diagnosis. In other samples classified as suspicious an overall benign pattern may be seen although an admixture of markedly atypical cells of malignant appearance is also present. Whereas the majority of equivocal lesions are subsequently found to be benign, most suspicious FNAC specimens (82% of excised abnormalities[37]) derive from malignant masses.

C5/Malignant

In smear classified as C5, sufficient material is present to be confident of the diagnosis and indeed the smears are often highly cellular. The cells show features typical of malignancy including discohesion, pleomorphism and an increase in size (Fig. 2.22). Nuclear atypicalities, particularly in Papanicolaou stained samples, such as chromatin clumping, and irregular nuclear membranes are evident. Necrotic debris and sometimes foamy macrophages may be seen in the background of the specimen. Other features may also be seen in individual cases such as intracytoplasmic lumina

or mucin pools in breast carcinomas showing lobular and mucinous features respectively.

DIAGNOSTIC PITFALLS

It is important to stress again the need for adequate clinical information on the FNAC request form so that false positive diagnoses such as the misdiagnosis of lactational change are avoided. Radiotherapy changes and hematomas may also produce worrisome cytological appearances. Fibroadenomas may result in cellular samples and show some epithelial pleomorphism, but the presence of stroma and abundant bare nuclei will provide clues to the correct diagnosis. Intramammary lymph nodes will also give cellular samples, but can be identified by the scanty cytoplasm and polymorphic nature of the cells. Lymphomas may be more difficult to recognize and immunohistochemistry with leucocyte common antigen (LCA) and anti-cytokeratin antibodies may be required for definite diagnosis (see Ch. 19). Apocrine cells and cells from papillomas, particularly if showing degenerative features, may appear atypical and false positive diagnoses from

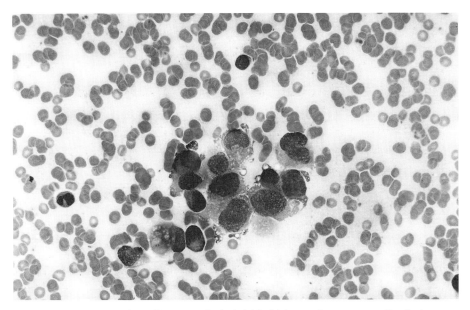

Fig. 2.22 An example of a malignant cytological yield which contains numerous discohesive epithelial cells which are large and show marked nuclear pleomorphism. Maygrunwald Giemsa ×400.

other lesions such as granulomatous mastitis can be avoided by caution and experience.

False negative diagnoses most commonly result from the aspirator failing to obtain samples from the lesion and are thus 'genuine' false negative results. In addition some tumors such as tubular carcinoma may have a markedly desmoplastic stroma and thus smears may be very scanty and insufficient cells obtained for definitive diagnosis. More rarely samples from low grade carcinomas or ductal carcinoma in situ (DCIS) may be missed by the cytopathologist; as described, these lesions may provide paucicellular smears and pleomorphism may also be relatively slight. It is prudent in these cases to classify the sample as suspicious rather than malignant and obtain a repeat FNAC sample or core or diagnostic biopsy.

NEEDLE CORE BIOPSY

INTRODUCTION

Although in the 1970s this mode of preoperative diagnosis was popular, needle core biopsy fell out of favor in the United Kingdom as a result of the widespread use of FNAC in association with the National Breast Screening Programme in the 1980s. Core biopsy has continued to be utilized for the diagnosis of symptomatic masses and, at the present time and with the introduction of new equipment, is re-emerging as a useful tool in preoperative diagnosis of screen detected lesions. The automated 'guns' for obtaining needle core biopsies are easier to use and have reduced patient discomfort, achieved a higher sampling success rate and better specimen quality than previous methods.[38] Although FNAC requires experience in both obtaining and interpreting the sample, core biopsy can be readily performed by clinicians and no or minimal additional training is necessary for histopathologists.

Histology samples from core biopsies also have the advantage that assessment of the presence of invasion can be made; if only in situ disease is identified, however, this does not exclude the possibility of invasion in a part of the lesion which has not been sampled (Fig. 2.23). The disadvantages of core biopsy include the need for local anesthetic and additional clinic time.

The reliability and reproducibility of core biopsy reports is extremely high[39] using both ultrasound and stereotaxic methods.[40,41] With an 18 gauge needle a 90% sensitivity and 100% specificity can

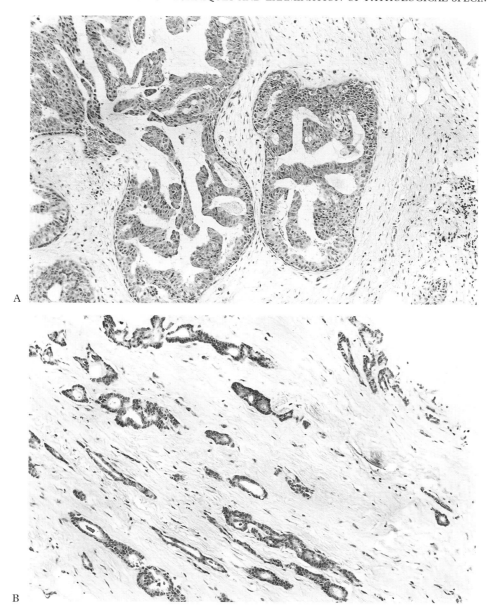

Fig. 2.23 Two core biopsy samples: one showing only ductal carcinoma in situ (A) the other showing an invasive carcinoma (B).

be obtained.[42] Similarly, a sensitivity of at least 89%[43,44] and specificity of 100% for suspicious masses has been reported with Trucut biopsy.[43] Use of 14 gauge core biopsy can produce even higher levels of sensitivity and specificity.[45]

TECHNIQUE

Both symptomatic and impalpable breast lesions can be sampled by a core biopsy technique. Although dedicated prone tables have been developed which allow core biopsies to be taken easily from screen-detected abnormalities,[45] some authors have reported obtaining samples successfully from up to 98% of suspicious cases using a regular mammographic table with an added stereotaxic device.[46] Despite the high success rate, in a proportion of cases non-representative or non-diagnostic material will be obtained with a needle core technique; this ranges from 6%[47] to 14.5%.[28]

As a result of this relatively high rate of 'missed' core biopsies there has been debate about the number of cores which should be obtained. Diagnostic accuracy is undoubtedly increased if more than one needle core biopsy is taken,[48] but some authors recommend taking very many biopsies. When at least five cores are sampled the biopsy result is reported to correspond to the subsequent excisional biopsy in 96% of benign conditions, 83% of malignant lesions and 90% of cases overall with a sensitivity of 85%.[49] When fewer samples than this are obtained, correlation with the excisional biopsy is less good; 81% of benign lesions, 79% of malignant tumors and 80% of cases overall correlated with the excision specimen providing a sensitivity of 84% in a series by Gisvold et al.[49] Similarly, other authors have reported that diagnosis could be made in 70% of lesions with one core of tissue, but taking two, three, four, five or six samples increased the diagnostic rate to 81%, 89%, 91%, 94% and 97% of cases respectively.[50] Thus taking five cores appears to provide the diagnosis in 99% of mass lesions and 87% of microcalcifications and, although taking more cores improves the yield in the latter cases to 92%,[50] patient discomfort is increased.

LABORATORY HANDLING

Once obtained, the cores are either placed on card and X-rayed, if taken for the diagnosis of mammographic calcifications, or placed directly into fixative if derived from mass lesions. Specimen X-ray of the core in cases of microcalcification is invaluable in demonstrating the presence, features and site of the abnormality within the sample and should be sent to the laboratory with the tissue sample (Fig. 2.24). The cores are there routinely processed. We recommend histological examination at three levels through the paraffin block with standard hematoxylin and eosin stains. Further assessment including histochemical and immunohistochemical stains can be utilized, if required, at a later time.

In particular clinical circumstances core biopsy technique may be the best method of diagnosis; definitive diagnosis of mammographically detected microcalcifications for example, may be made by core biopsy. Core biopsy may also be utilized if initial FNAC is inadequate or greatly at variance with the clinical findings; although only approximately 45% of repeat FNAC samples are useful, 90% of subsequent cores provide clinically significant information.[51]

In particular, core biopsy may be significantly better than FNAC in the diagnosis of some low grade or 'special type' cancers and also lobular carcinomas.[52] These tumors can be difficult to diagnose definitively on cytological preparations in part due to their low yield of cells and partly to the subtle cytological features of malignancy present. Tubular, cribriform and lobular breast cancers may, for example, be diagnosed as malignant in only 30% to 40% of cases by FNAC although inclusion of the suspicious category (C4) can increase positive diagnosis to 60% to 70%;[53] core biopsy may be advantageous in these cases.

As noted above, core biopsy is particularly useful in the definitive diagnosis of calcifications (Fig. 2.24). However, the number of cases in which the core biopsy contains the mammographic microcalcifications varies from 40%[54] to up to 93%.[55] In addition to the assessment of several levels through the core, the biopsies should be examined under polarized light to avoid missing mammographic calcifications which may be due to calcium oxalate.[56] Von Kossa histochemical stains have also been reported to demonstrate calcifications not visible with hematoxylin.[57] Nevertheless, in up to 22% of cases,[54] although present in the specimen X-ray, microcalcification cannot be found in the histological specimen. It is believed that, in at least some of these cases, the calcification has shattered from the block on sectioning. It may still, however, be possible to reach a diagnosis in some specimens in the absence of calcification.

Conversely, in up to 13% of cases no calcifications are seen on X-ray, but histological microcalcifications are present.[54] In these latter cases it must be determined whether the histological calcification is representative of that seen in the mammogram

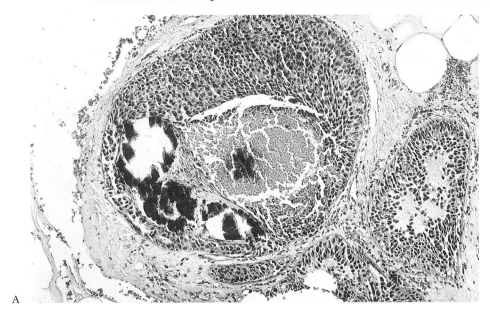

A

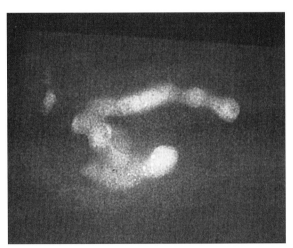

B

Fig. 2.24 Tissue diagnosis of areas of microcalcification can be made accurately by core biopsy. In this example of high grade DCIS (Fig. 2.24A) the biopsy X-ray (Fig. 2.24B) confirms the presence of appropriate microcalcification in the biopsy sample.

and if there is doubt, repeat biopsy should be recommended; if for example, small foci of benign microcalcification are identified when mammographically suspicious rod-shaped/linear calcification is seen, further investigation is mandatory.

COMPLICATIONS AND PITFALLS

Clinical complications from core biopsy are rare and usually minimal; up to 19% of women develop hematomas but this is very rarely clinically significant.[58] The most common adverse reaction of significance is a vasovagal attack which

is said to occur in up to 11% of procedures.[48] Case reports of other very rare complications have been described including the development of a milk fistula after core biopsy.[59] Difficulties for the histopathologist may occur if multiple cores are taken in identifying the site from which the biopsies were derived although this is very rare; four lesions (three masses and one cluster of microcalcifications) disappeared after core biopsy in a series of 113 cases by Hann et al[55] and removal of the entire focus of malignancy has been described.[60] Seeding of malignant cells along the track of core biopsy has also been reported[61] and this may occur more commonly than previously believed;

for example, malignant seeding was seen in two out of 47 consecutive cases of Trucut biopsy.[62] The clinical significance of the feature is not known and epithelial displacement, both benign and malignant, has also been reported after FNAC and other needling procedures.[63,64] Tracking of cells along the core or needle site may however cause diagnostic difficulties and the seeding of benign epithelium may mimic carcinoma. Care must therefore be taken in the interpretation of unusual deposits of epithelial cells adjacent to the site of previous core biopsy.

Core or FNAC?

At the present time, there is an ongoing debate regarding the optimal method of obtaining a preoperative diagnosis. Some groups maintain that FNAC is less invasive and as reliable as core biopsy whilst others recommend core biopsy, particularly as it provides additional architectural information. We believe that the mode of preoperative diagnosis can be tailored according to the clinical features and that each technique may be more useful than the other in specific circumstances. Thus in the diagnosis of microcalcifications core biopsy is advantageous, providing definite identification of the presence and nature of microcalcific foci. In addition core may be particularly useful in the diagnosis of low grade malignancies and invasive lobular carcinoma. Performing both core biopsy and FNAC increases the yield of definite preoperative diagnosis, although it also increases the laboratory workload.

In one of the few studies which has assessed both FNAC and core biopsy, Cheung et al found that FNAC was diagnostic in approximately 79% of cancers and in 72% of benign lesions.[65] Core biopsy was diagnostic in a larger proportion (83%) of cancers but in a smaller number (62%) of benign lesions. Although the percentage of non-representative samples will vary according to the type of lesions sampled and is thus difficult to compare, the number of non-diagnostic samples in this series by FNAC and Trucut biopsy was 27% and 33% respectively. In our experience, the introduction of core biopsy dramatically increased the preoperative diagnosis of DCIS from 35% to 80% of cases, but did not significantly improve preoperative diagnosis of mass lesions over FNAC alone.[66]

FROZEN SECTION

Frozen section examination of breast lesions is widely used in some units where definitive preoperative diagnosis is not sought or is believed to be unreliable. In many series it has been found to be a reliable technique for perioperative diagnosis of symptomatic masses with clinically significant discrepancies in diagnosis in only approximately 3% of cases.[67] The sensitivity and specificity of frozen section diagnoses in a representative series by Bianchi et al were 91.7% and 99.2% respectively.[68] False positive diagnoses are rare and frozen section is a highly accurate method of rapid histological diagnosis.

As with FNAC interpretation, however, significant training and experience in the histopathological diagnosis of frozen sections is required so that false positive and false negative diagnoses are minimized. Nevertheless in some cases the diagnosis should be deferred to await paraffin section examination; the proportion of cases in which this is necessary varies in the literature from 3%[69] to 33%.[68]

Discrepancies between frozen section diagnosis and paraffin section features, although rare, are most commonly caused by either misinterpretation by the pathologist or the presence of a focal or missed lesion.[67,70,71] Over-diagnosis of malignancy may be caused by 'sclero-elastotic lesions'[72] and lesions which mimic, and are thus misinterpreted as, invasive lobular carcinoma.[73] On occasions inflammatory infiltrates may be especially difficult to distinguish from invasive lobular carcinoma and caution is necessary before this diagnosis is made. False negative diagnosis may be a particular problem with DCIS where the accuracy may be as low as 27%, largely as a result of errors in selection of material.[70]

Whilst some authors suggest that frozen section diagnosis of mammographically detected lesions is as accurate as in symptomatic practice (approximately 98%[74]) it is generally agreed that frozen section examination of screen-detected lesions is not recommended.[75] In exceptional circumstances its use may be warranted,[76] but false diagnosis increases with diminishing size of the lesion. The use of frozen sections to examine small lesions (less than 1 cm or impalpable) may also result in the loss of much of the neoplastic tissue[77,78] leaving only limited or poorly fixed/prepared material for full histopathological assessment in paraffin material at a later date. As described above, DCIS may be particularly difficult to diagnose accurately on frozen section and this technique is not advised for the examination of microcalcifications.[79]

EXAMINATION OF PATHOLOGICAL SPECIMENS

INTRODUCTION

Increasing numbers of breast biopsies are performed for screen-detected, impalpable lesions and the widespread use of needle localization 'marker' biopsies and associated greater surgical biopsy workload has led to greater scrutiny of the way breast specimens are handled in the laboratory. The surgical technique for diagnostic and excision biopsies differ not only in size but also in nature.

An excision biopsy is composed of a cylinder of tissue from the dermis extending to the deep margin of the breast whilst a diagnostic biopsy includes only the area of interest without concern for the margin of surrounding uninvolved breast parenchyma. The histopathological determination of distance to individual excision margins in the latter specimens is therefore not of great significance, whilst in the former the accurate assessment and measurement of completeness of excision is mandatory. Each breast specimen thus requires handling according to the type of surgical procedure performed and the clinical and mammographic abnormality present.

SYMPTOMATIC LESIONS: EXCISION OF BENIGN ABNORMALITIES AND DIAGNOSTIC BIOPSY OF PALPABLE MASSES

The increased use of the triple approach to diagnosis, with the option of leaving benign lesions in place, has led to a reduction in the need for, and use of, surgical biopsy for benign conditions. When electively excising a benign lesion (or if performing a diagnostic biopsy on a palpable lesion), surgeons are now endeavoring to remove the lesion with the minimum amount of surrounding breast parenchyma; usually less than 20 grams of tissue is resected, thus ensuring the minimum cosmetic defect.

If a discrete lesion is seen macroscopically which corresponds to the clinical description of the lesion, this area should be sampled. If no macroscopic lesion is identified it is often possible to block the entirety of these small specimens after serially slicing at 3–5 mm intervals. Microscopic examination of the entirety of every grossly benign breast biopsy is not, however, cost effective. Where no discrete lesion is seen on macroscopic examination it is best to concentrate sampling on the fibrous parenchymal component of the breast tissue.[80] Schnitt and Wang found that over 75% of microscopically invisible carcinomas or areas of atypical hyperplasia could be identified by taking five tissue blocks and the vast majority were identified if ten blocks were sampled.[80] There appears therefore to be no significant value in taking more than ten blocks from a benign specimen in the first instance and the probability of detecting a significant abnormality in the fatty tissue portion of a benign breast biopsy is exceptionally low.

As noted above the assessment of specific excision margins is usually irrelevant in these small specimens as the lesion will inevitably be close to the edges of the tissue sampled. In our routine practice we do not specifically identify individual margins in such specimens; re-excision is mandatory should a malignant tumor be identified in these samples.

MAMMOGRAPHIC SCREENING LESIONS: MARKER/WIRE LOCALIZATION BIOPSIES

Screen-detected lesions may be particularly difficult to interpret histologically and careful handling and optimum fixation is vital. The specimen must not be incised before reaching the laboratory.

The surgeon should mark the external surface in order to obtain proper orientation. For this purpose we believe that sutures are preferable to metal staples which may retract into the specimen becoming impossible to recognize, and may also obscure microcalcifications. For each unit it is helpful to establish a code of orientation for the sutures (which should be indicated on the requested form); for example, it is our practice to use a short suture to indicate the superior margin, a long suture the lateral margin and a medium length stitch the medial edge of the biopsy (Fig. 2.25). It is, however, important that these are long enough to be easily identified after the specimen has been 'inked' which may obscure very short dark sutures. After surgical excision the specimen, with the guide wire in situ, should be X-rayed so that it can be determined whether the relevant lesion has been resected.

Frozen section examination is generally inappropriate to assess clinically impalpable breast lesions. Extremely rarely it may be justified so that a firm diagnosis of invasive carcinoma can be made and definitive surgery can be carried out in one operation. This should only be attempted if definitive preoperative diagnosis has proved impossible. In addition the mammographic abnormality must be clearly identified on macroscopic

examination and large enough to allow an adequate proportion of the lesion to be fixed and processed without prior freezing. Previously frozen and then routinely processed samples are invariably and notoriously difficult to interpret reliably. Tissue for estrogen receptor (ER) determination by ligand binding assay should be snap frozen in liquid nitrogen within 30 minutes of excision; we now, however, routinely assess ER status on formalin-fixed, paraffin-embedded sections.[81] If sent to the laboratory 'fresh' the specimen should be examined within 2–3 hours, but the intact specimen may be examined in the fresh or in the fixed state.

To demonstrate adequacy of excision, the entire surface of the specimen should be painted with marker pigments so that the edges of the sample can be easily determined microscopically; India ink, alcian blue, radiolucent pigments or dyed gelatin are suitable materials. External marking is facilitated by prior removal of surface lipid by dipping the specimen in alcohol and drying and by subsequent external fixation by an acid fixative. The specimen can then be dried and incised in the fresh state if required without penetration of the pigment.

It cannot be stressed enough that good fixation is vital to preserve the degree of morphological detail needed to diagnose borderline lesions and to report features of prognostic significance, particularly histological grade and vascular invasion in invasive carcinomas. Small specimens may be fixed whole, but larger ones should be examined and incised/sliced if possible within 2–3 hours of excision to allow optimum penetration of fixative.

The specimen should be weighed and measured and then serially sliced at intervals of up to 4 mm. The slices are then carefully inspected. Palpation may also be informative. The size, color, contour and consistency of any macroscopic lesion are recorded. The macroscopic measurement of lesions should be checked later on histological sections; the true extent of the abnormality is not always apparent by naked eye. If the macroscopic and microscopic measurements are conflicting, the histological dimensions should be accepted as the true size. Adequacy of excision of lesions should also be assessed by naked eye and the distance to the margins re-measured microscopically.

Specimen orientation

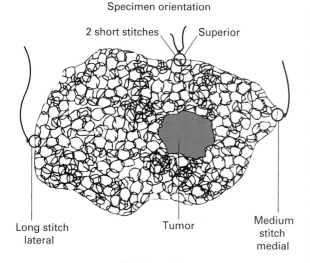

Left breast biopsy

Fig. 2.25 Orientation of surgical specimens requires intraoperative marking of specimens, preferably using a standardized annotation system.

Unless a lesion obviously accounting for the radiological abnormality is identified on inspection of the specimen slices, further X-ray examination should be performed. Blocks should then be taken from the areas corresponding to the mammographic abnormalities in addition to any other macroscopically suspicious zones (Fig. 2.26). For reviews see Anderson (1989),[82] Armstrong and Davies (1991),[83] Elston and Ellis (1990)[84] and Schnitt and Connolly (1992).[85] This method of specimen slice radiography allows precise correlations to be made between the mammographic, specimen and slice X-rays and histological appearances. It gives a very high level of confidence that the histological sections produced are representative of the mammographic lesion originally identified in the screening mammograms. It has been demonstrated that block selection on the basis of radiographic abnormality has a very high level of detection of clinically significant abnormalities and a considerable reduction in the amount of tissue processed.[86]

However, this optimum method is time-consuming and a number of shorter, one stage, methods have been reported; for reviews see Anderson (1989),[82] Armstrong and Davies (1991)[83] and Elston and Ellis (1990).[84] We do not recommend that tissue is simply taken from around the guide wire, which may not necessarily

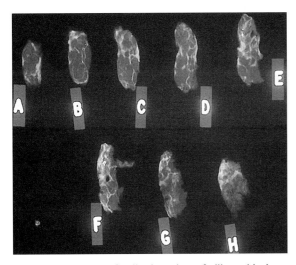

Fig. 2.26   An X-ray of a sliced specimen facilitates block selection from diagnostic mammographic localization specimens by identifying those slices of tissue which contain the mammographic lesion.

be very close to the mammographic abnormality. Whichever method is chosen, the pathologist must be satisfied that the pathological changes responsible for radiological abnormalities have been identified in the sections; it may be necessary to consult with the radiologists to be certain of this. If there is doubt, it is helpful to re-X-ray the residual unblocked tissue and/or the paraffin blocks. Thus any residual tissue should be stored until the mammographic changes have been definitively characterized histologically.

Rarely the mammographic abnormality cannot be identified either in the specimen slices or in the histological sections. This may result when the lesion produces only architectural change in the clinical mammogram but may also occur when the surgical localization of the abnormality has been unsuccessful. Pathological examination should be thorough even in the latter cases and the findings communicated to the surgeon. Repeat mammography can subsequently be used to determine whether the lesion is still present in the breast.

It is not possible to be dogmatic regarding the precise number of blocks which should be taken. This clearly depends on the size and number of lesions present. If the specimen is small it is often simplest to block and examine all the tissue. For malignant tumors in excess of 20 mm in maximum extent, at least three or four blocks of the tumor are desirable. A minimum of one block should include the edge of the tumor and, if possible, the nearest excision margin to enable measurement of this distance, in millimeters, on the histological sections.

For larger biopsies which cannot be blocked in toto, it is advisable to sample some radiologically and macroscopically apparently normal breast tissue. In this way the detection of small occult cancers, particularly in situ carcinoma, and atypical proliferative lesions can be increased. The incidental detection of such abnormalities in unscreened women depends on the number of blocks taken. Additional sampling is more effective if restricted to fibrous parenchyma rather than adipose tissue.[80,86] The extent of sampling, both of biopsies containing benign mammographic abnormalities and breast parenchyma adjacent to malignant lesions, will depend largely on local resources.

Large blocks and sections are used in some laboratories where they are found to be of value in identifying screen-detected lesions and determining their size, adequacy of excision and distance to the margins of the specimen.[87,88] They particularly facilitate orientation by obviating the need for mental reconstruction of the specimen from several sections; fewer large blocks are required. Adequate fixation and good cytological detail may, however, be difficult to achieve and large sections are technically more difficult to cut and also to store. The use of large blocks depends on local preference and is not essential.

THERAPEUTIC/WIDE LOCAL EXCISION SPECIMENS

Such specimens arise from patients with a pre-operative diagnosis of carcinoma, achieved through the triple approach assessment, who have been deemed suitable for conservation therapy and who have chosen local excision. The surgeon aims to achieve excision with an adequate surrounding margin of uninvolved breast tissue; these specimens are thus usually larger than a diagnostic excision biopsy. As discussed above, the surgeon resects a cylinder of breast tissue from the dermis to the deep fascia, unless there is macroscopic gross involvement of the superficial or deep margins. We routinely utilize intraoperative specimen X-rays and thus assess the distance of the tumor mass to the radial (not superficial or deep) edges of the tissue taken (see Ch. 22). Should the lesion be seen to be close to a margin on specimen radiograph, re-excision can be immediately directed to the appropriate area. The additional, separate specimen is also submitted for histological examination having been orientated by appropriate sutures by the surgeon.

The main specimen is orientated using the standard convention of sutures in our unit: a long suture marks the lateral border, medium the medial edge and short the superior margin of the tissue, as noted above and shown in Fig. 2.25. As also described above, the specimen excision surfaces are marked; we use India ink for this purpose. The tumor is then incised in the fresh state in a cruciate fashion (Fig. 2.27) to ensure rapid

fixation of a number of faces of the tumor and to allow fresh tumor samples to be taken, if required.

After fixation, the specimen is sampled; a series (usually four) of tumor blocks for prognostic factor evaluation (histological grade, type, size and vascular invasion) are taken which include the peripheral margin of the tumor (Figs 2.27 and 2.28). Further blocks (usually four in number) are taken to include tumor and parts of the radial excision margin to allow measurement of distance to margins. In a smaller specimen the blocks of the periphery of the tumor may also encompass the radial resection margins of the biopsy. Shave blocks from the external surface are also taken (Fig. 2.28). Unless the tumor extends extremely close to, or overtly involves, the superficial or deep excision margins these are not separately sampled for the reasons given above.

RE-EXCISION SPECIMENS

Those patients who have had a previous diagnostic biopsy which contained carcinoma or a therapeutic excision with an involved margin may have re-excision of the cavity and surrounding tissue. Selection of blocks may be difficult in these specimens and it is essential that the specimen is accurately orientated by the surgeon and this detail communicated to the pathologist. The extent of sampling of the specimen depends on the amount of tissue resected, but it is currently our policy to concentrate on shave excision blocks from the peripheral radial margins. The cavity margin is also sampled (but not exhaustively) to determine whether residual carcinoma is present.

MASTECTOMY SPECIMENS

Mastectomy specimens should ideally be examined and incised within 2 hours of removal to allow adequate penetration of fixative. We currently restrict this to incision of the tumor immediately after resection in a cruciate manner, as described above, and slice the breast more extensively after fixation. Alternatively others favor slicing the entire breast in the fresh state, from the deep surface in the sagittal plane at about 10 mm inter-

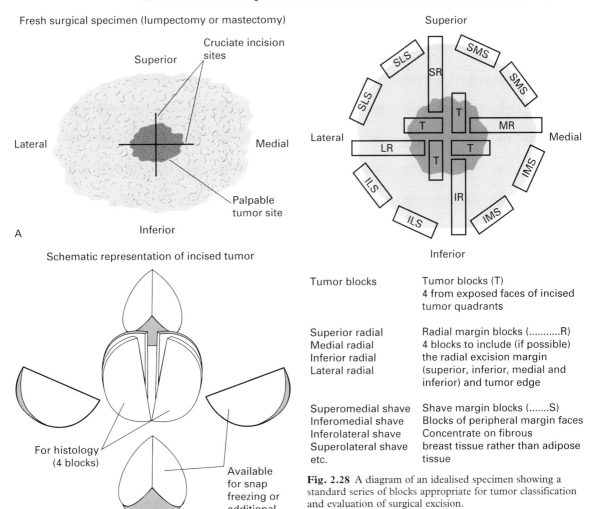

Fig. 2.27 In our unit tumors are incised in the fresh state in a cruciate manner to allow optimum fixation of a number of faces of the tumor and to allow sampling of fresh tissue.

Tumor blocks	Tumor blocks (T) 4 from exposed faces of incised tumor quadrants
Superior radial Medial radial Inferior radial Lateral radial	Radial margin blocks (..........R) 4 blocks to include (if possible) the radial excision margin (superior, inferior, medial and inferior) and tumor edge
Superomedial shave Inferomedial shave Inferolateral shave Superolateral shave etc.	Shave margin blocks (.......S) Blocks of peripheral margin faces Concentrate on fibrous breast tissue rather than adipose tissue

Fig. 2.28 A diagram of an idealised specimen showing a standard series of blocks appropriate for tumor classification and evaluation of surgical excision.

vals after measuring the dimensions of the specimen. The slices are either left joined by the skin or may be separated completely and arranged in order. The site and maximum diameter of the main lesion should be measured and the distance from the nearest margin of excision determined as for biopsies (see above).

Blocks of tumor should be taken to include the periphery of the mass, as described above, and must always be sufficient to represent the maximum extent of the lesion noted macroscopically. If tumor is suspected to reach an excision margin macroscopically this must be sampled; painting with India ink or pigments may again be helpful. If the margins of a previous therapeutic excision specimen have been involved and the patient has been required to convert to mastectomy, blocks should be taken from the biopsy cavity wall. This can be identified by an area of fat necrosis, scarring or hematoma according to the time since biopsy.

The whole breast slices should be examined by careful inspection and palpation and sections taken from any suspicious areas, noting the quadrant from which they are located. In addition 'random' blocks from the fibrous tissue of each quadrant and from the nipple should be examined.

AXILLARY SPECIMENS

Axillary specimens received either alone or with mastectomy or biopsy specimens should be examined thoroughly in order to maximize the lymph node yield. This is usually achieved by slicing the specimen thinly with subsequent careful inspection and palpation. Clearing agents or Bouin's solution may increase lymph node yield but are both time-consuming and expensive and are not, in our opinion, necessary. If axillary contents, rather than sampled lymph nodes, are obtained the specimen can be divided into three levels if the surgeon has marked the specimen appropriately.

All lymph nodes received must be examined histologically and the report should record both the total number of nodes and the number containing metastatic deposits. Lymph nodes less than 5 mm in maximum extent should be embedded in their entirety. A single section of a lymph node which clearly contains metastatic tumor is adequate. We believe that other lymph nodes should be sliced and examined individually in separate blocks. It is our practise to examine a slice of lymph node for each 5 mm of the maximum extent; thus two slices of a 10 mm lymph node and three slices of a 15 mm lymph node are assessed microscopically. Detection of metastatic deposits can be increased by examination at two or more levels of the paraffin blocks or through use of immunocytochemistry; this is, however, both time consuming and expensive and we do not routinely perform these further procedures.

REFERENCES

1. Lamb J, Anderson TJ, Dixon MJ, Levack PA. Role of fine needle aspiration cytology in breast cancer screening. J Clin Pathol 1987; 40: 705–709.
2. Negri S, Bonetti F, Capitanio A, Bonzanini M. Preoperative diagnostic accuracy of fine-needle aspiration in the management of breast lesions: comparison of specificity and sensitivity with clinical examination, mammography, echography, and thermography in 249 patients. Diagn Cytopathol 1994; 11: 4–8.
3. Martelli G, Pilotti S, Coopmans de Yoldi G et al. Diagnostic efficacy of physical examination, mammography, fine needle aspiration cytology (triple-test) in solid breast lumps: an analysis of 1708 consecutive cases. Tumori 1990; 76: 476–479.
4. Vetto J, Pommier R, Schmidt W et al. Use of the 'triple test' for palpable breast lesions yields high diagnostic accuracy and cost savings. Am J Surg 1995; 169: 519–522.
5. Sibbering DM, Burrell HC, Evans AJ et al. Mammographic sensitivity in women under 50 presenting symptomatically with breast cancer. The Breast 1995; 4: 127–129.
6. Stavros T, Thickman D, Rapp CL, Dennis MA, Parker SH, Sisney GA. Solid breast nodules: use of sonography to distinguish between benign and malignant lesions. Radiology 1995; 196: 123–134.
7. Ciatto S, Rosselli Del Turco M, Catarzi S, Morrone D. The contribution of ultrasonography to the differential diagnosis of breast cancer. Neoplasma 1994; 41: 341–345.
8. Fornage BD, Lorigan JG, Andry E. Fibroadenoma of the breast: sonographic appearances. 1989; 172: 671–675.
9. Ciatto S, Morrone D, Catarzi S et al. Radial scars of the breast: review of 38 consecutive mammographic diagnoses. Radiol 1993; 187: 757–760.
10. Finlay ME, Liston JE, Lunt LG, Young JR. Assessment of the role of ultrasound in the differentiation of radial scars and stellate carcinomas of the breast. Clin Radiol 1994; 49: 52–55.
11. Sonnerfeld MR et al. Lobular carcinoma in situ: mammographic-pathologic correlation of results of needle directed biopsy. Radiol 1991; 181: 363–367.
12. Rubin E, Mazue MT, Urist MM, Maddox WA. Clinical, radiographic and pathological correlation of atypical ductal hyperplasia, ductal carcinoma in situ and ductal carcinoma in situ with microinvasion. Breast 1993; 2: 21–26.
13. Stomper PC, Connolly JL. Ductal carcinoma in situ of the breast: correlation between mammographic calcification and tumour subtype. AJR Am J Roentgenol 1992; 159: 483–485.
14. Evans A, Pinder SE, Wilson ARM et al. Ductal carcinoma in situ of the breast: correlation between mammographic and pathologic findings. AJR Am J Roentgenol 1994; 162: 1307–1311.
15. Holland R, Hendricks JHCL, Verbeek ALM, Mravunac M, Schuurrmans Stekhoven JH. Extent, distribution and mammographic/histological correlations of breast ductal carcinoma in situ. Lancet 1990; 335: 519–522.
16. Checcherini AFA, Evans AJ, Pinder SE, Wilson ARM, Ellis IO, Yeoman LJ. Is ipsilateral mammography worthwhile in Paget's disease of the breast? Clin Radiol 1996; 51: 35–38.
17. Burrell HC, Pinder SE, Wilson ARM et al. The positive predictive value of mammographic signs: a review of 425 non-palpable breast lesions. Clin Radiol 1996; 51: 277–281.

18. De Nunzio MC, Evans AJ, Pinder SE et al. Correlations between the mammographic features of prevalent round screen detected invasive breast cancer and pathological prognostic factors. Breast 1997; 6: 146–149.

19. Cornford EJ, Wilson ARM, Athanassiou E et al. Mammographic features of invasive lobular cancer and invasive ductal carcinoma of the breast: a comparative analysis. Br J Radiol 1995; 68: 450–453.

20. Leiberman AJ, Lewis M, Kruse B. Tubular carcinoma of the breast: mammographic appearance. AJR Am J Roentgenol 1993; 160: 263–265.

21. Stutz JA, Pinder SE, Ellis IO et al. The radiological appearances of invasive cribriform carcinoma of the breast. Clin Radiol 1994; 49: 693–695.

22. Chopra S, Evans AJ, Pinder SE et al. Pure mucinous breast cancer-mammographic and ultrasound findings. Clin Radiol 1996; 51: 421–424.

23. Liberman L, Dershaw DD, Kaufman RJ et al. Angiosarcoma of the breast. AJR Am J Roentgenol 1992; 183: 649–654.

24. Guidelines for cytology procedures and reporting in breast cancer screening. Sheffield: NHSBSP Publications, 1993. NHSBSP Publication No. 22.

25. Fessia L, Botta G, Arisio R, Verga M, Aimone V. Fine-needle aspiration of breast lesions: role and accuracy in a review of 7,495 cases. Diagn Cytopathol 1987; 3: 121–125.

26. Esteban JM, Zaloudek C, Silverberg SG. Intraoperative diagnosis of breast lesions. Comparison of cytologic with frozen section technics. Am J Clin Pathol 1987; 88: 681–688.

27. De Rosa G, Boschi R, Boscaino A et al. Intraoperative cytology in breast cancer diagnosis: comparison between cytologic and frozen section techniques. Diagn Cytopathol 1993; 9: 623–631.

28. Dahlstrom JE, Jain S, Sutton T, Sutton S. Diagnostic accuracy of stereotaxic core biopsy in a mammography breast cancer screening programme. Histopathology 1996; 28: 537–541.

29. Layfield LJ, Glasgow BJ, Cramer H. Fine-needle aspiration in the management of breast masses. Pathol Annu 1989; 24: 23–62.

30. Adye B, Jolly PC, Bauermeister DE. The role of fine-needle aspiration in the management of solid breast masses. Arch Surg 1988; 123: 37–39.

31. Preece PE, Hunter SM, Duguid HL, Wood RA. Cytodiagnosis and other methods of biopsy in the modern management of breast cancer. Semin Surg Oncol 1989; 5: 69–81.

32. Lee KR, Foster RS, Papillo JL. Fine needle aspiration of the breast. Importance of the aspirator. Acta Cytol 1987; 31: 281–284.

33. Hunt CH, Wilson S, Pinder SE, Elston CW, Ellis IO. United Kingdom national audit of breast fine needle aspiration cytology in 1990–1991. Organization and level of activity. Cytopathology 1996; 7: 316–325.

34. Howat AJ, Stringfellow HF, Briggs WA, Nicholson CM. Fine needle aspiration cytology of the breast: A review of 1,868 cases using the Cytospin method. Acta Cytol 1994; 38: 939–944.

35. Guidelines for cytology procedures and reporting on fine needle aspirates of the breast. Cytology Subgroup of the National Coordinating Committee for Breast Cancer Screening Pathology. Cytopathology 1994; 5: 316–334.

36. Matthews P, Pinder SE, Elston CW, Ellis IO. Audit of

37. Matthews P, Pinder SE, Elston CW, Ellis IO. Suspicious fine needle aspiration cytology of the breast — an audit of use and outcome. J Pathol 1996; 178: 23A.

38. McMahon AJ, Lutfy AM, Matthew A et al. Needle core biopsy of the breast with a spring-loaded device. Br J Surg 1992; 79: 1042–1045.

39. Parker SH, Burbank F, Jackman RJ et al. Percutaneous large-core breast biopsy: a multi-institutional study. Radiology 1994; 193: 359–364.

40. Parker SH, Lovin JD, Jobe WE, Burke BJ, Hopper KD, Yakes WF. Nonpalpable breast lesions: stereotactic automated large-core biopsies. Radiology 1991; 180: 403–407.

41. Parker SH, Jobe WE, Dennis MA et al. US-guided automated large-core breast biopsy. Radiology 1993; 187: 507–511.

42. Vega A, Garijo F, Ortega E. Core needle aspiration biopsy of palpable breast masses. Acta Oncol 1995; 34: 31–34.

43. Cusick JD, Dotan J, Jaecks RD, Boyle W Jr. The role of Tru-Cut needle biopsy in the diagnosis of carcinoma of the breast. Surg Gynecol Obstet 1990; 170: 407–410.

44. Minkowitz S, Moskowitz R, Khafif RA, Alderete MN. TRU-CUT needle biopsy of the breast. An analysis of its specificity and sensitivity. Cancer 1986; 57: 320–323.

45. Parker SH. Percutaneous large core breast biopsy. Cancer 1994; 74: 256–262.

46. Caines JS, McPhee MD, Konok GP, Wright BA. Stereotaxic needle core biopsy of breast lesions using a regular mammographic table with an adaptable stereotaxic device. AJR Am J Roentgenol 1994; 163: 317–321.

47. Dronkers DJ. Stereotaxic core biopsy of breast lesions. Radiology 1992; 183: 631–634.

48. Vega A, Arrizabalaga R, Garijo F, Guerra I. Nonpalpable breast lesion. Stereotaxic core needle aspiration biopsy with a single pass. Acta Radiol 1995; 36: 117–121.

49. Gisvold JJ, Goellner JR, Grant CS et al. Breast biopsy: a comparative study of stereotaxically guided core and excisional techniques. AJR Am J Roentgenol 1994; 162: 815–820.

50. Liberman L, Dershaw DD, Rosen PP, Abramson AF, Deutch BM, Hann LE. Stereotaxic 14-gauge breast biopsy: how many core biopsy specimens are needed? Radiology 1994; 192: 793–795.

51. Carty NJ, Ravichandran D, Carter C, Mudan S, Royle GT, Taylor I. Randomized comparison of fine-needle aspiration cytology and biopty-cut needle biopsy after unsatisfactory initial cytology of discrete breast lesions. Br J Surg 1994; 81: 1313–1314.

52. Sadler GP, McGee S, Dallimore NS et al. Role of fine-needle aspiration cytology and needle-core biopsy in the diagnosis of lobular carcinoma of the breast. Br J Surg 1994; 81: 1315–1317.

53. Lamb J, Anderson TJ. Influence of cancer histology on the success of fine needle aspiration of the breast. J Clin Pathol 1989; 42: 733–735.

54. Liberman L, Evans WR, Dershaw DD et al. Radiography of microcalcifications in stereotaxic mammary core biopsy specimens. Radiology 1994; 190: 223–225.

55. Hann LE, Liberman L, Dershaw DD, Cohen MA,

equivocal fine needle aspiration cytology (FNAC) — use and outcome. J Pathol 1996; 178: 6A.

Abramson AF. Mammography immediately after stereotaxic breast biopsy: is it necessary? AJR Am J Roentgenol 1995; 165: 59–62.

56. Tornos C, Silva E, el-Naggar A, Pritzker KP. Calcium oxalate crystals in breast biopsies. The missing microcalcifications. Am J Surg Pathol 1990; 14: 961–968.

57. Symonds DA. Use of the von Kossa stain in identifying occult calcifications in breast biopsies. Am J Clin Pathol 1990; 94: 44–48.

58. Harlow CL, Schackmuth EM, Bregman PS, Zeligman BE, Coffin CT. Sonographic detection of hematomas and fluid after imaging guided core breast biopsy. J Ultrasound Med 1994; 13: 877–882.

59. Schackmuth EM, Harlow CL, Norton LW. Milk fistula: a complication after core breast biopsy. AJR Am J Roentgenol 1993; 161: 961–962.

60. Mikhail RA, Nathan RC, Weiss M et al. Stereotactic core needle biopsy of mammographic breast lesions as a viable alternative to surgical biopsy. Ann Surg Oncol 1994; 1: 363–367.

61. Harter LP, Curtis JS, Ponto G, Craig PH. Malignant seeding of the needle track during stereotaxic core needle breast biopsy. Radiology 1992; 185: 713–714.

62. Grabau DA, Andersen JA, Graversen HP, Dyreborg U. Needle biopsy of breast cancer. Appearance of tumour cells along the needle track. Eur J Surg Oncol 1993; 19: 192–194.

63. Youngson BJ, Cranor M, Rosen PP. Epithelial displacement in surgical breast specimens following needling procedures. Am J Surg Pathol 1994; 18: 896–903.

64. Youngson BJ, Liberman L, Rosen PP. Displacement of carcinomatous epithelium in surgical breast specimens following stereotaxic core biopsy. Am J Clin Pathol 1995; 103: 598–602.

65. Cheung PS, Yan KW, Alagaratnam TT. The complementary role of fine needle aspiration cytology and Tru-cut needle biopsy in the management of breast masses. Aust NZ J Surg 1987; 57: 615–620.

66. Litherland JC, Evans AJ, Wilson ARM et al. The impact of core biopsy on preoperative diagnosis rate of screen detected cancers. Clin Rad 1996; 51: 562–565.

67. Torp SH, Skjorten FJ. The reliability of frozen section diagnosis. Acta Chir Scand 1990; 156: 127–130.

68. Bianchi S, Palli D, Ciatto S et al. Accuracy and reliability of frozen section diagnosis in a series of 672 nonpalpable breast lesions. Am J Clin Pathol 1995; 199–205.

69. Caya JG. Accuracy of breast frozen section diagnosis in the community hospital setting: a detailed analysis of 628 cases. Wis Med J 1991; 90: 58–61.

70. GhandurMnaymneh L, Porto R, Moezzi M. The changing presentation of carcinoma of the breast and its impact on the reliability of the frozen section diagnosis. Breast Dis 1992; 5: 235–242.

71. Jakic-Razumovic J, Cacic M, Krizanac S, Boric I. Frozen section analysis of breast biopsy specimens. Acta Med Croatica 1993; 47: 75–79.

72. Dalla Palma P. Pathological problems of intraoperative diagnosis in sclero-elastotic lesions of the breast. Eur J Gynaecol Oncol 1988; 9: 94–97.

73. Underwood JC, Parsons MA, Harris SC, Dundas SA. Frozen section appearances simulating invasive lobular carcinoma in breast tissue adjacent to inflammatory lesions and biopsy sites. Histopathology 1988; 13: 232–234.

74. Ferreiro JA, Gisvold JJ, Bostwick DG. Accuracy of frozen-section diagnosis of mammographically directed breast biopsies: Results of 1,490 consecutive cases. Am J Surg Pathol 1995; 19: 1267–1271.

75. Fechner RE. Frozen section examination of breast biopsies. Practice parameter. Am J Clin Pathol 1995; 103: 6–7.

76. Rosen PP. Pathological assessment of nonpalpable breast lesions. Semin Surg Oncol 1991; 7: 257–260.

77. Eskelinen M, Collan Y, Puittinen J, Valkamo E. Frozen section diagnosis of breast cancer. Acta Oncol 1989; 28: 183–186.

78. Hou MF, Huang TJ, Lin HJ et al. Frozen section of diagnosis of breast lesions. Kao Hsiung I Hsueh Ko Hsueh Tsa Chih 1995; 11: 621–625.

79. Tinnemans JG, Wobbes T, Holland R et al. Mammographic and histopathologic correlation of nonpalpable lesions of the breast and the reliability of frozen section diagnosis. Surg Gynecol Obstet 1987; 165: 523–529.

80. Schnitt SJ, Wang HH. Histologic sampling of grossly benign breast biopsies. How much is enough? Am J Surg Pathol 1989; 13: 505–512.

81. Goulding H, Pinder S, Cannon P et al. A new immunohistochemical antibody for the assessment of estrogen receptor status on routine formalin-fixed tissue samples. Hum Pathol 1995; 26: 291–294.

82. Anderson TJ. Breast cancer screening: principles and practicalities for histopathologists. In: Anthony PP, MacSween RNM, ed. Recent advances in histopathology. Edinburgh: Churchill Livingstone, 1989; vol 14, pp. 46–61.

83. Armstrong JS, Davies JD. Laboratory handling of impalpable breast lesions: A review. J Clin Pathol 1991; 44: 89–93.

84. Elston CW, Ellis IO. Pathology and breast screening. Histopathology 1990; 16: 109–118.

85. Schnitt SJ, Connolly JL. Processing and evaluation of breast excision specimens. A clinically oriented approach. Am J Clin Pathol 1992; 98: 125–137.

86. Owings DV, Hann L, Schnitt SJ. How thoroughly should needle localization breast biopsies be sampled for microscopic examination? A prospective mammographic/pathologic correlative study. Am J Surg Pathol 1990; 14: 578–583.

87. Gibbs NM. Comparative study of the histopathology of breast cancer in a screened and unscreened population investigated by mammography. Histopathol 1985; 9: 1307–1318.

88. Gibbs NM, Armstrong JS, Davies JD. Laboratory handling of impalpable breast lesions. J Clin Pathol 1991; 44: 524.

I. O. Ellis and C. W. Elston

3

Classification of benign breast disease

The pathological and clinical classification of breast disease and in particular benign breast disease is hampered by a failure to use common terminology both within individual medical disciplines and between disciplines, leading to confusion and difficulties of comparison between some published studies. The Royal College of Pathologists[1-3] and American Society of Pathology[4,5] have produced guidelines on reporting breast disease which support this view and propose virtually identical systems of classification of benign conditions which pathologists are encouraged to adopt. In the following chapters on benign breast disease we mirror these classifications. Benign breast tumors are presented according to the major accepted groupings of fibrocystic change, fibroadenoma and variants, sclerosing lesions, papillary lesions, epithelial proliferative disease, inflammatory conditions and the rare and unusual in a miscellaneous section.

Studies of diagnostic reproducibility between pathologists have shown a poor concordance when there is no consensus on classification methodology[6] but good agreement when pathologists are encouraged to adopt the same diagnostic descriptions and are offered training.[7,8] We have endeavored to use widely accepted definitions and descriptions for the common benign conditions and would encourage readers to adhere to such terminology.

Attempts have been made to simplify classification of benign breast disease and the most notable has been the introduction of the concept of 'Aberrations of Normal Development and Involution'.[9,10] This concept is based on the view that most benign conditions can be explained as

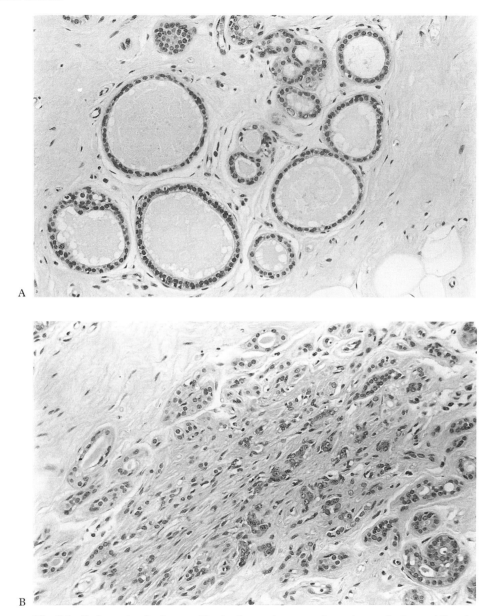

Fig. 3.1 Various microfocal areas of benign breast changes such as microcystic change (A) and sclerosing adenosis (B) are very common findings and can be classified as minimal alteration. Hematoxylin–eosin × 185.

minor aberrations of the normal processes of development (fibroadenoma and juvenile hypertrophy), cyclical change (mastalgia and nodularity), and involution (cyst formation and sclerosing adenosis). In contrast the condition duct ectasia is believed to be a primary event resulting from duct leakage and inflammation. Epithelial hyperplasia and papillomas are regarded as more complex conditions which may have an association with cyclical and involutional changes. Although a laudable attempt to unify terminology and assist management of many common breast conditions we share the views of Anderson[11] that specific benign conditions should be recognized and classified separately to improve knowledge of their significance. We have adopted the term 'minimal alteration (ANDI)' used by Anderson[11] to describe microfocal areas of adenosis, apocrine metaplasia, sclerosed lobules, and microcysts (<1 mm) seen in isolation or in combination, and use standard terminology to describe more established benign lesions.

The major challenge to pathologists in the arena of benign breast disease is the need to improve consistency of recognition of the range of epithelial proliferative lesions and their boundary with low grade in situ malignancy. Again studies have show poor reproducibility,[6,8] but the results of one study where clear guidelines and training were given[7] suggest that acceptable levels of agreement can be achieved between enthusiastic are trained observers. The significance of such lesions in terms of risk for subsequent development of breast cancer is now generally accepted[12] and it rests with diagnostic pathologists to explore these lesions and develop classification methods which are reproducible and have clinical relevance.

REFERENCES

1. Royal College of Pathologists Working Group. Pathology Reporting in Breast Cancer Screening. J Clin Pathol 1991; 44: 710–725.
2. National Coordinating Committee for Breast Screening Pathology. Pathology Reporting in Breast Cancer Screening. Second ed. Sheffield NHS Breast Screening Programme, 1995.
3. Royal College of Pathologists Working Group and UK National Breast Screening Programme. Pathology Reporting in Breast Cancer Screening. Sheffield: NHS Breast Screening Programme, 1990.
4. Hutter RVP. Goodbye to 'fibrocystic disease'. New Eng J Med 1985; 312: 179–181.
5. Hutter RVP. Consensus meeting. Is fibrocystic disease of the breast precancerous? Arch Pathol 1986; 110: 171–173.
6. Rosai J. Borderline epithelial lesions of the breast. Am J Surg Pathol 1991; 15: 209–221.
7. Schnitt SJ, Connolly JL, Tavassoli FA et al. Interobserver reproducibility in the diagnosis of ductal proliferative breast lesions using standardised criteria. Am J Surg Pathol 1992; 16: 1133–1143.
8. Sloane JP, Ellman R, Anderson TJ et al. Consistency of histopathological reporting of breast lesions detected by breast screening: Findings of the UK national external quality assessment (EQA) scheme. Eur J Cancer 1994; 10: 1414–1419.
9. Hughes LE, Mansel RE, Webster DJT. Aberrations of normal development and involution (ANDI): A new perspective on pathogenesis and nomenclature of benign breast disorders. Lancet 1987; i: 1316–1319.
10. Hughes LE, Mansel RE, Webster DJT. Benign disorders and diseases of the breast. In: London: Baillière Tindall, 1989; pp. 93–101.
11. Anderson TJ. Classifying benign breast changes. Lancet 1988; i: 240–241.
12. Connolly JL, Schnitt SJ. Benign breast disease, resolved and unresolved issues. Cancer 1993; 71: 1187–1189.

Fibrocystic change

INTRODUCTION

The term fibrocystic change refers to a variety of morphological features which are believed to represent an exaggerated physiological response in breast tissue. The current terminology reflects this and has replaced previous terms such as 'fibrous mastopathy', 'mammary dysplasia' and 'fibrocystic disease', in which a pathological process is implied. The changes seen include gross and microscopic cysts, apocrine metaplasia and blunt duct adenosis. At one end of the spectrum they merge with minor changes including microcyst formation, fibrosis, lobular involution and minor degrees of sclerosing adenosis or blunt duct adenosis which may be regarded as normal morphological variations, or aberrations of normal development and involution.[1] At the other end of the spectrum, they should be distinguished from specific entities in which a dominant histological process is present, such as sclerosing adenosis, which may have different clinicopathological implications (Ch. 7).

In view of its importance in determining breast cancer risk, the presence or absence of epithelial hyperplasia and its character should be reported separately.[2,3] For this reason, although a frequent component of fibrocystic change, epithelial hyperplasia is discussed separately in Chapter 5.

The microscopic features of each component will be described separately but the pathogenesis, clinical features, macroscopic features, management and prognostic implications will be considered for the entity as a whole.

This chapter also includes two further epithelial alterations which may be seen as an incidental finding in breast tissue, namely focal lactational change and clear cell metaplasia.

CLINICAL FEATURES

Both clinical[4,5] and autopsy[6] studies show that morphological features of fibrocystic change affect women between 20 and 50 years of age, but with the majority occurring between 40 and 50 years. In her study of 225 post mortems, Frantz reported visible cysts of 1 mm or more in diameter in 18.6% and microscopic changes in 34%.[6] However, of those with visible cysts, only one had palpable gross cysts. Thus, the majority of women with morphological changes are likely to be asymptomatic and there is poor correlation between histology and symptoms. Where present, symptoms usually subside within a year or two of the menopause unless estrogen replacement therapy is administered. Symptomatic women may also give a history of menstrual abnormalities, early menarche and late menopause, are often nulliparous or have a history of spontaneous abortions and are unlikely to use an oral contraceptive which appears to have a protective effect.[7]

Some women may present with smooth, discrete breast lumps which may or may not be fluctuant and which are identified as cysts on aspiration. Non-fluctuant, 'tension cysts' may resemble a carcinoma clinically. Sudden pain, probably following leakage of cyst contents causing chemical irritation, may draw attention to a cyst. Alternatively, they may be discovered incidentally during clinical examination or mammography. Cysts are frequently multiple and recur. In Haagensen's series of 1998 patients with cystic disease followed up for a minimum of 5 years, approximately half had a single cyst, a third had from three to five and the remainder developed more than five.[4]

Another group of patients present with breast pain and nodularity which are often cyclical and it is in this group of patients that the correlation between symptoms and morphological features is especially poor. Vorherr has divided these clinical features into three phases.[5] In the earliest phase, women in their mid-twenties to early thirties complain of premenstrual breast pain, tenderness and swelling of about one week's duration which subside on menstruation. Later, pain and tenderness increase in both intensity and duration and the breast tissues become denser and nodular. In the final phase, usually in women in their forties, the symptoms may be permanent and the palpable lumps and cysts larger. In approximately 20% of patients, axillary lymphadenopathy and tenderness are observed. Cyst formation and microcalcification may be identified on ultrasound and imaging investigations.

It must be stressed again that there is little correlation between the symptoms described in the foregoing paragraph and the morphological changes to be described below, particularly in the earliest phases.

MACROSCOPIC FEATURES

The changes are usually multifocal and bilateral but localized accentuation may result in the removal of a clinically palpable lump. In grossly evident cases, involved areas are usually ill-defined and consist of firm fibro-fatty tissue within which there are multiple blue-domed cysts which are usually 1–2 mm in diameter but which may be several centimeters across. The smaller cysts may contain thin straw-colored fluid but larger cysts more usually contain thicker, darker fluid and often have a thick, fibrous lining.

MICROSCOPIC FEATURES

The term fibrocystic change refers to a number of morphological patterns which are often seen in combination but will be described separately. In addition to the changes described below, foci of sclerosing adenosis and of epithelial hyperplasia may be seen but are discussed elsewhere.

CYSTS

The cyst lining is variable but two main types are recognized; those lacking an epithelial lining or lined by attenuated epithelium and myoepithelium (Fig. 4.1), and those lined by apocrine type

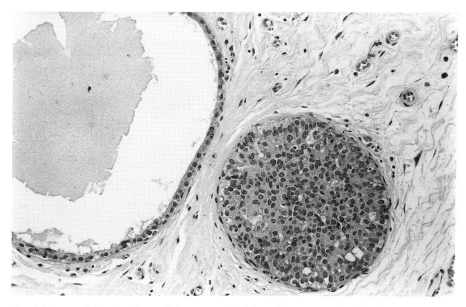

Fig. 4.1 Part of the wall of a small breast cyst lined by a thin attenuated epithelial and myoepithelial layer. Note the adjacent duct space showing epithelial hyperplasia.

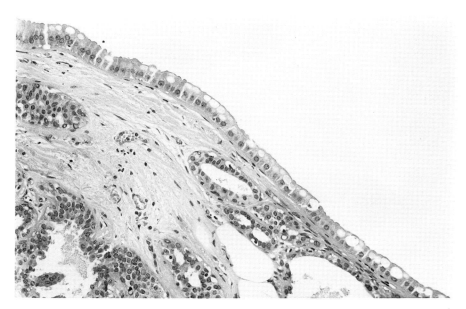

Fig. 4.2 Part of the wall of an apocrine cyst lined by a layer of plump epithelial cells of apocrine morphology. Hematoxylin–eosin × 185.

epithelium in which the cells are large, often columnar, and have abundant granular eosinophilic cytoplasm and a basally located nucleus (Fig. 4.2). The cytoplasmic granules show sudan black and PAS diastase resistant positivity[8] and the cytoplasm may protrude into the lumen as apical snouts. Apocrine cell nuclei often have a prominent round nucleolus and occasional enlarged nuclei are seen. Such 'apocrine atypia' is thought to reflect tetraploidy[9] (Fig. 4.3) (see also Ch. 5). The apocrine cells may form small papillary clusters and, occasionally, more complex

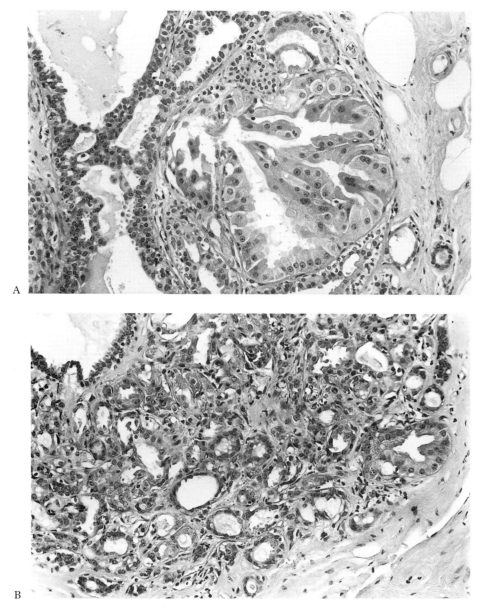

Fig. 4.3 Apocrine epithelial cells can show benign atypia in the form of nuclear enlargement, some pleomorphism and nucleolar prominence (A). This may involve an area of sclerosing adenosis (B) and can be mistaken for an invasive adenocarcinoma. Hematoxylin–eosin × 185.

architectural patterns (Fig. 4.4). The surrounding stroma is often sclerotic and may contain a chronic inflammatory cell infiltrate secondary to cyst rupture.

Examination of cyst fluid has revealed a high content of electrolytes, proteins, including immunoglobulins, and hormones such as calcitonin, prolactin and androgens. The separation of cysts into two diffcrent types on the basis of their epithelial lining is reflected in differences in the composition of the cyst fluid. Apocrine cysts have been found to contain a lower ratio of sodium to potassium than cysts lined by attenuated epithelium whose electrolyte composition more closely approximates to that of plasma.[10] A group of protcins termed 'gross cystic disease fluid proteins' (GCDFP) and first described by Pearlman et al[11]

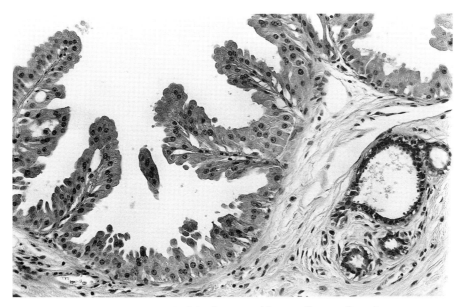

Fig. 4.4 Apocrine metaplastic epithelial cells arranged in a papillary configuration. Hematoxylin–eosin × 185.

has been isolated from cysts and some of these, for example, GCDFP-15, localize immunohistochemically to apocrine epithelium.[12,13]

It has also been suggested that the two types of cyst may show a different pattern of clinical behavior. Dixon et al have suggested that patients who have cysts containing fluid with a high level of potassium (i.e. apocrine cysts) appear more likely to have multiple cysts at presentation and to develop further cysts,[14] although this has been disputed by Ebbs and Bates.[15] Page and Dupont have noted that flattened cysts are larger than apocrine cysts, suggesting that cysts lined by flattened epithelium represent the late stage of development in which the active secretory element is no longer present.[16]

APOCRINE METAPLASIA

This is a frequent finding in the breast and appears to increase in frequency with increasing age. In both the autopsy study of Frantz[6] and that of Wellings and Alpers[17] no apocrine metaplasia was seen in the 13- to 19-year age group whereas this change was identified in over half of those above 30 years. It is usually associated with cysts (see above) but other benign processes such as

sclerosing adenosis, papillomas and fibroadenomas may also be involved[18–20] in which instances, particularly sclerosing adenosis, the histological appearances can closely mimic invasive carcinoma[20] (Fig. 4.3). Confusingly, the term 'apocrine adenosis' has been applied both to apocrine metaplasia occurring in lobules or sclerosing lesions[19] and to a different lesion, also showing apocrine differentiation, which occurs in association with a type of adenomyoepithelioma[21] and was previously termed adenomyoepithelial adenosis by Kaier and associates.[22]

The light microscopical features (Figs 4.2, 4.3, 4.4) are described above and resemble those seen in oncocytes. Ultrastructural examination has been performed by several groups of workers.[23–26] They describe abundant mitochondria which differ from those of oncocytes in possessing few or incomplete cristae which do not extend into the central area; in oncocytes the cristae are usually well developed and complete. Microvilli are also described along the luminal margin.

BLUNT DUCT ADENOSIS

'Blunt duct adenosis' is the term used by Foote and Stewart[27] and Azzopardi[28] to describe an extremely common change which is dismissed by some as a normal morphological variation.[4] Other terms used include 'columnar alteration of lobules',[29] 'hyperplastic terminal groupings',[30] 'columnar metaplasia'[31] and 'atypical lobules type A'.[32] It is often seen either as a chance finding or in association with other changes in fibrocystic change and is not identifiable macroscopically. Microcalcification of luminal secretions can occur resulting in its detection by mammography.[33]

Microscopically, the normal luminal epithelial layer of individual TDLUs is replaced by a single layer of taller columnar epithelial cells with basal nuclei and apical cytoplasmic snouts (Fig. 4.5). Nuclei may be enlarged, but there is no atypia. Instead of the normal rounded acinar configuration, there are larger, irregularly branching, blind ended duct-like structures (Fig. 4.5). Myoepithelial cells and basement membrane are readily apparent. There is often associated mild stromal proliferation.

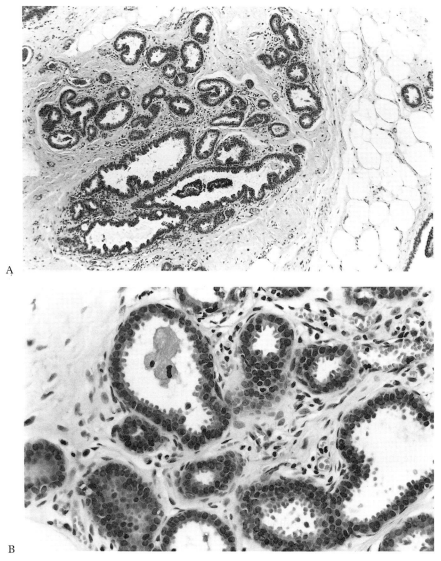

A

B

Fig. 4.5   An example of blunt duct adenosis in which the terminal duct lobular unit is expanded with the acinar units taking on a more expanded 'ductal' configuration (A). The glandular spaces are lined by tall columnar epithelial cells (B). Hematoxylin–eosin, A × 125; B × 400.

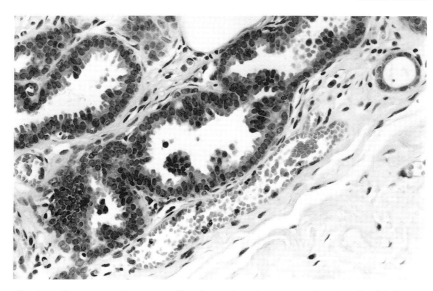

Fig. 4.6 Gynecomastoid micropapillary hyperplasia is a term used to describe this form of mild epithelial proliferation which can be found in association with blunt duct adenosis. Hematoxylin–eosin × 400.

A form of epithelial hyperplasia which resembles the pattern seen in the male breast as a manifestation of gynecomastia (Fig. 4.6) may be present in association with blunt duct adenosis and other forms of fibrocystic change. It is not currently recognized to carry any significant risk of subsequent development of breast cancer and should not be confused with other more well described forms of epithelial hyperplasia.[34] The term micropapillary gynecomastoid hyperplasia has been used to describe this lesion (see also Ch. 5).

PATHOGENESIS

In the normal breast, proliferation of fibrous tissue and epithelial development are brought about by estrogens whereas progestogens, together with prolactin, modulate this process and induce development of ductal and lobular structures. Clinical observations suggest a role for hormonal imbalance in the development of fibrocystic change. Thus, the changes are most common in the middle and late reproductive period and regress after the menopause unless estrogen replacement therapy is administered. These observations suggest a relative excess of estrogen and depletion of progestogen may have an etiological role but

are difficult to confirm. One approach is to measure the levels of individual hormones in serum. However, there are problems with such studies; firstly, the action of hormones on the breast is likely to involve a complex series of interactions and the action of an individual hormone is unlikely to be directly related to its plasma concentration; secondly, there is poor correlation between symptoms and morphological changes (see above). This aside, several investigators have identified hormonal imbalances in clinically evident disease. Sitruk-Ware and colleagues described a relative excess of estrogen and depletion of progesterone in symptomatic women thought to be caused by luteal phase insufficiency,[35] but others have been unable to confirm this[36] and attention has turned to the role of prolactin. Cole and colleagues described significantly elevated prolactin levels in cyst patients compared with controls or other patients with benign disease.[37] Kumar and co-workers have shown that the peak secretion of prolactin in response to thyrotrophin releasing hormone is higher in patients with cyclical breast pain and nodularity than in matched controls[38] suggesting a disturbance in hypothalamic control of hormone secretion.

Whatever the underlying hormonal mechanisms may be, cysts are believed to develop from an exaggerated process of lobular involution[1,8,39] with progression of microcysts to gross cysts through expansion or coalescence. Following their observations using serial sectioning and a subgross sampling technique respectively, Vilanova et al in 1983[40] and Wellings and Alpers in 1987[17] have suggested that apocrine metaplasia of the terminal duct lobular unit is the initial event, with microcysts developing as a result of the secretory activity of these cells.

DIFFERENTIAL DIAGNOSIS

At one end of the spectrum, the morphological features of fibrocystic change must be differentiated from normal variations. To this end, an arbitrary size cut-off may be used to separate normal cystic lobular involution and abnormal cyst formation. Alternatively, fibrocystic change may be diagnosed when the morphological features are considered sufficiently advanced to account reasonably for symptoms.[41] At the other end of the spectrum, the lobule-derived cysts may be confused with duct ectasia. Differentiating features include the linear configuration, surrounding elastica and inspissated eosinophilic secretions of ectatic ducts as opposed to the round or oval structure, lack of elastica, often empty lumina or homogeneous pale contents and frequent apocrine metaplasia of cysts.

Apocrine metaplasia is generally easily recognized. However, Carter and Rosen have drawn attention to the combination of apocrine atypia and sclerosing lesions (atypical apocrine sclerosing lesions)[20] which can cause confusion with invasive carcinoma (Fig. 4.3B). The recognition of a myoepithelial component and of the apocrine nature of the cells should enable the correct diagnosis to be made. Immunostaining for GCDFP-15 may aid identification of apocrine differentiation; however, positive staining is reported in a high proportion of breast carcinomas.[42,43]

PROGNOSIS AND MANAGEMENT

Medical treatment is based on reducing the hormonal imbalance frequently present. Combined oral contraceptive preparations are reported to halt progression and relieve symptoms in 70–90%[44] and use of progestogen-only preparations during the luteal phase of the menstrual cycle to result in improvement in 80%.[44] Tamoxifen has also been used with success.[45] Other treatments include danazol which, though successful in alleviating symptoms, is associated with substantial adverse side effects.[5]

Cysts are very common, and although most are asymptomatic,[6] Haagensen estimates that 7% of women will develop one or more palpable cysts.[4] Management of palpable cysts is usually by aspiration. As the incidence of intracystic carcinoma is very low in comparison to the frequency of such cysts, cytological examination of cyst fluid is not regarded as worthwhile unless the aspirate is uniformly bloodstained or a residual mass is present. Exceptionally, recurrent large cysts and multiple cysts causing disfiguration or discomfort or the presence of an intracystic lesion will prompt excision.

The relationship of fibrocystic change to the development of cancer has been extensively investigated, with confusing and conflicting results. The majority of women with fibrocystic changes are asymptomatic and even those with palpable cysts are rarely biopsied but diagnosed and treated by aspiration alone. Several studies in which women with palpable cysts were treated mainly by aspiration have recorded a slight increase in the risk of developing cancer subsequently, ranging from 1.77 to 5.7 times the expected normal incidence.[4,46–52] The higher figure was identified by Bodian and co-workers in a group of women requiring 10 or more aspirations;[52] overall, these workers found a relative risk around double that of the general population. Thus, gross cystic disease appears to be associated with a mild to moderately increased risk, with carcinoma often developing only after many years.[4,51]

Such studies, while assessing the risks for the majority of women with palpable cysts, cannot identify the relative contribution of the various components of fibrocystic change to that risk. For this, biopsy is required and there have been a number of studies assessing relative risks in the admittedly small proportion of women who do undergo biopsy. One of the largest was performed by Dupont and Page[53] who demonstrated that the majority of women undergoing biopsy for benign breast disease were at no increased risk for the development of cancer. They did, however, identify epithelial hyperplasia, particularly atypical hyperplasia, as a risk factor; that risk being increased further in the presence of a positive family history. Women with non-proliferative changes had a relative risk of 0.89 overall and women with non-proliferative changes, but gross cysts had a relative risk of 1.5 increasing to 3.0 in the presence of a positive family history. This is compared to a relative risk of 3.5 in those with atypical hyperplasia and no family history and 8.9 in those with both atypical hyperplasia and a positive family history. Several subsequent studies, using similar diagnostic criteria for the assessment of hyperplasia and atypia, have resulted in similar conclusions[54–56] (see Ch. 5).

In 1986, the Cancer Committee of the College of American Pathologists reviewed the available evidence and issued a consensus statement subdividing patients with benign breast disease into three major risk categories.[2] Cysts, apocrine metaplasia and mild epithelial hyperplasia (without atypia) fell into category I (no increased risk), moderate or florid hyperplasia into category II (1.5–2 × risk) and the presence of any atypical hyperplasia placed the patient into category III (5 × risk).

There still remains considerable controversy about the risks associated with apocrine metaplasia and gross cysts. Using a subgross sampling technique on whole breasts, Wellings and Alpers identified a statistically significant association between ipsilateral or contralateral carcinoma and apocrine metaplasia,[17] although they did not interpret this as indicating an increased risk if apocrine metaplasia is found in biopsy material.[57] Furthermore, in assessing risks associated with gross cysts, several groups have suggested that cyst type may be important, with cancer occurring more frequently in women who have previously had an apocrine cyst rather than a flattened cyst as identified on the basis of cyst fluid composition.[58,59] This may also explain why those women requiring multiple aspirations for gross cystic disease have been identified as having a higher relative risk for the development of cancer than those undergoing a single biopsy or aspiration,[4,50,52] in that apocrine cysts are more likely to be multiple or recurrent.

The relevance of apocrine atypia as described above is also at present unclear. Page and Anderson have suggested it is a purely benign phenomenon[41] whereas others have suggested it may be a direct precursor of some forms of carcinoma, particularly apocrine carcinoma and medullary carcinoma.[4] Given the current state of knowledge, we do not currently believe there is sufficient evidence to recommend close follow up or surveillance for patients in whom the only form of epithelial proliferation is of an apocrine type as described above (see also Ch. 5 and Ch. 14).

FOCAL LACTATIONAL CHANGE

Lactational changes are occasionally seen in women who are neither pregnant nor lactating. Frantz described the changes in around 3% of women at autopsy[6] and Kaier and Andersen described a similar incidence in resected breast tissue.[60]

The microscopical changes seen are identical to those seen in pregnancy and lactation (see Ch. 1) but are focal. Affected lobules may consist of dilated acini lined by plump, vacuolated cells (Fig. 4.7) and containing abundant PAS positive secretory material. Alternatively, affected acini may be lined by degenerate-appearing hobnail cells showing minimal cytoplasmic vacuolation and containing enlarged irregular or pyknotic nuclei (Fig. 4.8). Such acini contain little secretion but often contain detached cells.

It has been suggested that the appearances represent persistent lactational changes following pregnancy. However, it is unlikely that such changes would persist for up to 48 years, the longest reported interval since last pregnancy.[6] Furthermore, several cases have been reported in nulliparous women[60] and in men,[61,62] indicating an alternative etiological mechanism in at least some cases. It is known that several therapeutic drugs can induce this change. For example, Huseby and Thomas described lactational changes in women taking exogenous estrogens for advanced breast cancer[63] and reported cases of the change

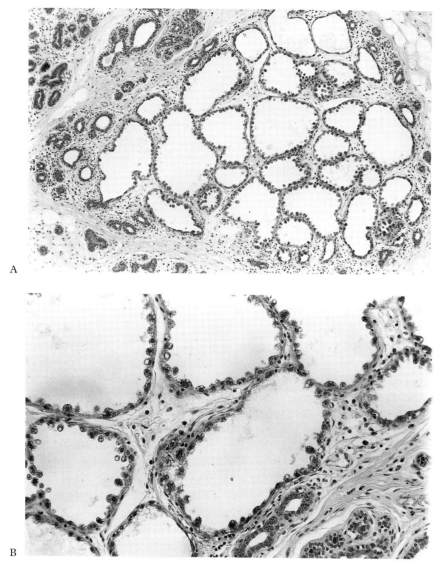

Fig. 4.7   Focal lactational change involving and enlarging a lobular unit (A). The epithelial cells show a lactational type of cytoplasmic vacuolation (B). Hematoxylin–eosin, A × 57; B × 400.

in men have also been associated with exogenous estrogen administration.[61,62] Other therapeutic agents have also been implicated. Wellings and colleagues found lactational changes to be more common in breasts from patients treated with digitalis, dilantin and reserpine[32] and Hooper et al describe abnormal lactation in patients taking major tranquilizers, particularly thioridazine,[64] and probably related to stimulation of prolactin secretion. Not all cases are associated with exogenous hormones or therapeutic agents, however, and Kaier and Andersen supported a third etiological possibility, previously proposed by Foote and Stewart,[27] that some lobules may show 'selective susceptibility' to endogenous hormones.[60]

Focal lactational change is an entirely benign incidental microscopic phenomenon with no known associated risk for the development of cancer.

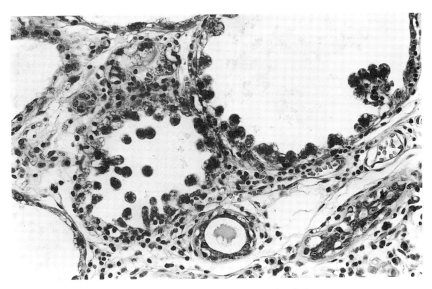

Fig. 4.8 The epithelial cells in some forms of focal lactational change may appear atypical with large darkly staining nuclei. Hematoxylin–eosin × 400.

CLEAR CELL METAPLASIA

This change, described by Barwick, Kashgarian and Rosen in 1982,[65] was identified in 1.6% of a series of 934 biopsies reviewed by Vina and Wells.[66]

Microscopically, there is partial or complete involvement of, usually multiple, lobules within an affected area. The change may also affect areas of sclerosing adenosis. The epithelial cells contain abundant clear or occasionally foamy or vacuolated cytoplasm (Fig. 4.9) with sparse PAS positive granules. Vina and Wells also describe Alcian blue positivity.[66] Nuclei are small, without atypia. These cells may extend into adjacent ductules and are distinguished from myoepithelial cells by their

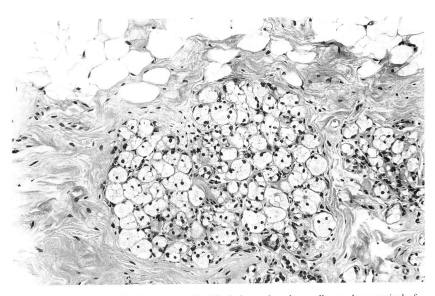

Fig. 4.9 The acinar epithelial cells in this lobule have abundant cell cytoplasm typical of clear cell change. Hematoxylin–eosin × 100.

lack of positive immunohistochemical staining for S-100 protein or actin.

One of the cases in the series of Tavassoli and Yeh[62] was studied by transmission electron microscopy and showed empty rounded spaces within the cytoplasm which replaced cytoplasmic organelles and gradually compressed the nucleus to one side. Similar vacuolation was seen, but to a lesser extent, in neighboring myoepithelial cells. The lack of any identifiable secretory material was thought to be due to processing effects.[62]

Clear cell change has been thought, on morphological grounds, to be related to focal lactational change, due to the presence of secretory granules ultrastructurally[65] and some further support for this was provided by Tavassoli and Yeh who described two patients with coexistent lactational and clear cell change.[62] However, Vina and Wells dispute this on the basis of different immunohistochemical phenotypes and instead suggest the change represents eccrine metaplasia.[66]

The maintenance of the overall lobular architecture and presence of myoepithelial cells should prevent any confusion with clear cell carcinoma and, like focal lactational change, clear cell change appears to be a benign phenomenon with no premalignant connotation.

REFERENCES

1 Hughes LE, Mansel RE, Webster DJT. Aberrations of normal development and involution (ANDI): A new perspective on pathogenesis and nomenclature of benign breast disorders. Lancet 1987; (ii): 1316–1319.

2 Hutter RVP. Consensus meeting. Is fibrocystic disease of the breast precancerous? Arch Pathol 1986; 110: 171–173.

3 National Coordinating Committee for Breast Screening Pathology. Pathology reporting in breast cancer screening, 2nd edn. Sheffield: NHS Breast Screening Programme Publications, 1995.

4 Haagensen CD. Diseases of the breast. Philadelphia: WB Saunders, 1986.

5 Vorherr H. Fibrocystic breast disease: Pathophysiology, pathomorphology, clinical picture and management. Am J Obstet Gynecol 1986; 154: 161–179.

6 Frantz VK, Pickren JW, Melcher GW, Auchincloss HJ. Incidence of chronic cystic disease in so-called normal breasts. A study based on 225 postmortem examinations. Cancer 1951; 4: 762–783.

7 Pastides H, Kelsey JL, LiVolsi VA, Holford TR, Fischer DB, Goldenberg IS. Oral contraceptive use and fibrocystic breast disease with special reference to its histopathology. J Natl Cancer Inst 1983; 71: 5–9.

8 Azzopardi JE. Problems in breast pathology. London: WB Saunders, 1979; pp 60–72.

9 Izuo M, Okagaki T, Richard RM, Lattes R. DNA content in 'apocrine metaplasia' of fibrocystic disease complex and breast cancer. Cancer 1971; 27: 643–650.

10 Dixon JM, Miller WR, Scott WN, Forrest APM. The morphological basis of human breast cyst populations. Br J Surg 1983; 70: 604–606.

11 Pearlman WH, Giueriguian JD, Sawyer ME. A specific progesterone-binding component of human breast cyst fluid. J Biol Chem 1973; 248: 5736–5741.

12 Bundred NJ, Miller WR, Walker RA. An immunohistochemical study of the tissue distribution of the breast cyst fluid protein, Zn-a2 glycoprotein. Histopathology 1987; 11: 603–610.

13 Mazoujian G, Haagensen DEJ. The immunopathology of gross cystic disease fluid proteins. NY Acad Sci 1990; 586: 188–197.

14 Dixon JM, Scott WN, Miller WR. Natural history of cystic disease: Importance of cyst type. Br J Surg 1985; 72: 190–192.

15 Ebbs SR, Bates T. Breast cyst type does not predict the natural history of cyst disease or breast cancer risk. Br J Surg 1988; 75: 702–704.

16 Page DL, Dupont WD. Are breast cysts a premalignant marker? Eur J Cancer Clin Oncol 1986; 22: 635–636.

17 Wellings SR, Alpers CE. Apocrine cystic metaplasia: Subgross pathology and prevalence in cancer-associated versus random autopsy breasts. Hum Pathol 1987; 18: 381–386.

18 Bussolati G, Cattani MG, Gugliotta P, Patriarca E, Eusebi V. Morphologic and functional aspects of apocrine metaplasia in dysplastic and neoplastic breast tissue. Ann NY Acad Sci 1986; 464: 262–274.

19 Simpson JF, Page DL, Dupont WD. Apocrine adenosis — a mimic of mammary carcinoma. Surg Pathol 1990; 3: 289–299.

20 Carter DJ, Rosen PP. Atypical apocrine metaplasia in sclerosing lesions of the breast: A study of 51 patients. Mod Pathol 1991; 4: 1–5.

21 Eusebi V, Casadei GP, Bussolati G, Azzopardi JG. Adenomyoepithelioma of the breast with a distinctive type of apocrine adenosis. Histopathology 1987; 11: 305–315.

22 Kaier H, Nielsen B, Paulsen S, Soresen IM, Dyreborg V, Blichert-Toft M. Adenomyoepithelial adenosis and low grade malignant adenomyoepithelioma of the breast. Virchows Arch A 1984; 405: 55–67.

23 Archer F, Omar M. The fine structure of fibroadenoma of the human breast. J Pathol 1969; 99: 113–117.

24 Ahmed A. Apocrine metaplasia in cystic hyperplastic mastopathy. Histochemical and ultrastructural observations. J Pathol 1975; 115: 211–214.

25 Pier WJ, Garancis JC, Kuzma JF. The ultrastructure of apocrine cells. In intracystic papilloma and fibrocystic disease of the breast. Arch Pathol 1970; 89: 446–452.

26 Ozello L, ed. Ultrastructure of the human mammary gland. Symmers SC, ed. Pathology Annual; Vol 6. London: Butterworth, 1971; pp 1–59.

27 Foote FW, Stewart FW. Comparative studies of cancerous versus non-cancerous breasts. Basic morphological characteristics. Ann Surg 1945; 121: 6–53.

28 Azzopardi JG. Problems in breast pathology. London: WB Saunders, 1979; pp 25–32.

29 Page DL, Anderson TJ. Diagnostic histopathology of the breast. Edinburgh: Churchill Livingstone, 1987; pp 86–88.

30 Gallagher HS. Sources of uncertainty in interpretation of breast biopsies. Breast 1976; 2: 12–15.

31 Bonser GM, Dossett JA, Jull W. Human and experimental breast cancer. London: Pitman Medical, 1961; pp 336–347.

32 Wellings SR, Jensen HM, Marcum RG. An atlas of subgross pathology of the human breast with special reference to possible precancerous lesions. J Natl Cancer Inst 1975; 55: 231–273.

33 Barnard NJ, George BD, Tucker AK, Gilmore OJA. Histopathology of benign non-palpable breast lesions identified by mammography. J Clin Pathol 1988; 41: 26–30.

34 Tham KT, Dupont WD, Page DL, Gray FG, Rogers LW. Micro-papillary hyperplasia with atypical features in female breasts, resembling gynaecomastia. Progr Surg Pathol 1989; 10: 101–109.

35 Sitruk-Ware R, Sterkers N, Mauvais-Jarvis P. Benign breast disease I: Hormonal investigation. Obstet Gynecol 1979; 53: 457–460.

36 Walsh PV, Bulbrook RO, Stell PM, Wang DY, McDicken IW, George WD. Serum progesterone concentration during the luteal phase in women with benign breast disease. Eur J Cancer Clin Oncol 1984; 20: 1339–1343.

37 Cole EN, Sellwood RA, England PC, Griffiths K. Serum prolactin concentrations in benign breast disease throughout the menstrual cycle. Eur J Cancer 1977; 13: 597–603.

38 Kumar S, Mansel RE, Hughes LE et al. Prolactin response to thyrotropin-releasing hormone and dopaminergic inhibition in benign breast disease. Cancer 1984; 53: 1311–1315.

39 Hayward JL, Parks AG. Alterations in the microanatomy of the breast as a result of changes in the hormonal environment. In: Currie AR, ed. Endocrine aspects of breast cancer. Edinburgh: Churchill Livingstone, 1958; pp 133–134.

40 Vilanova JR, Simon R, Alvarez J, Rivera-Pomar JM. Early apocrine change in hyperplastic cystic disease. Histopathology 1983; 7: 693–698.

41 Page DL, Anderson TJ. Cysts and apocrine change. In: Page DL, Anderson TJ, eds. Diagnostic histopathology of the breast. Edinburgh: Churchill Livingstone, 1987; pp 43–50.

42 Wick MR, Lillemoe TJ, Copland GT, Swanson PE, Manivel JC, Kiang DT. Gross cystic disease fluid protein-15 as a marker for breast cancer: Immunohistochemical analysis of 690 human neoplasms and comparison with alpha-lactalbumin. Hum Pathol 1989; 20: 281–287.

43 Haagensen DE. Is cystic disease related to breast cancer. Am J Surg Pathol 1991; 15: 687–694.

44 London RS, Sundaram GS, Goldstein PJ. Medical management of mammary dysplasia. Obstet Gynecol 1982; 59: 519–523.

45 Ricciardi I, Iannaruberto A. Tamoxifen-induced regression of benign breast lesions. Obstet Gynecol 1979; 54: 80–84.

46 Jones BM, Bradbeer JW. The presentation and progress of macroscopic breast cysts. Br J Surg 1980; 67: 669–671.

47 Harrington E, Lesnick G. The association between gross cysts of the breast and breast cancer. Breast 1981; 7: 113–117.

48 Bundred NJ, Mansel RE. Clinical factors influencing the risk of breast cancer in women with gross cysts. Br J Clin Pract 1989; 43: 103–105.

49 Ciatto S, Biggeri A, Del Turco MR, Bartoli D, Iossa A. Risk of breast cancer subsequent to gross cystic disease. Eur J Cancer 1990; 26: 555–557.

50 Bundred NJ, West RR, Dowd JO, Mansel RE, Hughes LE. Is there an increased risk of breast cancer in women who have had a breast cyst aspirated? Br J Cancer 1991; 64: 953–955.

51 Devitt JE, To T, Miller AB. Risk of breast cancer in women with cysts. Can Med Assoc J 1992; 147: 45–49.

52 Bodian CA, Lattes R, Perzin KH. The epidemiology of gross cystic disease of the breast confirmed by biopsy or by aspiration of cyst fluid. Cancer Detect Prevent 1992; 16: 7–15.

53 Dupont WD, Page DL. Risk factors for breast cancer in women with proliferative breast disease. N Engl J Med 1985; 312: 146–151.

54 London SJ, Connolly JL, Schnitt SJ, Colditz GA. A propective study of benign breast disease and the risk of breast cancer. JAMA 1992; 267: 941–944.

55 Dupont WD, Parl FF, Hartmann WH et al. Breast cancer risk associated with proliferative breast disease and atypical hyperplasia. Cancer 1993; 71: 1258–1265.

56 McDivitt RW, Stevens JA, Lee NC, Wingo PA, Rubin GL, Gersell D. Histologic types of benign breast disease and the risk for breast cancer. The Cancer and Steroid Hormone Study Group. Cancer 1992; 69: 1408–1414.

57 Wellings SR, Alpers CE. Hum Pathol (Letter) 1988; 19: 121–122.

58 Dixon JM, Lumsden AB, Miller WR. The relationship of cyst type to risk factors for breast cancer and the subsequent development of breast cancer in patients with breast cystic disease. Eur J Cancer Clin Oncol 1985; 21: 1047–1050.

59 Bradlow HL, Fleischer M, Breed CN, Chasalow FI. Biochemical classification of patients with gross cystic disease. Ann NY Acad Sci 1990; 586: 12–16.

60 Kaier HW, Andersen JA. Focal pregnancy-like changes in the breast. Acta Path Microbiol Scand A 1977; 85: 931–947.

61 Schwartz IS, Wilens SL. The formation of acinar tissue in gynecomastia. Am J Pathol 1963; 43: 797–807.

62 Tavassoli FA, Yeh I-T. Lactational and clear cell changes of the breast in non-lactating, non-pregnant women. Am J Clin Pathol 1987; 87: 23–29.

63 Huseby RA, Thomas LB. Histological and histochemical alterations in normal breast tissues of patients with advanced breast cancer being treated with estrogenic hormones. Cancer 1954; 145: 54–74.

64 Hooper JHJ, Welch VC, Shackelford RT. Abnormal lactation associated with tranquilizing drug therapy. JAMA 1961; 178: 133–134.

65 Barwick KW, Kashgarian M, Rosen PP. 'Clear-cell' change within duct and lobular epithelium of the human breast. Pathol Annu 1982; 17: 319–328.

66 Vina M, Wells CA. Clear cell metaplasia of the breast: a lesion showing eccrine differentiation. Histopathology 1989; 15: 85–92.

Epithelial hyperplasia

INTRODUCTION

The theoretical and practical underpinnings of definition and clinical utility of epithelial hyperplasia derive from two sources. First and foremost is the recognition of a cluster of patterns of epithelial cell increase which are frequently present in breast biopsies. This approach is in opposition to those who would impose pre-conceived categories of cytological or histological pattern to breast epithelial proliferations. The second major underpinning of our approach is to link reproducibly recognizable patterns of epithelial hyperplasia with epidemiological outcomes so that guidelines for clinical management can be developed.

The term hyperplasia is used as it signifies an increase in cell number for whatever reason, be it from an increase in cell proliferation or a decrease in cell subtraction. The latter occurs normally in the human breast by programed cell death (apoptosis), and apoptosis and mitoses occur in the latter half of the menstrual cycle.[1] Common patterns of hyperplasia have been identified by other names in the past including 'epitheliosis' and 'papillomatosis'. Both terms have suffered from a lack of precise definition that has resulted in their general abandonment in current histopathological practice. Specifically, epitheliosis has been used to describe some very worrying lesions and indeed some lesser examples of ductal carcinoma in situ have been included within that definition.[2] It was Wellings and Jensen[3] who first tried to extract us from such general terms which were in wide use in the 1970s. Their use of numbers to define a progression of changes (their A series included ductal pattern lesions) attempted to take cytological and histological pattern criteria together to define them in a sequence of escalating concern which was also correlated with the subgross appearance of lobular units. This system was further enhanced in the 1980s by attempting to define more precisely the atypical end of the spectrum (recognized in the Wellings and Jensen system as number 4, just short of carcinoma in situ). These criteria separating the atypias from ductal carcinoma in situ are quite different from the criteria separating the atypical lesions from ordinary hyperplasia.[4] Criteria were not placed in a continuous scale, but were focused specifically at identifying the borderline between the common hyperplastic lesions and carcinoma in situ.[5–6] This was done primarily to foster interobserver agreement (without the availability of a borderline category, different observers might assign an individual case either to the benign proliferative lesions or carcinoma in situ) and to link the specific diagnosis of atypical lesions to useful clinical implication. Such a specific linkage to clinical outcomes is a requirement for the acceptance of any borderline category as noted by Azzopardi.[7] The major theoretical underpinning to the identification of a group of proliferative lesions of the most common or usual type in the breast, is to recognize the typical characteristics of these lesions. The term 'disease' may be applied to the better developed lesions because they have been regularly linked to a slightly increased risk of breast cancer. They are proliferative lesions and have been termed 'proliferative disease without atypia' or 'proliferative disease of usual or common type'. Thus, without coining a new term, the intent has been to use phrases that have intrinsic utility and general reference. They are then capable of being stratified by the level of risk of later carcinoma development which they identify.

The term 'ductal' continues to be applied to these lesions as a counterpoint to the lobular pattern proliferative lesions discussed in Chapter 6. This is understandable and recognizes a long history of an attempt to dichotomize all proliferative lesions in the breast into lobular and ductal, recognizing a few other special types.[8] Considering that the majority if not all of these lesions occur within the lobular unit or terminal ducts which enter the lobular unit, it is quite inappropriate to term these lesions 'intra-ductal'. We retain use of the word 'ductal' however, as it has become the standard term for those lesions that are non-lobular and corresponds to specific patterns and cytologic criteria. Thus, with the understanding that 'ductal' refers to patterns and appearances of cells, and not their location or site of origin, the term continues to be a useful one.

The introduction of this system of classification has engendered an appropriate inquiry into its utility and reproducibility. When the criteria outlined here are used, agreement is quite impressive (over 90%), even when the most difficult lesions clustered at the borderline are chosen for study.[9] In addition, the originally identified levels of breast cancer risk for the 10–15 year period of time after biopsy[5–6] have been reproduced by subsequent epidemiological cohort studies using the same histological criteria.[10–12]

EPITHELIAL HYPERPLASIA OF USUAL TYPE (DUCTAL)

MILD HYPERPLASIA

This category was originally proposed to describe lesser forms of hyperplasia indicating a minimally increased number of cells above the basement membrane. Usually, in such cases there are whole lobular units or occasional acini where cells are more than two layers thick between the basement membrane and the lumen. Thus, the cell number above the basement membrane is greater than two and may be recognized as increased or hyperplastic. Such lesions are readily recognized as not reaching any indication of atypia by the low power scanning view of the microscope (Fig. 5.1). When cells are increased in number more than four above the basement membrane, and the cells tend to cross the space, then the next category of moderate and florid hyperplasia of usual type is recognized.[13] This is a fairly readily reproducible endpoint. We would further recommend that in general, if there are very few areas where cells seem to approach the more advanced category below, this 'mild' lesser category be recognized. In other words, when in doubt, include the case in question in the mild category which recognizes no

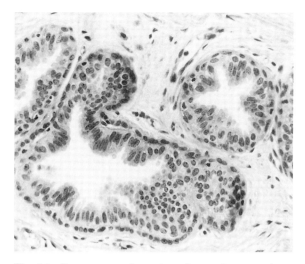

Fig. 5.1 Basement membrane-bound spaces[3] representing acini within a lobular unit are present. Note cells increased in number above the region of the cell basement membrane and above layers of rounded myoepithelial cells best seen at lower left. The cells are increased in number to three and perhaps four, but much of the increase in number is artefact of sectioning. This is the common form of hyperplasia of mild variety. From Page and Anderson, Diagnostic Histopathology of the Breast, Churchill Livingstone, 1988.[2] Hematoxylin–eosin × 225.

increased risk of later breast cancer (see Clinical Implications section below).

The major purpose for recognizing mild hyperplasia is that it gives confines of definition to the categories of moderate and florid hyperplasia described below. The definitions used for mild and moderate hyperplasia are largely those of Wellings and Jensen[2–3] for their A series lesions (categories 2 and 3) which are 'ductal' pattern lesions.

Columnar alteration of lobular units

It is often difficult to separate a very mild degree of increased cell number relative to the basement membrane from situations in which the cells are enlarged, elongated and prominent. Indeed, sometimes they appear pseudo-stratified. Active cells which are enlarged and present within prominent lobular units often with slightly dilated acini or spaces has been one of the changes termed 'blunt duct adenosis' in the past. We have called this lesion columnar alteration of lobules[14] recognizing the columnar nature of these cells while

others have termed this appearance hyperplastic terminal groupings. Figure 5.1 has such an appearance in areas without cell increase.

MODERATE AND FLORID HYPERPLASIA

The changes that we term moderate and florid hyperplasia are the most common epithelial lesions in the female breast that have recognized clinical significance.[11] Indeed, these lesions, although presenting many different faces, can be recognized as having a basic cohesion and commonality in presentation.

As noted above, examples of moderate and florid hyperplasia distend the spaces in which they occur and regularly have cells crossing those spaces (Fig. 5.2). Note that a space not otherwise specified merely means a circle bounded by a basement membrane in the breast and could be an element of a lobular unit or a duct. When cells cross such a space and form intercellular spaces within the bigger area, these latter may be termed secondary spaces. The importance of the formation and shape of these secondary spaces is intrinsic to the understanding of the differential diagnosis of hyperplastic lesions. The major features of moderate and florid hyperplasia are noted in Table 5.1. Other elements have been detailed, particularly in the exhaustive description of those changes termed 'epitheliosis' by Azzopardi,[7] but features that most reliably separate these lesions from more worrying patterns are emphasized here as defining.

The cytological features of these lesions are characteristically variable. Although recognizing

Table 5.1 Criteria for epithelial hyperplasia of usual type

Cytology	Varied nuclear shape and chromatin pattern with rounded nuclei mixed with elongated, often asymmetrical nuclei.
Orientation and placement of cells	Cell placement tends to be disordered and varied in regard to distance between nuclei and orientation one to another. Cytoplasmic borders are often indistinct and cells frequently exhibit streaming or swirling patterns of parallel cell placement.
Intercellular spaces	Shapes of spaces between cells are irregular in size and shape, frequently slit like.

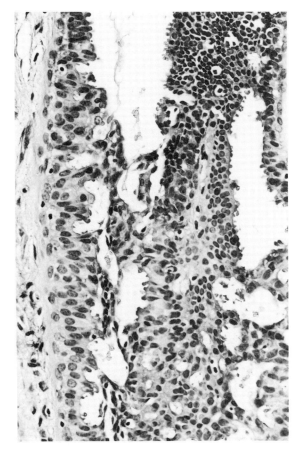

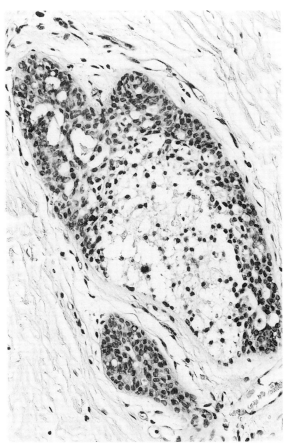

Fig. 5.2 A cross-section, largely longitudinal, of spaces with a mild and focally moderate increase in cell number. Note where the cells are increased four or more cells above the basement membrane that they tend to arch across and meet other cell groupings. This is mild to moderate hyperplasia of usual type without atypia. Hematoxylin–eosin × 210.

Fig. 5.3 Commonly, ordinary hyperplasia is punctuated by the presence of foam cells which are seen here in abundance above layers of mildly increased cell numbers characterizing mild hyperplasia. Hematoxylin–eosin × 160.

that fixation artefacts can render cells more uniformly dense or vacuolated, there are considerable variations in cell shape and size that distinguish the great majority of these lesions (Figs 5.3–5.7). In particular, there tends to be marked variation in nuclear shape and chromatin distribution, and familiarity with the variability of these patterns will help to avoid misinterpretation as something more ominous.[9]

Cell placement in florid hyperplasia is characteristic in three separate ways:

1. In general the cells have a haphazard and irregular relationship to each other.
2. The intercellular or secondary spaces formed by these proliferations are irregular in size and shape, and most characteristically, noncircular, elongated and often slit-like.

3. Despite the characteristic of irregularity, cell placement is not irregularly irregular, but often exhibits small areas where the cells tend to be parallel to each other, especially within larger lesions. We have termed this phenomenon of regional uniformity of cell orientation 'swirling', but the same pattern of cell placement was termed 'streaming' by Azzopardi.[7] What is particularly interesting about this phenomenon is that it is probably linked to the maintenance of cell polarity and specific attachments across cell membranes.[15] Lesions that lose this appearance of cell to cell

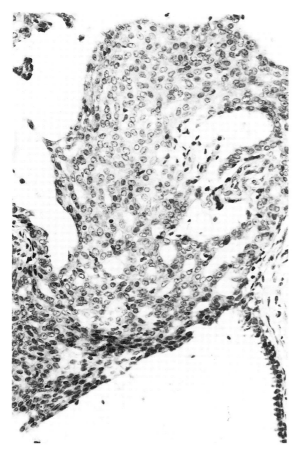

Fig. 5.4 Florid hyperplasia exhibits irregularity of cell placement and considerable variation of secondary spaces in regard to shape and size. Hematoxylin–eosin × 160.

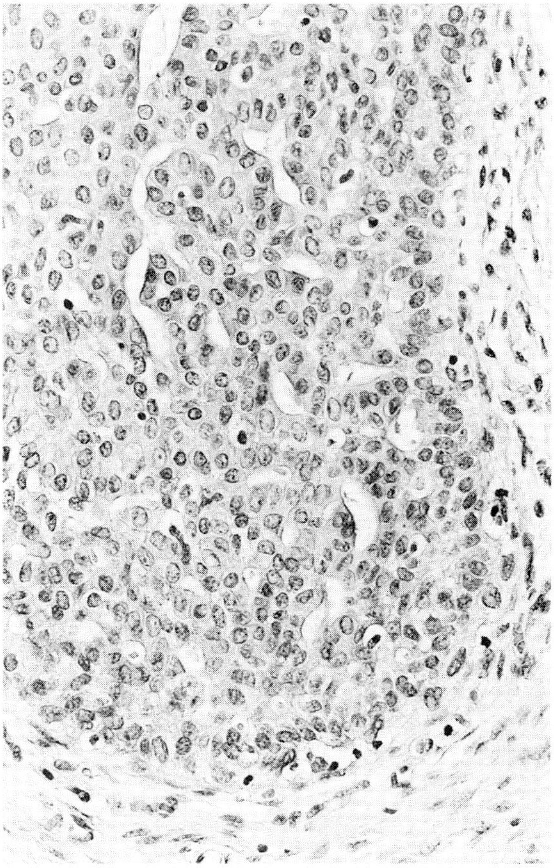

Fig. 5.5 Medium power view of florid hyperplasia exhibiting numerous small slit-like and irregular spaces interspersed throughout the lesion. Again, note irregularity of cell placement and nuclear variability. Hematoxylin–eosin × 210.

adhesion often represent more advanced examples that are truly atypical.

Although necrosis is characteristic of advanced, high grade ductal carcinoma in situ, occasionally one may see necrosis in the middle of larger examples of florid hyperplasia. These areas of necrosis are regularly confined to a small number of foci and are never present extensively throughout the lesion.

Juvenile papillomatosis — recognizes the localized occurrence of quite extreme examples of cyst formation in company with complex patterns of hyperplasia and sclerosis.[16–17] As stated in the original paper proposing this term: 'Although the individual microscopic features were not unique to this entity, the constellation did prove remarkable'. Thus, while the diagnosis serves as a practical clustering of histological findings, it is evident that the definition is imprecise and invites misuse. In addition, examples of this constellation of findings are not limited solely to young women. The circumscription of some of these cases is so remarkable that they almost simulate a fibroadenoma in the sharpness of demarcation from adjacent normal breast tissue. The association of these changes with breast cancer risk is unknown although suggestive.

Gynecomastoid hyperplasia

This phrase was coined in order to recognize a

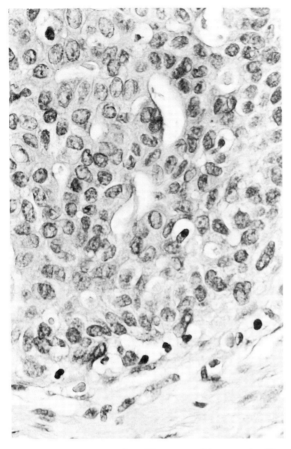

Fig. 5.6 Higher power from Figure 5.5 with serpentine-like and rounded secondary spaces between the hyperplastic cells. Hematoxylin–eosin × 415.

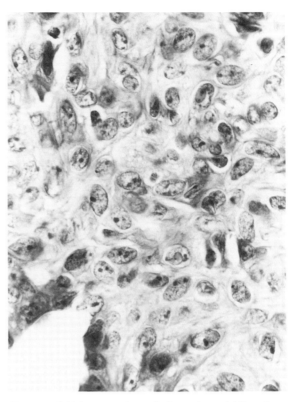

Fig. 5.7 A high power view to indicate the variability of nuclear pattern in both chromatin distribution and shape which characterizes ordinary hyperplasia of the moderate and florid types. From Page and Anderson, Diagnostic Histopathology of the Breast, Churchill Livingstone, 1988.[2] Hematoxylin–eosin × 800.

pattern of hyperplasia within the female breast which is remarkably similar to that seen in approximately one quarter of cases of gynecomastia in men.[18] The association of these changes with breast cancer risk is no more than that recognized by moderate or florid hyperplasia of usual type and may even be less if present in solitary form. The reason this term has some utility is because the change can mimic micropapillary atypical ductal hyperplasia, and thus be over-diagnosed as indicating a moderately elevated risk of later breast cancer development.

The histological and cytological alterations which recognize this pattern are quite specific. Small, papillary-like clusters of cells without fibro-vascular stalks surmount a more usual appearing epithelium (Fig. 5.8). The underlying epithelium is usually two, although sometimes three, cells

thick above the basement membrane and tends to have more vesicular nuclei. The characteristic papillary clusters of cells often taper toward the lumen, and have small, pyknotic nuclei which tend to be arranged around the outer edge of the papillary structure. The variability of nuclear features within these clusters is characteristic, denying the first requirement of atypical hyperplasia. In some patterns of hyperplasia, the papillary fronds achieve confluence, with irregular, typically elongated spaces between the fronds and the underlying cells. In such cases criteria of usual hyperplasia are met without the need to recognize them as a special pattern.

Compact dense hyperplasia

We have chosen to separate a subset of florid

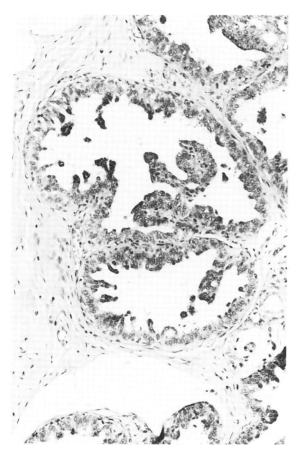

Fig. 5.8A   At this low power, these dilated spaces may be disturbing because of micropapillary patterns, but since these are regularly placed and tend to taper toward the lumen, they represent the gynecomastoid variant of ordinary hyperplasia. Hematoxylin–eosin × 105.

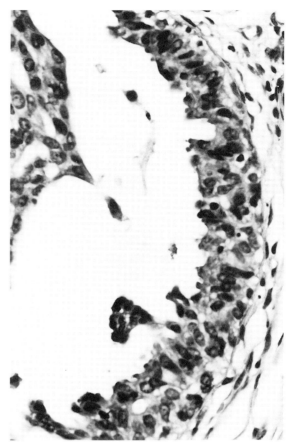

Fig. 5.8B   Higher power view of gynecomastoid pattern hyperplasia demonstrates the characteristic pyknotic nuclei of the tapering bars in these angulated micropapillae which are placed above more usual appearing epithelial cells. The latter are often increased in number by three to four in thickness as present here. Hematoxylin–eosin × 315.

hyperplasia cases with the descriptive phrase compact dense hyperplasia. We believe this represents a useful designation as it recognizes a group of lesions that can be particularly worrying in appearance although there is no suggestion that they imply a level of risk any different from that associated with florid hyperplasia. Such lesions characteristically consist of expanded acini containing a proliferation of small, closely packed cells with a minimal amount of cytoplasm (Fig. 5.9). The nuclei tend to be small and irregular, but often have more uniformity than is typically seen in cases of florid hyperplasia. These lesions can be the cause of considerable difficulty in the setting of suboptimal histological preparations (particularly sections 10 microns thick or greater) or at the

time of frozen section analysis. The histopathologist must be aware of this specific problem and diagnose florid hyperplasia without atypia. Whether one recognizes the descriptive term 'compact' or not is irrelevant.

Cystic hypersecretory hyperplasia

This form of hyperplasia has been recognized relatively recently and is characterized by cystically dilated acini and duct spaces lined by epithelial cells exhibiting prominent secretory features.[19] These expanded spaces contain a homogeneous eosinophilic substance that has tinctoral qualities not unlike that of thyroid colloid (Fig. 5.10). This lesion has been reported to be associated with

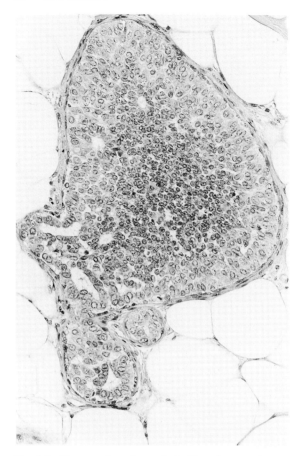

Fig. 5.9 Compact dense hyperplasia. Note the central crowding of the cellular proliferation showing minimal cytoplasm. Although suggestive of solid ADH or solid low grade (non-comedo) ductal carcinoma in situ, the cells are sufficiently varied in cellular placement and nuclear features to deny this diagnosis. Hematoxylin–eosin × 160.

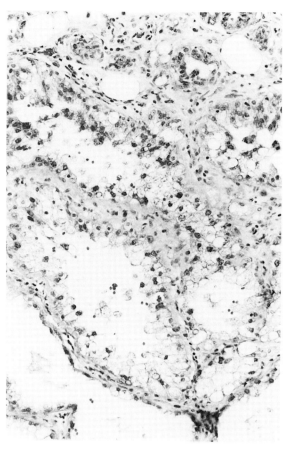

Fig. 5.10A Cystic hypersecretory hyperplasia is so-named because of its resemblance to lactating breast which is seen here. Note the bubbly cytoplasm, protrusion of cytoplasm apically as well as apical protrusions of nuclei. Hematoxylin–eosin × 125.

an increased risk for the development of breast cancer, but it is unclear whether the level of risk is independent of other lesions with which cystic hypersecretory hyperplasia has been associated. In particular, several of the reported cases have been seen in association with coexisting areas of invasive carcinoma.[20] Thus, while cystic hypersecretory hyperplasia may prove to be an increased risk lesion in itself, we believe that the level of attendant risk associated with this diagnosis should be dependent upon evaluating the epithelium within the lesion according to the same criteria used for other hyperplastic lesions of the breast.[21] In our experience these lesions frequently, but not

uniformly contain areas of atypical hyperplasia supporting the concept that there is a spectrum of attendant risk. Therefore, when appropriate we qualify this diagnosis by noting the presence or absence of atypia. Not infrequently, breast epithelium will exhibit secretory features without cystic dilatation of the involved space. This is most frequently manifest as single or few lobular units with fully developed features of lactation. In such cases the presence of secretory change is noted, but there is no recognized association with increased breast cancer risk (Fig. 5.11).

One pattern rarely found in proliferative lesions is worthy of note because of its mimicry of atyp-

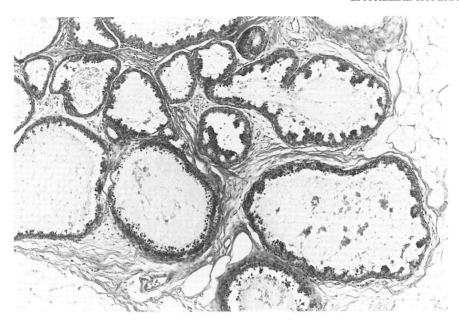

Fig. 5.10B Well developed example of cystic hypersecretory hyperplasia, with greatly dilated spaces, characteristic epithelial changes, and accumulation of intraluminal eosinophilic secretions. Hematoxylin–eosin × 120.

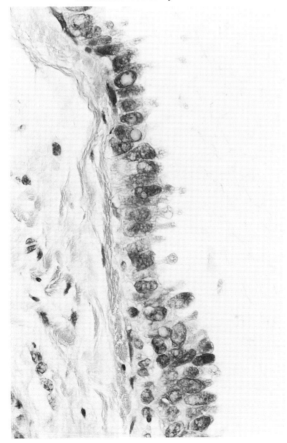

Fig. 5.10C High power view of Figure 5.10B showing typical apical cytoplasmic alterations of cystic hypersecretory change. Hematoxylin–eosin × 470.

ical ductal hyperplasia or low grade ductal carcinoma in situ under the low power of the microscope. This lesion has been called collagenous spherulosis (see also Ch. 11) by Clement et al,[22] and Wells[23] and others have shown that these sharply round spaces are characterized by having basement membrane material within them, particularly type IV collagen (Fig. 5.12). The secondary spaces defined between collections of cells are worrying for low grade ductal carcinoma in situ at low power examination because of their extreme precision of roundness. With several of them present in one space it is obvious why the pattern criteria for a worrying lesion are met. However, the cells defining the spaces regularly have varied cell placement and appearance which would deny atypical ductal hyperplasia or a more advanced diagnosis such as low grade (non-comedo) ductal carcinoma in situ.

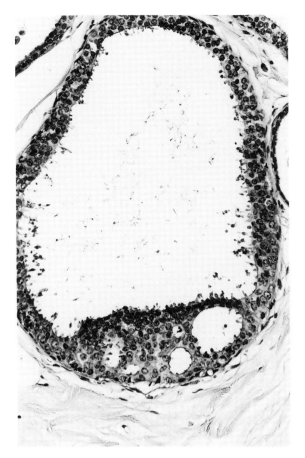

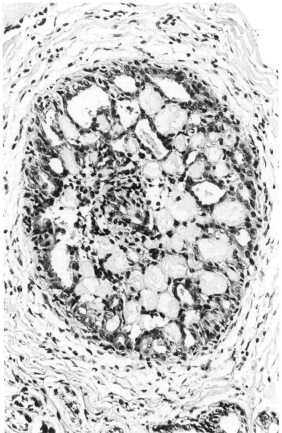

Fig. 5.11 Secretory change with mild hyperplasia. Note that the apical portions of the cells have prominent snouts with focal elongation and tapering. Although concerning for atypical hyperplasia there is considerable variability of cell placement and the secondary spaces are irregularly formed. Hematoxylin–eosin × 160.

Fig. 5.12 This example of so-called collagenous spherulosis shows the rigid rounded concretions lightly stained in this example. The nuclei and cells in between the spheres are tapered. Thus despite the resemblance to DCIS because of the sharply defined spaces, the cell population is not suspicious. Hematoxylin–eosin × 300.

ATYPICAL DUCTAL HYPERPLASIA

MORPHOLOGICAL CRITERIA

Standard 'ductal'-type lesions

When specifically defined, atypical ductal hyperplasia (ADH) recognizes an increased risk for the subsequent development of invasive carcinoma in either breast. This epidemiologically documented relationship is greatly different from that which is seen following diagnosis of small examples of ductal carcinoma in situ (DCIS). The diagnosis of DCIS implies not only a greatly increased relative risk for invasive carcinoma, but also implicates the specific region of the breast from which

the biopsy was taken. It is this difference that gives clinical utility to the diagnosis of ADH. Several recent studies using a constellation of histological features and defined criteria for pattern and lesion extent have confirmed the reproducibility of this approach.

The development of terms related to atypical hyperplasia, specifically defined, has taken place in the background of a long-standing and appropriate recognition that there are two patterns of advanced in situ proliferative lesions in the human female breast. These patterns were originally recognized because of their regular association with patterns of invasive carcinoma, and have been termed 'lobular' and 'ductal' for over 50 years.

Thus, despite the amazing diversity of patterns of cellular proliferation in the breast, there is a fundamental dichotomy which was recognized early in histological analysis. These histological patterns and cytological characteristics predominate over considerations of site of origin or site of presentation of these lesions. The first is unknown, and both patterns may involve either ducts or lobules. Thus, despite the fact that they are misnomers to some extent, they have become firmly and appropriately entrenched in the practice of histopathology.

When specifically defined, atypical hyperplasia of ductal pattern (ADH) may be recognized as indicating the very least (minimal) examples of low grade (non-comedo) ductal carcinoma in situ, thus providing a backdrop and a focus point for precision in diagnosis and the fostering of inter-observer agreement. The definition of ADH recognizes the confluence of cytological and histological pattern criteria[4] (Fig. 5.13). The criteria which were originally proposed for ADH have largely remained unaltered with one beneficial exception, that of overall size of the lesion as suggested by Tavassoli and Norris.[24] This utilization of combined histological and cytological criteria is also employed in the definition of specific lesions in other organ systems with non-invasive proliferations similar to carcinoma in situ;[25] and many publications in the last 10 years have addressed the issues inherent in the introduction of new diagnostic terms: criteria; assess-ment of reliability and reproducibility; and clinical outcome linkage.

This approach to classification of hyperplastic lesions of the breast has been accepted by several professional groups around the world, but not by all. The lack of universal acceptance of these criteria does not detract from the clinical utility derived from their validation by repeated, formal epidemiological studies.[10–11] Those who choose not to adopt these criteria should refrain from using the phrase atypical hyperplasia diagnostically to indicate a medically meaningful increased risk, because ADH links specific morphological criteria to an epidemiologically determined risk for invasive breast cancer. Without this linkage, the phrase loses the validity derived from scientifically-conducted studies that used the specific criteria.[4]

The identification of ADH, specifically defined, has as its upper boundary the most minimal lesions recognized as ductal carcinoma in situ, i.e., the low grade (non-comedo) lesions, largely cribriform in pattern. The lower boundary of ADH is defined by examples of florid hyperplasia with focal areas of cellular uniformity and even placement of cells (Fig. 5.14). The histological criteria for ADH (see Table 5.2) begin with a requirement for a group of cells of uniform placement and cytology. In most cases the cells also exhibit nuclear hyperchromasia, and will show some combination of patterns as detailed in Table 5.2 (Figs 5.15–5.23). For most examples of ADH, the extent of the lesion is the main determinant of

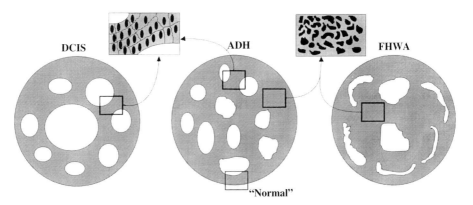

Fig. 5.13 Defining criteria for the separation of ductal carcinoma in situ, atypical ductal hyperplasia, and common patterns of florid hyperplasia. See discussion of atypical ductal hyperplasia, standard type. Modified from Page and Rogers.[4] FHWA indicates florid hyperplasia without atypia.

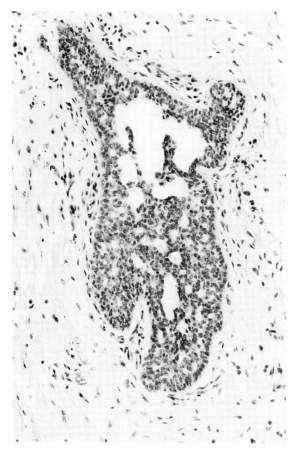

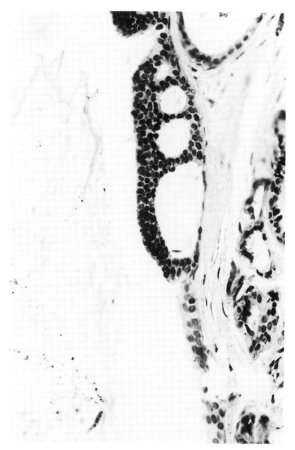

Fig. 5.14 This is a difficult case, to demonstrate that diagnosis of atypical ductal hyperplasia is sometimes not straightforward. We believe that the diagnosis is suggested here, but that there is sufficient variability of intercellular orientation and the secondary space formation to deny that designation with certainty. Hematoxylin–eosin × 125.

Fig. 5.15 Atypical ductal hyperplasia is well demonstrated in this example with an arch of similar appearing hyperchromatic cells sharply separated from adjacent cells below which have a more vesicular nucleus and a greater amount of cytoplasm. Hematoxylin–eosin × 250.

Table 5.2 Histological criteria for the recognition of atypical ductal hyperplasia (ADH) (specifically defined)

Distinguishes from usual hyperplasia	{ 1. Uniform population 2. Patterns of non-comedo DCIS	
	3. Extent of change a. to basement membrane-bound spaces b. overall dimension (2–3 mm)	} Distinguishes from low grade DCIS

what separates ADH from DCIS. The first two criteria separate ADH from proliferative disease of usual type. Thus hyperplastic epithelial lesions fall within a spectrum with three defined points of diagnostic reference (Fig. 5.13):

1. DCIS features sharply defined cellular groups with smooth and similarly shaped luminal borders within a basement membrane-bound larger space. The cytological features require a uniform cell population as seen in the inset of Fig. 5.13 which is regularly present throughout the entire space and at least one other basement membrane-bounded space. This last rule is not illustrated, but obviously includes a requirement of extensiveness or overall size.

2. ADH has groups of cells like those of low grade DCIS, and some suggestion of the sharply sculpted secondary spaces, but these are not fully developed through the entire involved primary space. Also, there is usually a portion of the space with normal appearing cells as noted by the lower

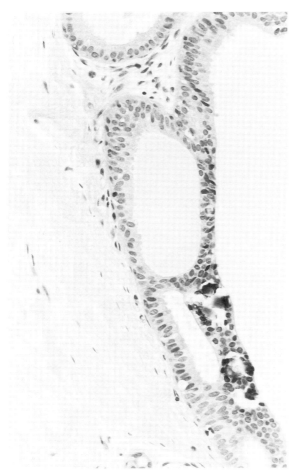

Fig. 5.16 Here the usual appearance of palisaded cells with a large apical cytoplasmic compartment (left) is contrasted to the even placement of smaller nuclei in the arch which make the diagnosis of atypical ductal hyperplasia. Note two lamellar calcifications in the central arch. Hematoxylin–eosin × 200.

inset in Fig. 5.13. These latter cells are usually polarized perpendicular to the basement membrane, and have different nuclear patterns from those in the central lesion (Figs 5.16 and 5.18B).

3. FHWA (florid hyperplasia without atypia) is the most densely cellular and extensive of the examples of proliferative disease without atypia. Irregularity of secondary spaces, often slit-like and variability of the nuclei (seen in above inset in Fig. 5.13) are the hallmarks of these lesions.

The concept inherent in ADH is clear as it creates a borderline between diagnoses of ductal carcinoma in situ and the common mammary

hyperplasias. The utility of a borderline category is evident; the diagnosis of ductal carcinoma in situ becomes better defined and more reproducible, and it gives recognition and clinical meaning to the observed spectrum of hyperplastic lesions of the breast as determined by follow-up studies. This has satisfied the understandable request of Azzopardi[7] that the utilization of the term atypical hyperplasia should have specific clinical meaning.

Logically one might believe that any 'atypical' or unusual patterns of hyperplasia could be termed atypical hyperplasia. However, practical implementation of this approach quickly becomes untenable due to the many varieties and iterations of usual hyperplasia in the breast and the need for specific reproducible definitions with sufficient numbers of cases that can be validated epidemiologically by numerous investigators. Therefore we have not encouraged extensive subgroup analysis of usual hyperplasia patterns, but have recognized a number of subgroups due to their frequent misidentification with ADH. It is for this reason that we have recognized two specific types of hyperplasia and applied the descriptive terms 'compact' and 'gynecomastoid'. We also recognize apocrine patterns[26] and hypersecretory patterns[21] of hyperplasia which have been described as 'atypical', and which therefore require discussion to separate them from the specifically defined examples with extensive follow-up studies linking them to a moderate level of breast cancer risk.

A comment about the identification of atypical hyperplasia by fine needle aspiration cytology is appropriate here since there has been a reticence to accept the fact that specifically defined ADH is not easily transferable to single cell analysis.[27] Recent studies have made the point strongly that the usual criteria for cytological atypia do not recognize the combined architectural and cytological criteria of specifically diagnosed ADH.[28] The combined criteria may be identified in some cytological samples that contain large clusters and three dimensional groups of cells.[29]

Atypical hyperplasia of mixed type

The diagnostic phrase or descriptive suggestion that a hyperplastic alteration qualifies as 'atypical'

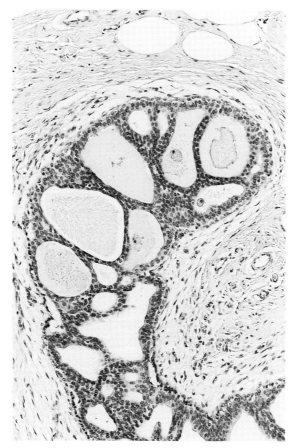

Fig. 5.17A   Well-developed example of extensive atypical ductal hyperplasia. Note considerable uniformity of the cell population focally along with well-formed and rigid appearing arches. At low power this lesion is quite worrying for low grade (non-comedo) ductal carcinoma in situ. Hematoxylin–eosin × 80.

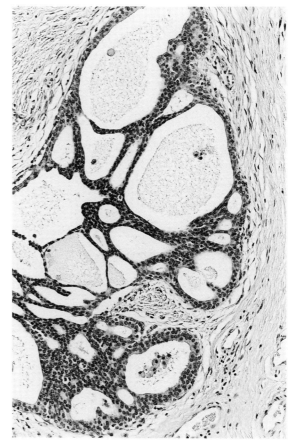

Fig. 5.17B   A second area from the same case again demonstrates extensive cell uniformity and well-defined arch formation. Note however that focally there is tapering of the arches and that there is clearly a second population of ordinary breast epithelial cells present focally adjacent to basement membrane. Hematoxylin–eosin × 80.

and is of mixed type or pattern accepts the fact that qualities of both atypical lobular hyperplasia (see Ch. 6) and ADH are present. It is an uncommon situation; in our original study only 10 cases in over 10 000 benign biopsies had separate areas of both major types of atypical hyperplasia[5] (Fig. 5.24). Similarly uncommon is the intermixture of cytological and architectural patterns of lobular neoplasia as detailed in Chapter 6, and those discussed here. Essentially, these occurrences are so rare and so varied that we do not attempt to describe the patterns that are virtually unique to individual cases. Rather, we take practical guidance from the fact that the coexistence of both patterns of atypical hyperplasia does not

seem to add to the magnitude of breast cancer risk identified by either alone.[5] Thus we can say that both are present and that the clinical implications are unchanged from having either alteration in isolation.

Apocrine ADH

Hyperplastic lesions of the human breast with apocrine cytology are frequent. One of the problems in understanding apocrine features is that they may present in classic or variant forms. Most of the variant forms would include loss of either a deeply acidophilic cytoplasm or loss of the characteristic nuclear features.[30]

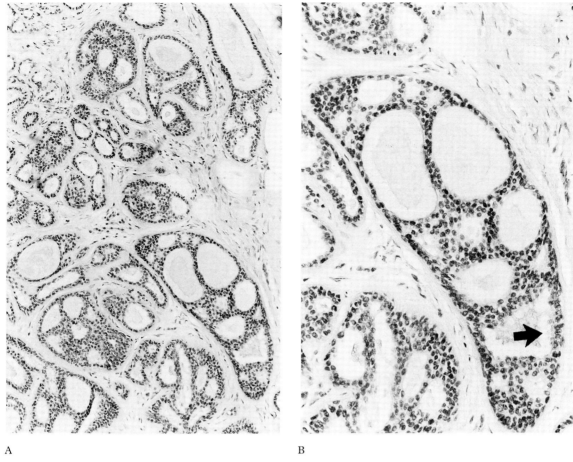

A

B

Fig. 5.18   (A) and (B) (See caption overleaf).

When present in classic forms, apocrine cells have an abundant, finely granular and eosinophilic cytoplasm with a somewhat large, exquisitely rounded nucleus, usually containing a prominent, through not greatly enlarged nucleolus. Occasional large nuclei are probably due to tetraploidy.[31] These cells frequently line cysts, particularly smaller ones. They may be cuboidal, but they are frequently seen in a characteristic columnar arrangement with an apical 'snout' characteristic of apocrine secretion. Frequently, these cells surmount delicate fibrovascular papillary cores or, most commonly, are present themselves in a papillary arrangement of several to many cells in depth or length. When these are regularly arranged they are fairly common in occurrence and are of no concern. It is when apocrine cells become arborescent in a complex fashion that they begin to mimic patterns otherwise accepted as atypical hyperplasia or even low grade carcinoma in situ (Figs 5.25, 5.26) (see also Ch. 14). This is a difficult area in which little precise work has been done. Our approach is to deny the atypical character of these proliferations if they are confined in distribution and even more particularly if they contain the characteristic nuclei of ordinary apocrine change.[26] When the nuclei tend to have the patterns of hyperchromasia seen in the low grade carcinomas in situ of ductal type, we will then consider a designation of possible atypical hyperplasia. When such changes are extensive, and the cell population is quite uniform, then we consider the possibility that this may be analogous to the lower grade ductal carcinomas in situ.[32]

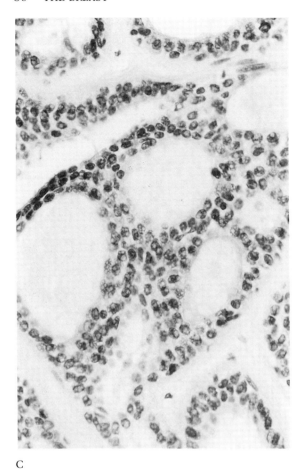

C

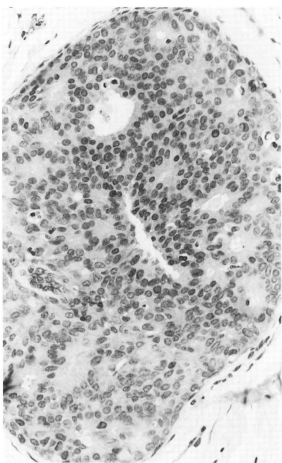

Fig. 5.18 (A) shows the low power appearance of a suspicious ductal lesion present within a focus of adenosis. Again the uniformity of the cell population and crisply demarcated spaces suggest the diagnosis of low grade (non-comedo) DCIS at low power. An intermediate power photomicrograph shown in (B) demonstrates that focally there is a secondary population of cells which deny the diagnosis of ductal carcinoma in situ (note arrow). The high power shown in (C) represents a small portion of the lesion which, *if seen in greater extent*, would qualify this lesion as a low grade (non-comedo) ductal carcinoma in situ. The overall size of this lesion (less than 2 to 3 mm) and the lack of involvement of more than one space with a completely uniform population of cells establishes the diagnosis of atypical ductal hyperplasia. Hematoxylin–eosin, A × 80, B × 160, C × 315.

Fig. 5.19 Atypical ductal hyperplasia is diagnosed here because the pattern of micro-rosettes or microglands of so-called solid DCIS is present centrally. The diagnosis of DCIS is denied because the cells around the outer portion of the space are quite different with more cytoplasm and more vesicular nuclei. Thus, the same cell population does not make up the entire basement membrane-bound space. Hematoxylin–eosin × 250.

ADH within combined stromal/epithelial proliferations (or: presenting in unusual locations)

The occurrence of patterns either defining or reminiscent of atypical hyperplasia within regionally defined lesions such as fibroadenoma, papil-loma, the nipple area,[33] radial scar[34] or ductal adenoma present special problems in histological differential diagnosis. The major problems attending this presentation of histological patterns is that once diagnosed, the clinical importance is not clear. Indeed, even the presence of a limited (less than several mm in extent) form of carcinoma in situ within these regionally defined lesions is of questionable clinical importance. It is this realization of the lack of direct linkage between these patterns and clinical relevance which mandates conservation with regard to the diagnosis of atypia

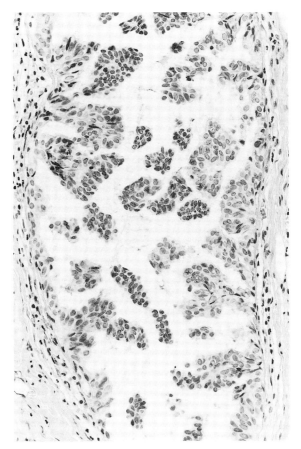

Fig. 5.20 This is an unusual case of micropapillary pattern atypical ductal hyperplasia. Note that the papillae are largely blunted and focally tapered. The blunt pattern is characteristic of DCIS of micropapillary type. However, there is a second population of cells around the entire space above the basement membrane which denies the diagnoses of ductal carcinoma in situ. Such cases are treacherous because portions of a well-developed micropapillary DCIS may look like this and the specimen must be carefully examined. Hematoxylin–eosin × 160.

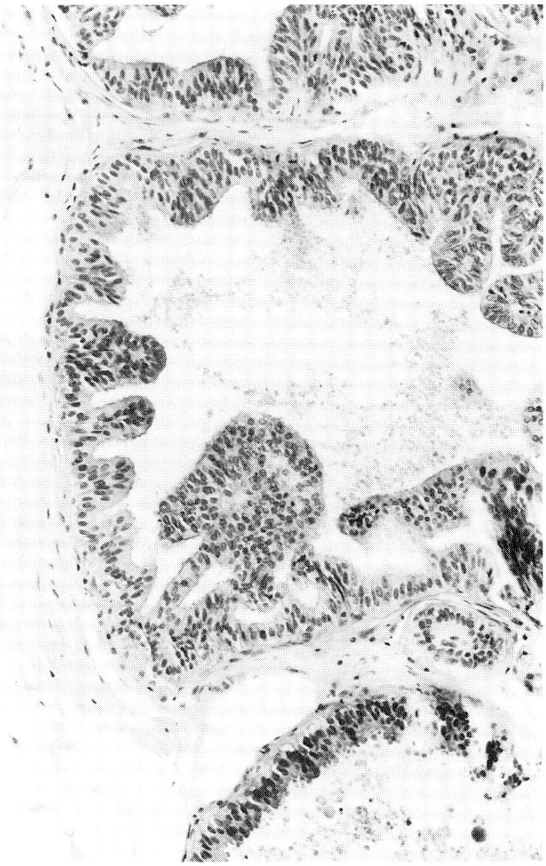

Fig. 5.21 Another example of atypical ductal hyperplasia with a papillary-like pattern but without central fibrovascular cores. This was almost the full extent of this lesion so that atypical ductal hyperplasia could be diagnosed with certainty. Such appearances should prompt a search for the possibility of more worrying lesions elsewhere. Hematoxylin–eosin × 105.

and carcinoma in situ in these settings. In any case, it is important to attempt to be consistent in the application of histological and cytological diagnoses in the breast, and one should not avoid making the diagnosis when the criteria are clearly present.

Basically, we try to transfer the approach used in the diagnosis of atypical ductal hyperplasia within the breast parenchyma to these special settings within papillomas, etc. This includes evaluation of the extent or size of the lesion, a point that was originally recognized in our own criteria

where an atypical ductal hyperplastic lesion may have the appearance of ductal carcinoma in situ, but does not qualify as such because it does not extend completely throughout the population of cells in two basement membrane-bound spaces. It is very common for these small lesions to have adjacent areas which are not fully involved, characterized by polarized cells bordering the lumen and maintaining largely the appearance seen in the normal breast with only two cells above the basement membrane. It is also clear that the entire extent of these lesions is usually no more than

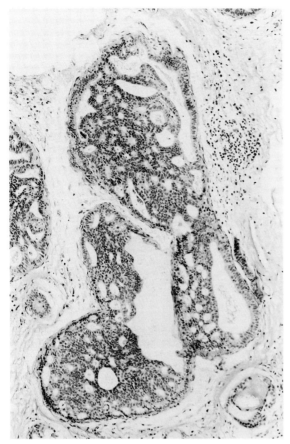

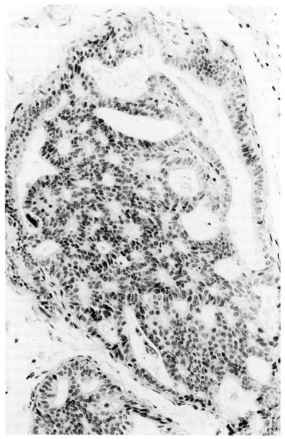

Fig. 5.22A   This low power view demonstrates an extremely well-developed example of atypical ductal hyperplasia. Although focally the lesion closely resembles DCIS, even at low power the maintenance of a normally polarized population of cells can be appreciated. Hematoxylin–eosin × 80.

Fig. 5.22B   Higher magnification of Figure 5.22A; the normal cell population is more clearly demonstrated. Hematoxylin–eosin × 160.

2–3 mm in size and usually several spaces are present which are only partially involved.[35]

We think that the criterion developed by Tavassoli and Norris[23] recognizes lesions of precisely the same type by establishing a 2–3 mm diameter as a lower limit for the diagnosis of DCIS. Transferring these criteria into quite unusual configurations of stroma and epithelium presents obvious difficulties. However, the recognition that a uniform population of neoplastic-appearing cells needs to be present over an area approaching 2–3 mm in size gives rough confines of definition to this process. It also seems evident to us that microfoci (2 mm or less in diameter) of ductal carcinoma in situ within these larger

defined lesions probably has no more significance than atypical hyperplasia,[35] supporting a conservative posture (Fig. 5.18). When the extent of these uniform cellular populations is greater than 4 and certainly 8 mm, ductal carcinoma in situ is diagnosed with confidence. This is particularly true if the ductal carcinoma in situ also has the histological patterns (cribriform, etc) which are so prominently displayed in more characteristic lesions. However, most of these cases have a more solid pattern, regularly lack the microglandular or rosette-like features seen in some solid examples of ductal carcinoma in situ, and present obvious problems in differential diagnosis as noted above. It should be emphasized that none of these fine

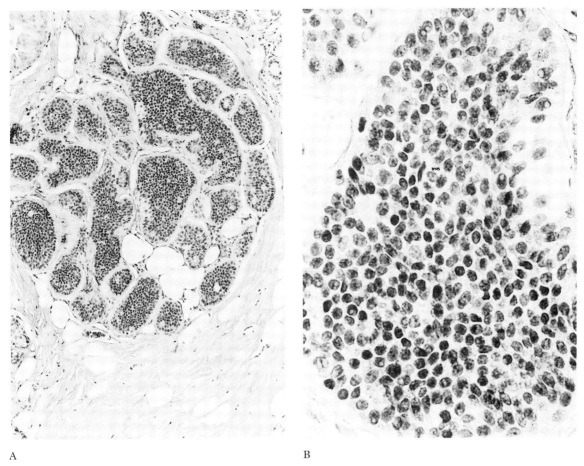

A   B

Fig. 5.23 (A) Low power view of a distended and enlarged lobular unit which is suggestive of low grade, solid (non-comedo) DCIS. (B) A higher power view, shows that while there is some uniformity of cells there is continued irregularity of cell placement and several well-formed small micro acini. In addition a population of cells is present along one basement membrane that is clearly different from the more disturbing cells. We would diagnose this lesion as an example of solid atypical ductal hyperplasia. Hematoxylin–eosin, A × 80, B × 415.

points of differential diagnosis relate to obvious examples of cell populations with the advanced nuclear atypia of high grade or comedo DCIS.

MOLECULAR STUDIES OF ADH

The characterization of hyperplastic lesions of the human female breast by modern molecular markers and indicators of specific biological activity is in its infancy. In general these markers have found little if any alteration from normal breast for epithelial hyperplasia of usual type with regard to the presence of proliferative, genetic or other malignancy-associated alterations. The majority of such changes have been described in the ductal carcinomas in situ,[36–38] and therefore are not a subject for this chapter. It is interesting, however, that the low grade (non-comedo) ductal carcinomas in situ are often without associated genetic or proliferative changes of malignancy and more resemble the related ADH lesions.[39]

Specifically, the characterization of these lesions with regard to proliferation was first done by Meyer in the late 1970s[40] who examined normal breast tissue and a few proliferative lesions with tritiated thymidine labelling. He found that in the usual hyperplasias the cells undergoing DNA

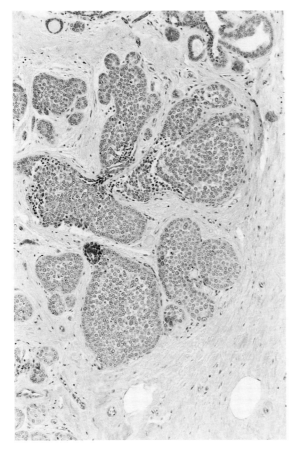

Fig. 5.24A This low power view of a distended lobular unit has an appearance similar to that seen in lobular carcinoma in situ, although the tendency for smaller outlines to be present at outer portions would be unusual for that diagnosis. Hematoxylin–eosin × 80.

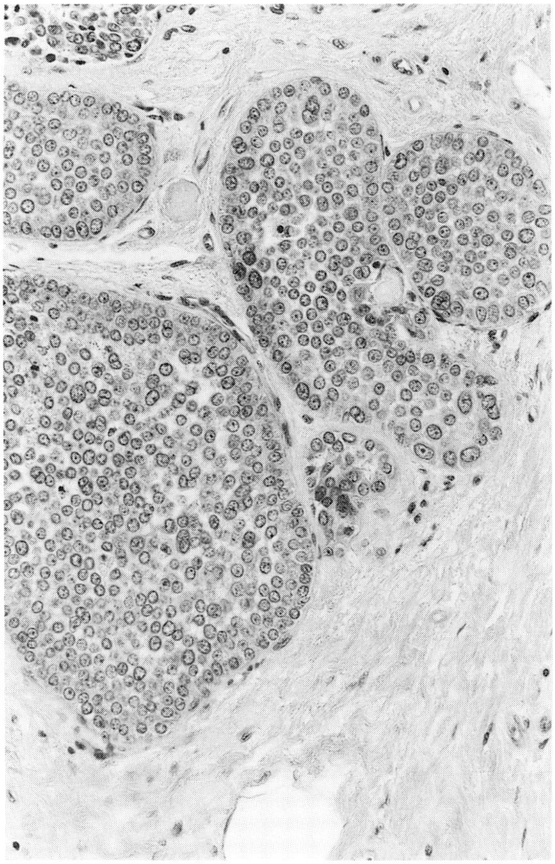

Fig. 5.24B Here at high power we notice that the centrally placed cells are very much like those of lobular neoplasia (see Ch. 6). However the cells present around the outside present a confusing cue because their regular placement is more like that of the ductal series of atypical lesions. Hematoxylin–eosin × 160.

synthesis were approximately the same in lesional tissue as they were in the other parts of the breast. He also found that proliferation was primarily related to the age of the patient as well as the menstrual cycle. Proliferation of breast epithelium was found to take place in the latter half of the menstrual cycle and this work was confirmed by Anderson and Ferguson.[1,41] Potten et al[42] have also studied the effect of age and menstrual cycle on activity in the breast and noted great variability between patients and within different areas of the breast in individual patients.

Few studies have been carried out concerning oncogenes, tumor suppressor genes, or growth factors and their receptors in proliferative diseases of the breast. These have not been particularly helpful or revealing up to the present time with regard to characterizing different lesions or determining likely clinical outcomes. p53 overexpression has been sought, as has c-erbB-2 expression in proliferative lesions from the usual type through atypical hyperplasia to different categories of ductal carcinoma in situ. It seems quite evident that overexpression is virtually confined to comedo and high grade ductal carcinomas in situ. Neither O'Malley et al[39] nor Umekita et al[43] found p53 expressed in ordinary hyperplasias, ductal carcinoma in situ of low grade or atypical ductal hyperplasias by immunocytochemistry. Mutated p53 has only been found in the high grade DCIS

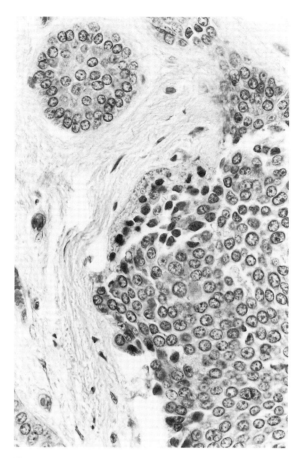

Fig. 5.24C At high power we complete this mixed pattern case in which it might be appropriate to diagnose both lobular and ductal atypical hyperplasia. Cells with almost no cytoplasm look more like those of the ductal series of atypical ductal hyperplasia. We often diagnose such cases as mixed pattern atypical hyperplasia. See clinical correlations (p. 86 and Fig. 5.27). Hematoxylin and eosin × 320.

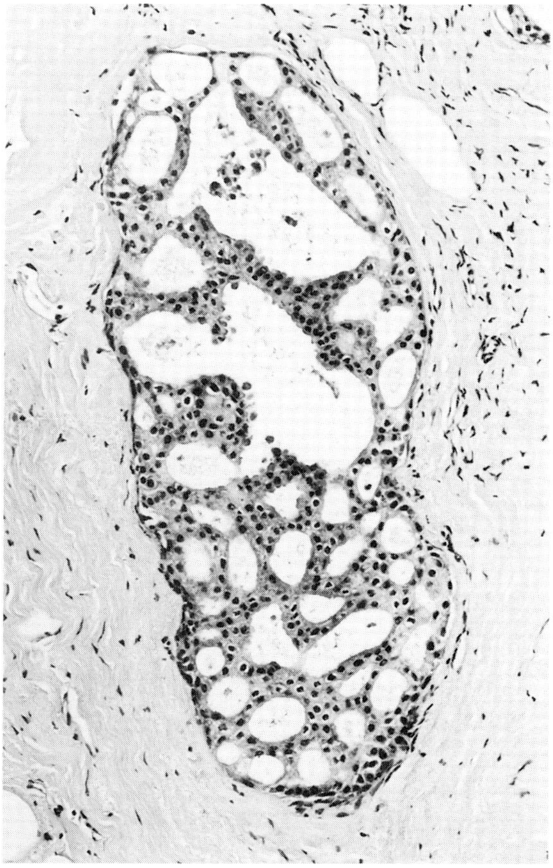

Fig. 5.25 These apocrine proliferations with rigid arches and bars present particularly difficult differential problems because they frequently do not completely recapitulate the pattern seen in other atypical ductal lesions. When cases are this complex and are less than about 4 mm in greatest extent, we recognize them as a variant of atypical hyperplasia with apocrine cytology. Hematoxylin–eosin × 105.

lesions by the above authors as well as by Poller et al.[38] The oncogene c-erbB-2 has not been found to be overexpressed in hyperplastic lesions including ADH,[44] and is absent in low grade (non-comedo) DCIS.[37,45] Parham and Jankowski[46] assessed transforming growth factor alpha semi-quantitatively in normal tissue, ordinary hyper-plasia, atypical hyperplasia, and cases of DCIS. They found no reliable differences between the various hyperplastic and neoplastic categories; however all were elevated in expression of trans-forming growth factor alpha with regard to normal ductal structures.

Ploidy has been evaluated in lesions of usual hyperplasia and atypical ductal hyperplasia in several studies.[47–49] The general conclusion is that some of the atypical lesions are aneuploid, while some remain diploid. No follow-up studies have been conducted to determine the clinical utility of these findings.

There has been some attempt to characterize the hyperplasias with regard to different types of keratins, but this has not been defining. There have also been several studies with actin related proteins that demonstrated that the cells in the myoepithelial position are regularly positive and other cells even within epithelial proliferative lesions are regularly negative or rarely positive.[50]

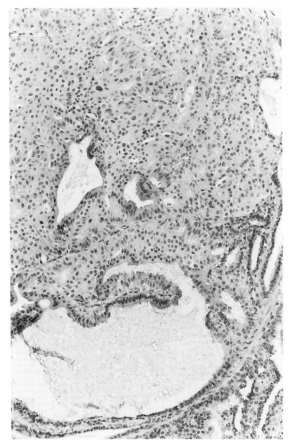

Fig. 5.26 Within a region of a papilloma these rigid arches and bars with focal microcalcifications suggest and indeed document the presence of atypical hyperplasia. Their extent is important with regard to determining their clinical relevance, and if less than 4 mm in greatest extent are diagnosed as atypical hyperplasia. Hematoxylin–eosin × 80.

Two studies[50–51] have shown that some S100 positivity may be seen within the epithelial proliferative lesions but this does not seem helpful with regard to differential diagnosis or further biological characterization of these proliferative lesions.

CLINICAL IMPLICATIONS

The milder examples of hyperplasia have been shown to have no clinical importance. They are probably more common in cancer-associated breasts as pointed out by Jensen et al.[52] However,

in follow-up studies, these milder changes have not been shown to be associated with a reliably increased risk of breast cancer in comparable women.[6,10–11,53] Moderate and florid hyperplasia were found to be present in approximately 30% of benign breast biopsies in the premammographic area and are an indicator of slightly increased cancer risk. This magnitude of risk should not be regarded as one indicating a great deal of concern on the part of an individual patient. The relative risk elevation is in the range of 60% over that of comparable women. In the age group in which this change is usually found, the late premenopausal and perimenopausal years, the risk in absolute terms is not greatly increased and would change from approximately 1.5 to 2 per thousand per year to 2 or 3 per/1000/year in high risk countries for a women in her mid-40s. Thus, in absolute terms this is not a magnitude of difference readily transferable into any clinical regimen or recommendation differing from that of comparable women. Additional support for minimizing the level of concern for this mild elevation of risk is the knowledge that the risk indicated by these lesions falls with time; 10–15 years after a biopsy demonstrating such lesions, these women return to approximately the same risk as that of comparable women without such changes,[54–55] although the study of Marshall et al did not find risk falling at long periods after biopsy.[56]

The relative risk of developing a subsequent invasive breast cancer following diagnosis of a small low grade (non-comedo) ductal carcinoma in situ (not otherwise treated except by the diagnostic biopsy) is approximately 10-fold greater than that of control populations of women.[57] This translates into an absolute risk of about 25% over the next 10–15 years of the woman's life. For atypical ductal hyperplasia in the absence of family history the relative risk is approximately 4-fold greater than comparable women and the absolute risk applied to an individual woman approaches 10% over the same time period. For women with atypical ductal hyperplasia and a positive family history the relative and absolute risks closely approximate to those of a microscopic, low grade ductal carcinoma in situ. One important point to note is that while the risk implications for atypical ductal hyperplasia are

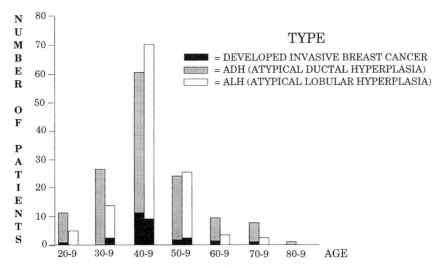

Fig. 5.27 Age at time of biopsy and number of women with each atypical lesion in each age group. The number actually developing carcinoma is indicated and represents incidence of subsequent invasive carcinoma over a 15-year period of follow-up. Modified from Page et al.[5]

bilateral, the diagnosis of ductal carcinoma in situ predicts the development of an invasive carcinoma in the same breast as that from which the original biopsy was obtained. This difference in risk implications would strongly suggest that ADH is currently proven as a marker for increased breast cancer risk only, while DCIS is a true precursor lesion of invasive breast carcinoma.[57] Minor examples of DCIS as recognized in an important follow-up study of Eusebi et al[58] indicate a risk of carcinoma after biopsy closer to that of ADH.

A final point about the relevance of breast cancer risk assignment from histological patterns, and ADH specifically, is to emphasize the importance of the patient's age in this process. The simplified scheme of risk assignment portrayed above is appropriate for perimenopausal women in the high risk geographical areas of the world, predominantly North America and Europe. The reason for this circumscription of reference is evident from the data which has been derived from such women. Figure 5.27 is taken from data for women with 15 years of follow-up after biopsies demonstrating specific patterns of atypical hyperplasia. The majority of women studied are between 35 and 55 years of age at time of biopsy. Thus risk assignment to both younger[59] and older women is carried out with little or no depth of understanding because of the dearth of evidence.

REFERENCES

1. Anderson TJ, Ferguson DJP, Raab GM. Cell turnover in the 'resting' human breast: the influence of parity, contraceptive pill, age and laterality. Br J Cancer 1982; 46: 376–382.

2. Page DL, Anderson TJ, Rogers LW. Epithelial hyperplasia. In: Page DL, Anderson TJ, eds. Diagnostic histopathology of the breast. Edinburgh: Churchill Livingstone, 1988; 120–156.

3. Wellings SR, Jensen HM, Marcum RG. An atlas of subgross pathology of the human breast with special reference to possible precancerous lesions. J Natl Cancer Inst 1975; 55: 231–273.

4. Page DL, Rogers LW. Combined histologic and cytologic criteria for the diagnosis of mammary atypical ductal hyperplasia. Hum Pathol 1992; 23: 1095–1097.

5. Page DL, Dupont WD, Rogers LW, Rados MS. Atypical hyperplastic lesions of the female breast. A long-term follow-up study. Cancer 1985; 55: 2698–2708.

6. Dupont WD, Page DL. Risk factors for breast cancer in women with proliferative breast disease. N Engl J Med 1985; 312: 146–151.

7. Azzopardi J. Problems in breast pathology. Philadelphia: Saunders, 1979; 266–273.

8. Fechner RE, Mills SE. Breast Pathology: Benign

proliferations, atypias, and in situ carcinomas. Chicago: American Society of Clinical Pathologists, 1990.

9. Schnitt SJ, Connolly JL, Tavassoli FA et al. Interobserver reproducibility in the diagnosis of ductal proliferative breast lesions using standardised criteria. Am J Surg Pathol 1992; 16: 1133–1143.

10. Dupont WD, Parl FF, Hartmann WH et al. Breast cancer risk associated with proliferative breast disease and atypical hyperplasia. Cancer 1993; 71: 1258–1265.

11. London SJ, Connolly JL, Schnitt SJ, Colditz GA. A prospective study of benign breast disease and risk of breast cancer. JAMA 1992; 267: 941–944.

12. Palli D, Rosselli del Turco M et al. Benign breast disease and breast cancer: A case-control study in a cohort in Italy. Int J Cancer 1991; 47: 703–706.

13. Hutter R. Consensus meeting. Is 'fibrocystic disease' of the breast precancerous? Arch Pathol Lab Med 1986; 110: 171–173.

14. Page DL, Anderson TJ. Columnar Alteration of Lobules. In: Page DL, Anderson TJ, eds. Diagnostic histopathology of the breast. Edinburgh: Churchill Livingstone, 1988; 86–88.

15. Simpson JF, Page DL. Altered expression of a structural protein (fodrin) within epithelial proliferative disease of the breast. Am J Pathol 1992; 141: 285–289.

16. Rosen PP, Cantrell B, Mullen DL, DePalo A. Juvenile papillomatosis (Swiss cheese disease) of the breast. Am J Surg Pathol 1980; 4: 3–12.

17. Dehner LP. The continuing evolution of our understanding of juvenile papillomatosis of the breast. Am J Clin Pathol 1990; 93: 713–731.

18. Tham KT, Dupont WD, Page DL et al. Micro-papillary hyperplasia with atypical features in female breasts, resembling gynecomastia. Prog In Surg Pathol 1989; 10: 101–109.

19. Guerry P, Erlandson RA, Rosen PP. Cystic hypersecretory hyperplasia and cystic hyperpsecretory duct carcinoma of the breast: Pathology, therapy, and follow-up of 39 patients. Cancer 1988; 61: 1611–1620.

20. Jensen RA, Page DL. Cystic hypersecretory carcinoma: what's in a name? Arch Pathol Lab Med 1988; 112: 1176.

21. Page DL, Kasami M, Jensen RA. Hypersecretory hyperplasia with atypia in breast biopsies: what is the proper level of clinical concern? Pathology Case Reviews 1996; 1: 36–40.

22. Clement PB, Young RH, Azzopardi JG. Collagenous spherulosis of the breast. Am J Surg Pathol 1987; 11: 411–417.

23. Wells CA, Wells CW, Yeomans P et al. Spherical connective tissue inclusions in epithelial hyperplasia of the breast ('collagenous spherulosis'). J Clin Pathol 1990; 43: 905–908.

24. Tavassoli FA, Norris HJ. A comparison of the results of long-term follow-up for atypical intraductal hyperplasia and intraductal hyperplasia of the breast. Cancer 1990; 65: 518–529.

25. Hamilton PW, Allen DC, Watt P. A combination of cytological and architectural morphometry in assessing regenerative hyperplasia and dysplasia in ulcerative colitis. Histopathol 1990; 16: 59–68.

26. Page DL, Dupont WD, Jensen RA. Papillary apocrine change of the breast associated with atypical hyperplasia and risk of breast cancer. Cancer Epidemiol, Biomarkers and Prev 1996; 5: 29–32.

27. Page DL, Dupont WD. Proliferative breast disease: Diagnosis and implications. Science 1991; 253: 915.

28. Stanley MW, Henry SM, Zera R. Atypia in breast fine-needle aspiration smears correlates poorly with the presence of a prognostically significant proliferative lesion of ductal epithelium. Hum Pathol 1993; 24: 630–635.

29. Sneige N, Staerkel GA. Fine-needle aspiration cytology of ductal hyperplasia with and without atypia and ductal carcinoma in situ. Hum Pathol 1994; 25: 485–492.

30. Raju U, Zarbo RJ, Kubus J, Schultz DS. The histologic spectrum of apocrine breast proliferations: analysis. Hum Pathol 1993; 24: 173–181.

31. Izuo M, Okagaki T, Richart RM, Lattes R. DNA content in 'apocrine metaplasia' of fibrocystic disease of the breast. Cancer 1971; 27: 643–650.

32. O'Malley FP, Page DL, Nelson EH, Dupont WD. Ductal carcinoma in situ of the breast with apocrine cytology: Definition of a borderline category. Hum Pathol 1994; 25: 164–168.

33. Rosen PP, Caicco JA. Florid papillomatosis of the nipple. A study of 51 patients, including nine with mammary carcinoma. Am J Surg Pathol 1986; 10: 87–101.

34. Sloane JP, Mayers MM. Carcinoma and atypical hyperplasia in radial scars and complex sclerosing lesions: Importance of lesion size and patient age. Histopathol 1993; 23: 225–231.

35. Page DL, Salhany KE, Jensen RA, Dupont WD. Subsequent breast carcinoma risk after biopsy with atypia in a breast papilloma. Cancer 1996; 78: 258–266.

36. Allred DC, Clark GM, Molina R et al. Overexpression of HER-2/neu and its relationship with other prognostic factors change during the progression of in situ to invasive breast cancer. Hum Pathol 1992; 23: 974–979.

37. Allred DC, O'Connell P, Fuqua S. Biomarkers in early breast neoplasia. J Cell Biochem 1993; 53: 125–131.

38. Poller DN, Roberts EC, Bell JA et al. p53 Protein expression in mammary ductal carcinoma in situ: Relationship to immunohistochemical expression of oestrogen receptor and c-erbB-2 protein. Hum Pathol 1993; 24: 463–468.

39. O'Malley FP, Vnencak-Jones CL, Dupont WD et al. p53 Mutations are confined to comedo type ductal carcinoma in situ of the breast. Lab Inv 1994; 71: 67–72.

40. Meyer JS. Cell proliferation in normal human breast ducts, fibroadenomas, and other ductal hyperplasias as measured by tritiated thymidine, effects of menstrual phase, age, and oral contraceptive hormones. Hum Pathol 1977; 8: 67–81.

41. Ferguson DJP, Anderson TJ. Morphological evaluation of cell turnover in relation to the menstrual cycle in the 'resting' human breast. Br J Cancer 1981; 44: 177–181.

42. Potten CS, Watson RJ, Williams CT et al. The effect of age and menstrual cycle upon proliferative activity of the normal human breast. Br J Cancer 1988; 58: 163–168.

43. Umekita Y, Takasaki T, Yoshida H. Expression of p53 protein in benign epithelial hyperplasia, atypical ductal hyperplasia, non-invasive and invasive mammary carcinoma: An immunohistochemical study. Virchows Archiv A Pathol Anat Histopathol 1994; 424: 491–494.

44. Lodato RF, Maguire HC, Greene MI et al. Immunohistochemical evaluation of c-erbB-2 oncogene expression in ductal carcinoma in situ and atypical ductal hyperplasia of the breast. Mod Pathol 1990; 3: 449–454.

45. Visscher DW, Sarkar FH, Crissman JD. Correlation of DNA ploidy with c-erbB-2 expression in preinvasive and invasive breast tumors. Anal Quant Cytol Histol 1991; 13: 418–424.

46. Parham DM, Jankowski J. Transforming growth factor alpha in epithelial proliferative diseases of the breast. J Clin Pathol 1992; 45: 513–516.

47. Crissman JD, Visscher DW, Kubus J. Image cytophotometric DNA analysis of atypical hyperplasias and intraductal carcinomas of the breast. Arch Pathol Lab Med 1990; 114: 1249–1253.

48. Norris HJ, Bahr GF, Mikel UV. A comparative morphometric and cytophotometric study of intraductal hyperplasia and intraductal carcinoma of the breast. Anal Quant Cytol Histol 1987; 10: 1–9.

49. Teplitz RL, Butler BB, Tesluk H et al. Quantitative DNA patterns in human preneoplastic breast lesions. Anal Quant Cytol Histol 1990; 12: 98–102.

50. Raju U, Crissman JD, Zarbo RJ, Gottlieb C. Epitheliosis of the breast: An immunohistochemical characterization and comparison to malignant intraductal proliferations of the breast. Am J Surg Pathol 1990; 14: 939–947.

51. Bassler R, Katzer B. Histopathology of myoepithelial (basocellular) hyperplasias in adenosis and epitheliosis of the breast demonstrated by the reactivity of cytokeratins and S100 protein. An analysis of heterogenic cell proliferations in 90 cases of benign and malignant breast diseases. Virchows Archiv A Pathol Anat Histopathol 1992; 421: 435–442.

52. Jensen HM, Rice JR, Wellings SR. Preneoplastic lesions in the human breast. Science 1976; 191: 295–297.

53. McDivitt RW, Stevens JA, Lee NC et al. Histologic types of benign breast disease and the risk for breast cancer. Cancer 1992; 69: 1408–1414.

54. Dupont WD, Page DL. Relative risk of breast cancer varies with time since diagnosis of atypical hyperplasia. Hum Pathol 1989; 20: 723–725.

55. Page DL, Jensen RA. Evaluation and management of high risk and premalignant lesions of the breast. World J Surg 1994; 18: 32–38.

56. Marshall LM, Hunter DJ, Connolly JL, et al. Risk of breast cancer associated with atypical hyperplasia of lobular and ductal types. Cancer Epidemiol Biomarkers Prev 1997; 6: 297–301.

57. Page DL, Dupont WD. Anatomic Markers of Human Premalignancy and Risk of Breast Cancer. Cancer 1990; 66: 1326–1335.

58. Eusebi V, Foschini MA, Cook MG et al. Long-term follow-up of in situ carcinoma of the breast with special emphasis on clinging carcinoma. Sem Diagn Pathol 1989; 6: 165–173.

59. Eliasen CA, Cranor ML, Rosen PP. Atypical duct hyperplasia of the breast in young females. Am J Surg Pathol 1992; 16: 246–251.

Lobular neoplasia

Atypical lobular hyperplasia and lobular carcinoma in situ

INTRODUCTION

Foote and Stewart, in 1941, described the histological features and assigned the term *lobular carcinoma in situ* (LCIS) to a characteristic proliferation within breast lobules.[1] Their description was limited to well-developed examples, and as such, LCIS is a well-established histopathological entity. Early studies did not specifically report on histologically similar, but less well-developed examples.[2] These lesser examples have been termed *atypical lobular hyperplasia* (ALH), although only recently have there been strict histological criteria for its diagnosis.[3–4] The term lobular neoplasia (LN) has been used to denote the full spectrum of proliferation of the characteristic cell type within acini, ranging from atypical lobular hyperplasia (ALH) to lobular carcinoma in situ (LCIS).[5] The term lobular neoplasia is appealing due to the absence of the word 'carcinoma'; however, we prefer the designations LCIS and ALH because the former term is well established in the literature, and the latter term implies a lower risk for developing carcinoma. In a discussion of both entities, lobular neoplasia is an acceptable inclusive term, and will be used in this chapter in that context.

MICROSCOPIC APPEARANCES

The defining cell type present in lobular neoplasia is round, cuboidal, or polygonal, often with clear or light cytoplasm. Nuclei are round to oval, cytologically bland, with an occasional small nucleolus. Hyperchromatism and mitotic figures are not

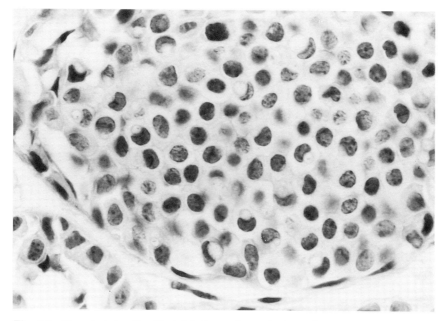

Fig. 6.1 Characteristic cells of both lobular carcinoma in situ and atypical lobular hyperplasia. The neoplastic cells have round, regular, uniform, nuclei, and clear cytoplasm. Frequently, cytoplasmic clear vacuoles are present. Hematoxylin–eosin × 600.

features of lobular neoplasia, but may be seen rarely. Cells are very evenly placed within the involved spaces, and cellular monotony is the rule. Helpful, though neither invariably present nor required for the diagnosis, is the presence of cytoplasmic clear vacuoles (Fig. 6.1).[6] These vacuoles are clear when stained with Hematoxylin and eosin, and accentuated with Alcian Blue and/or PAS stains.[7] By ultrastructural analysis, these vacuoles are actually microvilli-lined intracytoplasmic lumina.[7] Identification of these intracytoplasmic vacuoles in cells obtained from a fine-needle aspiration strongly suggests the diagnosis of lobular neoplasia.[8]

The preceding description is referable to both LCIS and ALH; it is the degree of involvement of breast lobules upon which distinction between the two is made (Fig. 6.2). The normal acinus is the point of reference for determining the presence of any type of hyperplasia. Accepting two cells as the normal number lining an acinus, the presence of three or more cells above the basement membrane defines hyperplasia. The diagnosis of LCIS requires that (1) the involved acini are populated exclusively by the characteristic cells (2) these

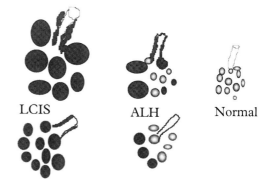

LCIS   ALH   Normal

Fig. 6.2 Morphological criteria for diagnosis of LCIS. More than half of the acini within a lobular unit are distended and distorted, and no central lumina are present. ALH is diagnosed when these changes are less well developed. Although pagetoid spread of neoplastic cells into adjacent ducts is more frequently seen in LCIS, it may be present in ALH (modified from Page, Kidd, Dupont et al,[25] courtesy of LW Rogers).

cells, fill, distend, and distort at least one half of the acini within the lobular unit (Figs 6.3 and 6.4). ALH is diagnosed when (1) fewer than half of the acini are expanded and distorted, (2) filling is incomplete, i.e., interspersed, intercellular spaces

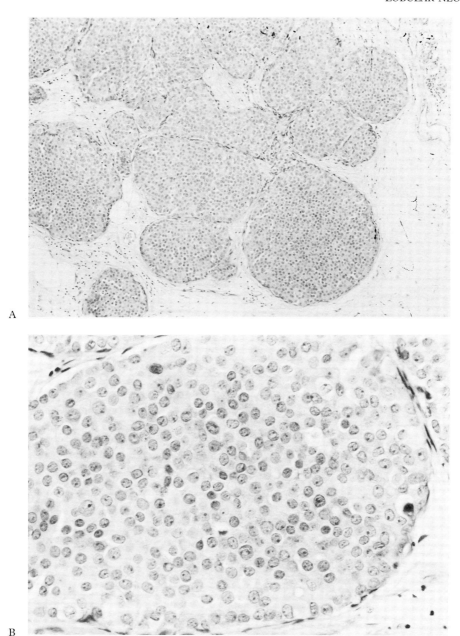

A

B

Fig. 6.3 Lobular carcinoma in situ. (A) Virtually all the acini of this lobular unit are distended, filled and distorted by (B) characteristic neoplastic cells. Hematoxylin–eosin, A × 125; B × 480.

remain or (3) other cell types are intermixed (Figs 6.5–6.8).

Note that the diagnosis of lobular neoplasia rests on finding the characteristic cells within lobules. Not infrequently cytologically identical cells may focally involve ducts, a condition termed 'pagetoid' involvement.[1] Just above the basement membrane, there is a proliferation of neoplastic cells which tends to undermine the normal lining epithelial cells (Figs 6.9–6.11). The difficulty arises when only pagetoid involvement is identified, without the more characteristic lobular

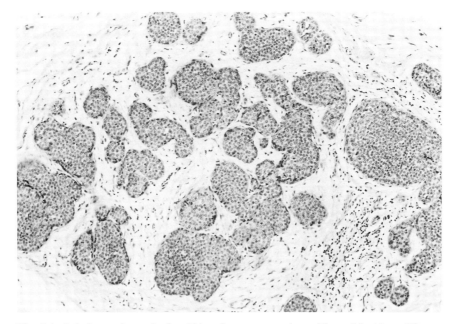

Fig. 6.4 Lobular carcinoma in situ. Although not as extensive as Figure 6.3, this qualifies as LCIS because more than half of the acini of this lobular unit are filled and distorted. Hematoxylin–eosin × 75.

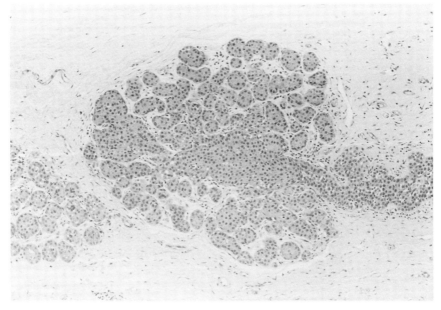

Fig. 6.5 Atypical lobular hyperplasia. Filling is complete, but distension is minimal in this example, with only a few acini qualifying. Hematoxylin–eosin × 125.

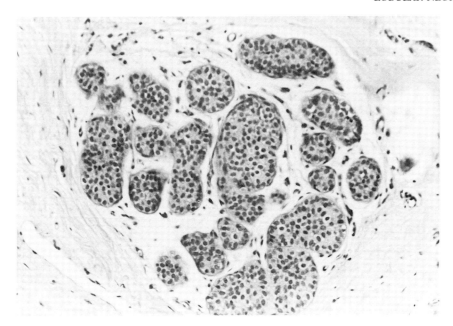

Fig. 6.6   Atypical lobular hyperplasia. Although the characteristic cells are present within acini, distension and distortion of more than half of the acini are not present. Hematoxylin–eosin × 200.

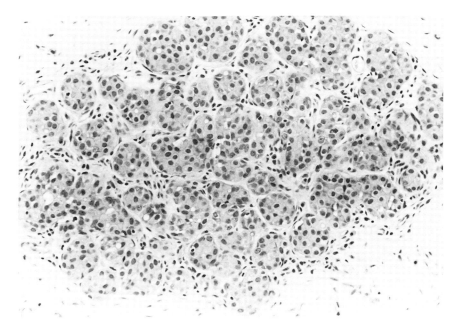

Fig. 6.7   ALH. Neoplastic cells are present without the distention required for LCIS. The majority of the lumina are intracytoplasmic, compared to Figure 6.8. Hematoxylin–eosin × 200.

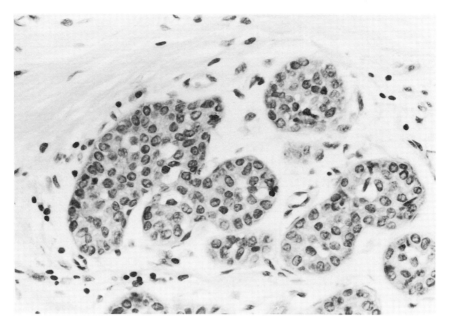

Fig. 6.8   ALH. Note residual (extracellular) space within acini and second cell population. Hematoxylin–eosin × 250.

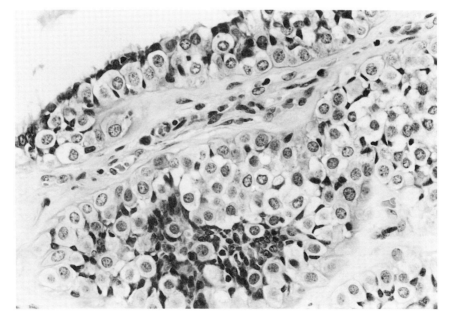

Fig. 6.9   Characteristic cells of lobular neoplasia grow beneath luminal epithelium (so-called pagetoid growth pattern) of lactiferous sinus. Note remaining normal epithelium (lower centre, upper left). Hematoxylin–eosin × 480.

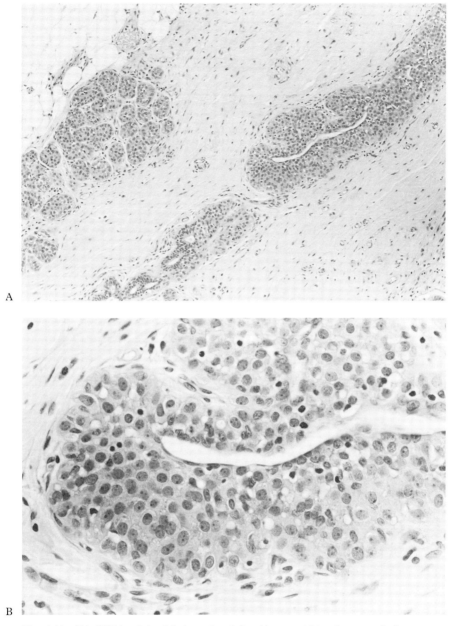

Fig. 6.10 (A) ALH involving lobular unit at left, with pagetoid involvement of adjacent duct (right). Note partial involvement of the space at lower centre. (B) Higher power of (A) showing the proliferation of neoplastic cells above the basement membrane, and lifting the residual luminal epithelial cells. Hematoxylin–eosin, A × 125; B × 450.

changes. In this instance, a careful search within the breast for lobular involvement by LCIS or ALH is indicated. Pagetoid involvement is more common and its presence more extensive in LCIS than ALH. Its presence in association with LCIS

does not affect risk implications; however when ductal involvement is associated with ALH (Fig. 6.10), the subsequent risk is increased to a level intermediate between ALH and LCIS.[9]

Following the above guidelines, the diagnosis

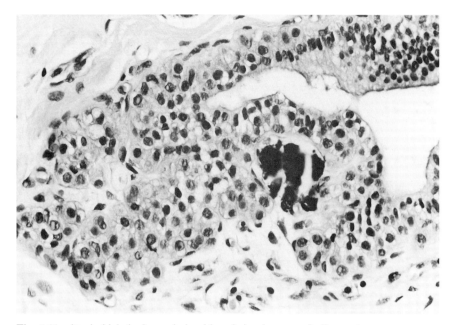

Fig. 6.11   Atypical lobular hyperplasia with early involvement of adjacent duct. Microcalcification (right of center) is an unusual finding in lobular neoplasia. Hematoxylin–eosin × 450.

of LCIS is based on the presence of a single population of characteristic cells filling the acini of a lobular unit, with distension and distortion of more than half of the acini. In practical terms, full distension of acini as required for a diagnosis of LCIS translates to eight or more cells being present across the diameter of an acinus. Most examples of LCIS are not difficult to recognize when these diagnostic guidelines are followed.

DIFFERENTIAL DIAGNOSIS

The distinction of LCIS from some types of ductal carcinoma in situ (DCIS) may in rare cases be difficult. The mere presence of a diagnostic category of 'low nuclear grade, solid pattern (non-comedo) ductal carcinoma in situ' should indicate that the patterns so-defined might overlap or closely approximate those seen in lobular carcinoma in situ. This is because in each case there is a filling of distended, basement membrane-bound spaces by cells without defining intercellular spaces giving cribriform or papillary formations. Indeed, the coincidence of similar histological and

cytological criteria, or their overlapping, can give rise to situations in which both diagnoses must be made in order to explain the patterns which are present[10] (see also Ch. 14 p. 263 and p. 270). If there is only a suggestion of a ductal pattern, there will be present in some spaces, at least small secondary glandular-like spaces within the solid masses of cells. These may be rosette-like and are a feature of many so-called solid non-comedo DCIS (Fig. 6.12). A very subtle, but defining and important feature is the placement of the cells and their relations with each other at the plasma membrane. The cells of lobular neoplasia have been said to have a somewhat 'dishevelled' pattern, but this is better relayed as an absence of the more sharp definition of cell membranes usually seen in ductal carcinoma in situ. That is to say that in DCIS the circumference of the cell wall is sharply defined and cells appear to be arranged as several linear segments, rather than in LCIS where (although difficult to understand) it would almost seem that the rounded cytoplasmic compartment defined by each cell has no relationship to adjacent cells. The cytoplasm is clear in most of these cases of solid DCIS as well as in

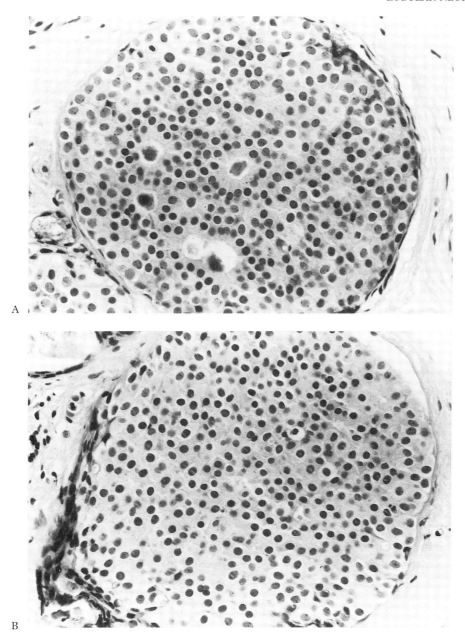

Fig. 6.12 (A) Cytological features of this carcinoma in situ closely resemble those seen in LCIS, including several intracytoplasmic lumina. The cellular placement, including the formation of microglands is diagnostic of solid (or neuroendocrine) type ductal carcinoma in situ. The same cytological features are seen in an adjacent space (B) without microgland formation. Hematoxylin–eosin, A, B × 450.

LCIS and presents no helpful discerning criterion except in the case of the intracytoplasmic lumina or vesicles so characteristic of lobular neoplasia. However, it must be recalled that occasionally when a completely ductal pattern is present, these intracytoplasmic lumina may be present as well.[11] The final criterion which is helpful in making this difficult histological differential diagnosis is the low-power view which is so characteristically lobulo-centric in LCIS because of a regular dilatation of the acini within lobular units. This may be contrasted to the more common appearance of DCIS in which dilatation and distortion of the same structures are more haphazard, producing a general distortion of lobular units and ducts and not just the acini within lobular units (see also Ch. 14).

Another difficult differential diagnosis occurs when DCIS extends into individual acini without destruction of lobular architecture (Fig. 6.13). This growth pattern has been termed 'cancerization of lobules' by Azzopardi.[12] Careful attention to cytological features and to architectural patterns

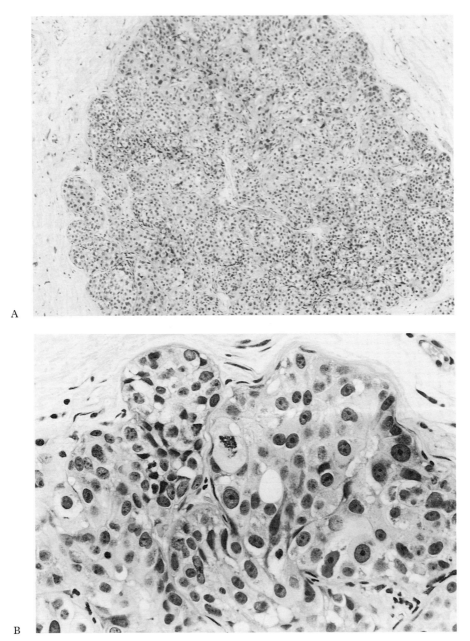

A

B

Fig. 6.13 (A) Lobular unit involved by ductal carcinoma in situ. (B) Cytological features are too pleomorphic to consider LCIS. Hematoxylin–eosin, A × 125; B × 520.

will facilitate the distinction from lobular neo-plasia. However, there are occasions when features of both DCIS and LCIS cannot be denied and in this instance, as stated above, both should be diagnosed.

Although not a frequent occurrence, lobular neoplasia may be found within those lobular alter-ations of the breast that commonly produce a mass. Sclerosing adenosis (SA)[13-14] and fibro-adenoma[14-16] may occasionally contain foci of

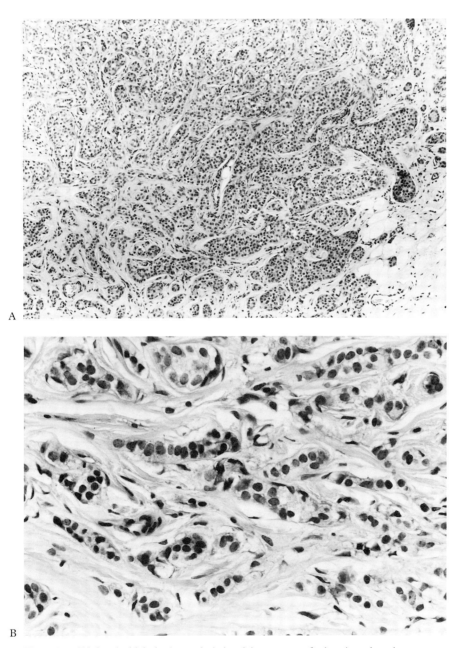

Fig. 6.14   (A) Atypical lobular hyperplasia involving an area of sclerosing adenosis. Distinction from LCIS is based on lack of distention and distortion of involved spaces. (B) Central area of sclerosing adenosis involved by ALH. Compressed glands should not be interpreted as invasive carcinoma. Hematoxylin–eosin, A × 75; B × 450.

otherwise characteristic lobular neoplasia. Fechner has described lobular neoplasia within sclerosing adenosis as a potential source of confusion with invasive carcinoma (Fig. 6.14).[13] Jensen et al showed a nearly 3-fold increased incidence of ALH in biopsy specimens containing sclerosing adenosis compared with those biopsies without SA, but only one of 21 such specimens had ALH within the sclerosed lobular units.[17] This observation of a favored association of ALH and sclerosing adenosis in the same biopsy specimen should spur the pathologist to look diligently for ALH in cases of sclerosing adenosis. The relative risk for such patients may be greater than that attending either of these entities individually (six to seven times that of the general population) as determined from a single study.[17] Risk implications for lobular neoplasia within a fibroadenoma (Fig. 6.15) are not known for certain, but probably are no greater than when lobular neoplasia is seen in the usual setting.[18]

CLINICAL FEATURES AND INCIDENCE

The clinical features of LCIS and ALH are similar

and are listed below. The incidence is greatest before the menopause, with a dramatic decrease thereafter — less than 10% of patients with LCIS are postmenopausal.[5] Lobular neoplasia characteristically affects both breasts in a multifocal, multicentric pattern. If LCIS is found in a breast biopsy, more than half of cases will contain residual LCIS within the ipsilateral breast, and if the contralateral breast is extensively biopsied, more than one-third will contain LCIS;[20] it is evident from this that the disease does not affect both sides completely equally. Involvement is greatest within the breast in the areas containing the most breast parenchyma, i.e., beneath the nipple and in the upper, outer quadrant.[21-22] There is no mass associated with LCIS; the discovery of LCIS or ALH is incidental in a biopsy performed for another reason. No specific mammographic features of LN are described,[23] although adjacent breast tissue sometimes will contain microcalcifications.[24]

FEATURES OF LCIS AND ALH

1. Multifocal, multicentric, bilateral;

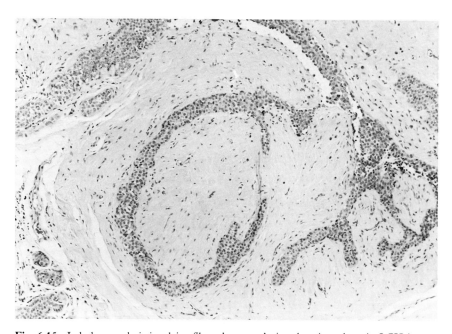

Fig. 6.15 Lobular neoplasia involving fibroadenoma. As in sclerosing adenosis, LCIS is not diagnosed in this setting without full distention and distortion of involved spaces (see text). Hematoxylin–eosin × 75.

2. Decreasing incidence after the menopause;
3. Non-palpable, grossly not visible;
4. Incidental even to mammography;
5. Slight association with adjacent calcification;
6. Risk indicators of developing invasive carcinoma.

This incidental nature of discovery of lobular neoplasia within a biopsy makes accurate assessment of incidence within the general population difficult. Only about one-quarter of patients with LCIS (and even fewer with ALH) subsequently develop an invasive carcinoma (see below), indicating that most examples must remain clinically silent,[25] because residual disease in the rest of the breast is highly likely.[20] And because the vast majority of diagnoses of LCIS or ALH are in premenopausal women, lobular neoplasia probably regresses after the menopause. Since there are no clinical or mammographic signs linked to lobular neoplasia, we may assume that the incidence of lobular neoplasia within the general population is equivalent to the incidence in breast biopsies. Thus, if one or two percent of otherwise benign breast biopsies contain LN, the general population may be assumed to have a similar incidence.[26] The apparent incidence of lobular neoplasia appears to have increased in the last 20–30 years for several reasons: (1) mammographic detection of calcifications which have a slight association with adjacent LCIS, (2) lower threshold of suspicion resulting in more biopsies performed, (3) more complete histological sectioning and examination of tissue by pathologists.

LOBULAR NEOPLASIA AS A RISK INDICATOR

As stated above, lobular neoplasia encompasses a histological spectrum with LCIS representing one extreme. It is now widely accepted that there is also a spectrum of risk that parallels histological extent of involvement.[25] Until 1978 the clinical implications of LCIS were not well characterized. Two separate institutions, in that year, reported their experience with patients having LCIS in a biopsy, with no further treatment.[5,19] Long-term follow-up showed that these patients were at an increased risk for developing a subsequent invasive carcinoma. The term ALH was later instituted in order to place diagnostic boundaries on the spectrum of lobular neoplasia, separating lesser examples of lobular neoplasia and resulting in more precise clinical implications.[3-4]

Since the first reports, there have been several studies of lobular neoplasia and its risk implications, with only one group stratifying cancer risk by separating marked examples (LCIS) from lesser examples (ALH).[4,25] Table 6.1 compares the findings of the various follow-up studies of lobular neoplasia; these studies are included here because they are the best documented and most often cited.[4-5,19,25,27-28] Two recent reports have divided the spectrum of lobular neoplasia into well-developed examples and lesser ones, using a numerical system.[29,30] Both studies found a smaller risk for the less well-developed examples that we diagnose as ALH.

Despite differences in terminology and in the

Table 6.1 Comparison of various reported studies of lobular neoplasia and follow-up results

Study	No of cases	Average age at biopsy	% LCIS or LN	% IBC	Relative risk	Follow-up in years	% IBC/years of follow -up
Page et al[25]	44[a]	45	0.5	23	9.0	18	1.27
Wheeler et al[27]	32	44	0.8	12.5[b]		17.5	0.7
Rosen et al[19]	99[c]	45	1.3	36.4	9.0	24	1.52
Andersen[28]	47	46	1.5	21.3	12.0	15	1.42
Haagensen et al[15]	211	46	3.8	17.0[d]	7.2	14	1.21
Page et al[4]	126[e]	46	1.6	12.7	4.2	17	0.75

[a,e]From the same Nashville cohort of patients, source of two separate reports on LCIS and ALH, respectively.
[b]Four of 32 total cases (one of 25 ipsilateral breast plus three of 32 contralateral breasts).
[c]Follow-up was not available for 15 patients.
[d]The risk is even lower, since 23% of those developing carcinoma developed only DCIS.

number of cases, there are remarkable similarities among these studies. Most consistent are the average age at biopsy and the relative risk of subsequent development of an invasive carcinoma. An obvious difference is in the incidence of lobular neoplasia, ranging from 0.5%[25] up to 3.8%[5] of otherwise benign breast biopsies. Series with a higher incidence of lobular neoplasia concomitantly have a lower percentage of patients developing an invasive carcinoma.[5] Both of these observations could be explained by the inclusion of lesser examples that we would recognize as ALH. Indeed, if we include all patients in the Nashville cohort that were the subject of two separate reports, namely ALH and LCIS, the incidence of lobular neoplasia would be 2.1% of 223 breast biopsies[4,25] with only 15% of patients later developing an invasive carcinoma.

Another difference in these studies of lobular neoplasia relates to the time to development of invasive carcinoma. In the Page et al study of LCIS, two-thirds of those developing an invasive carcinoma did so within the first 15 years after biopsy.[25] In contrast, more than half the invasive carcinomas in the Rosen et al study developed after 15 years.[1,19] Despite these differences, the relative risk figures are not dissimilar. With a median follow-up of 5 years, Ottesen et al reported an 11% incidence of development of invasive carcinoma after LCIS alone, supporting the idea that the risk is greatest within the first 10 or 15 years.[31]

Atypical lobular hyperplasia has important implications not only from the point of view of whether risk assessments have been somewhat 'diluted' by the inclusion of these lesser examples. By recognizing and diagnosing ALH, we are assigning a moderately increased risk of subsequent development of carcinoma, of four to five times that of the general population.[3–4] By applying strict histological criteria to separate LCIS and ALH, Page et al[4] have shown that the risk implications of ALH are approximately half the magnitude of LCIS. A further important consideration in risk assessment for patients with ALH is the influence of a positive family history, i.e., a first degree relative (mother, sister, or daughter) with breast carcinoma. Patients having ALH, but no family history, have an 8% to 10% risk of developing invasive carcinoma within 10 to 15 years.

However, in a patient having ALH and a first degree relative with breast carcinoma, the risk increases to 20% within 10 to 15 years, equivalent to LCIS.[3–4] A positive family history does not further affect risk in patients with LCIS.[25]

In discussions of risk assessment, two aspects must be considered, relative risk and absolute risk. Relative risk statements are used to compare groups and must be interpreted in terms of a carefully pre-established denominator. Thus, understanding the magnitude of relative risk of ALH (four to five times) presupposes understanding of a comparison group and its risk (general population). Absolute risk is the likelihood of an individual patient or group of patients developing a disease process within a given period of time, expressed as percentage.[32] A patient with ALH has an absolute risk of approximately 8% of developing an invasive carcinoma during the subsequent 10 to 15 years. For a patient with LCIS, this absolute risk is approximately 17 to 20%. These suggested ranges of risks are most relevant to women in their fifth decade and progressively less relevant to younger and older women. Specifically, for older women (over age 55 or postmenopausal) the risk after LN or ALH[4,33] decreases.

The studies summarized in Table 6.1 are in agreement that the diagnosis of LCIS indicates an increased relative risk of developing carcinoma of about 10 times that of the general population. By applying strict histological criteria, a more refined assessment of risk can be assigned, with ALH recognizing a risk half that of LCIS.[4,25] These risk figures are best used during the first 10 to 15 years after biopsy, with their implications less clear after that time.[25,32] Clinically, LCIS is becoming accepted as an anatomical risk indicator, although management remains varied.[22] High risk lesions such as LCIS offer an ideal situation for breast cancer prevention trials, as reviewed by Morrow.[34]

The risk of developing an invasive carcinoma applies to both breasts, with a slight preponderance of subsequent carcinomas developing in the breast from which LCIS was diagnosed.[25,27] In the Page et al (1991) series, five carcinomas developed in the ipsilateral breast, three in the contralateral breast, and one patient developed bilateral invasive carcinomas.[25] The types of invasive carcinomas developing vary among the reviewed series. In the series of Page et al, predominantly invasive lobular carcinoma or a variant thereof developed. Of the ten carcinomas, three were pure lobular, four were a variant of lobular, two were tubular carcinomas, and only one was of no special type (ductal).[25] In other series, the majority of developing carcinomas were ductal[26–27] or predominantly lobular.[5,28]

Careful examination of a biopsy specimen for an invasive component associated with LCIS cannot be overemphasized. Fortunately, this occurrence is not common, but must be borne in mind, especially since it may take the subtle form of invasive lobular carcinoma. Distinguishing the latter from an inflammatory infiltrate may sometimes be difficult, and is facilitated by the use of an Alcian Blue/PAS stain or by the use of immunohistochemistry to detect epithelial differentiation.[35] Intracytoplasmic lumina will be so demonstrated in at least a small percentage of cells in 70–80% of invasive lobular carcinomas and this finding will positively differentiate infiltrating carcinoma from mast cells or macrophages.[36]

REFERENCES

1. Foote F, Stewart F. Lobular carcinoma in situ: a rare form of mammary carcinoma. Am J Pathol 1941; 17: 491–496.
2. McDivitt RW, Hutter RVP, Foote FW, Stewart F. In situ lobular carcinoma: a prospective follow-up study indicating cumulative patient risks. JAMA 1967; 201: 96–100.
3. Dupont WD, Page DL. Risk factors for breast cancer in women with proliferative disease. N Engl J Med 1985; 312: 146–151.
4. Page DL, Dupont WD, Rogers LW, Rados MS. Atypical hyperplastic lesions of the female breast. A long-term follow-up study. Cancer 1985; 55: 2698–2708.
5. Haagensen CD, Lane N, Lattes R, Bodian C. Lobular neoplasia (so-called lobular carcinoma in situ) of the breast. Cancer 1978; 42: 737–769.
6. Quincey C, Raitt N, Bell J, Ellis IO. Intracytoplasmic lumina — a useful diagnostic feature of adenocarcinomas. Histopathol 1991; 19: 83–87.
7. Battifora H. Intracytoplasmic lumina in breast carcinoma, a helpful histopathologic feature. Arch Pathol 1975; 99: 614–617.
8. Salhany KE, Page DL. Fine-needle aspiration of mammary lobular carcinoma in situ and atypical lobular hyperplasia. Am J Clin Pathol 1989; 92: 22–26.
9. Page DL, Dupont WD, Rogers LW. Ductal involvement by cells of atypical lobular hyperplasia in the breast: a long-term follow-up study of cancer risk. Hum Pathol 1988; 19: 201–207.
10. Page DL, Anderson TJ, Rogers LW. Carcinoma in situ. In: Diagnostic histopathology of the breast. Page DL, Anderson TJ, eds. Edinburgh: Churchill Livingstone, 1987; 181.
11. Fisher ER, Brown R. Intraductal signet ring carcinoma: a hitherto undescribed form of intraductal carcinoma of the breast. Cancer 1985; 55: 2533–2537.
12. Azzopardi JG. Problems in breast pathology. London: W.B. Saunders, 1979; 203.
13. Fechner RE. Lobular carcinoma in situ in sclerosing adenosis. Am J Surg Pathol 1981; 5: 233–239.
14. Haagensen CD, Lane N, Lattes R. Neoplastic proliferation of the epithelium of the mammary lobules: adenosis, lobular neoplasia, and small cell carcinoma. Surg Clin North Am 1972; 52: 497–524.
15. Pick PW, Iossifides IA. Occurrence of breast carcinoma within a fibroadenoma, a review. Arch Pathol Lab Med 1984; 108: 590–594.
16. Diaz NM, Palmer JO, McDivitt RW. Carcinoma arising within fibroadenomas of the breast, a clinicopathologic study of 105 patients. Am J Clin Pathol 1991; 95: 614–622.
17. Jensen RA, Page DL, Dupont WD, Rogers LW. Invasive breast cancer risk in women with sclerosing adenosis. Cancer 1989; 64: 1977–1983.
18. Dupont WD, Page DL, Parl FF. Breast cancer risk associated with fibroadenomas. Lab Invest 1990; 62: 28A.
19. Rosen PP, Lieberman PH, Braun DW Jr et al. Lobular carcinoma in situ of the breast: detailed analysis of 99 patients with average follow-up of 24 years. Am J Surg Pathol 1978; 2: 224–251.
20. Rosen PP, Braun DW Jr, Lyngholm B et al. Lobular carcinoma in situ of the breast: preliminary results of treatment by ipsilateral mastectomy and contralateral breast biopsy. Cancer 1981; 47: 813–819.
21. Lambird PA, Shelley WM. The spatial distribution of lobular in situ mammary carcinoma. JAMA 1969; 210: 689–693.
22. Shack RB, Page DL. The patient at risk for breast cancer: pathologic and surgical considerations. Prospect Plast Surg 1988; 2: 43–59.
23. Sonnenfeld MR, Frenna TH, Weidner N, Meyer JE. Lobular carcinoma in situ: mammographic-pathologic correlation of results of needle-directed biopsy. Radiol 1991; 181: 363–367.
24. Pope T, Fechner R, Wilhelm M et al. Lobular carcinoma in situ of the breast: mammographic features. Radiol 1988; 168: 63–66.
25. Page DL, Kidd TE Jr, Dupont WD et al. Lobular neoplasia of the breast: higher risk for subsequent invasive cancer predicted by more extensive disease. Hum Pathol 1991; 22: 1232–1239.
26. Bartow SA, Pathak DR, Black WC et al. Prevalence of benign, atypical, and malignant breast lesions in populations at different risk for breast cancer. Cancer 1987; 60: 2751–2760.
27. Wheeler JE, Enterline HT, Roseman JM et al. Lobular

carcinoma in situ of the breast: long-term follow-up. Cancer 1974; 34: 554–563.

28. Andersen JA. Lobular carcinoma in situ: a long-term follow-up in 52 cases. Acta Pathol Microbiol Scand 1974; 82: 519–533.

29. Bodian CA, Perzin KH, Lattes R. Lobular neoplasia: long term risk of breast cancer and relation to other factors. Cancer 1996; 78: 1024–1034.

30. Fisher ER, Costantino J, Fisher B et al. Pathologic findings from the National Surgical Adjuvant Breast Project (NSABP) protocol B-17. Five year observations concerning lobular carcinoma in situ. Cancer 1996; 78: 1403–1416.

31. Ottesen GL, Graversen HP, Blichert-Toft M et al. Lobular carcinoma in situ of the female breast: short-term results of a prospective nationwide study. Am J Surg Pathol 1993; 17: 14–21.

32. Dupont WD, Page DL. Relative risk of breast cancer varies with time since diagnosis of atypical hyperplasia. Hum Pathol 1989; 20: 723–725.

33. Marshall LM, Hunter DJ, Connolly JL et al. Risk of breast cancer associated with atypical hyperplasia of lobular and ductal types. Cancer Epidem Biomarkers Prevent 1997; 6: 297–301.

34. Morrow M. Pre-cancerous breast lesions: implications for breast cancer prevention trials. Int J Radiation Oncology Biol Phys 1992; 23: 1071–1078.

35. Cardoso de Almeida PC, Pestana CB. Immunohistochemical markers in the identification of metastatic breast cancer. Br Cancer Res Treat 1992; 21: 201–210.

36. Dixon JM, Anderson TJ, Page DL et al. Infiltrating lobular carcinoma of the breast. Histopathol 1982; 6: 149–161.

Sclerosing lesions

GENERAL INTRODUCTION

A number of benign breast lesions are characterized by a combination of epithelial proliferation and stromal fibrosis and sclerosis often resulting in the formation of a mass lesion. They have many overlapping features and their importance lies partly in the fact that they may be mistaken clinically, mammographically and histologically for carcinoma. Thus, we have included sclerosing adenosis, microglandular adenosis and radial scar/complex sclerosing lesion in this chapter. A further entity with overlapping morphological features is the so-called ductal adenoma; however, we consider this to be a sclerosed intraduct papilloma and the reader is referred to Chapter 8 for a description of this lesion.

SCLEROSING ADENOSIS

INTRODUCTION

Before discussing the entity sclerosing adenosis, it is first worth considering the term 'adenosis' which, when unqualified, has been used to refer to any benign alteration of glandular elements and as such we feel is both diagnostically unhelpful and confusing. We agree with Page and Anderson[1] that adenosis is not a diagnostic term, but rather a descriptive one which should always be qualified further as, for example, in the entities sclerosing adenosis and microglandular adenosis to be discussed in this chapter and blunt duct adenosis as discussed in Chapter 4. For the same reasons we would also avoid the term 'fibroadenosis' and instead refer to fibrocystic change with a description of the components present in a given case (see Ch. 4).

Sclerosing adenosis refers to a benign entity composed of disordered epithelial, myoepithelial and connective tissue elements arising predominantly from the terminal duct lobular unit. It covers a spectrum of lesions ranging from a microscopic alteration of lobules which may be considered a normal variation,[2] to a microscopic component of fibrocystic change (Ch. 4) and, more rarely, a mass lesion which may be palpable and which has been termed 'adenosis tumour'[3–5] but is probably more appropriately referred to as 'nodular sclerosing adenosis'.[6–7] As stated in the general introduction to this chapter, the importance of this lesion lies in the fact that, particularly when presenting as a mass, it may be mistaken clinically, radiologically and histologically as carcinoma.[5]

CLINICAL FEATURES

In many cases sclerosing adenosis occurs as an incidental finding in breast tissue removed for other reasons. Asymptomatic, impalpable lesions are also being detected with increasing frequency by mammography following the introduction of screening programs for breast cancer since both the parenchymal deformity and the microcalcifications seen mammographically may be indistinguishable from those seen in carcinoma.[8–9]

The clinicopathological features of the palpable masses have been well described previously.[5,10–13] Patients with a clinically palpable mass are generally younger, often pre- or perimenopausal, but with an age range of 20–70 years. The mass is usually solitary, although Heller and Flemming have reported multiple[11] and Haagensen and colleagues bilateral[13] masses. It may be ill-defined and can be somewhat fixed within the breast, but fixation to skin or deep fascia are seldom seen. Pain and tenderness are not uncommon in contrast with carcinoma and may be related to perineural infiltration.

MACROSCOPIC APPEARANCES

There are no distinctive gross appearances in the diffuse microscopic form, the breast tissue either appearing normal or showing features of associated fibrocystic change. The nodular type forms a firm, lobulated but often ill-defined mass varying in size from 0.5 to 5 cm. A nodular and whorled appearance may be appreciated if the cut surface is examined with a hand lens.[14] A distinctive granularity has been emphasized by some[10–11,13] although Nielsen found this in only about a quarter of the 27 cases in her series.[5] Areas with closely packed tiny cysts are also described[5] and although inconstant macroscopic features, the presence of granularity and cysts is a useful clue to the diagnosis as both are exceptional in tubular carcinoma.

MICROSCOPIC APPEARANCES

Sclerosing adenosis may occur in three forms: tiny foci in an otherwise normal breast, especially in the perimenopausal age group (Fig. 7.1A and B); larger though still microscopic areas as part of the spectrum of fibrocystic change (Fig. 7.2A and B); or it may form a nodular mass (Fig. 7.3A and B). In each case a disorderly proliferation of acini and intralobular stromal cells results in distortion and expansion of lobules, with an overall whorled appearance. However, even in the nodular form in which the distorted lobules merge to form a definite mass lesion the lobulocentric architecture is maintained. This lobular or 'organoid' configuration is best appreciated on low power examination. At higher magnification microtubular structures may be seen but the distorted compressed acini frequently show obliteration of their lumina (Figs 7.1B, 7.3B). Epithelial and myoepithelial elements may proliferate separately but two-layered structures are usually evident at least focally; their identification may be facilitated by immunostaining of the myoepithelial component with anti-smooth muscle actin (Figs 7.4, 7.5). The centre of a lesion is often more cellular, reflecting earlier stages of development whereas sclerosis predominates at the periphery and it is here that the distorted tubular structures are often more readily appreciated (Figs 7.3A, 7.6). Nuclei are small and regular without atypia and mitotic figures are infrequent (Figs 7.3B, 7.7B). The luminal

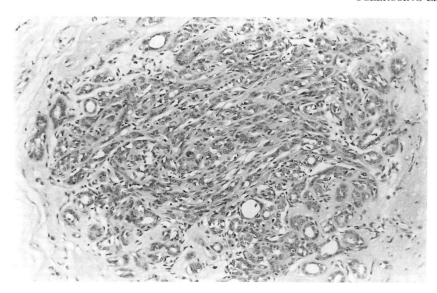

Fig. 7.1A Sclerosing adenosis. In this example the process involves a single lobule only. A number of other lobules in this biopsy showed the same features, but no nodular lesion was identified. Hematoxylin–eosin × 125.

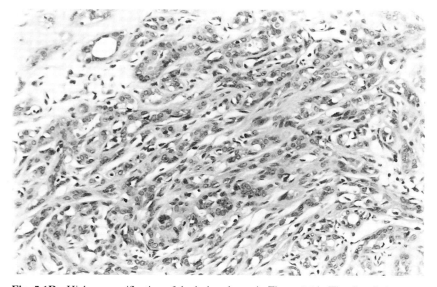

Fig. 7.1B Higher magnification of the lesion shown in Figure 7.1A. The disorderly proliferation of epithelial and stromal cells is well seen. Hematoxylin–eosin × 185.

spaces of the microtubular structures frequently show microcalcification (Fig. 7.7A and B) which appears as tiny clusters in mammograms (see Ch. 2). A small proportion (around 2%) of cases show extension of benign acini into perineural and vascular spaces,[15–17] a finding that should not be regarded as indicative of malignancy in the absence of confirmatory features. Apocrine meta-

plasia may be present and may show cytological atypia.[18–19] Similarly, both ductal carcinoma in situ and lobular neoplasia (Fig. 7.8) have been recorded in the nodular form of sclerosing adenosis[5,20–23] and may be mistaken for invasive carcinoma unless the lobular configuration and presence of myoepithelial cells are noted. Lobular neoplasia in particular requires a cautious approach and a

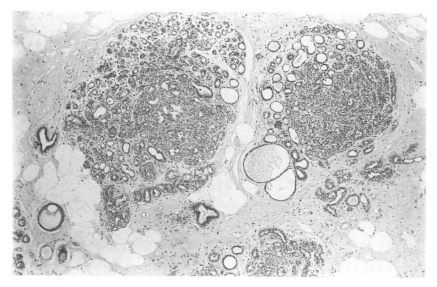

Fig. 7.2A   Fibrocystic change with associated sclerosing adenosis involving two adjacent lobular units. Hematoxylin–eosin × 57.

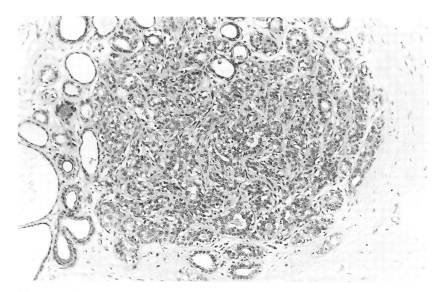

Fig. 7.2B   Sclerosing adenosis. Microcystic change is seen around the periphery of the involved lobule. Same case as Figure 7.2A. Hematoxylin–eosin × 125.

diagnosis of lobular carcinoma in situ is only made if all the criteria are fully satisfied (see Ch. 6).[1]

PATHOGENESIS

Symmers considered sclerosing adenosis to represent an abnormal pattern of age-related regression or postlactational involution and suggested that the frequent associated history of menstrual disturbance or abnormal obstetric and lactational history implicates an underlying disorder of ovarian function in its pathogenesis.[24] Others consider it to be a proliferative process[14,25] and this is supported by the many well-documented cases of perineural invasion.[15–16] Histologically,

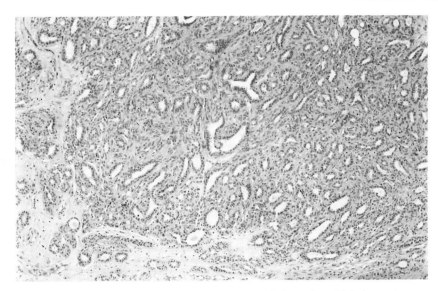

Fig. 7.3A Nodular sclerosing adenosis. Note the rounded margin and lobulocentric structure. Hematoxylin–eosin × 100.

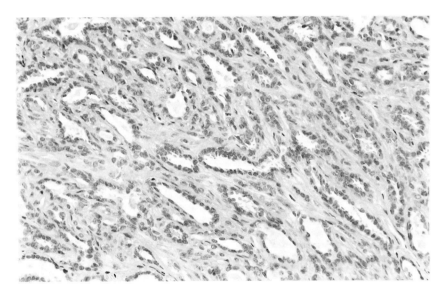

Fig. 7.3B Higher magnification of the lesion shown in Figure 7.3A. Microtubular structures are set within a proliferation of stromal cells. Hematoxylin–eosin × 185.

both proliferative and involutional changes are seen, suggesting that both processes may occur. Using stereomicroscopic techniques, Tanaka and Oota[25] have shown that the process of epithelial hyperplasia originates not only in lobules, but also by a process of budding from small and medium sized ducts. Azzopardi came to the same conclusion following step sectioning of a series of cases.[14]

We consider the processes occurring to represent, at one end of the spectrum, a normal physiological tissue response resulting in the microscopic alteration of lobules which may be considered a normal variation, to, at the other end of the spectrum, an abnormal response in which the features of sclerosing adenosis are dominant and which may be associated with a slightly increased risk for

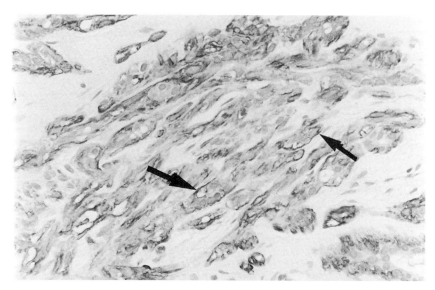

Fig. 7.4   Sclerosing adenosis. Myoepithelial cells in obliterated microtubules are identified by immunoreactivity to actin (arrowheads). Immunostaining for anti-smooth muscle actin × 400.

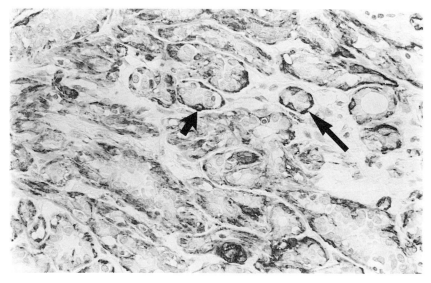

Fig. 7.5   Another example of sclerosing adenosis in which myoepithelial cells are identified in both open (large arrowhead) and closed (small arrowhead) tubular structures. Immunostaining for anti-smooth muscle actin × 400.

the subsequent development of carcinoma (see below).[26] The similar but less florid appearances seen as one of the components of fibrocystic change may be regarded as an exaggerated but not strictly pathological tissue response and fall somewhere between these two extremes.

DIFFERENTIAL DIAGNOSIS

The nodular form can be confused clinically, mammographically and histologically with carcinoma, especially the tubular type. The lobulocentric configuration of sclerosing adenosis

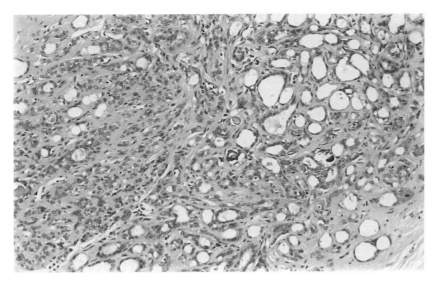

Fig. 7.6 Sclerosing adenosis. Another example of the nodular type. The center is to the left and the tubular structures at the periphery are to the right of the field. Hematoxylin–eosin × 125.

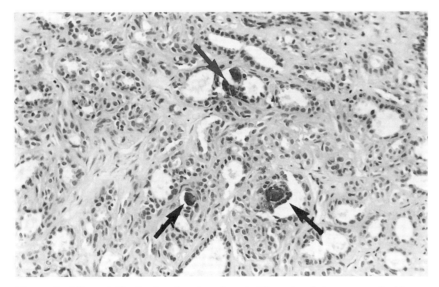

Fig. 7.7A Microcalcification in sclerosing adenosis. Three tiny foci are present in this field (arrowheads). Hematoxylin–eosin × 185.

should, however, be readily apparent on low power examination, whereas higher magnification will show the distorted microtubules with an identifiable two layered epithelial-myoepithelial cell lining. In contrast, invasive tubular carcinoma contains separate tubular structures with clear lumina lined by a single layer of epithelial cells set in a characteristic desmoplastic stroma. Lesions showing atypical apocrine metaplasia may also be mistaken for invasive carcinoma, but recognition of the above benign features and of the apocrine nature of the epithelial cells should prevent this. Similarly, lesions with coexistent ductal carcinoma in situ or lobular neoplasia may closely

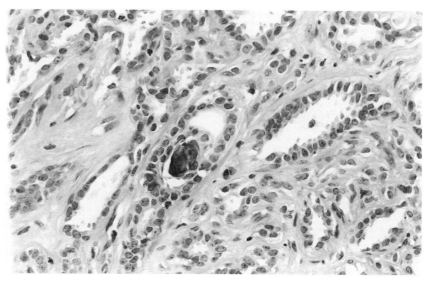

Fig. 7.7B Microcalcification in sclerosing adenosis. At this magnification a focus of calcification can be identified clearly within a tubular lumen. Same case as Figure 7.7A. Hematoxylin–eosin × 400.

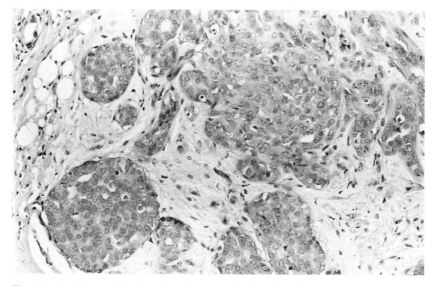

Fig. 7.8 Lobular neoplasia in sclerosing adenosis. This field is from the periphery of the lesion; several lobular acini are involved by a proliferation of small, regular epithelial cells. The pattern fulfils the criteria for a diagnosis of lobular carcinoma in situ. Hematoxylin–eosin × 185.

mimic invasive carcinoma and require careful appraisal. In this respect immunostaining for smooth muscle actin, S-100 protein, type IV collagen and laminin, as well as a periodic acid Schiff stain with diastase digestion to identify the myoepithelial cells and intact basal lamina respec-

tively, may be helpful in excluding an invasive component.[23,27]

The other main differential diagnosis histologically is radial scar/complex sclerosing lesion. Low power examination should identify the architectural complexity of the complex sclerosing lesion,

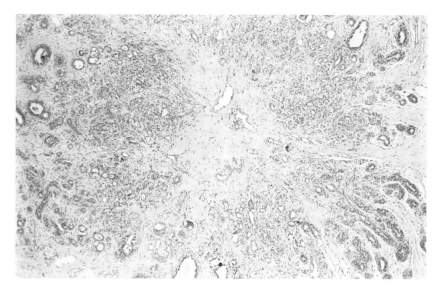

Fig. 7.9A   Nodular sclerosing lesion with central fibrosis. Hematoxylin–eosin × 57.

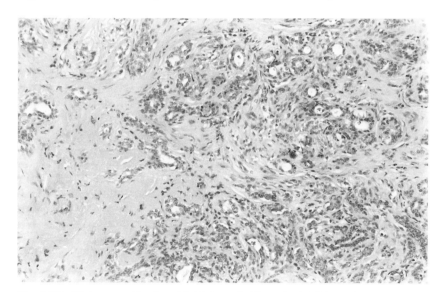

Fig. 7.9B   Higher magnification of field shown in Figure 7.9A. This confirms that the lesion is composed predominantly of sclerosing adenosis which merges with central fibrosis and entrapped epithelial structures (to the left of the field). Because of this it is better designated as sclerosing adenosis than as a complex sclerosing lesion. Hematoxylin–eosin × 125.

with loss of lobular orientation and a prominent central elastotic scar, in contrast with the maintenance of a lobular pattern in sclerosing adenosis. However, central elastosis with entrapped tubules is occasionally seen in sclerosing adenosis (Fig. 7.9A and B)[5] and, conversely, foci of sclerosing adenosis are frequently found in complex sclerosing lesions. This suggests that the two lesions may represent the ends of a spectrum of proliferative changes. Thus, for practical purposes, it is probably sensible to categorize an individual lesion on the basis of the predominant pattern.

The differential diagnosis of sclerosing lesions is summarized in Table 7.1.

Table 7.1 Differential diagnosis of sclerosing lesions

Tubular carcinoma	Sclerosing adenosis	Microglandular adenosis	Radial scar
Infiltrative, often stellate architecture	Lobulocentric architecture	Infiltrative, disorderly architecture	Complex, stellate architecture
Desmoplastic stroma. Central elastosis frequent	Often central cellularity with sclerotic periphery	Fibrotic stroma	Variable stromal cellularity
Well formed angulated tubules	Distorted, compressed tubules. Frequent obliterated lumina	Uniform round tubules	Distorted tubules
Abundant eosinophilic cytoplasm often with apical snouts	Infrequent apical snouts	Clear, vacuolated or granular epithelial cytoplasm. No apical snouts	No apical snouts
Absent myoepithelial cells	Prominent admixed myoepithelial cells	Occasional myoepithelial cells described	Myoepithelial cells seen
Patchy, incomplete basement membrane	Uniform basement membrane	Prominent basement membrane	Basement membrane seen
Intraluminal secretion or microcalcification may be seen	Intraluminal microcalcification may be seen	Intraluminal colloid-like material which may be calcified	Intraluminal secretion uncommon. Microcalcification may be seen
Frequent associated low grade cribriform or micropapillary DCIS	May be associated apocrine metaplasia. Associated DCIS and lobular neoplasia rare but described	Atypical features rarely described (see text)	Associated cysts, sclerosing adenosis, epithelial hyperplasia and rarely in situ or invasive carcinoma

PROGNOSIS AND MANAGEMENT

Lesions presenting as masses are usually excised, although there is some evidence to suggest that such lesions may regress after the menopause.[3] The relationship between sclerosing adenosis and cancer risk has been difficult to define. Although Dupont and Page had reported a slightly increased risk for invasive breast cancer in patients with sclerosing adenosis when analyzed in combination with other proliferative lesions,[28] the consensus statement of the Cancer Committee of the College of American Pathologists, following careful review of the literature available at the time, placed sclerosing adenosis in the 'no increased risk' category.[29] However, more recent work by Jensen et al has again suggested a slightly increased risk (relative risk 1.5–2.0), independent of the presence of atypical hyperplasia or a positive family history.[26] In this study, 349 women with sclerosing adenosis were followed for an average of 17 years. Strict histological criteria were applied which required well developed examples where affected areas were approximately double the size of adjacent 'normal' lobules and had at least 50% of their acini involved by the sclerosing process.

This study also supported a previous assertion by Haagensen et al[3] of an association between sclerosing adenosis and lobular neoplasia, as sclerosing adenosis and atypical lobular neoplasia were found to occur together almost three times more commonly than would be expected by chance. The authors therefore suggest that the identification of sclerosing adenosis in a biopsy specimen should prompt a careful search for co-existent lobular neoplasia. The occurrence of lobular neoplasia within sclerosing adenosis has been referred to in the section on differential diagnosis above.

The clinical significance of apocrine atypia in sclerosing adenosis is uncertain, but it is of interest that Simpson et al,[18] in a review of 55 cases, identified a positive association between apocrine adenosis and atypical hyperplasia, both ductal and lobular. They suggest that the discovery of apocrine atypia in a sclerosing lesion should prompt a careful search for atypical hyperplasia. (These authors use the term apocrine adenosis to refer to apocrine metaplasia occurring in glands within any recognizable, albeit deformed, lobular units, including those of sclerosing adenosis. This is in contrast with the use of the same term by Eusebi et al[30–31] to refer to a specific lesion previously described as 'adenomyoepithelial adenosis'[32] which is associated with a type of adenomyoepithelioma and referred to below in the section on microglandular hyperplasia and also in Chapter 16). Whether apocrine atypia in this setting is by itself a marker of increased relative risk remains unknown and we would agree with Carter and Rosen[19] that careful follow-up of women who have had such lesions excised is to be recommended until more is known of their natural history.

MICROGLANDULAR ADENOSIS

INTRODUCTION

Microglandular adenosis (MGA) is a rare proliferation of small duct-like structures which may be confused with invasive tubular carcinoma.[33–36]

CLINICAL FEATURES

Small foci of MGA may be present as an incidental finding in breast tissue removed for other reasons but the majority present as a palpable mass which may be several centimeters in diameter. The majority of patients are aged between 45 and 60 years at presentation, but the age range extends from the mid-20s to over 80 years. Mammographic features are not specific but may be suspicious of carcinoma.[34–36]

MACROSCOPIC APPEARANCES

The macroscopic appearances are nondescript and similar to those of fibrocystic change, consisting of an ill-defined area of fibro-fatty tissue which may measure up to 20 cm in diameter, although usually only 3–4 cm.

MICROSCOPIC APPEARANCES

The classical appearances are of a disorderly proliferation of small round acinar structures, apparently infiltrating between normal ducts and lobules and extending into adipose tissue (Fig. 7.10A, B and C). In contrast with sclerosing adenosis the growth pattern is not lobulocentric and there is no intervening spindle cell component. The acini appear to be lined by a single layer of epithelial cells which have clear (vacuolated) or finely granular, eosinophilic cytoplasm and lack apical snouts. Mitoses are absent or rare and there

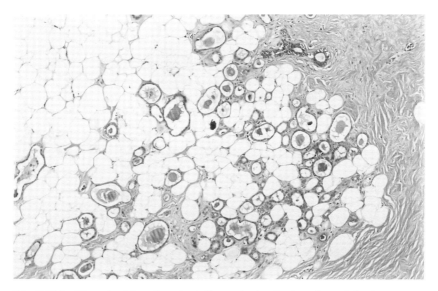

Fig. 7.10A Microglandular adenosis. A disorganized collection of rounded acinar structures without a discernible lobular architecture is present within adipose tissue. A normal duct is present at the top right of the field. Hematoxylin–eosin × 100.

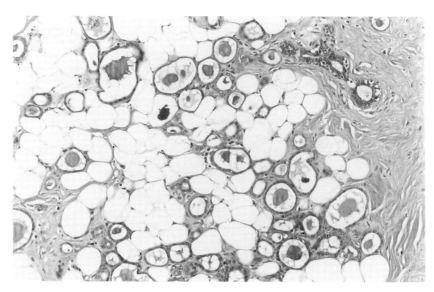

Fig. 7.10B   Higher magnification of the field shown in Figure 7.10A. Many acini contain a luminal secretion. Note the lack of a spindle cell stromal component. Hematoxylin–eosin × 125.

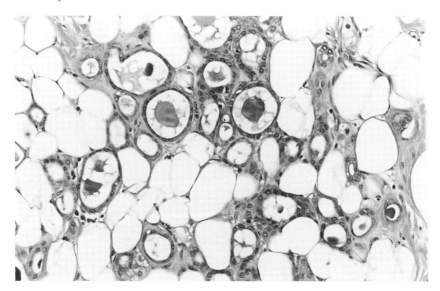

Fig. 7.10C   Another view of the area shown in Figure 7.10A and B. The acini appear to be lined by a single layer of regular epithelial cells; there is no nuclear atypia and mitoses are not seen. Hematoxylin–eosin × 185.

is no nuclear atypia. The glands often contain PAS positive, diastase-resistant, eosinophilic, colloid-like material which may rarely be calcified. Alcian Blue positivity is variable. Myoepithelial cells are characteristically said to be absent (Fig. 7.10D);[31,33–37] however, as discussed below, cases are described in which there is an identifiable, albeit inconspicuous, myoepithelial cell component[38] which may be highlighted by immunostaining for smooth muscle actin (Fig. 7.11A, B and C). The glandular proliferation may be accompanied by a hypocellular, dense collagenous stroma and the glands are surrounded by PAS positive basement membrane material, although delineation of this from the surrounding fibrocollagenous stroma may be difficult and

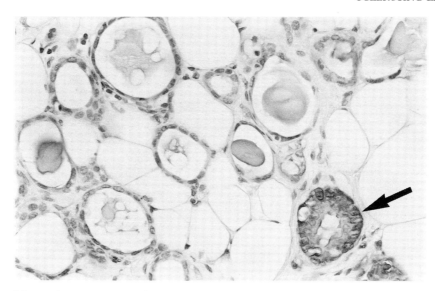

Fig. 7.10D The absence of a myoepithelial layer in this lesion is demonstrated by actin immunostaining. The identification of actin positive cells in the normal ductule at the bottom right serves as an internal control (arrowhead). Immunostaining for anti-smooth muscle actin × 400.

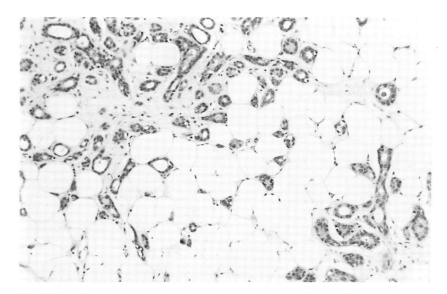

Fig. 7.11A Microglandular adenosis. In this example the acini are small but rounded and appear to infiltrate diffusely within fibrous stroma and adipose tissue. Hematoxylin–eosin × 125.

require immunostaining for laminin[31] or even electron microscopy.[36]

Occasional examples of MGA, particularly the rare recurrent examples, may show atypical features with a more complex architectural arrangement, including glandular budding and the development of a cribriform architecture, together with stratification of the lining epithelium and cytological abnormalities, including nuclear enlargement, chromatin clearing and the presence of nucleoli.[6,36,39–40] The significance of such features is discussed below.

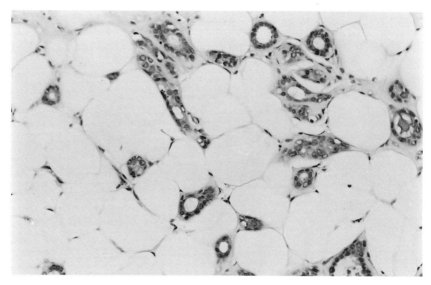

Fig. 7.11B   Higher magnification of field shown in Figure 7.11A. Note the apparent single layer of epithelial cells. Hematoxylin–eosin × 185.

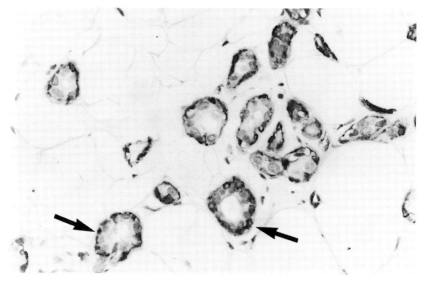

Fig. 7.11C   A definite, if incomplete, layer of myoepithelial cells is identified in the tubules (arrowheads) in this example of microglandular adenosis. Same case as Figure 7.11A and B. Immunostaining for anti-smooth muscle actin × 400.

PATHOGENESIS

Microglandular adenosis has been considered to be a proliferation of epithelial cells only; characteristically the proliferating tubules are said to lack a myoepithelial cell layer. However, Kay in 1985[41] and Diaz et al in 1991[38] described cases in which myoepithelial cells were seen and we too have identified similar cases (Fig. 7.11A, B and C). Tavassoli regards such cases as a distinct form of adenosis termed secretory adenosis.[36] However, we would argue that sclerosing adenosis and microglandular adenosis in fact form two ends of a spectrum defined by the relative prominence of myoepithelial cells. Against this argument is the recent finding of Tavassoli and Bratthauer[37] that the proliferating cells in MGA express S-100 protein whereas those in sclerosing adenosis and secretory adenosis do not. These authors suggest that the epithelial cells in MGA correspond to an S-100 positive epithelial cell type that is often present in small numbers in normal breast. In contrast, Diaz et al[38] found variable immunostaining for S-100 protein and, unlike Tavassoli and Bratthauer, also identified S-100 positivity in a proportion of tubular carcinomas. Clearly, further studies are required to resolve these issues.

DIFFERENTIAL DIAGNOSIS

The most important differential diagnosis is invasive tubular carcinoma, particularly the sclerosing variant (see Ch. 15). Tubular carcinoma differs from microglandular adenosis by its usual stellate configuration with central elastosis and characteristic desmoplastic stroma. The glandular structures in tubular carcinoma are irregular in outline, often with angular protrusions, and are lined by a single layer of cells with abundant eosinophilic cytoplasm, often forming characteristic apical snouts, in contrast with the generally uniform, round glands lined by clear or vacuolated cells of MGA. Intraluminal secretion is less common in tubular carcinoma. Finally, cribriform or micropapillary intraduct carcinoma often accompanies tubular carcinoma but not MGA. These features are summarized in Table 7.1.

MGA may also be confused with the tubulolobular variant of invasive lobular carcinoma.[42] However, close inspection of the tissue sections in the latter will reveal not only small tubular structures, but also cords of cells more characteristic of classical lobular carcinoma. The demonstration of myoepithelial cells where possible will also count against a diagnosis of carcinoma.

Sclerosing adenosis is distinguished from MGA by its lobulocentric architecture and the prominence of myoepithelial cells, although as discussed previously, we believe that the two conditions may be related and form opposite ends of a spectrum.

A recently described entity may also enter the differential diagnosis; termed 'apocrine adenosis' by Eusebi and co-workers[30] and previously referred to as 'adenomyoepithelial adenosis' by

Kaier and associates,[32] it occurs in association with, or as a precursor to, adenomyoepithelioma. It is distinguished from microglandular adenosis by the presence of prominent myoepithelial cells and by positive immunohistochemical staining for gross cystic disease fluid protein (GCDFP)-15, a marker of apocrine differentiation[31] (see also Ch. 16).

PROGNOSIS AND MANAGEMENT

Palpable lesions are usually excised and rarely recur, but recurrence has been associated with the development of atypical features as described above.[6,39] These atypical features have been found by Rosenblum et al[39] and James et al[40] in a small number of cases in which in situ or invasive carcinoma has developed in MGA. Thus, careful histological sampling is indicated, particularly in atypical lesions. It has been suggested that such lesions be widely excised and followed up in the same way as atypical hyperplasias.[39]

Carcinoma arising within MGA is reported to have distinct morphological and possibly prognostic features; Rosenblum et al[39] described marked secretory activity in the carcinomatous epithelium in three of their eight cases, clear cells in six cases and heavily granulated cells in four; James et al[40] found immunoreactivity for S-100 protein in seven of eight cases examined, although this is a relatively non-specific finding and has been described in other types of breast carcinoma.[38,43] These authors also suggest a relatively favorable prognosis despite histopathological and immunohistochemical features usually associated with a poor outcome.[40] However, because of the infiltrative nature of MGA and the difficulty in establishing the extent of carcinoma in this setting they advocate mastectomy with axillary node dissection in such cases.

RADIAL SCAR/COMPLEX SCLEROSING LESION

INTRODUCTION

A variety of descriptive terms has been used to describe these distinctive lesions, including 'rosette-like lesions',[44] 'sclerosing papillary proliferations',[45] 'benign sclerosing ductal proliferation',[46] 'infiltrating epitheliosis'[14] and 'indurative mastopathy',[47] with the term 'radial scar' initially introduced in the German literature ('strahlige Narben')[48] now the most widely used.[6,49–50] These lesions vary in size and as larger examples are more likely to have a complex structure with associated epithelial hyperplasia, Page and Anderson[50] have suggested the term radial scar (RS) be used for those lesions measuring 1–9 mm and complex sclerosing lesion (CSL) for those which are 10 mm or more. With the development of breast screening programs, these lesions are being detected more frequently as it is virtually impossible to distinguish them from small invasive carcinomas mammographically.[49]

CLINICAL FEATURES

RS/CSL has been reported to occur over a wide age range but is most common in pre- and perimenopausal women. Both autopsy studies and examination of surgical mastectomy specimens have shown them to be common, multiple and frequently bilateral. The lowest incidence reported is 1.7% in the series of Andersen and Gram.[51] However, these authors examined only a small number of tissue blocks from surgically resected benign breast specimens. The highest, 28%, was reported by Nielsen et al[52] following extensive sampling of breasts from a series of 83 consecutive, unselected autopsies. In this series 67% were multicentric and 43% bilateral.[52] The lesions are usually but not always impalpable[53] and are identified either as an incidental finding in breast tissue removed for other reasons or are detected mammographically during breast screening, in which case they usually appear as small spiculated structures (see Ch. 2), although microcalcification may also be present.[54]

MACROSCOPIC APPEARANCES

The smaller lesions may not be visible to the naked eye. Larger lesions may mimic carcinoma macroscopically due to their stellate architecture with central puckering, firm texture and pale yellow flecks of elastosis. Cysts are occasionally seen in the periphery.

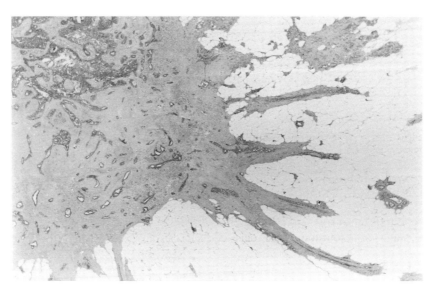

Fig. 7.12A Complex sclerosing lesion. This low power view shows a spiculate mass lesion with a central fibrous core and radiating arms at the periphery. The lesion measured 18 mm in maximum diameter. Hematoxylin–eosin × 23.

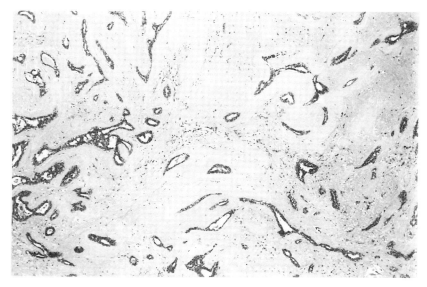

Fig. 7.12B Higher magnification of field shown in Fig. 7.12A. Entrapped tubules are seen within the fibroelastotic stroma. Hematoxylin–eosin × 57.

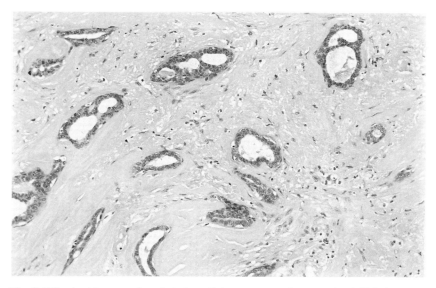

Fig. 7.12C At this power the relatively acellular stroma can be appreciated. Tubules are mainly elongated and oval rather than rounded.

MICROSCOPIC APPEARANCES

These depend on both the plane of section of the lesion and its stage of evolution. The classic appearance of a stellate or radial arrangement of parenchymal structures around a central fibroelastotic core represents a well developed lesion (Fig. 7.12A, B and C and Fig. 7.13A and B). Earlier lesions are composed of a small group of radiating ductules or tubules in a cellular connective tissue stroma (Fig. 7.14A and B) which includes abundant myofibroblasts.[55] As central sclerosis and elastosis develop, entrapped tubules become compressed and distorted and may give rise to confusion with invasive carcinoma (Figs 7.12C, 7.14B). However, careful examination, possibly aided by immunostaining for anti-smooth muscle actin, will confirm the double, epithelial-

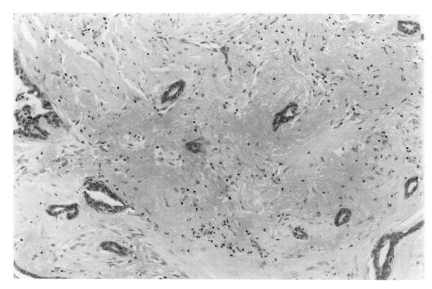

Fig. 7.13A Central part of another complex sclerosing lesion. Scanty entrapped tubules are seen within a dense fibroelastic stroma. Hematoxylin–eosin × 125.

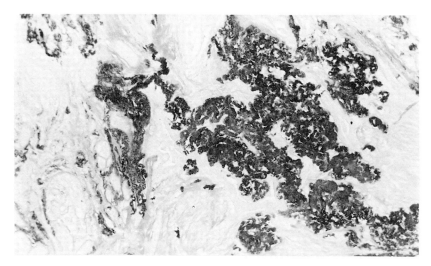

Fig. 7.13B Tangled elastic fibers in the stroma at the center of a complex sclerosing lesion. Same case as Fig. 7.13B. Elastic-Van Gieson × 125.

myoepithelial cell lining of the benign ductules (Fig. 7.15B). Cystic change is frequently observed in the ductular structures of the radiating arms (Figs 7.14A, 7.16) and microcalcification is also common (Figs 7.17, 7.19B). As the lesions become more complex, a variety of other features are frequently seen, including foci of sclerosing adenosis, papilloma formation and variable degrees of epithelial hyperplasia (Fig. 7.18A, B and C). The latter must be evaluated carefully for the presence of atypical ductal hyperplasia (Fig. 7.19A and B), lobular neoplasia and in situ carcinoma (Fig. 7.20) as all three together with invasive carcinoma may arise in association with RS/CSL,[56–57] particularly in the larger lesions. In a study of 126 radial scars and complex sclerosing lesions from 91 women, Sloane and Mayers[57] found 27 containing atypical hyperplasia and/or carcinoma; these were especially likely to occur in lesions measuring more than 7 mm in diameter

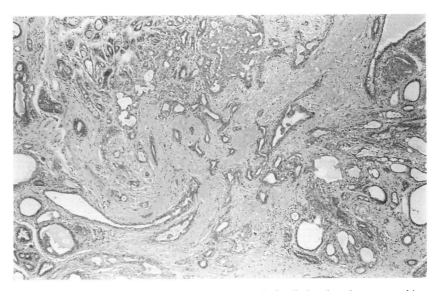

Fig. 7.14A Radial scar. This small lesion is composed of radiating ductules entrapped in fibroelastic stroma. Extensive fibrocystic change was present in the adjacent breast tissue; microcysts are seen at the bottom right of the field. This was an incidental finding in a wide local excision specimen for carcinoma. Hematoxylin–eosin × 57.

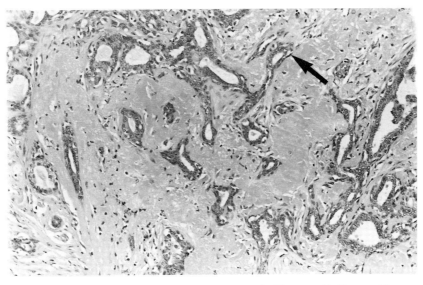

Fig. 7.14B Higher magnification of radial scar shown in Figure 7.14A. Even at this power a double layered epithelium can be identified in the ductules (arrowhead), a point of distinction from tubular carcinoma. Hematoxylin–eosin × 125.

and in women older than 50 years. Not unexpectedly, they were also the lesions which were more likely to have been detected mammographically as part of a breast screening program. The association between sclerosing lesions and ductal hyperplasia is considered further in Chapter 5 and lobular neoplasia in Chapter 6.

PATHOGENESIS

Wellings and Alpers[58] suggested that RS/CSL may begin as a reaction to unknown injury which heals as focal areas of fibrosis and elastosis. With contraction of this fibroelastic core, the surrounding ducts and lobules are pulled into the charac-

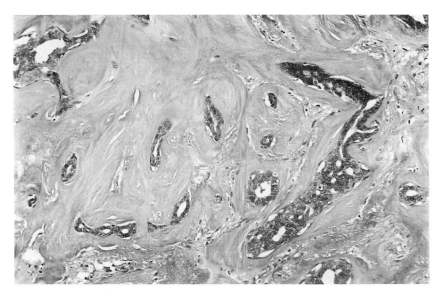

Fig. 7.15A Central part of another radial scar/complex sclerosing lesion. In this example identification of a myoepithelial layer is made difficult by fixation artefact. Hematoxylin–eosin × 57.

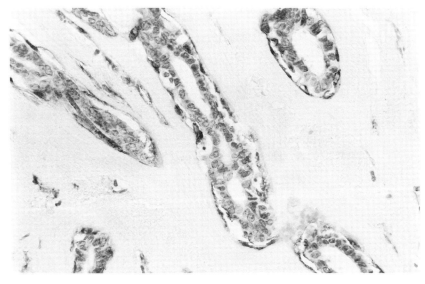

Fig. 7.15B A myoepithelial layer is identified in the entrapped ductules of this lesion by immunostaining for actin. Same case as Figure 7.15A. Immunostaining for anti-smooth muscle actin × 400.

teristic radial conformation. Proliferative changes may be present in these surrounding structures already or may develop subsequently. An association with duct ectasia has been suggested by some[46,48,51] and Hamperl[48] emphasized duct obliteration as an important histogenetic factor, describing remnants of epithelium of the satellite ducts which are often seen in the central parts of radial scars. The illustrations he used suggest development of the infiltrating tubules from these remnants.

Duct ectasia is not always identified in breasts containing radial scars however[52] and tiny lesions are often seen as part of the spectrum of fibro-

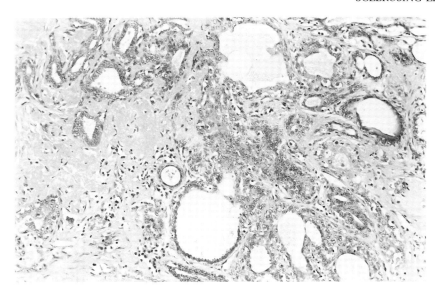

Fig. 7.16 Complex sclerosing lesion. The central part of the lesion is at the top left where tubular structures and fibroelastic stroma are seen. Fibrocystic change is present around the periphery. Hematoxylin–eosin × 125.

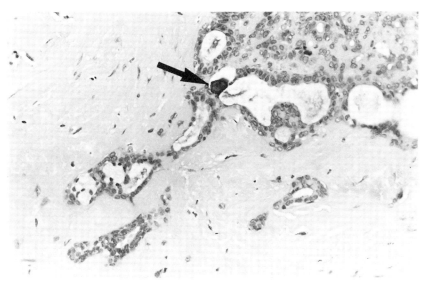

Fig. 7.17 Complex sclerosing lesion. A focus of microcalcification is present in the lumen of an entrapped tubular structure (arrowhead). Hematoxylin–eosin × 185.

cystic change (Fig. 7.14A and B). Indeed, several investigators confirm a significant positive association between RS/CSL and fibrocystic change.[44,46,51–52] For example, in their study of breasts from 83 consecutive unselected female autopsies, Nielsen and co-workers found radial scars in 43% of breasts with fibrocystic change but only 17% of those without.[52] On the basis of such evidence, we believe radial scars are one of the manifestations of fibrocystic change.

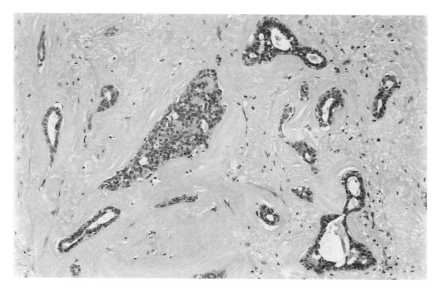

Fig. 7.18A   Complex sclerosing lesion with minimal epithelial hyperplasia. Hematoxylin–eosin × 125.

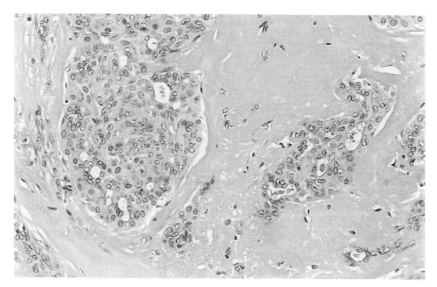

Fig. 7.18B   A moderate degree of epithelial hyperplasia of usual type is seen in this complex sclerosing lesion. Hematoxylin–eosin × 125.

DIFFERENTIAL DIAGNOSIS

The histological differentiation from nodular sclerosing adenosis has already been discussed. The most important differential diagnosis is tubular carcinoma. As mentioned in the foregoing section, the double cell lining of the entrapped, distorted tubular structures will confirm their benign nature, but its identification may require the use of immunostaining for actin. Another helpful feature is the flattened, elongated outline of the entrapped tubules in contrast with the round or oval structures of tubular carcinoma. Furthermore, the desmoplastic stroma of tubular carcinoma is quite different to the dense, poorly cellular stroma of the RS/CSL. (See Table 7.1 for a summary of these features.)

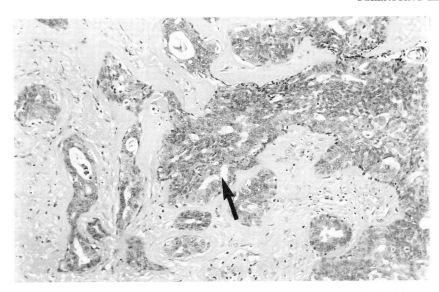

Fig. 7.18C   In this complex sclerosing lesion there is florid epithelial hyperplasia without atypia. Note the peripheral slit-like lumina in the central ductule (arrowhead). Hematoxylin–eosin × 125.

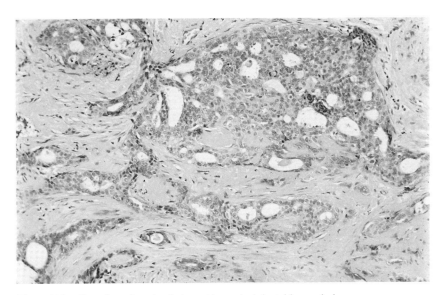

Fig. 7.19A   Complex sclerosing lesion with atypical ductal hyperplasia. Hematoxylin–eosin × 125.

PROGNOSIS AND MANAGEMENT

Because of the difficulty in differentiating them from carcinomas mammographically, all scar lesions should be excised and carefully examined for the presence of epithelial atypia or carcinoma. The possible pre-neoplastic nature of RS/CSL has been the subject of considerable debate. Linell et al described naked tubular structures scattered in fatty tissue in some radial scars and regarded this as evidence for the development of tubular carcinoma from these lesions,[56] a possibility previously raised by Hamperl.[48] Further supportive evidence for the pre-neoplastic nature of RS/CSL was

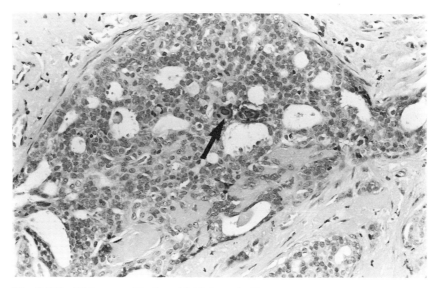

Fig. 7.19B Higher magnification of field shown in Figure 7.19A. There is an imperfect cribriform structure within the epithelial proliferation with some roman bridges, but the changes are insufficiently developed for a diagnosis of low grade ductal carcinoma in situ. Microcalcification is also seen (arrowhead). Hematoxylin–eosin × 185.

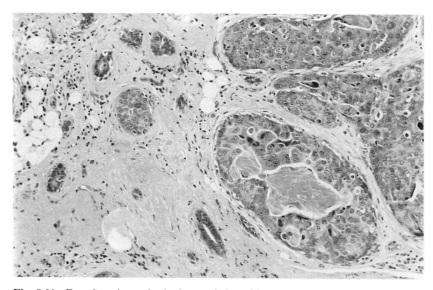

Fig. 7.20 Ductal carcinoma in situ in association with a complex sclerosing lesion. Entrapped ductules and a fibroelastic stroma are seen to the left of the field and high grade ductal carcinoma in situ of comedo type to the right. Hematoxylin–eosin × 125.

provided by Wellings and Alpers who found a significantly higher proportion of radial scars in breasts containing cancer or contralateral to cancer-containing breasts than in breasts obtained from a random autopsy series.[58] However, neither Nielsen et al in their autopsy series[52] nor Anderson and Battersby in their study of surgically resected breast tissue were able to confirm this[59] and the latter authors concluded that tissue sampling and diligence of search has more influence on the frequency of detection of radial scars than any association with cancer. These authors also searched for but were unable to provide evidence to support Linell's concept of the development and progression of radial scars into invasive carcinomas. Finally, two studies in which follow up information is available fail to show an increased incidence of subsequent development of carcinoma following the removal of a radial scar.[45,51]

Nevertheless, there is no doubt that both in situ and invasive carcinomas do occur in association with RS/CSLs.[55-56] However, on the basis of the available evidence, we conclude that RS/CSLs are not, in themselves, premalignant or associated with an increased cancer risk. They may contain foci of atypical hyperplasia, in which case the risk may be increased, although this would not be expected to be any greater than that associated with atypical hyperplasia occurring outwith RS/CSL (see also Ch. 5).

REFERENCES

1. Page DL, Anderson TJ. Adenosis. In: Page DL, Anderson TJ, eds. Diagnostic histopathology of the breast. Edinburgh: Churchill Livingstone, 1987; 51–61.
2. Hughes LE, Mansell RE, Webster DJT. Aberrations of normal development and involution (ANDI): A new perspective on pathogenesis and nomenclature of benign breast disorders. Lancet 1987; ii: 1316–1319.
3. Haagensen CD, Lane N, Lattes R. Neoplastic proliferation of the epithelium of the mammary lobules. Surg Clin N America 1972; 52: 497–524.
4. Linell F, Ljunberg O. Atlas of breast pathology. 1st ed. Copenhagen: Munksgaard, 1984.
5. Nielsen BB. Adenosis tumour of the breast — a clinico-pathological investigation of 27 cases. Histopathol 1987; 11: 1259–1275.
6. Tavassoli FA. Benign lesions. In: Tavassoli FA, ed. Pathology of the breast. Norwalk: Appleton and Lange, 1992; 79–153.
7. Ellis IO, Elston CW. Tumors of the breast. In: Fletcher CDM, ed. Diagnostic histopathology of tumors. Churchill Livingstone, 1995; 635–690.
8. MacErlean DP, Nathan BE. Calcification in sclerosing adenosis simulating malignant breast calcification. Br J Radiol 1972; 45: 944–945.
9. Roebuck EJ. Clinical radiology of the breast. Oxford: Heinemann Medical, 1990.
10. Urban JA, Adair FE. Sclerosing adenosis. Cancer 1949; 2: 625–634.
11. Heller EL, Fleming JC. Fibrosing adenomatosis of the breast. Am J Clin Pathol 1950; 20: 141–146.
12. Dawson EK. Fibrosing adenosis. Edinb Med J 1954; 61: 391–401.
13. Haagensen CD, Bodian C, Haagensen DE. Breast carcinoma — risk and detection. Philadelphia: WB Saunders, 1981.
14. Azzopardi JG. Overdiagnosis of malignancy. In: Problems in breast pathology. Azzopardi JG, ed. Philadelphia: WB Saunders, 1979; 167–191.
15. Taylor HB, Norris HJ. Epithelial invasion of nerves in benign diseases of the breast. Cancer 1967; 20: 2245–2249.
16. Davies JD. Neural invasion in benign mammary dysplasia. J Pathol 1973; 109: 225–231.
17. Eusebi V, Azzopardi JG. Vascular infiltration in benign breast disease. J Pathol 1976; 118: 9–16.
18. Simpson JF, Page DL, Dupont WD. Apocrine adenosis — a mimic of mammary carcinoma. Am J Surg Pathol 1990; 3: 289–299.
19. Carter DJ, Rosen PP. Atypical apocrine metaplasia in sclerosing lesions of the breast: a study of 51 patients. Mod Pathol 1991; 4: 1–5.
20. Fechner RE. Lobular carcinoma in situ in sclerosing adenosis. Am J Surg Pathol 1981; 5: 233–239.
21. Chan JKC, Ng WF. Sclerosing adenosis cancerized by intraductal carcinoma. Pathol 1987; 19: 425–428.
22. Oberman HA, Markey BA. Non-invasive carcinoma of the breast presenting in adenosis. Mod Pathol 1991; 4: 31–35.
23. Rasbridge SA, Millis RR. Carcinoma in situ involving sclerosing adenosis: a mimic of invasive breast carcinoma. Histopathol 1995; 27: 269–273.
24. Symmers W St C. The Breasts. In: Symmers W St C, ed. Systemic pathology 2nd ed, vol 4. Edinburgh: Churchill Livingstone, 1978; 1791–1796.
25. Tanaka Y, Oota K. A stereomicroscopic study of the mastopathic female breast. I. Three dimensional studies of abnormal duct evolution and their histologic entity. Virchows Arch (A) Pathol Anat 1970; 349: 195–214.
26. Jensen RA, Page DL, Dupont WD, Rogers LW. Invasive breast cancer risk in women with sclerosing adenosis. Cancer 1989; 64: 1977–1983.
27. Eusebi V, Collina G, Bussolati G. Carcinoma in situ in sclerosing adenosis of the breast: an immunocyto-chemical study. Semin Diagn Pathol 1989; 6: 146–152.
28. Dupont WD, Page DL. Risk factors for breast cancer in women with proliferative breast disease. N Engl J Med 1985; 312: 146–151.
29. Hutter RVP. Consensus meeting. Is 'fibrocystic disease' of the breast precancerous? Arch Pathol Lab Med 1986; 110: 171.
30. Eusebi V, Casadei GP, Bussolati G, Azzopardi JG. Adenomyoepithelioma of the breast with a distinctive type of apocrine adenosis. Histopathol 1987; 11: 305–311.
31. Eusebi V, Foschini MP, Betts CM et al. Microglandular adenosis, apocrine adenosis, and tubular carcinoma of the breast. An immunohistochemical comparison. Am J Surg Pathol 1993; 17: 99–109.
32. Kaier H, Nielsen B, Paulsen S et al. Adenomyoepithelial adenosis and low grade malignant myoepithelioma of the breast. Virchows Arch A 1984; 405: 55–67.
33. Clement PB, Azzopardi JG. Microglandular adenosis of

the breast: a lesion simulating tubular carcinoma. Histopathol 1983; 7: 169–180.

34. Rosen PP. Microglandular adenosis. A benign lesion simulating invasive mammary carcinoma. Am J Surg Pathol 1983; 7: 137–144.

35. Millis RR, Eusebi V. Microglandular adenosis of the breast. Adv Anat Pathol 1995; 2: 10–18.

36. Tavassoli FA, Norris HJ. Microglandular adenosis of the breast: a clinicopathologic study of 11 cases with ultrastructural observations. Am J Surg Pathol 1983; 158: 731–737.

37. Tavassoli FA, Bratthauer GL. Immunohistochemical profile and differential diagnosis of microglandular adenosis. Mod Pathol 1993; 6: 318–322.

38. Diaz NM, McDivitt RW, Wick MR. Microglandular adenosis of the breast. An immunohistochemical comparison with tubular carcinoma. Arch Pathol Lab Med 1991; 115: 578–582.

39. Rosenblum MK, Purrazella R, Rosen PP. Is microglandular adenosis a precancerous disease? A study of carcinoma arising therein. Am J Surg Pathol 1986; 10: 237–245.

40. James BA, Cranor ML, Rosen PP. Carcinoma of the breast arising in microglandular adenosis. Am J Clin Pathol 1993; 100: 507–513.

41. Kay S. Microglandular adenosis of the female mammary gland: Study of a case with ultrastructural observations. Hum Pathol 1985; 16: 637–640.

42. Weidner N. Benign breast lesions that mimic malignant tumours: Analysis of five distinct lesions. Semin Diagn Pathol 1990; 7: 90–101.

43. Dwarakanath S, Lee AKC, Dellelis RA et al. S-100 protein positivity in breast carcinomas: a potential pitfall in diagnostic immunohistochemistry. Hum Pathol 1987; 18: 1144–1148.

44. Semb C. Fibroadenomatosis cystica mammae. Acta Chir Scand 1928; 10 (suppl): 1–484.

45. Fenoglio C, Lattes R. Sclerosing papillary proliferations in the female breast. A benign lesion often mistaken for carcinoma. Cancer 1974; 33: 691–700.

46. Tremblay G, Buell RH, Seemayer TA. Elastosis in benign sclerosing ductal proliferations of the female breast. Am J Surg Pathol 1977; 1: 1155–1158.

47. Rickert RR, Kalisher L, Hutter RVP. Indurative

mastopathy: A benign sclerosing lesion of the breast with elastosis which may simulate carcinoma. Cancer 1981; 47: 561–571.

48. Hamperl H. Strahlige Narben und obliterierende mastopathie. Beitrage zur pathologischen histologie der mamma. XI. Virchows Arch (A) Pathol Anat 1975; 369: 55–68.

49. Andersen JA, Carter D, Linell F. A symposium on sclerosing duct lesions of the breast. Pathol Ann 1986; 21: 145–179.

50. Page DL, Anderson TJ. Radial scars and complex sclerosing lesions. In: Page DL, Anderson TJ, eds. Diagnostic histopathology of the breast. Edinburgh: Churchill Livingstone, 1987; 112–113.

51. Andersen JA, Gram JB. Radial scar in the female breast: A long-term follow-up study of 32 cases. Cancer 1984; 53: 2557–2560.

52. Nielsen M, Jensen J, Andersen JA. An autopsy study of radial scar in the female breast. Histopathol 1985; 9: 287–295.

53. Wallis MG, Devakumar R, Hosie KB et al. Complex sclerosing lesions of the breast can be palpable. Clin Radiol 1993; 48: 319–320.

54. Barnard NJ, George BD, Tucker AK, Gilmore OJA. Histopathology of benign non-palpable breast lesions identified by mammography. J Clin Pathol 1988; 41: 26–30.

55. Battersby S, Anderson TJ. Myofibroblast activity of radial scars. J Pathol 1985; 147: 33–40.

56. Linell F, Ljungberg O, Anderssen I. Breast carcinoma: Aspects of early stages, progression and related problems. Acta Pathol Scand (suppl) 1980; 272: 1–233.

57. Sloane JP, Mayers MM. Carcinoma and atypical hyperplasia in radial scars and complex sclerosing lesion: importance of lesion size and patient age. Histopathol 1993; 23: 225–231.

58. Wellings SF, Alpers CE. Subgross pathologic features and incidence of radial scars in the breast. Hum Pathol 1984; 15: 475–479.

59. Anderson TJ, Battersby S. Radial scars of benign and malignant breasts: Comparative features and significance. J Pathol 1985; 147: 23–32.

Papillary lesions

INTRODUCTION

No concensus has been reached regarding the terminology of the papillary lesions of the breast. Different authors use similar terms for different lesions and other lesions have a variety of names. Thus whilst some authors refer to 'juvenile papillomatosis' and others to 'papillomatosis' these lesions may also be classified as 'multiple peripheral papillomas'. These differences make accurate interpretation of published series difficult. We do not favor the use of the term 'juvenile papillomatosis' as, although multiple papillomas are most frequently seen women under 30 years of age,[1] this disease also occurs, albeit less commonly, in older women.

In addition, terms are used by some authors such as 'atypical papilloma' for those lesions showing focal epithelial atypia similar to that of atypical ductal hyperplasia (ADH) or loss of a myoepithelial layer in less than one-third of the papillary fronds. These experts would classify a lesions as 'carcinoma arising in a papilloma' if these areas comprise more than one-third of the lesion but less than 90%.[2] The clinical significance of these lesions has not however been determined and, given the good prognosis of encysted (intracystic) carcinoma, may be unnecessary and elaborate. We do not use these terms and if the papillary lesion shows overt features of malignancy, no matter what the proportion, it would be classified as either in situ or invasive papillary carcinoma, as appropriate.

The papillary lesions of the breast form a spectrum of disease and to a large extent the prognosis depends on the number of lesions and the presence of associated epithelial proliferation. We consider invasive papillary carcinoma, however, to be a separate entity which is covered in Chapter 15 and will not be further discussed here.

DUCT PAPILLOMA

Duct papillomas are true benign neoplasms which show monoclonality[3] and which are most commonly solitary peri- or sub-areolar in situation. These lesions have previously been classified as 'central' papillomas. 'Peripheral' lesions which are associated with the terminal-duct-lobular unit are also relatively common and are often multiple.[4,5,6] Some authors refer to these multiple lesions as 'papillomatosis' or 'juvenile papillomatosis' and these lesions do often occur in younger women in the fourth decade of life. We do not, however, recommend the latter term as multiple peripheral papillomas may occur in patients of many ages and the term 'juvenile' implies patients other than the women in their thirties.

CLINICAL FEATURES

Patients with papillomas most commonly present with single duct nipple discharge, which may be blood-stained or, less frequently, with a symptomatic mass. With the advent of breast screening programs, however, these lesions may also be identified as mammographic masses, dilated ducts,[7] microcalcifications or nodularity.[8] Patients are most commonly between 35 to 60 years of age, but papillomas have been described in all age groups including young children[9,10] and may also arise in men.

MACROSCOPIC APPEARANCES

The majority of duct papillomas measure less than 2–3 mm in diameter and are therefore difficult or impossible to see macroscopically; in most cases no gross abnormality is noted by the pathologist. In these samples multiple blocks may be required to identify a microscopic abnormality. Less frequently debris or blood can be seen within a

dilated duct within a specimen of fibro-fatty tissue or larger papillomas up to 1–2 cm in maximum dimension may be identified macroscopically as nodular solid masses within a cystic duct.

MICROSCOPIC APPEARANCES

Microscopically papillomas are composed of epithelium covering a fronded fibrovascular core attached by a stalk to the duct wall (Fig. 8.1). The surface epithelium is cuboidal or may be columnar in morphology (Fig. 8.2). The epithelium may be stratified but should not be more than four cells in depth. Metaplastic apocrine change is often identified in benign papillomas, but is rarely seen in papillary carcinomas and may be a useful feature. Squamous metaplasia may also, less commonly, be identified. A second inner myoepithelial layer is always present (Fig. 8.2). This myoepithelial cell layer may be incomplete, but it may also, more rarely, form a major part of the epithelial proliferation. The presence of this layer can be confirmed immunohistochemically by positive alpha smooth muscle actin reactivity.

Architecturally the multiple fronds of the papilloma may extend into several adjacent duct spaces. Occasionally the base may be sessile. In the case of single, central duct papillomas the adjacent duct structures are essentially unremarkable, although dilated and cystic. More rarely the duct space may contain hemorrhagic debris and macrophages.

Multiple papillomas are usually found in smaller peripheral ducts, but show essentially similar features to single lesions. They may frequently be associated with part of a focal or more diffuse epithelial proliferative process (Fig. 8.3). Multiple papillomas may therefore be accompanied by almost any type of epithelial lesion, including usual type hyperplasia, atypical ductal hyperplasia, lobular neoplasia or ductal carcinoma in situ. Cardenosa and Eklund, for example, found associated atypical ductal hyperplasia in 43% of cases of multiple peripheral papillomas.[8]

Papillomas may undergo central fibrosis with entrapment of tubular structures which may mimic carcinoma and these lesions may be referred to as sclerosing papillary lesions or sclerosed

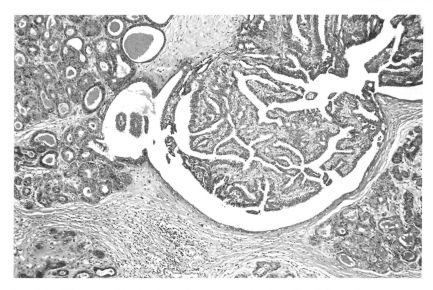

Fig. 8.1   A low magnification view of a papilloma showing a fronded growth pattern supported by fibrovascular cores. Hematoxylin–eosin × 57.

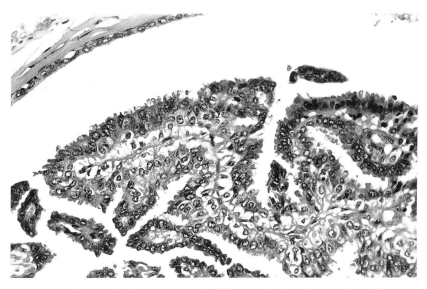

Fig. 8.2   Benign papillomas are composed of fibrovascular fronds covered by a bilayer consisting of myoepithelial cells under a surface epithelial layer. Hematoxylin–eosin × 185.

papillomas or, if fibrosis is a less dominant feature, ductal adenoma (Fig. 8.4) (see below). Whilst these have been separately classified by some authors we believe that they are a form of benign papilloma and do not warrant a separate categorization. A central area with hyalinization is often seen simulating a radial scar. The wall of the duct

may also be fibrotic and the lesion may be mistaken macroscopically for a solid mass rather than an intracystic lesion. The entrapped tubular structures may be misinterpreted as invasive carcinoma, but a myoepithelial layer is still apparent microscopically or with the use of actin immunohistochemical stains.

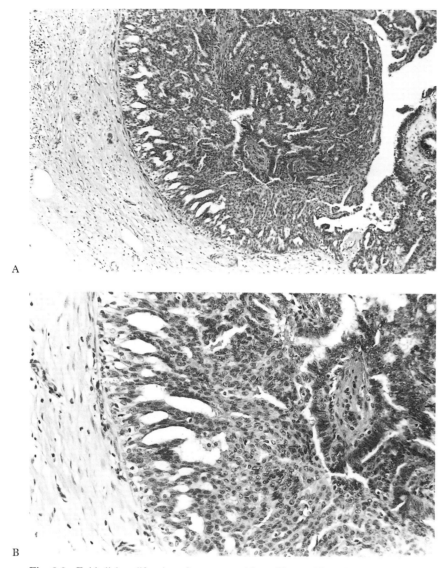

Fig. 8.3 Epithelial proliferation often occurs with papillomas (A) and may be of usual (non-atypical) type or show features of atypical ductal hyperplasia. In this example there is florid usual type epithelial hyperplasia (B). Hematoxylin–eosin, A × 57; B × 185.

DIFFERENTIAL DIAGNOSIS

Good reproducibility in the diagnosis of papillomas has been reported.[11] However distinguishing a large benign papilloma from an encysted papillary carcinoma may on occasions cause diagnostic difficulties.[4] In these cases the use of immunohistochemistry can be invaluable; the former shows an obvious myoepithelial layer with smooth muscle actin whilst in the latter myoepithelial cells are focally absent or very sparse.

As described, large sclerosed papillomas may bear foci of periductal fibrosis or central scarring in which entrapped epithelial structures are seen. These must be interpreted with care in order to avoid overdiagnosis of malignancy, but retain a myoepithelial layer which can again be demonstrated with smooth muscle actin immunostaining.

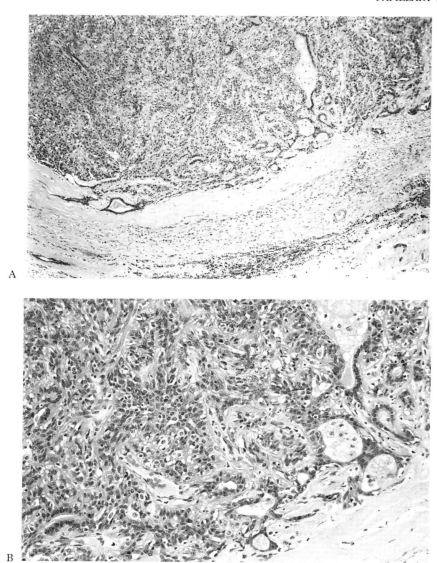

Fig. 8.4 Papillomas may undergo degenerative changes resulting in fibrosis and hyalinization which can entrap epithelial tubular structures mimicking invasion. Loss of the dominant papillary architecture and duct space are features used to classify such lesions as ductal adenomas. Hematoxylin–eosin, A × 57; B × 185.

Multiple peripheral papillomas are associated in some cases with an associated atypical epithelial proliferation amounting to atypical ductal hyperplasia (ADH) or ductal carcinoma in situ (DCIS) and interpretation of the epithelial component of these lesions must be performed with care. A thorough search for any associated atypical hyperplasia or DCIS should thus be made before an unequivocally benign diagnosis is issued.

Occasionally some of the individual fronds (Fig. 8.5) or the entire papilloma may become torted and a hemorrhagic infarcted mass may be the only evidence of the underlying pathology within a cytically dilated duct. Interpretation of the remaining viable tissue may be possible and

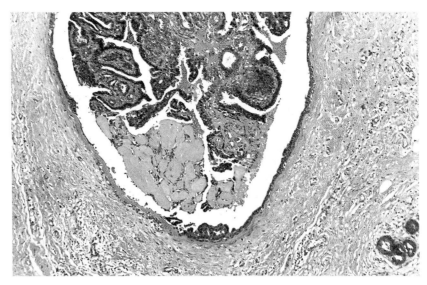

Fig. 8.5 A small duct papilloma showing focal hyaline degeneration most probably as a consequence of infarction of a papillary frond. Hematoxylin–eosin × 57.

can be used to make the diagnosis, but rarely this is impossible. If the whole of the lesion is infarcted care must be taken to avoid over-diagnosis of malignancy and if there is significant doubt we recommend a benign rather than malignant diagnosis is made.

PROGNOSIS

Carter described 64 women who had had locally excised papillomas; 6% were found to have recurred and 6% of women developed carcinoma subsequently, two-thirds of which were invasive.[5] The true relationship between papillomas and subsequent invasive carcinoma is, however, difficult to determine accurately in view of the associated epithelial proliferative lesions often present. It appears likely that the risk carried by women with benign papillary disease varies according to the pattern and number of tumors. There is little or no evidence that those patients with single central papillomas have a significant increased risk of developing breast carcinoma.[12] Multiple papillomas may, however, be associated with concurrent ADH and/or DCIS and thus carry an increased risk of subsequent malignancy.[4,5,6,8]

In a report of 41 patients with multiple papillomas, Rosen et al found that 15% were bilateral and in 58% of cases a family history of breast carcinoma was obtained.[1] Although 10% of women in this series developed subsequent breast carcinoma, this only occurred in those with recurrent and bilateral disease, all of whom had a positive family history of breast cancer. None of those women with unilateral, non-recurrent multiple papillomas developed carcinoma.

A recent study showed loss of heterozygosity (LOH) of 16q in 67% of cases of intracystic papillary carcinoma but in none of 11 papillomas.[13] LOH of 18q was, however, seen in 27% of papillomas and the authors suggested that this chromosome may be implicated in malignant transformation of these lesions.[14] Indeed very rarely papillomas have been described as showing overt malignant transformation and carcinosarcoma arising in a papilloma has been reported.[15]

DUCTAL ADENOMA AND SCLEROSING PAPILLARY LESIONS

The term ductal adenoma was introduced by Azzopardi and Salm to describe a solid benign lesion, usually occurring in association with one of the main breast ducts[16] with a sclerosing adeno-matous or papillary structure. As more cases have been described it has become clear that there is considerable overlap in the morphological appear-ances with sclerosing duct papilloma, sclerosing adenosis and complex sclerosing lesion[17,18] but the central location in the breast is a distinguishing feature in most cases. The majority are thought to evolve by sclerosis of duct papillomas.[18]

CLINICAL FEATURES

Ductal adenoma is uncommon and can occur at any age after puberty, but the majority have been found in women over the age of 45. Most present as a solitary palpable mass close to the nipple, although some lesions may be peripheral.

MACROSCOPIC APPEARANCES

Grossly most ductal adenomas appear as well-defined pale brown or gray nodules measuring up to 3 cm in diameter. In some cases a clear asso-ciation with a duct lumen or a cystic structure can be identified.

MICROSCOPIC APPEARANCES

The microscopical appearances are varied, depending in large measure on the amount of associated fibrosis. Single or multiple adenoma-tous nodules are seen, composed of two-layered epithelium: luminal secretory cells and a basal myoepithelium. This structure can be confirmed by immunostaining for anti-smooth muscle actin.[18,19] In some cases the epithelial proliferation has a papillary configuration. The lesion is sur-rounded by dense fibrosis (Fig. 8.4) which often contains fragmented elastic tissue, presumably derived from the original duct, parts of which may be discernible. A minority of duct adenomas have a central stellate sclerosing appearance. Apocrine change is frequently seen within the epithelial component and this may exhibit a pattern of nuclear atypia.

DIFFERENTIAL DIAGNOSIS

Ductal adenomas are benign lesions and care must be taken not to overdiagnose malignancy. This is particularly the case if entrapped tubules are found (Fig. 8.4) and where there is apparent epithelial atypia. As noted above there is consid-erable overlap in the morphological features with sclerosing adenosis and complex sclerosing lesion and in some cases it may be impossible to make a firm distinction.[17]

NIPPLE ADENOMA

The term nipple adenoma[17,20,21] does not delineate a specific entity, but has been used to describe any mass lesion of the nipple which is benign. Other nomenclature including erosive adenosis, erosive adenomatosis, papillary adenoma [22,23] and florid or sub-areolar duct papillomatosis[24–27] has been used for this lesion which shows a variety of histo-logical appearances. However all these terms refer to an entity composed of an exuberant prolifera-tion of epithelial structures which exhibit both papillary and adenomatous patterns.

Adenomas of the nipple may occur at any age after puberty, with a peak in the perimeno-pausal era. Lesions have rarely been described in men.[28] They present clinically as nipple discharge or as a small firm nodule beneath the nipple. The latter may be reddened and even crusted, mimic-king the appearances of Paget's disease.

MACROSCOPIC APPEARANCES

The pathologist usually receives all or part of the nipple and areola, depending on the size of the lesion, which rarely measures more than 1 to 1.5 cm. The nodule is ill-defined and firm, but has no specific distinguishing features.

MICROSCOPIC APPEARANCES

The microscopical features are variable but consist in essence of a diffuse papillary ductular epithelial proliferation, often intermingled with adenomatous areas (Fig. 8.6). The epithelium is two-layered with a variable degree of secretory epithelial hyperplasia, mainly of usual type (Fig. 8.7). Normal ductular and lobular structures may be included within the lesion. A cellular stroma accompanies the proliferative process, and at the periphery a pseudo-infiltrative pattern of entrapped tubules may be seen. This, together with a tendency towards nuclear hyperchromatism, may lead the unwary into a mistaken diagnosis of malignancy.

DIFFERENTIAL DIAGNOSIS

Adenoma of the nipple must be distinguished from the rare entity of syringomatous adenoma of nipple [29] (see Ch. 11). In this latter lesion there is an infiltrate of tubular structures amongst lacti-

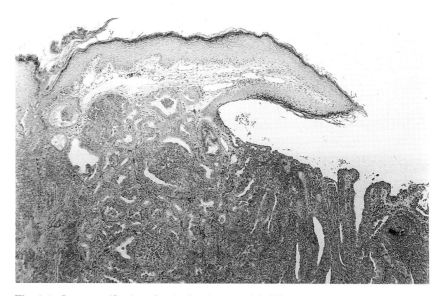

Fig. 8.6 Low magnification of a nipple adenoma with diffuse papillary and adenomatous areas. Hematoxylin–eosin × 23.

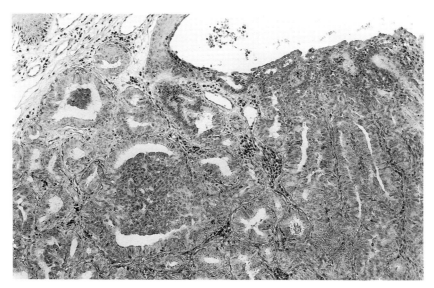

Fig. 8.7 High power magnification of a nipple adenoma (Fig. 8.6) with epithelium showing usual type hyperplasia. Hematoxylin–eosin × 100.

ferous ducts in contrast to the intraductal papillary proliferation of nipple adenoma.

As indicated above, the pseudo-infiltrative pattern in nipple adenoma may raise the possibility of a malignant process. The regularity of the epithelial structures throughout the lesion and absence of the characteristic features of ductal carcinoma in situ favor a benign process, as does the presence of a two-layered epithelium. Atypical intraductal hyperplasia has however been identified in association with nipple adenoma[30] and careful sampling is important. Indeed, although the risk is low, there are some reports of an association with carcinoma.[27,30,31] Jones and Tavassoli reported five examples of concurrent nipple duct adenoma and carcinoma (four invasive and one intraduct).[30] The patients, ranging from 48 to 70 years of age all presented with symptoms typical of nipple adenoma: mass, nipple distortion with discharge or nipple erosion mimicking Paget's disease.

ENCYSTED PAPILLARY CARCINOMA/ INTRACYSTIC PAPILLARY CARCINOMA/ IN SITU PAPILLARY CARCINOMA

Encysted papillary carcinoma and intracystic papillary carcinoma are synonymous terms and refer to lesions with the underlying structure of a papilloma. The majority of these lesions are well defined and have a surrounding collagenous fibrous 'capsule' thus producing the 'encysted' appearance.[32–36] Papillary carcinoma in situ is a comparable disease comprising an in situ malignant epithelial proliferative process occurring in a lesion with the underlying structure of a papilloma[5,37,38] (see also Ch. 14). The capsule in papillary carcinoma in situ is less pronounced than in a typical 'encysted' papillary carcinoma but the lesion is essentially homologous.

CLINICAL FEATURES

These lesions are reported to comprise approximately 1–2% of all breast carcinomas[39] and occur in women of all ages but are more common in the older population. Lesions occurring in the male breast have also been described.[40–43]

These tumors present most frequently as masses or as nipple discharge which may be blood-stained, although with the advent of screening programs they may be detected mammographically as either a well-defined mass[44] or microcalcifications. As with papillomas the lesions may be single and solitary or peripheral and multifocal; the latter may not be palpable and are most commonly identified as a result of breast screening.

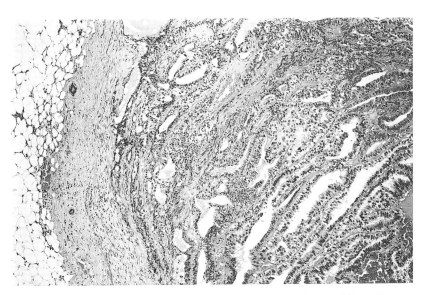

Fig. 8.8 Low power magnification of an encysted papillary carcinoma with a well-defined fibrous 'capsule'. Hematoxylin–eosin × 57.

MACROSCOPIC APPEARANCES

These lesions are usually larger than papillomas on excision and can be seen by naked eye examination of the specimen as well-circumscribed areas of firm tissue. Residual cystic areas may be visible, containing fluid, which is often brown, or blood stained. Size at presentation may vary but is usually between 1–3 cm.

MICROSCOPIC APPEARANCES

Encysted papillary carcinomas are usually well-defined, round in shape and often have a surrounding dense collagenous fibrous capsule (Fig. 8.8). The underlying tumor has a papillary structure with fibrovascular cores evident. These are covered at least focally by a normal bilayer of myoepithelium and surface epithelium. Classically the

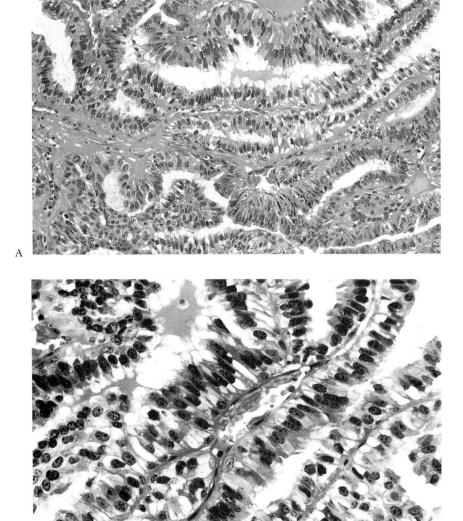

A

B

Fig. 8.9A,B Medium and high power magnification of an encysted papillary carcinoma with columnar epithelial cells arranged perpendicular to the papillary stalk. Note the absence of a myoepithelial cell population covering the fibrovascular fronds. Hematoxylin–eosin, A × 185; B × 400.

neoplastic cells in papillary carcinoma in situ are closely packed and tall and columnar in type and arranged perpendicular to the papillary stalk (Fig. 8.9). The nuclei are oval, basally placed and are either pale or hyperchromatic. In some tumors a loss of polarization of these neoplastic cells is present.

A most important feature is the lack of the normal myoepithelial layer in at least some of the tumor. In many cases, particularly larger tumors, there is associated extensive hyalinization or fibrosis of fibrovascular fronds.

The classic description of papillary carcinomas by Kraus and Neubecker[37] includes the presence of micropapillary and cribriform ductal carcinoma in situ within the definition. In our experience associated carcinoma in situ of a variety of types may be seen. This is frequently of micropapillary

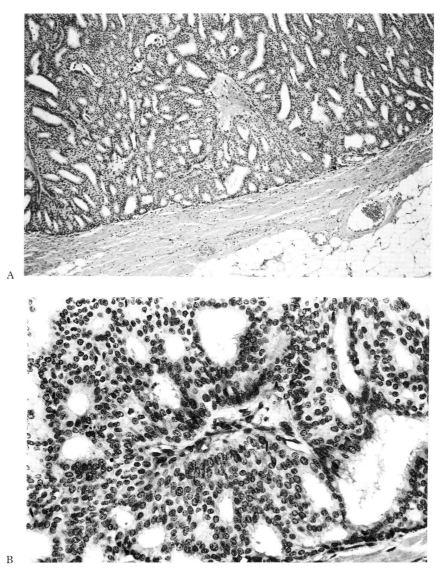

Fig. 8.10A,B Low grade DCIS, here with a cribriform growth pattern, may also form part or the majority of the in situ epithelial malignancy in encysted papillary carcinoma. Hematoxylin–eosin, A × 57; B × 185.

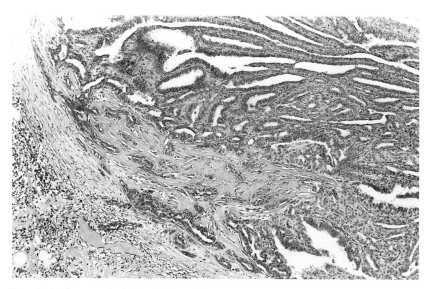

Fig. 8.11 Entrapped tubules within the fibrous capsule of an encysted papillary carcinoma should not be interpreted as coexisting invasive carcinoma. Hematoxylin–eosin × 57.

and cribriform morphology and is present either in isolation or in combination with some of the above features (Fig. 8.10).

Microscopic examination of the adjacent tissue for extension of the in situ process into adjacent ducts is also important as local recurrence after conservation therapy is high when this feature is present. Because of the distinction and differences in clinical presentation and prognosis between the variants of DCIS some prefer to accept the stricter criteria laid down by Carter[45] for the classification of papillary carcinoma in situ.

DIFFERENTIAL DIAGNOSIS

It has been reported that the elevated carcino-embryonic antigen (CEA) content of the cyst fluid around an encysted carcinoma may be of help in diagnosis[46] but we do not routinely perform this assay. Although associated invasive carcinoma may occur, as with benign papillomas, epithelial elements may become entrapped in the adjacent fibrous tissue component or 'capsule' of these lesions which may mimic invasion (Fig. 8.11). We recommend that invasion is not diagnosed in encysted papillary carcinomas which bear epithelial elements within the capsule and unless invasion is seen into the surrounding normal breast tissue we dismiss such foci.

PROGNOSIS

The prognosis of papillary carcinoma in situ following conservation therapy is extremely good if there is no extension of ductal carcinoma in situ beyond the fibrous capsule.[45] In a recent series the 10-year survival rate in series was 100%, and the 10-year disease-free survival rate 91%.[47] Mastectomy had however been performed in 72% of these patients.

REFERENCES

1. Rosen PP, Kimmel M. Juvenile papillomatosis of the breast. A follow-up study of 41 patients having biopsies before 1979. Am J Clin Pathol 1990; 93: 599–603.
2. Tavassoli FA. Papillary lesions. In: Tavassoli FA, ed. Pathology of the Breast. Connecticut: Appleton and Lange, 1992; pp. 193–228.
3. Noguchi S, Motomura K, Inaji H, Imaoka S, Koyama H. Clonal analysis of solitary intraductal papilloma of the

breast by means of polymerase chain reaction. Am J Pathol 1994; 144: 1320–1325.

4. Papotti M, Gugliotta P, Ghiringhello B, Bussolati G. Association of breast carcinoma and multiple intraduct papillomas: A histological and immunohistochemical investigation. Histopathology 1984; 8: 963–975.

5. Carter D. Intraduct papillary tumours of the breast. A study of 78 cases. Cancer 1977; 39: 1689–1692.

6. Ohuchi N, Abe R, Kasai M. Possible cancerous change of intraduct papillomas of the breast. Cancer 1984; 54: 605–611.

7. Woods ER, Helvie MA, Ikeda DM, Mandell SH, Chapel KL, Adler DD. Solitary breast papilloma: Comparison of mammographic, galactographic, and pathologic findings. Am J Roentgenol 1992; 159: 487–491.

8. Cardenosa G, Eklund GW. Benign papillary neoplasms of the breast: Mammographic findings. Radiology 1991; 181: 751–755.

9. Rosen PP. Papillary duct hyperplasia of the breast in children and young adults. Cancer 1985; 56: 1611–1617.

10. Betta PG, Merlini E, Seymandi PL. Juvenile papillomatosis of the breast in a 2½-year-old female infant after exposure to an estrogen ointment. Breast Dis 1993; 6: 207–210.

11. Bodian CA, Perzin KH, Lattes R, Hoffmann P. Reproducibility and validity of pathologic classifications of benign breast disease and implications for clinical applications. Cancer 1993; 71: 3908–3913.

12. Page DL, Dupont WD. Premalignant conditions and markers of elevated risk in the breast and their management. Surg Clin North Am 1990; 70: 831–851.

13. Tsuda H, Uei Y, Fukutomi T, Hirohashi S. Different incidence of loss of heterozygosity on chromosome 16q between intraductal papilloma and intracystic papillary carcinoma of the breast. Jap J Cancer Res 1994; 85: 992–996.

14. Tsuda H, Fukutomi T, Hirohashi S. Pattern of gene alterations in intraductal breast neoplasms associated with histological type and grade. Clin Cancer Res 1995; 1: 261–267.

15. Pitt MA, Wells S, Eyden BP. Carcinosarcoma arising in a duct papilloma. Histopathology 1995; 26: 81–84.

16. Azzopardi JG, Salm R. Ductal adenoma of the breast: A lesion which can mimic carcinoma. J Pathol 1984; 144: 15–23.

17. Page DL, Anderson TW. Diagnostic Histopathology of the Breast. Edinburgh: Churchill Livingstone, 1987.

18. Lammie GA, Millis RR. Ductal adenoma of the breast. A review of fifteen cases. Hum Pathol 1989; 20: 903–908.

19. Gusterson BA, Sloane JP, Middwood C et al. Ductal adenoma of the breast — a lesion exhibiting a myoepithelial/epithelial phenotype. Histopathol 1987; 11: 103–110.

20. Handley RS, Thackray AC. Adenoma of the nipple. Br J Cancer 1962; 16: 187–194.

21. Ahmed A. Diagnostic Breast Pathology. Edinburgh: Churchill Livingstone, 1992.

22. Haagensen CD. Diseases of the Breast. Philadelphia: Saunders, 1986.

23. Perzin KH, Lattes R. Papillary adenoma of the nipple (florid papillomatosis, adenoma, adenomatosis). A clinico-pathologic study. Cancer 1972; 29: 996–1009.

24. Jones DB. Florid papillomatosis of the nipple ducts. Cancer 1955; 8: 315–319.

25. Doctor VM, Sirsat MV. Florid papillomatosis (adenoma) and other benign tumours of the nipple and areola. Br J Cancer 1971; 25: 1–9.

26. Bhagavan BS, Patchefsy A, Koss LG. Florid subareolar duct papillomatosis (nipple adenoma) and mammary carcinoma: Report of three cases. Hum Pathol 1973; 4: 289–295.

27. Rosen PP, Caicco AA. Florid papillomatosis of the nipple. A study of 51 patients, including nine with mammary carcinoma. Am J Surg Pathol 1986; 10: 87–101.

28. Moulin G, Darbon P, Balme B, Frappart L. Adenomatose erosive du mamelon. A Propos de 10 cas avec etude immunohistochimique. Ann Dermatol Venereol 1990; 117: 537–545.

29. Rosen PP. Syringomatous adenoma of the nipple. Am J Surg Pathol 1983; 7: 739–745.

30. Jones MW, Tavassoli FA. Coexistence of nipple duct adenoma and breast carcinoma: A clinicopathologic study of five cases and review of the literature. Modern Pathol 1995; 8: 633–636.

31. Gudjonsdottir A, Hagerstrand I, Ostberg G. Adenoma of the nipple with carcinomatous development. Acta Pathol Microbiol Scand (A) 1971; 79: 676–680.

32. Gatchell FG, Dockerty MB, Clagett OT. Intracystic carcinoma of the breast. Surg Gynaecol Obstet 1958; 106: 347–352.

33. Czernobilsky B. Intracystic carcinoma of the female breast. Surg Gynaecol Obstet 1967; 124: 93–98.

34. McKittrick JE, Doane WA, Failing RM. Intracystic papillary carcinoma of the breast. Am J Surg 1969; 35: 195–202.

35. Hunter CE Jr, Sawyers JL. Intracystic papillary carcinoma of the breast. South Med J 1980; 73: 1484–1486.

36. Squires JE, Betshill WLJ. Intracystic papillary carcinoma of the breast: A correlation of the cytomorphology, gross pathology, microscopic pathology and clinical data. Acta Cytol 1981; 25: 267–271.

37. Kraus FT, Neubecker RD. The differential diagnosis of papillary tumours of the breast. Cancer 1962; 15: 444–455.

38. Murad TM, Swaid S, Pritchett P. Malignant and benign papillary lesions of the breast. Hum Pathol 1977; 8: 379–390.

39. Framarino Dei Malatesta ML, Piccioni MG, Felici A et al. Intracystic carcinoma of the breast. Our experience. Europ J Gynaecol Oncol 1992; 13: 40–44.

40. Motzkus A, Friedrich M. Intrazystisch Wachsendes, Proliferierendes Papillom der Mamma beim Mann. Akt Radiol 1994; 4: 268–270.

41. Leblan I, Pierucci F, Cholley JP et al. Carcinome papillaire intra-kystique du sein chez l'homme. Sein 1995; 5: 294–301.

42. Fallentin E, Rothman L. Intracystic carcinoma of the male breast. J Clin Ultrasound 1994; 22: 118–120.

43. De Rosa G, Giordano G, Boscaino A, Terracciano L, Donofrio V, De Dominicis G. Intracystic papillary carcinoma of the male breast. A case report (Histochemical, immunohistochemical and ultrastructural study). Tumori 1992; 78: 37–42.

44. Soo MS, Williford ME, Walsh R, Bentley RC, Kornguth PJ. Papillary carcinoma of the breast: Imaging findings. Am J Roentgenol 1995; 164: 321–326.

45. Carter D, Orr SL, Merino MJ. Intracystic papillary carcinoma of the breast. After mastectomy, radiotherapy or excisional biopsy alone. Cancer 1983; 52: 14–19.

46. Matsuo S, Eto T, Soejima H et al. A case of intracystic carcinoma of the breast: The importance of measuring carcinoembryonic antigen in aspirated cystic fluid. Breast Cancer Res Treat 1993; 28: 41–44.

47. Lefkowitz M, Lefkowitz W, Wargotz ES. Intraductal (intracystic) papillary carcinoma of the breast and its variants: A clinicopathological study of 77 cases. Human Pathol 1994; 25: 802–809.

Fibroadenoma and related conditions

GENERAL INTRODUCTION

The inclusion together of some of the entities described in this chapter may at first sight seem somewhat arbitrary, but they are all either related pathogenetically or share so closely in the differential diagnosis of fibroadenoma that their common grouping has some merit in clinicopathological terms.

FIBROADENOMA

INTRODUCTION

Although it is tempting to dismiss fibroadenomata as relatively unimportant lesions because they rarely cause serious clinical problems, they cannot be regarded too lightly. They are extremely common, and in an age of increasing breast awareness, since they invariably present as a palpable mass, may cause considerable anxiety in patients until the correct diagnosis of benignity is established. They may pose diagnostic problems in assessment of fine needle aspiration cytology (FNAC) and those lesions which have not presented clinically may be detected in mammographic screening, where carcinoma is an important differential diagnosis.

CLINICAL FEATURES

Fibroadenoma is one of the commonest causes of a breast lump in the female breast[1-2] (see also Ch. 12), but the true incidence is almost impossible to determine because so many lesions go undetected clinically especially in younger women. Deschênes[3] found a prevalence of 8.3 per 1000 in a population of Canadian women aged 40–59 in the first round of mammographic screening. Frantz[4] estimated an overall prevalence of only 10% from a study of just over 200 autopsies but Parks,[5] in a detailed micro-anatomical study of 100 breast biopsies and 50 autopsy cases, found that they are much more common; although he did not supply numerical data he suggested that microscopical fibroadenoma may actually be present in most female breasts. This is, perhaps, unlikely and Bartow[6] could only identify microscopical fibroadenomas in 17% of autopsies in 519 women.

Fibroadenomas may present clinically at any age, but the peak incidence is in the third decade.[7] Hughes and colleagues[2] have defined four clinical subgroups:

1. Small palpable superficial lesions which measure less than 5 mm in diameter, and may remain unchanged for many years.

2. The most common type, making up approximately 80% of clinical cases, which grow to 1–3 cm in diameter before becoming static.

3. Juvenile or giant fibroadenomas, which are rare, and undergo very rapid growth up to 15–20 cm. These are discussed in more detail on page 160.

4. Uncommon lesions (approximately 10%) measuring 4–5 cm in diameter, which may be found at any age but occur mainly in the perimenarchal and perimenopausal age groups.

Clinically most fibroadenomas in younger women present as small, discrete, firm, mobile masses which are painless. In older age groups, particularly in the premenopausal era, the presence of a fibroadenoma may be obscured by a general increase in adipose tissue, or by the presence of fibrocystic change giving rise to a diffuse 'lumpiness'. Following the introduction of breast screening programs such cases are being detected with increasing frequency by mammography. Although there is no evidence that fibroadenomas *develop* after the menopause, pre-existing lesions may become palpable in elderly women as the breast mass diminishes and the breasts become pendulous.

In the majority of cases presenting clinically fibroadenomas are solitary, but 10–20% are multiple.[1,7–8] In some patients the lesions may be bilateral, and more rarely several fibroadenomas develop in succession. It has been suggested that fibroadenomas occur more frequently in black women,[9] but data based on hospital referral clinics should be interpreted with caution. Dent and Cant[8] in South Africa could find no racial differences in their clinical practice, but pointed out that they had been unable to carry out an accurate epidemiological study. Similarly, no racial predisposition was identified in an autopsy study from New Mexico.[6]

Vary rarely fibroadenomas may be familial and bilateral and multiple lesions have been described in a mother and daughter,[1] three siblings[10] and identical twins.[11] Fibroadenomas may also be a component of the Maffuci syndrome,[12] and Carney and Toorkey[13] have recently characterized a familial syndrome comprising endocrine overactivity, spotty pigmentation and myxomas in which a minority of subjects exhibit myxoid fibroadenomas.

MACROSCOPIC APPEARANCES

Fibroadenomas have a characteristic gross appearance (Fig. 9.1). They form sharply circumscribed, spherical or ovoid masses which are clearly distinct from the surrounding breast tissue. They are usually grey-white in color, but some lesions may have a pale yellow or brown appearance. In young women the majority of fibroadenomas are firm and rubbery to the touch, but in older women they may become hard due to sclerosis, and even calcified. The cut surface glistens and usually has a fine lobular structure; occasionally a myxoid appearance is noted. Although it is easy to 'shell out' a fibroadenoma from the adjacent structures they do not possess a true capsule.

MICROSCOPIC APPEARANCES

The major component of fibroadenomas is the stromal connective tissue element which surrounds, and is closely related to, a variable

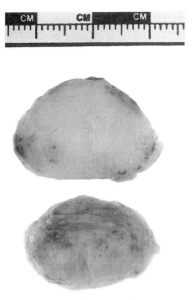

Fig. 9.1 Fibroadenoma. This lesion, from a 32-year-old female, shows the characteristic circumscribed gross appearance. The cut surface (above) is faintly lobulated. The nodule was 'shelled out' from the adjacent breast tissue.

number of epithelial structures (Fig. 9.2). In the majority of cases the stroma is loose and cellular and mitoses may occasionally be seen. The matrix may vary considerably, however, and some fibroadenomas have a distinctly myxoid structure. In

older lesions the stroma becomes progressively hyalinized and less cellular (Fig. 9.3). Focal calcification may occur (Fig. 9.4) and in some cases the whole lesion becomes calcified.

It is traditional to divide fibroadenomas into two types on the basis of the microscopical appearances, intracanalicular and pericanalicular. It must be stressed that both patterns may be present in the same lesion (Fig. 9.5), and indeed, the more thoroughly specimens are examined the greater the proportion in which this is found to be the case. In part the differences in appearance may be related to the plane in which the sections are taken. The terms are purely descriptive and carry no practical or prognostic significance.

The common *intracanalicular* pattern is so named because the connective tissue component forms irregularly rounded, cushion-like masses that invaginate the epithelial structures (the 'canaliculi'), which therefore appear as compressed, often slit-like spaces curving over and between the fibrous nodules (Fig. 9.6A and B). The complex picture that results is characteristic. The epithelium covering the fibrous ingrowth is two layered, but may undergo atrophy and disappear; usually, however, it remains well preserved where it lines the irregularly shaped spaces that occupy the angles between adjacent ingrowths. The connec-

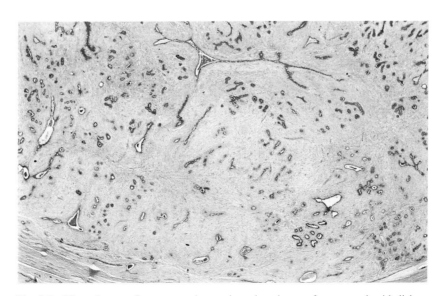

Fig. 9.2 Fibroadenoma. Low power view to show the mixture of stroma and epithelial elements. The edge of the lesion is at the lower margin of the photomicrograph. Hematoxylin–eosin × 23.

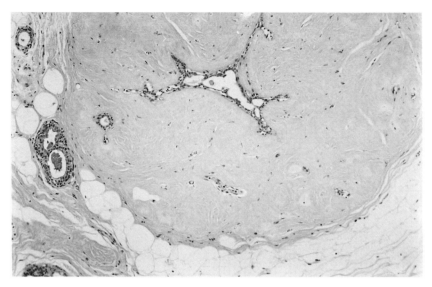

Fig. 9.3 Sclerosed fibroadenoma. Note the relative lack of epithelial structures. Incidental finding in breast tissue from a mastectomy specimen for carcinoma. Patient was a postmenopausal woman aged 54 years. Hematoxylin–eosin × 57.

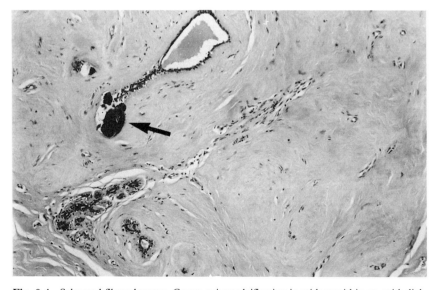

Fig. 9.4 Sclerosed fibroadenoma. Coarse microcalcification is evident within an epithelial cleft (arrowhead). The outline of other clefts is seen but the epithelium has undergone atrophy. This was an impalpable lesion, removed by diagnostic localization biopsy, in a woman aged 55 years. The microcalcification was detected at mammographic screening. Hematoxylin–eosin × 125.

tive tissue is usually loosely knit and moderately cellular, but is more frequently dense and hyaline than in the pericanalicular type.

It is characteristic of the *pericanalicular* pattern that the epithelial element consists of ductular structures, remarkably normal in appearance, but unduly numerous (Fig. 9.7A and B). Both epithelial and myoepithelial cells are present, as in the intracanalicular pattern, and the latter may be easily identified by the use of anti-smooth muscle

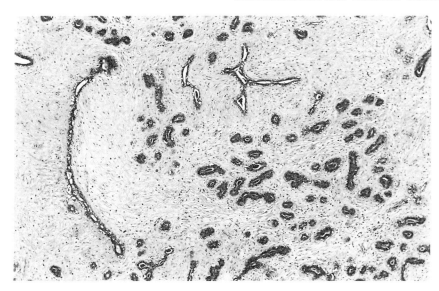

Fig. 9.5 Fibroadenoma. In this example there is a mixture of patterns, the intracanalicular on the left and the pericanalicular on the right. Hematoxylin–eosin × 57.

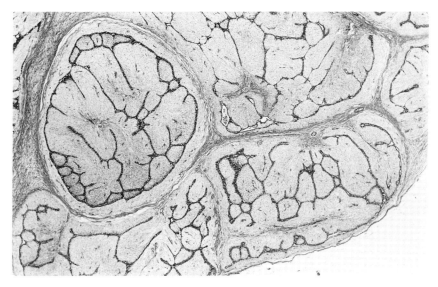

Fig. 9.6A Intracanalicular fibroadenoma. Note the lobulated structure. Hematoxylin–eosin × 23.

actin immunostaining (Fig. 9.7C). The connective tissue stroma is arranged in a concentric fashion around the ductules so that each is clearly separated from its neighbours.

Whilst the appearances described above are typical of the majority of fibroadenomas a range of other changes may also be observed. Epithelial hyperplasia is common (Fig. 9.8A and B) and tangential sectioning of ductular spaces may produce worrying patterns (Fig. 9.9). Mies and Rosen[14] reported a series of fibroadenomas in young women which exhibited 'severe atypical hyperplasia'. If their photomicrographs are representative the epithelial proliferation would probably not

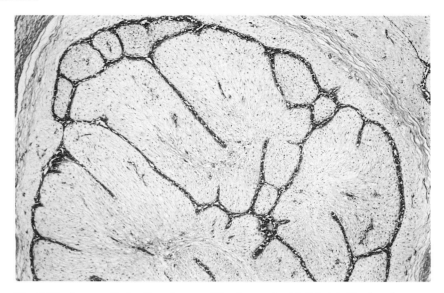

Fig. 9.6B Intracanalicular fibroadenoma. The elongated epithelial cleft-like ductular structures appear compressed by the cellular connective tissue stroma. Same case as Figure 9.6A. Hematoxylin–eosin × 57.

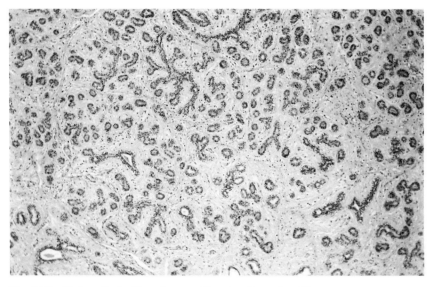

Fig. 9.7A Pericanalicular fibroadenoma. Hematoxylin–eosin × 57.

fulfil modern criteria for atypical ductal hyperplasia[15] and we agree with Fechner[16] that true atypical ductal hyperplasia is not seen in fibroadenomas. The association of lobular neoplasia and ductal carcinoma in situ with fibroadenoma is discussed below and in Chapter 6. Acinar hyperplasia in lobules and secretory change may be seen in fibroadenomas removed in late pregnancy or during lactation. Apocrine metaplasia is found in a significant minority of cases, with a recorded frequency of between 11 and 35%.[17–18] Blunt duct adenosis and fibrocystic change may also be present.[16–17] Sclerosing adenosis has been reported in less than 10% of fibroadenomas;[17–18] when present it is located entirely within the confines of the fibroadenoma. Care must be taken

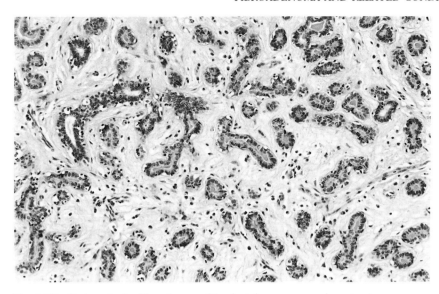

Fig. 9.7B Pericanalicular fibroadenoma. The ductules appear as acinar structures, surrounded by a concentric arrangement of stromal cells rather than invaginated as in the intracanalicular pattern. Compare with Figure 9.6B. Same case as Figure 9.7A. Hematoxylin–eosin × 125.

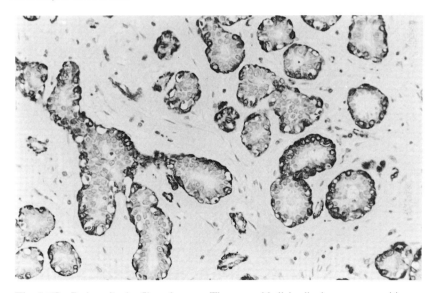

Fig. 9.7C Pericanalicular fibroadenoma. The myoepithelial cells show strong positive immunoreactivity for actin. Same case as Figure 9.7A and B. Immunostaining for anti-smooth muscle actin × 185.

not to mistake the appearances for infiltrating carcinoma. Squamous metaplasia occurs only rarely.[17]

Although many fibroadenomas exhibit a distinct increase in myxoid matrix, in a minority this appearance may dominate, transforming the lesion

to a gelatinous nodule. Tavassoli[18] has suggested anecdotally that this feature, occurring predominantly in women under the age of 40 years, is associated with a higher risk of recurrence; this observation clearly requires confirmation in a prospective study. Myxoid change is seen in an

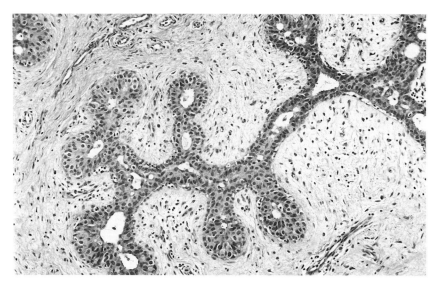

Fig. 9.8A Fibroadenoma in which there is a slight degree of epithelial hyperplasia. Hematoxylin–eosin × 125.

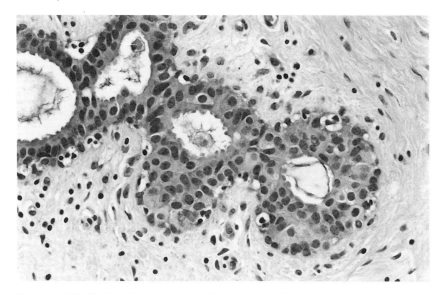

Figure. 9.8B Epithelial hyperplasia in a fibroadenoma. The epithelial cells are regular in appearance, with no atypical features. Same case as Figure 9.8A. Hematoxylin–eosin × 400.

extreme form in the rare syndrome described by Carney and Toorkey[13] in which myxomas may also be present in other organs. In older women, especially after the menopause, the stroma become relatively acellular and often hyalinized with atrophy of the epithelial elements. Fibroadenomas detected during mammographic screening usually come into this category. Although most fibro-adenomas diagnosed mammographically can be left in situ, they are sometimes removed because of suspicious microcalcification, which nearly always proves to be of dystrophic type, within the stroma or the epithelial clefts (Fig. 9.4). Some fibroadenomas become completely calcified in the elderly. Adipose tissue is occasionally present within the stroma[16,18] and osseous metaplasia has been reported as a rare occurrence.[19] Smooth muscle metaplasia is said to be extremely

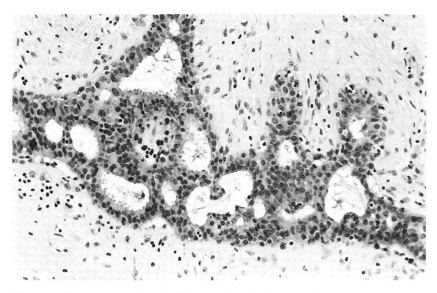

Fig. 9.9 Fibroadenoma with epithelial hyperplasia. In this example there are irregular spaces within the proliferative epithelium. They do not have the 'punched out' structure of a true cribriform pattern and these changes should not be diagnosed as atypical ductal hyperplasia. Hematoxylin–eosin × 125.

rare,[16,18,20] but this observation is based on routine light microscopic appearances, and the true incidence would be better assessed using immunostaining with anti-smooth muscle actin.

PATHOGENESIS

As the name implies, fibroadenomas have by long tradition been regarded as benign tumors of the breast. In the 19th century Sir Astley Cooper used the term 'chronic mammary tumor'[21] and in the current World Health Organization classification they are described as 'discrete benign tumors showing evidence of connective tissue and epithelial proliferation'.[22] Most standard textbooks of breast disease, both clinical and pathological, also place fibroadenomas firmly in the section on benign tumours.[1,16–18,23–24] Since they form discrete masses and malignancy is extremely rare, use of the broad term 'benign tumor' can be justified on pragmatic grounds, but most available evidence suggests that fibroadenomas are actually hyperplastic rather than neoplastic lesions.[2,8,25] They are composed of three different cell types, secretory epithelial, myoepithelial and stromal connective tissue cells, which is difficult to recon-

cile with the clonal theory of neoplasia. Furthermore, tiny microscopic foci having identical morphological appearances to fibroadenomas are seen frequently as an integral component of fibrocystic change (Fig. 9.10); these have been termed fibroadenomatoid hyperplasia[26] or fibroadenomatosis.[27] An elegant three dimensional model, constructed from drawings of serial histological sections of a tiny fibroadenoma, suggested that the lesion originated as an overgrowth of stromal connective tissue, compressing and invaginating a duct and leading to cyst formation and epithelial atrophy.[28] In a careful micro-anatomical study of over 150 breast specimens Parks[5] showed that fibroadenomas are extremely common, and suggested that they are almost certainly present in all breasts, which would be distinctly unusual for a neoplastic process. Both Parks[5] and Orcel and Douvin[29] have traced a morphological continuum from normal lobules, through hyperplastic lobules to fibroadenoma, and postulated that the latter are an exaggerated form of lobular hyperplasia. This is supported by morphometric studies[30] which have shown that both ductal epithelium and stroma participate in the proliferative process. Finally it has now been shown by Noguchi and colleagues,[31] in a study of 10 cases, that fibro-

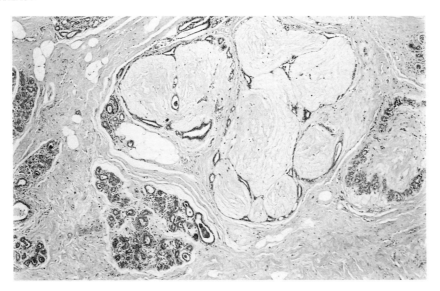

Fig. 9.10 Tiny fibroadenoma. Incidental finding in a breast biopsy in a woman aged 45 years. The lesion measures just over 1 mm in diameter; fibrocystic change was present in adjacent breast tissue. Hematoxylin–eosin × 57.

adenomas are composed of polyclonal epithelial and stromal cells, using restriction fragment length polymorphism (RFLP) of the X-chromosome-linked phosphoglycerokinase gene, a finding in keeping with a hyperplastic rather than a neoplastic process.

Fibroadenomas do not exhibit the continuous growth pattern of neoplastic lesions and rarely achieve more than 1–2 cm in size. The size stays constant until the menopause, following which they undergo atrophy with stromal hyalinization and occasionally calcification. These features point to a degree of hormone dependence similar to that of normal breast tissue, and indeed fibroadenomas may enlarge during pregnancy, undergo lactational change and revert to their previous size after the puerperium.

The precise etiology of fibroadenomas is unknown. The clinical data referred to above is strongly suggestive that hormonal influences play a central role in their development. Martin and colleagues[32] have proposed that they arise in patients with an imbalance between circulating estradiol and progesterone levels, resulting in unopposed estrogenic activity.[32–33] This view is based on observations of serum hormone levels and assessment of estrogen receptor protein in excised fibroadenomas. Insufficient numbers of cases have been studied to accept this theory unreservedly, and in any event it is difficult to reconcile with the data noted above concerning the recognized relative frequency of fibroadenomas. Further studies are clearly required.

DIFFERENTIAL DIAGNOSIS

Fibroadenomas must be distinguished from a number of lesions, but the most important, because of the therapeutic implications, is phyllodes tumor. Although the latter are seen more usually in an older age group, there is considerable overlap between the two entities at both ends of the age range. Size alone is of no value as a distinguishing feature; although most fibroadenomas are small and measure less than 2 cm in diameter, and many phyllodes tumors are larger than this, there is marked variation in the size range of both lesions. Nevertheless most problems are encountered with relatively large fibroadenomas in younger women, when the presence of leaf-like foci and hypercellular stroma raise the possibility of benign phyllodes tumor (Fig. 9.11A and B). Relative uniformity of stromal nuclei and

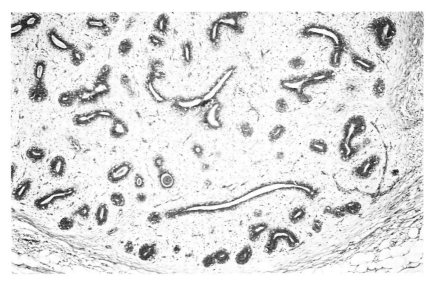

Fig. 9.11A   Fibroadenoma. In this field there is a predominantly intracanalicular pattern. The lesion measured 2.5 cm in diameter. Hematoxylin–eosin × 57.

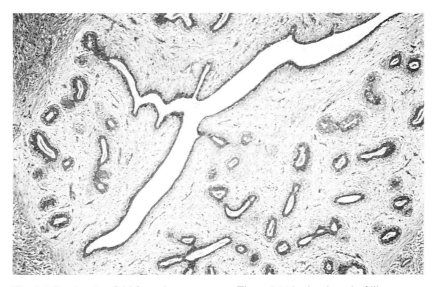

Fig. 9.11B   Another field from the same case as Figure 9.11A, showing a leaf-like pattern reminiscent of phyllodes tumor. Because stromal cellularity was only marginally increased and mitoses were infrequent a final diagnosis of fibroadenoma was issued. Hematoxylin–eosin × 57.

lack of mitoses would favor a diagnosis of fibro-adenoma. It may be impossible to make a clear distinction in some cases, and although we disagree with use of the term 'fibroadenoma phyllodes', as advocated by Tavassoli,[18] a cautious report may be necessary, especially if there is incomplete excision. We have encountered a small number of such borderline cases in consultation in which an initial diagnosis of fibroadenoma has been followed by recurrences with more typical features of phyllodes tumor, including one patient who eventually required mastectomy. In this context it is important to remember that a proportion of phyllodes tumors probably arises from a pre-existing fibroadenoma. This is discussed further on page 179 and a pertinent case is illustrated in Fig. 9.39A and B.

Distinction from tubular adenoma (see p. 161) should be relatively straightforward, since the latter is composed of tightly packed tubular structures, and lacks the relatively abundant stromal component of a fibroadenoma. In some fibroadenomas there are foci with a pronounced tubular structure; unless this is the dominant component the lesion should still be referred to as a fibroadenoma.

Fibromatosis is a rare lesion in the breast;[34–35] in some instances the fibroblastic proliferation may engulf residual ductular structures, producing a resemblance to fibroadenoma. The ill-defined, infiltrative edge, cellularity of stroma and relatively scant epithelial component are all features which would favour a diagnosis of fibromatosis, rather than fibroadenoma.

PROGNOSIS AND MANAGEMENT

The modern clinical management of patients with fibroadenoma is discussed in Chapter 12, but a number of points are pertinent here.

Until comparatively recently most lesions which were considered to be a fibroadenoma clinically were excised surgically. In the great majority of cases excision is curative, but in up to 10% of patients further lesions may develop.[2] Some of these 'recurrences' arise at the site of the original lesion and may be due to incomplete excision, but others are found in adjacent breast tissue in the ipsilateral breast or even in the contralateral breast, reflecting the fact that fibroadenomas are not infrequently multiple. Genuinely recurrent lesions should be excised because of the risk, albeit extremely low, of associated carcinoma (see below). There is an increasing trend amongst surgeons to adopt a more conservative approach to the management of patients with benign breast lumps, especially in younger women.[36–38] Our own policy is discussed in more detail in Chapter 12, but briefly we have found that it is perfectly safe to avoid surgery for presumed fibroadenoma,[39–40] using the triple approach of clinical examination, breast imaging and fine needle aspiration cytology,[41–42] especially for women under 30 years of age. Lesions are, of course, removed at the patient's request, but this only occurs in a minority of cases. A similar policy can be applied to impalpable lesions detected during mammographic screening.

It has been estimated that infarction occurs in approximately one in 200 clinically apparent fibroadenomas.[43–44] The majority of patients are either pregnant or lactating. The associated inflammatory reaction may produce a firm, fixed mass mimicking carcinoma clinically, and Pambakian and Tighe[45] have emphasized the dangers of misdiagnosis histologically on frozen section.

CARCINOMA ASSOCIATED WITH FIBROADENOMA

Carcinoma arising in association with fibroadenoma is a very rare event, but it is almost impossible to obtain an accurate estimate of the true frequency for the following reasons. No prospective, large scale, community-based, long-term follow-up studies have been performed; the true frequency of fibroadenoma itself is unknown because so many lesions are impalpable and detected only sporadically by mammography; many of the cases reported have been examples of lobular neoplasia (Fig. 9.12A and B), now regarded more as a risk lesion than established carcinoma. In a total of 8500 women aged 40–59 attending mammographic screening for the first time Deschênes[3] found carcinoma in two fibroadenomas (one ductal carcinoma in situ and one invasive ductal), an overall frequency of 0.02% (see also Ch. 5). Buzanowski-Konakry[46] identified five cases out of 4000 fibroadenomas reviewed retrospectively from a 43-year period, but all were of lobular type. A review of the literature in 1985 revealed 20 reported cases of carcinoma associated with fibroadenoma[47] and since then a further 105 cases, from personal consultation files, have been presented.[48] From these data it appears that over 50% of cases reported as carcinoma are, in fact, examples of lobular neoplasia, about a quarter are ductal carcinoma in situ, 5% are lobular neoplasia and ductal carcinoma in situ

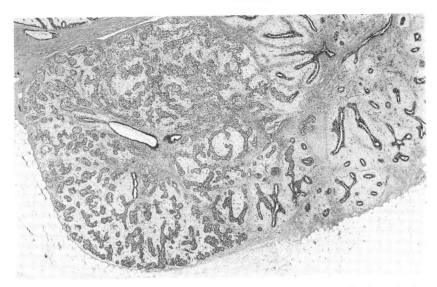

Fig. 9.12A   Fibroadenoma with associated atypical lobular hyperplasia. The hyperplastic epithelium is on the left and a typical intracanalicular pattern is seen on the right. Hematoxylin–eosin × 23.

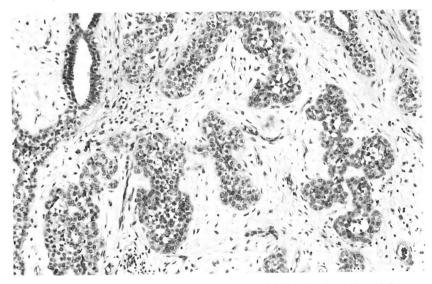

Fig. 9.12B   Higher magnification of field in Figure 9.12A showing the characteristic features of atypical lobular hyperplasia. Hematoxylin–eosin × 125.

combined and the rest invasive carcinoma of various types, but dominantly ductal NST and infiltrating lobular carcinomas. In up to a quarter of cases the in situ carcinoma is also present in adjacent breast tissue.

The prognosis for carcinoma arising in association with a fibroadenoma appears to be the same as for tumors of a similar morphological type

arising elsewhere in the breast.[47–48] Thus lobular neoplasia implies an increased risk for subsequent invasive carcinoma in either breast, whilst adequate local excision is usually curative for ductal carcinoma in situ (Fig. 9.13). For cases with invasive carcinoma the prognosis is related to prognostic factors such as tumor size, histological type and grade (see Ch. 18). Patient management

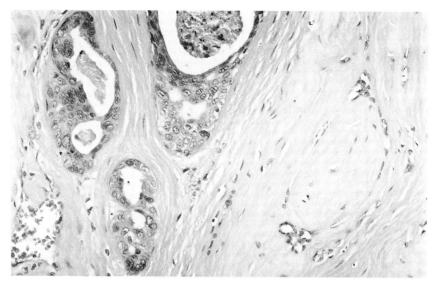

Fig. 9.13 Fibroadenoma with associated ductal carcinoma in situ. Much of the fibroadenoma appeared sclerosed (right hand side of field) whilst the epithelial spaces in approximately one third of the lesion were replaced by high grade ductal carcinoma in situ, comedo type (left hand side of field). From a woman aged 45 years who is alive and recurrence free 15 years after wide local excision. Hematoxylin–eosin × 185.

should reflect these clinical associations; breast conservation with long-term follow-up is suitable for both lobular neoplasia and ductal carcinoma in situ whilst more radical therapy *may* be appropriate for invasive carcinomas, depending on the prognostic index.

JUVENILE FIBROADENOMA

Considerable confusion has been produced by inconsistent use of the terms 'juvenile' and 'giant' fibroadenoma. The former has even been applied to lesions seen in middle aged and elderly women,[14] whilst the latter has been used, quite inappropriately, as a synonym for phyllodes tumor. In practice, virtually all juvenile fibroadenomas are large[49] and the term is best reserved for those lesions which occur in adolescence and have a very rapid growth rate. It has been estimated that between 5 and 10% of fibroadenomas in adolescents come into this category.[16,18,49] A preponderance of juvenile fibroadenoma has been noted in black females,[50–51] but this may be due to case selection bias.

Typically juvenile fibroadenoma forms a well-circumscribed, lobulated mass which may reach 15–20 cm in diameter, stretching the skin and distorting the nipple.[14,52] Growth is occasionally so rapid that the breast may double in size within a month,[53] which may lead to an erroneous clinical diagnosis of malignancy. They are usually solitary, but may be multiple and bilateral.[52]

The macroscopic and microscopic appearances of juvenile fibroadenoma differ little from those of ordinary fibroadenoma. The basic pericanalicular and intracanalicular growth patterns are seen, but the stroma is likely to be cellular rather than hyalinized. Epithelial proliferation is often florid,[52] and Mies and Rosen[14] used the presence of so-called atypical hyperplasia as a defining feature. However, judging by their illustrative photomicrography the epithelial proliferation in most of their cases would not nowadays be regarded as atypical hyperplasia as defined by Page and Rogers,[15] and even Mies and Rosen[14] conceded that the changes should be interpreted conservatively.

Complete local excision is advisable and even with very large lesions an excellent cosmetic result is usually obtained. Recurrence is uncommon after excision of solitary masses, but may occur in patients with multiple lesions.[52] Follow-up is not indicated except in the rare cases when the associated epithelial proliferation genuinely fulfils the criteria for atypical hyperplasia. There are two important entities in the differential diagnosis; unilateral juvenile hypertrophy and phyllodes tumor. In the former there is diffuse enlargement of the whole breast without a discrete mass. Phyllodes tumor is distinguished by the leaf-like pattern of the epithelial clefts and the cellularity of the stroma.

TUBULAR ADENOMA

INTRODUCTION

In the past the term 'adenoma' of breast was used rather indiscriminately, and most cases designated as such were, in fact, fibroadenomas with a prominent tubular component.[54] Indeed, Persaud[54] considered pure adenomas of the breast to be extremely rare. The entity of tubular adenoma was first defined with strict morphological criteria by Hertel, Zaloudek and Kempson in 1976.[55] They emphasized the well-circumscribed nature of the lesion, composed of closely packed tubular structures with little intervening stroma. They noted a strong association with previous or concurrent pregnancy and concluded that tubular adenoma and so-called lactational adenoma were related entities. This association with pregnancy was also observed by Tavassoli.[18] The true frequency in the community is unknown, because most reports have derived from referral centers. Hertel and colleagues[55] reported 28 cases from a 10-year period, during which they also saw 965 fibroadenomas. In a 15-year period at the Armed Forces Institute of Pathology a total of 142 tubular adenomas were diagnosed.[18] The age range is closely similar to that of fibroadenoma, and the great majority occur before the age of 40 years. Patients present with a firm, mobile, well-defined nodule in the breast which in a minority of cases is tender. About 40% have noted the lesion during pregnancy.

MACROSCOPIC APPEARANCES

In keeping with the clinical findings tubular adenomas form well-circumscribed, firm lesions, which measure between 1 and 4 cm in diameter, although the great majority are less than 2 cm. They are usually yellow or tan colored, with a finely nodular cut surface.[18,56]

MICROSCOPIC APPEARANCES

The lesions are sharply demarcated from the adjacent breast tissue, but lack a true fibrovascular capsule.[55] They are composed of closely packed tubular structures which are approximately the same size as the acini of the normal lobule. The tubules are lined by a single layer of secretory epithelial cells together with an outer layer of myoepithelial cells (Fig. 9.14A and B). The latter may be relatively flattened and indistinct in some cases, but is always present and can be readily identified using immunostaining with anti-smooth muscle actin. There is no nuclear atypia, but occasional mitoses may be observed. Tubular lumina may contain eosinophilic secretory material, and in a minority of lesions, particularly those associated with pregnancy, the epithelial cells show secretory vacuolation. The intervening stroma is sparse, consisting of a delicate fibrovascular network. Focal fibrosis is occasionally present, as is a chronic inflammatory infiltrate.

PROGNOSIS AND MANAGEMENT

Clinically, tubular adenomas are indistinguishable from fibroadenomas and they are therefore only diagnosed after excision biopsy has been performed. They are entirely benign and complete local excision is adequate therapy. Fechner et al[16] refer to two case reports in the literature of associated malignancy, but neither seems to be particularly convincing.

LACTATIONAL NODULES

It is not uncommon for women to discover a discrete breast lump during pregnancy or the puerperium and the nature of these lesions has been the subject of much debate. The term 'preg-

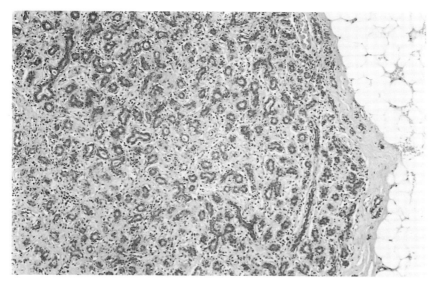

Fig. 9.14A Tubular adenoma. Note the nodular nature of the lesion and the dominant tubular structure. Hematoxylin–eosin × 100.

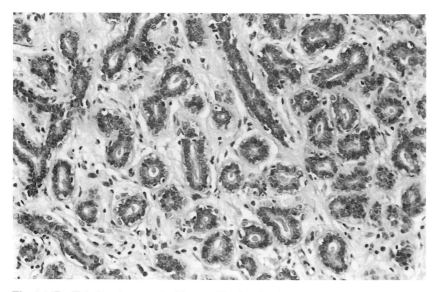

Fig. 9.14B Tubular adenoma. At this magnification the closely packed tubular structure is well seen; in this example the myoepithelial layer is prominent. Same case as Figure 9.16B. Hematoxylin–eosin × 125.

nancy or lactational adenoma' has been used to describe such lesions,[17–18,25,57–58] implying a distinct neoplastic entity associated with pregnancy. Others have suggested that they are simply fibroadenomas or tubular adenomas which have become modified by lactational changes.[54–55] Anecdotally, in our own experience, a substantial proportion of masses which *become palpable* during

pregnancy disappear after lactation ceases. They can probably be regarded as nodules of physiological lobular proliferation which are more prominent than the adjacent breast tissue and may then appear clinically to be a distinct mass. This view has recently been confirmed in a retrospective study carried out by Slavin and colleagues.[59] In a review of the morphological appearances of

30 lactational nodules they found seven fibro-adenomas, five tubular adenomas and six hamartomas, all of which showed superimposed secretory changes. However, the single biggest group were the 12 cases in which the features were those of localized lobular hyperplasia with no evidence of a specific pathological process. We agree with their view that these lesions should be recognized as a heterogeneous group, designated as lactational nodules, noting any underlying pathological process, but avoiding use of the term lactational adenoma.

MAMMARY HAMARTOMA

INTRODUCTION

Hamartomas are uncommon lesions which are composed of a discrete nodular collection of lobular structures, stroma and adipose tissue.[60–64] Prym[65] is usually credited with the first description of the entity, which he called mastoma, but it was Arrigoni and colleagues[60] who applied the term hamartoma. Although Linell[62] raised some reservations about the use of this terminology, it has now gained general acceptance and is included in the WHO classification of breast disease.[22] It is also probable that the entity originally designated as adenolipoma by Spalding,[66] and mostly reported in radiological journals[67–70] is closely related, if not the same lesion.[61,64] Similarly another variant composed of circumscribed nodules of lobular structures and stroma in which there is a prominent smooth muscle element has been designated muscular hamartoma.[71–73]

CLINICAL FEATURES

Hamartomas may occur at any age from the early teens to old age, but are found predominantly in the immediate premenopausal or perimenopausal age group.[60–62,64] They usually present with a single large palpable mass but, surprisingly, they may be impalpable and detected only on mammography. Clinically they may be confused with fibroadenoma or phyllodes tumor, and in pubertal patients the changes may mimic unilateral virginal hypertrophy. On mammography they appear as large, well-circumscribed mass lesions with a characteristic central lucency.

MACROSCOPIC APPEARANCES

Harmartomas vary considerably in size, measuring from as little as 1 cm up to 25 cm. They form well-circumscribed round to oval masses, which in some cases have a disc-like or lentiform shape. There is a firm, fleshy consistency and the lobulated appearance, characteristic of a fibroadenoma, is not seen (Fig. 9.15). They vary in color from gray to yellow, depending largely on the proportion of adipose tissue. Tiny cystic structures may be present.

MICROSCOPIC APPEARANCES

Histologically hamartomas lack a true capsule, although they are generally well-defined and separate easily from adjacent breast tissue. They are composed of a variable combination of connective tissue stroma and lobular structures (Figs 9.16, 9.17). The lobules may vary considerably in size and occasionally appear to merge, but within each lobule the structure is normal (Fig. 9.18) and acini are composed of the typical bilaminar epithelial and myoepithelial cell types. Ductular structures resembling subsegmental ducts are frequently seen; these may become ectatic and appear as cysts on cross-section (Fig. 9.19). Epi-

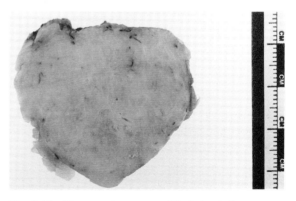

Fig. 9.15 Mammary hamartoma. The lesion is from a 42-year-old woman. Note the well-circumscribed margin and the homogeneous appearance of the cut surface.

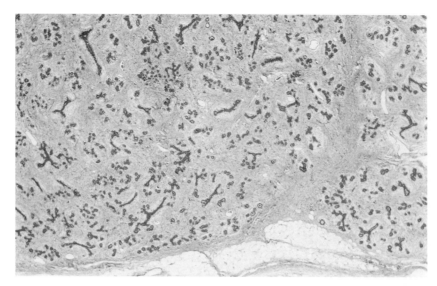

Fig. 9.16 Mammary hamartoma. Note the well-defined margin and the rather haphazard arrangement of ductular and lobular structures. Hematoxylin–eosin × 57.

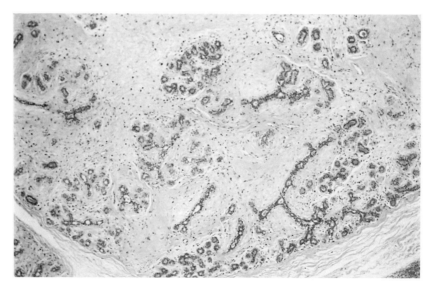

Fig. 9.17 Another example of mammary hamartoma demonstrating the relationship between epithelial and stromal elements. Hematoxylin–eosin × 57.

thelial hyperplasia is almost never a feature, although lobular neoplasia has been described in a single case designated as an adenolipoma,[68] and lobular neoplasia with infiltrating lobular carcinoma in one case of mammary hamartoma.[74] The stromal component varies in proportion, but is usually hyalinized and spreads into the lobules, often obliterating the specialized intralobular component (Fig. 9.20).[64] The amount of adipose tissue is also variable (Fig. 9.21); it may be entirely absent or occupy the great majority of the lesion as is the case in lesions described as adenolipomas. Smooth muscle is identified in a minority of hamartomas, using immunostaining with anti-smooth muscle antibody; rarely this is the dominant component (Fig. 9.22A, B and C).[71–73] Fisher

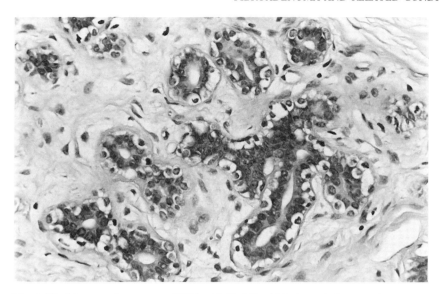

Fig. 9.18 Mammary hamartoma. Within this ill-defined lobular unit the normal structure of epithelial and myoepithelial cells is maintained. Hematoxylin–eosin × 185.

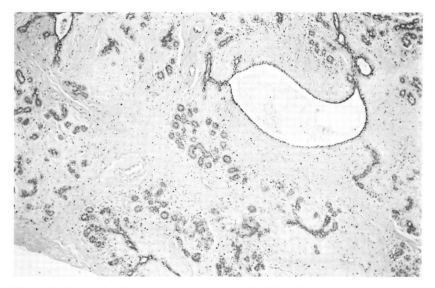

Fig. 9.19 Ectatic duct in a mammary hamartoma. Such 'cystic' structures are relatively common. Hematoxylin–eosin × 57.

et al[64] found changes of pseudo-angiomatous hyperplasia in nearly three quarters of their cases, but this phenomenon has not been recorded by others.

DIFFERENTIAL DIAGNOSIS

For relatively small lesions hamartomas must be distinguished from fibroadenoma. Both form firm, well-defined nodules clinically and benign cells should be obtained on fine needle aspiration cytology. Microscopically both are well-circumscribed, but the dominantly lobular structure and less cellular stroma favour the diagnosis of fibroadenoma. When larger lesions are encountered the differential diagnosis is wider and includes juvenile fibro-

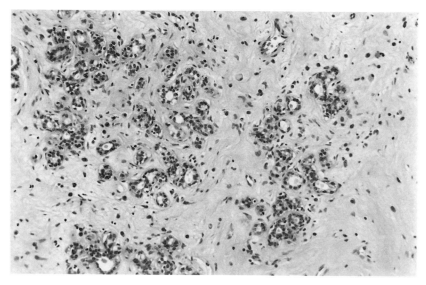

Fig. 9.20   The stromal fibrosis in this mammary hamartoma merges with the specialized intralobular stroma. Hematoxylin–eosin × 125.

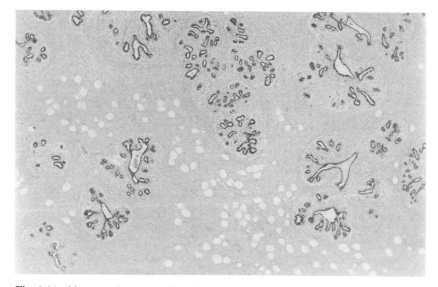

Fig. 9.21   Mammary hamartoma in which the stroma contains a small amount of adipose tissue, insufficient for the designation of adenolipoma. Hematoxylin–eosin × 57.

adenoma, unilateral virginal hypertrophy, and phyllodes tumor. Juvenile fibroadenomas differ little in structure from ordinary fibroadenoma.

Hamartomas may be massive and resemble virginal hypertrophy superficially, but the latter lacks the characteristic circumscription. Phyllodes tumor can be excluded by the presence of the

diagnostic leaf-like epithelial clefts, both macroscopically and, more obviously, microscopically.

PROGNOSIS AND MANAGEMENT

Hamartomas are entirely benign, with the

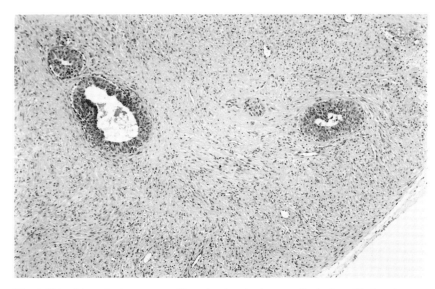

Fig. 9.22A Muscular hamartoma. Note the sharply circumscribed edge with ductular structures and associated cellular stroma. Hematoxylin–eosin × 100 (from a case kindly donated by Dr J Newman).

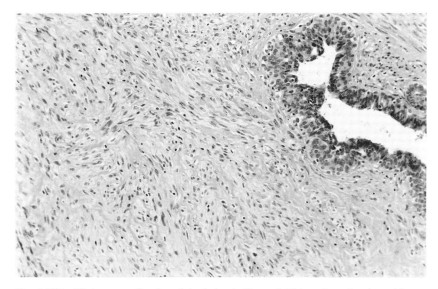

Fig. 9.22B Higher magnification of the lesion in Figure 9.22A to show the plump blunt-ended stromal nuclei. Hematoxylin–eosin × 125.

extremely rare exception of associated lobular carcinoma noted previously.[74] Smaller lesions will usually be managed in the same way as fibroadenomas, and local excision carried out if this is considered to be appropriate. Large lesions may cause considerable distortion of the breast, but these too can be managed by local excision with good cosmetic results. Rarely hamartoma is mistaken clinically for a sarcoma, especially if there are associated skin changes (stretching and even ulceration). In such cases fine needle aspiration cytology or wide bore needle biopsy can help to establish a benign diagnosis. In this way it should be possible to avoid mastectomy in the great majority of cases.

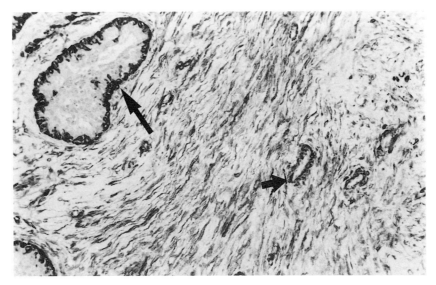

Fig. 9.22C   Strong positive actin immunoreactivity is seen in the stromal cells. Positive staining in myoepithelial cells (arrowhead) and arterioles (small arrowhead) serves as an internal control. Same case as Figure 9.22A and B. Immunostaining for anti-smooth muscle actin × 125.

PHYLLODES TUMOR

INTRODUCTION

These unusual, biphasic tumors of the breast have perplexed pathologists and clinicians alike since they were first recognized early in the 19th century. Ample witness to this is provided by the fact that over 60 different names have been applied to the lesion[75] since Müller first coined the term 'cystosarcoma phyllodes').[76] At this time sarcoma was a generic term for any fleshy mass and had not acquired the connotation of malignancy that it expresses now; phyllodes was chosen because of the leaf-like appearance of the cut surface on gross examination (phyllos = leaf, Greek). Such terminology is clearly inappropriate in a modern classification since the great majority of the lesions are benign (as indeed Müller himself emphasized), and it is of some concern that so many authors, especially in the United States, continue to use it. Equally inappropriate are the designation of serocystic disease, Brodie's tumor and giant fibroadenoma, since a minority are, in fact, malignant. We agree entirely with the view expressed in the WHO classification[22] that the broad term 'phyllodes tumor' should be used, qualified as benign or malignant according to the histological appearances where possible.

CLINICAL FEATURES

It is difficult to obtain an accurate estimate of the true incidence of phyllodes tumor because the majority of published studies are based on small numbers of patients from tertiary referral centers. Estimates range from 0.3 to 1% of primary breast tumors,[77–79] demonstrating that even with selection bias these tumors are uncommon. In a community based study in Nottingham we identified 32 patients with phyllodes tumor in the 15 years between 1975 and 1990;[80] during the same period over 6000 patients with breast cancer were treated, giving a frequency of about 0.5% for phyllodes tumor.

Although phyllodes tumor may occur at any age from 10 years to over 80 years,[81] in Europe and the United States they are seen predominantly in middle-aged or elderly patients. The average age at presentation is 45 to 50 years and they are rare under the age of 40. Thus patients with phyllodes tumor are in general 15 to 20 years older than those presenting clinically with fibroadenoma.

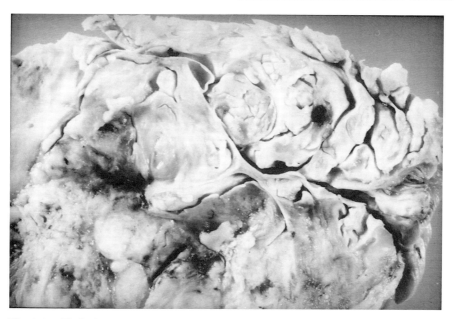

Fig. 9.23   Phyllodes tumor. The clefts are conspicuous and the resemblance to a compressed leaf bud is well seen.

However, they occur with much greater frequency in young women in the Far East.[82]

The majority of patients present with a unilateral breast mass. This may have been enlarging slowly for many years, often with more rapid growth shortly before seeking medical advice. Alternatively, tumors may exhibit a rapid growth rate from the onset of symptoms. Traditionally phyllodes tumors have always been regarded as very large lesions and indeed examples measuring as much as 40 cm have been recorded.[83] Nowadays it is our impression that more patients are presenting with smaller tumors than previously, perhaps due to the advent of mammographic screening and greater breast awareness, but the average size is still 5 cm.[80,84] Very large tumors may cause stretching of the overlying skin with predominance of superficial veins or, more rarely, actual ulceration. These clinical features are functions of size and not malignancy.

MACROSCOPIC APPEARANCES

Phyllodes tumors form firm, lobulated masses varying in size between 2 and 40 cm in diameter, with a reported average size of approximately 5 cm,[80,83–84] although rarely smaller lesions are encountered (see Fig. 9.40). They are usually well circumscribed with a clearly defined edge, but there is often a bosselated contour. The cut surface, which is usually yellowish grey in color, has a variable appearance. In larger lesions the characteristic whorled pattern is seen with visible clefts resembling a compressed leaf bud (Fig. 9.23). Smaller lesions may have a more solid, glistening mucinous appearance. In some cases the clefts are dilated and appear cystic. Foci of hemorrhage and necrosis are particularly associated with larger tumors.

MICROSCOPIC APPEARANCES

Histologically phyllodes tumors are composed of two dominant elements, clefts or cystic spaces lined by epithelial cells into which a cellular stroma projects in a leaf-like fashion (Figs 9.24–9.26). The epithelial element consists of the usual two layers of myoepithelial and secretory epithelial cells (Fig. 9.27). Metaplastic changes including apocrine and squamous epithelium are occasionally present. Focal epithelial hyperplasia is not unusual (Fig. 9.28), and may occasionally be

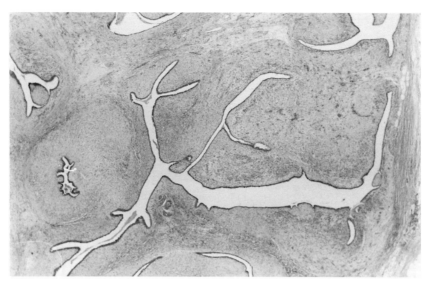

Fig. 9.24 Phyllodes tumor. The clefts are lined by epithelial cells and the leaf-like structures are formed by the cellular stroma. Hematoxylin–eosin × 23.

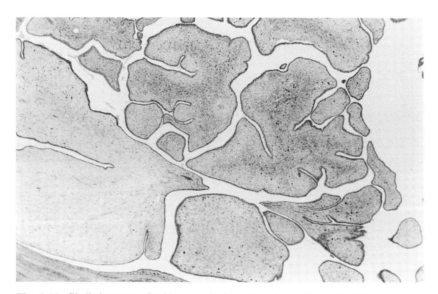

Fig. 9.25 Phyllodes tumor. In this example the pattern formed by the leaf-like clusters is rather complex. Hematoxylin–eosin × 23.

florid. Malignant epithelial change is extremely uncommon and will be discussed in a later section.

Given the basic biphasic morphological pattern of phyllodes tumor the appearances of the stromal element vary considerably from case to case, ranging from lesions which are difficult to distin-guish from cellular fibroadenoma to those with a highly pleomorphic stroma resembling a sarcoma.

In the great majority of cases the features are those of a benign process. Typically the stroma is more cellular and closely packed than in a fibroadenoma, but the spindle shaped fibroblastic cells do not exhibit nuclear pleomorphism and

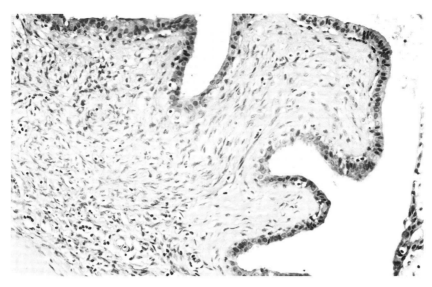

Fig. 9.26 Phyllodes tumor. The relationship between the epithelial and stromal elements is well seen in this example. Hematoxylin–eosin × 125.

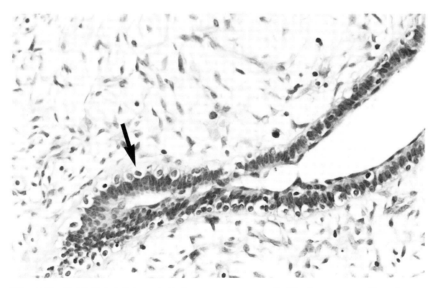

Fig. 9.27 Epithelial cleft in a phyllodes tumor, composed of both secretory cells and myoepithelial cells (arrowhead). Hematoxylin–eosin × 400.

mitoses are infrequent (Figs 9.26, 9.29). Appearances may vary within a lesion and areas of myxoid change and sparse stromal cellularity may be encountered with hyalinization (Figs 9.30, 9.31). As long as a basic cleft-like pattern is apparent such features do not exclude a diagnosis of phyllodes tumor. The lesions have a well-defined, circumscribed margin, although there is no true capsule (Fig. 9.32) and in keeping with the gross appearances the contour may have a nodular or bosselated appearance. The presence of occasional bizarre giant cells (Fig. 9.33A and B) should not be taken to indicate malignant change if the rest of the stromal cells appear entirely benign.

At the other end of the spectrum a minority of

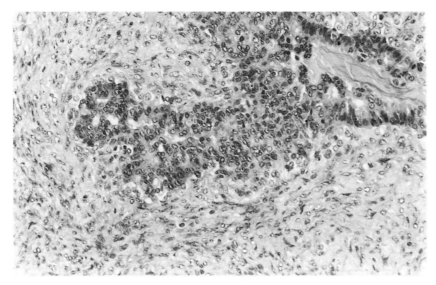

Fig. 9.28 Phyllodes tumor. Mild epithelial hyperplasia of usual type is present within the clefts of the lesion. Hematoxylin–eosin × 185.

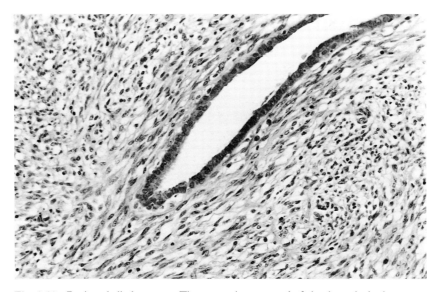

Fig. 9.29 Benign phyllodes tumor. The stroma is composed of closely packed, plump spindle cells with no nuclear pleomorphism. No mitotic figures are present. Hematoxylin–eosin × 185.

tumors show frankly sarcomatous change. There is an infiltrative rather than a pushing margin (Fig. 9.34) together with stromal hypercellularity and overgrowth in relation to the epithelial component (Figs 9.35, 9.36A). The fibroblastic cells display marked nuclear atypia and an increased mitotic count (Figs 9.36B and C, 9.37). In

particular, specific patterns such as liposarcoma, chondrosarcoma, osteosarcoma and rhabdomyosarcoma are clear indicators of malignancy[83-87] (Fig. 9.38). Single cases with areas resembling hemangiopericytoma[83] and malignant fibrous histiocytoma[88] have also been recorded.

There remains a group of tumors with inter-

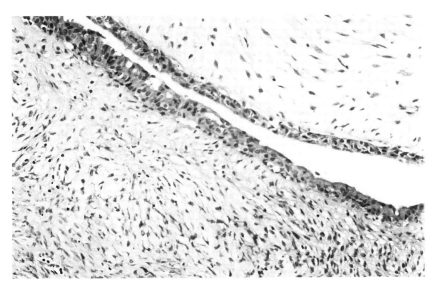

Fig. 9.30 Benign phyllodes tumor. In this lesion the stroma is relatively loose and the spindle cells are less plump than in the case illustrated in Figure 9.29, especially at the top right. Hematoxylin–eosin × 185.

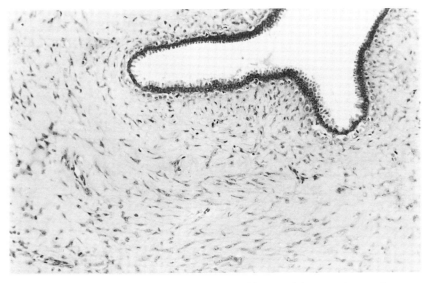

Fig. 9.31 Benign phyllodes tumor. The stroma in this area of the tumor is sparsely cellular and hyalinized. Note the characteristic epithelial cleft. Elsewhere the tumor showed greater cellularity. Hematoxylin–eosin × 125.

mediate features which pose problems for pathologists and clinicians alike in predicting the risk of local recurrence and metastatic malignant potential. A number of studies have addressed this issue[79,83–85,87,89–92] but no coherent pattern has emerged. There are a number of reasons for this, including the relatively small number of cases in each series, the varied database (most series being derived from secondary or tertiary referral centers) and the division of tumors into two groups, benign and malignant by some authors and three groups, benign, borderline and malignant by others. The

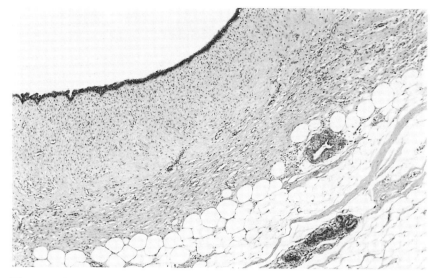

Fig. 9.32 Benign phyllodes tumor. The edge of the tumor is shown in this field; an epithelial cleft is to the top left and normal fatty breast tissue at the bottom right. Although the lesion is relatively well defined, no true capsule is present. Hematoxylin–eosin × 57.

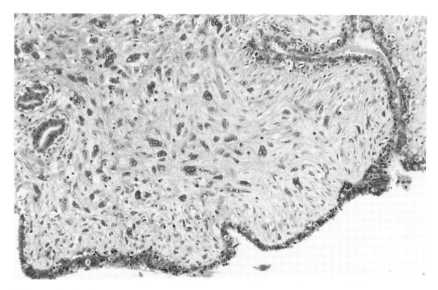

Fig. 9.33A Benign phyllodes tumor. Large, bizarre giant cells are present within the stroma. The adjacent stromal cells are entirely benign in appearance. Hematoxylin–eosin × 125.

importance of using several features to categorize phyllodes tumors was first shown by Norris and Taylor[85] who assessed the behavior of 94 cases in relation to tumor size, nature of tumor margin, degree of cellular atypia and mitotic counts. No single feature was reliable in predicting clinical outcome, but those tumors which were less than 4 cm in diameter, with pushing margins, minimal cellular atypia and fewer than three mitotic figures per 10 high power fields (field area not defined) were associated with a low risk of recurrence or death. Although Norris and Taylor[85] did not

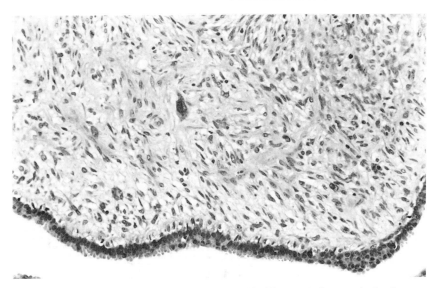

Fig. 9.33B   Higher magnification of case illustrated in Figure 9.33A to emphasize the benign stromal morphology despite the presence of tumor giant cells. Hematoxylin–eosin × 185.

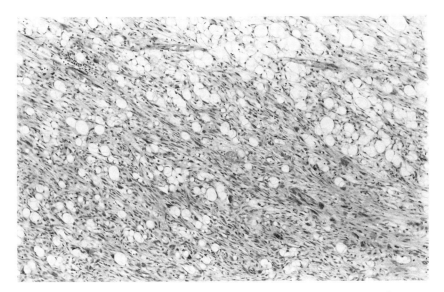

Fig. 9.34   Malignant phyllodes tumor. Diffuse infiltration of stromal cells into adjacent tissue is present at the tumor margin. Hematoxylin–eosin × 100.

attempt to classify individual tumors as benign or malignant most subsequent studies appear to have taken note of their findings in deriving criteria by which to make this distinction. Thus Pietrushka and Barnes,[83] based on an assessment of 42 cases, defined benign tumors as those with predominantly pushing margins, no or minimal stromal cell atypia and 0–4 mitoses per 10 high power fields. Malignant tumors had predominantly infiltrating margins, moderate to marked stromal atypia and 10 or more mitoses per 10 high power fields. They also recognized a borderline group with pushing or infiltrative margins, moderate stromal atypia and 5–9 mitoses per 10 high power

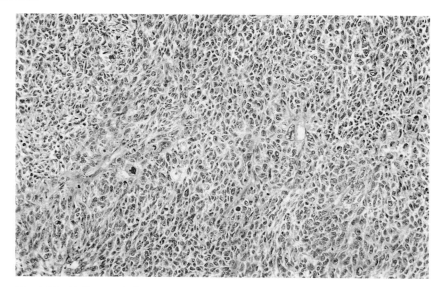

Fig. 9.35   Malignant phyllodes tumor. In this medium power view no epithelial elements are seen. The stroma is hypercellular and shows nuclear atypia. Hematoxylin–eosin × 125.

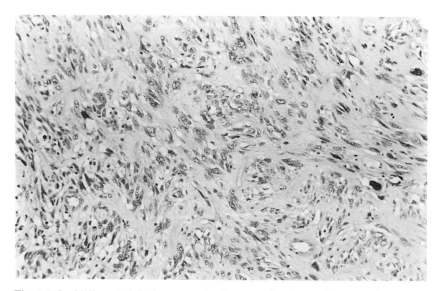

Fig. 9.36A   Malignant phyllodes tumor. Another example of stromal overgrowth. Although there is less cellularity no epithelial elements are visible in this field. Hematoxylin–eosin × 100.

fields. Hart[90] and Ward and Evans[91] used similar criteria, but introduced the presence of stromal overgrowth in relation to the epithelial elements, as a differential diagnostic feature implying poorer prognosis. Hawkins et al[84] have confirmed in another relatively small series that these features of infiltrative margins, stromal nuclear pleomor-

phism and increased mitotic count all predicted likelihood of metastasis, but the most powerful factor was stromal overgrowth. Murad et al[92] found that grading of the mesenchymal element, which included cellularity, atypia and mitotic counts, together with the presence of necrosis and more than one mesenchymal element, were the

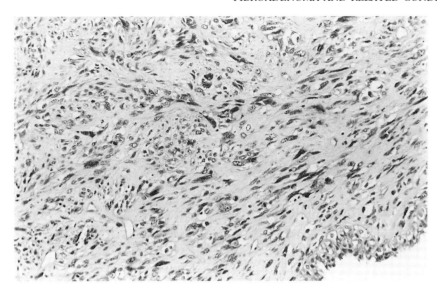

Fig. 9.36B Malignant phyllodes tumor. Even at this magnification the nuclear atypia of the stromal cells is apparent. Part of an epithelial cleft is seen at the bottom right. Same case as Figure 9.36A. Hematoxylin–eosin × 100.

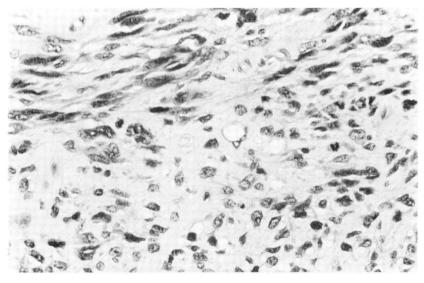

Fig. 9.36C Malignant phyllodes tumor. Higher magnification of another area of the tumor illustrated in Figure 9.36A and B to show marked nuclear pleomorphism. Hematoxylin–eosin × 400.

most useful features in predicting malignancy and more particularly metastasis. In contrast a number of studies have found no correlation between the morphological characteristics of phyllodes tumors and malignancy or recurrence.[79,89] In multivariate analysis Cohn-Cedermark et al[87] found that tumor necrosis and the presence of stromal elements other than fibromyxoid tissue were the only independent prognostic factors. Because of these inconsistencies Tavassoli[18] has proposed that the benign designation for phyllodes tumor be abandoned and the designations 'low grade' or 'high

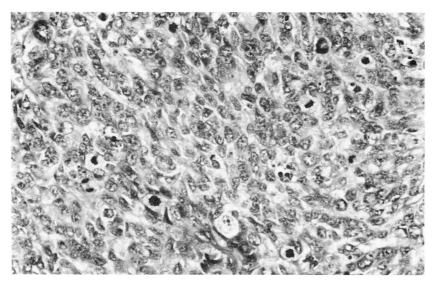

Fig. 9.37 Another malignant phyllodes tumor. There is marked nuclear pleomorphism and several mitotic figures are present in this field. Hematoxylin–eosin × 400.

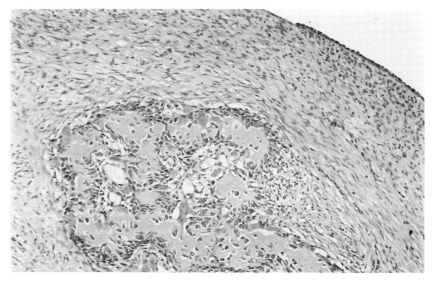

Fig. 9.38 Malignant phyllodes tumor. In this example the stroma shows the features of osteogenic sarcoma. Part of an epithelial cleft is seen at the top right. From a woman aged 52 years who died from metastatic disease. Hematoxylin–eosin × 125.

grade' cystosarcoma phyllodes be used. With respect we feel that this approach is completely unacceptable as it gives an entirely biased impression that the majority of phyllodes tumors are malignant, which, as has already been pointed out, is not the case. This highlights the problems associated with reporting series derived from tertiary referral centers and it is also clear that in many studies tumor recurrence alone is often equated with malignancy.

In order to overcome complete reliance on the morphological aspects of phyllodes tumor in predicting prognosis a number of groups have resorted to flow cytometric evaluation of DNA ploidy and proliferative activity, but results have been conflicting and inconclusive, due partly, no doubt, to the small number of cases studied. El-Naggar et al[93] found a striking association between DNA ploidy and natural history; the majority of their patients with aneuploid tumors developed recurrence, metastasis or tumor-related death, whilst all their patients with diploid tumors and low S-phase fractions were recurrence free. In contrast other studies have demonstrated that, although there is a general association between aneuploidy and traditional morphological features of malignancy there is no correlation with prognosis.[79,92,94–95] Only El-Naggar et al[93] and Palko et al[95] have found an association between S-phase fraction and prognosis. At the present time it must be concluded that neither DNA ploidy nor S-phase fraction, as determined by flow cytometry, adds to our ability to predict likely prognosis in phyllodes tumor.

In view of the uncertainties outlined above we have carried out our own community-based investigation into the correlation between tumor morphology and clinical outcome.[80] Semiquantitative criteria derived from those proposed by Pietrushka and Barnes[83] and Ward and Evans[91] were used to divide the tumors into three morphological categories, benign, borderline and malignant. In tumors designated as benign (22 cases, 68%) the margins were pushing, there was minimal stromal overgrowth, cellularity and pleomorphism and stromal mitotic counts were less than 10 per 10 fields (field area 0.152 mm^2). Malignant tumors (five cases, 16%) had infiltrative margins, marked stromal overgrowth, cellularity and pleomorphism with mitotic counts greater than 10 per 10 fields. A further five cases (16%) were classified as borderline because the features were intermediate with some but not all the characteristics of malignancy. We found that none of these morphological features was useful in predicting local recurrence, which was strongly related to completeness of local excision. All four recurrences in benign tumors (18%) and the single recurrence in a borderline tumor occurred in patients treated initially by local excision and were fully controlled by complete re-excision or mastectomy. There were no recurrences or metastases in patients treated initially by mastectomy for benign, borderline or malignant tumors. In

one patient with malignant phyllodes tumor, uncontrolled chest wall recurrences followed local excision (limited surgery carried out for medical reasons). None of the patients in this relatively small series developed metastases; anecdotally the only cases with metastatic disease which we have seen in consultation practice had definite morphological criteria of malignancy in the original primaries.

In summary, we believe that phyllodes tumors should be designated as benign or malignant, based on histopathological assessment of tumor margin, stromal overgrowth, pleomorphism and mitotic count, as described above. The borderline category is a useful one, which if used sensibly prevents overdiagnosis of malignancy and hence possible overtreatment.

PATHOGENESIS

Phyllodes tumors are distinctive fibroepithelial lesions which are derived from breast lobules. Their neoplastic rather than hyperplastic origin is confirmed by their clinical behavior, and they are composed of monoclonal stromal cells but polyclonal epithelial cells.[31] However, the precise pathogenesis remains obscure. There are two equally feasible possibilities, an origin in a pre-existing fibroadenoma or development de novo from the intralobular stroma and epithelium. The close histological similarity of many cases of benign phyllodes tumor to fibroadenoma suggest that the former is the more likely. This is supported by those rare cases in which it is possible to demonstrate both morphological patterns in the same lesion (Fig. 9.39A and B). Further supportive evidence is provided clinically by some patients who report the presence of small breast nodules for several years before sudden rapid growth stimulates them to seek medical advice. Furthermore, a minority of patients with phyllodes tumors have actually had histologically proven fibroadenomas removed previously from the same site. Noguchi and colleagues[96] have investigated three such cases using PCR-based trinucleotide repeat polymorphism of the X-chromosome-linked androgen receptor (AR). Interestingly they found that the stromal cells of

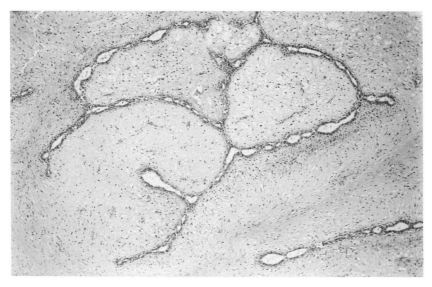

Fig. 9.39A Combined fibroadenoma and phyllodes tumor. In this field the lesion exhibits the pattern of an intracanalicular fibroadenoma. Hematoxylin–eosin × 57.

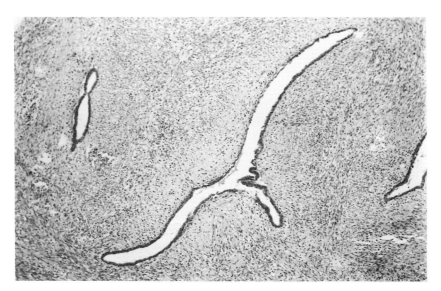

Fig. 9.39B Combined fibroadenoma and phyllodes tumor. Same case as Figure 9.39A showing the epithelial clefts and cellular stroma of a typical phyllodes tumor. The lesion, 5 cm in diameter, from the left breast of a 42-year-old woman, was accompanied by a further nodule in the same breast which had the histological features of a fibroadenoma. A fibroadenoma had been removed from each breast 6 years previously. Hematoxylin–eosin × 57.

both the phyllodes tumor and the previous fibroadenoma were monoclonal in each case, with inactivation of the same AR allele. This provides powerful, albeit anecdotal, evidence that at least some phyllodes tumors arise from a pre-existing fibroadenoma. Together with their previous study[31] Noguchi et al[96] also seem to have shown that there are two types of fibroadenoma, polyclonal and monoclonal, although unfortunately the morphological appearances are indistinguishable. Whether their suggestion that the PCR-based method for clonal analysis should be used pre-operatively on fine needle aspirates to make the distinction is a practical proposition remains to be seen. These findings clearly require confirmation, and they do not explain the pathogenesis of those tumors which arise in elderly women with no history of a pre-existing mass. The possibility remains that at least in some cases phyllodes tumors arise de novo.

DIFFERENTIAL DIAGNOSIS

At the benign end of the spectrum of morphological patterns of phyllodes tumor the main differential diagnosis is fibroadenoma, as discussed previously. It must be reiterated that although most phyllodes tumors are relatively large, size alone is of no value as a distinguishing feature since there is considerable overlap in range between the two entities (Fig. 9.40). The presence of a leaf-like pattern with deep epithelial clefts and hypercellular stroma favour phyllodes tumor. In the rare case where it is genuinely difficult to make a definite distinction the pathologist should err on the side of caution, especially if excision is incomplete, since the latter is associated with a high level of recurrence in phyllodes tumor.

Phyllodes tumors in which there is a relative overgrowth of the stromal element must be distinguished from fibromatosis and primary sarcoma of the breast, although both are extremely rare lesions. In fibromatosis (see Ch. 11) there is a bland infiltrative spindle cell proliferation with absent or scanty mitotic figures. When the stromal infiltrate surrounds existing lobules and ductular structures the appearances may bear a superficial resemblance to phyllodes tumor, but the characteristic epithelial clefts are not seen. In some malignant phyllodes tumors the stromal element may be so dominant that the lesion resembles a pure sarcoma. Adequate sampling is essential in such cases, especially where the lesion is very large; Tavassoli,[18] for example, recommends that one block is selected for every centimeter of maximum tumor diameter.

Care must also be taken with recurrent or metastatic lesions which have the morphological features of a pure sarcoma, and the original specimen should be examined for features which might identify it as a phyllodes tumor.

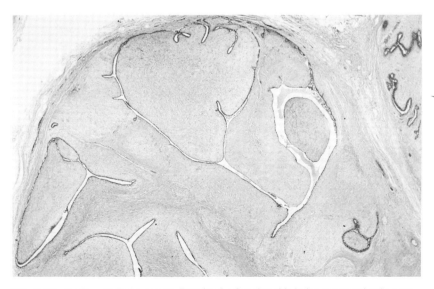

Fig. 9.40 Benign phyllodes tumor. Despite the fact that this lesion measured only 1 cm in diameter, the leaf-like clefted structure is diagnostic of a benign phyllodes tumor. Hematoxylin–eosin × 23.

PROGNOSIS AND MANAGEMENT

Phyllodes tumor has acquired an unwarranted reputation as a relatively malignant lesion in its behavior, due in great measure to the publication of selected series biased towards a poor outcome and based on relatively small numbers of cases, usually from tertiary referral centers. For example, an overall local recurrence rate of between 19 and 36% has been recorded, with a rate of metastatic disease of between 12 and 24% and mortality of 10 to 27% (Table 9.1). Such data should be interpreted with caution and it is surprising that Tavassoli,[18] in her recent textbook, reiterates the figure of 30% for the recurrence rate in phyllodes tumor without providing any supportive evidence. Much more appropriate data should be obtained if phyllodes tumor is divided into benign and malignant categories, as suggested previously. However, even when series are reported in this way there is an enormous variation in the propor-

tion of benign and malignant cases, ranging from 95% benign cases to 66% malignant cases (Table 9.2). The true frequency of benign or malignant phyllodes tumor can only be obtained from a community-based study. In our own study in Nottingham we found that 68% of the tumors satisfied the morphological criteria for benignity, 16% had borderline morphology and only a further 16% were malignant. Although the number of cases is small, these data, together with that from other studies,[89,97] suggest that the overall frequency of malignant phyllodes tumor is in fact less than 25%.

The data on local recurrence rates also require clarification. Most series report a figure of between 15 and 20% for local recurrence in benign phyllodes tumor (Table 9.2), but this is almost always related to the adequacy of the initial excision.[80,83] The rate is higher after wide local excision than following mastectomy, especially if inadequate attention is paid to excision margins.

Table 9.1   Overall recurrence, metastases and death rates for phyllodes tumor (no separate designation as benign or malignant)

Series	Center	Total number of cases	Recurrence rate	Metastases	Deaths
Treves and Sunderland, 1951[109]	Memorial Hospital, New York	77	18 (23%)	9 (12%)	8 (10%)
Norris and Taylor, 1967[85]	AFIP, Washington	94	28 (30%)	15 (17%)	15 (17%)
Ward and Evans, 1986[91]	MD Anderson, Houston	26	5 (19%)	5 (19%)	7 (27%)
Cohn-Cedermark, 1991[87]	Karolinska Institute, Stockholm	77	16 (21%)	16 (21%)	16 (21%)
Hawkins et al, 1992[84]	R Marsden Hospital, London	33	12 (36%)	8 (24%)	7 (21%)

Table 9.2   Recurrence, metastases and death rates for phyllodes tumor designated as benign, borderline or malignant

Series	Benign				Borderline				Malignant				Total
	No	Rec	Met	Death	No	Rec	Met	Death	No	Rec	Met	Death	
McDivitt et al, 1967[97]	59	10 (17%)	0	0	–	–	–	–	13	1 (8%)	0	0	72
Hajdu, Espinosa and Robbins, 1976[89]	150	28 (19%)	?	0	–	–	–	–	49	4 (8%)	?	?	199
Pietrushka and Barnes, 1978[83]	18	4 (22%)	0	0	5	1 (20%)	1	1	19	1 (5%)	3	3	42
Hart, Bower and Oberman, 1978[90]	12	2 (17%)	0	0	–	–	–	–	14	4* (29%)	3	2	26
Hines, Murad and Beal, 1987[107]	15	4 (27%)	0	0	–	–	–	–	10	6 (60%)	4	4	25
Salvadori et al, 1989[108]	24	1 (4%)	0	0	26	10 (38%)	1	1	21	3 (14%)	1	1	71
Moffatt et al, 1995[80]	22	4 (18%)	0	0	5	1 (2%)	0	0	5	1 (20%)	0	1†	32

No: number of cases.
Rec: number of recurrences.
Met: number with metastatic disease.
Deaths: number of deaths occurring.
*Multiple recurrences.
†Death from unrelated cause.

In any event, in benign phyllodes tumor it is our experience that local recurrences are controlled by further complete excision. A wide range of local recurrence has been recorded in malignant phyllodes tumor, from as little as 5% up to 60%, although in most series the figure is less than 10% (Table 9.2). This is almost certainly due to the greater use of mastectomy as primary treatment in these cases. In contrast with benign phyllodes tumor recurrent disease is rarely controlled by further surgery.

In the 300 cases of benign phyllodes tumor recorded in Table 9.2 none developed metastatic disease and no tumor-related deaths occurred. Relatively conservative management therefore seems appropriate. We recommend that benign phyllodes tumor should be treated by complete local excision, care being taken to remove a margin of normal breast tissue around the lesion. When complete excision is obtained in this way, (and the pathologist should sample margins very carefully) a low rate of recurrence can be expected. If margins are involved, immediate re-excision should be performed. Recurrent lesions are controlled adequately by further excision, or if necessary, by mastectomy. Mastectomy itself is a perfectly acceptable primary therapy in women with very large benign phyllodes tumors, especially in the elderly.

The management of malignant phyllodes tumor is more difficult. High rates of local recurrence have been recorded in some studies (Tables 9.1 and 9.2) and mastectomy therefore appears to be the primary treatment of choice. If local excision has been performed initially, say for diagnostic purposes, and the lesion proves to be a malignant phyllodes tumor, conversion to mastectomy is advisable. In our own small series[80] none of the four patients treated with mastectomy has suffered a recurrence, after long-term follow-up.

The mortality in malignant phyllodes tumor is difficult to estimate, because of the case selection bias referred to earlier. Thus the overall mortality in the series shown in Table 9.1 which included both benign and malignant cases was 17% whilst for those studies in Table 9.2 in which full data was available for malignant phyllodes tumor the mortality was 13%. This is, of course, considerably better than for patients with invasive carcinoma of histological grades 2 or 3[98] and belies the reputation of phyllodes tumor as a highly malignant lesion.

It is difficult to comment in detail on clinical outcome in phyllodes tumor of borderline morphology because of the small number of cases which have been reported. The local recurrence rate is between 20 and 33% with a very low mortality of under 6% (Table 9.2). We agree with Johnson[99] that it is a useful category in preventing overdiagnosis of malignancy and therefore potential overtreatment. It is clear that in cases labeled as borderline complete local excision is imperative, and that if this cannot be achieved by wide local excision, mastectomy should be performed.

CARCINOMA ASSOCIATED WITH PHYLLODES TUMOR

On an anecdotal basis both lobular neoplasia[81,100–102] and ductal carcinoma in situ[85,102–104] have been recorded. The association appears to be less common than with fibroadenoma, but similar rules apply. Lobular neoplasia is seen more often than ductal carcinoma in situ and the changes are usually also present in breast tissue adjacent to the lesion. Invasive carcinoma has been recorded even less frequently than in situ carcinoma in association with phyllodes tumor.[18,85,100–101,105–106] No specific type of infiltrating carcinoma predominates.[89,107–109]

REFERENCES

1. Haagensen CD. Adenofibroma. In: Haagensen CD, ed. Diseases of the breast. Philadelphia: Saunders, 1986a: 267–283.
2. Hughes LE, Mansel RE, Webster DJT. Fibroadenoma and related tumours. In: Hughes LE, Mansel RE, Webster DJT, eds. Benign disorders and diseases of the breast. London: Baillière Tindall, 1989; 59–73.
3. Deschênes L, Jacob S, Fabia J, Christen A. Beware of breast fibroadenomas in middle-aged women. Can J Surg 1985; 28: 372–374.
4. Frantz VK, Pickren JW, Melcher GW, Auchinloss J Jr. Incidence of chronic cystic disease in so-called 'normal breasts'. A study based on 225 post mortem examinations. Cancer 1951; 4: 762–783.
5. Parks AG. The micro-anatomy of the breast. Ann Roy Coll Surg, Engl 1959; 25: 235–251.
6. Bartow SA, Pathak DR, Black WC et al. Prevalence of benign, atypical and malignant breast lesions in populations at different risk for breast cancer. Cancer 1987; 60: 2751–2760.
7. Foster ME, Garrahan N, Williams S. Fibroadenoma of the breast. J Roy Coll Surg, Edinb 1988; 33: 16–19.
8. Dent DM, Cant PJ. Fibroadenoma. World J Surg 1989; 13: 706–710.
9. Funderburk WW, Rosero E, Leffall LD. Breast lesions in blacks. Surg Gynec Obstet 1972; 135: 58–60.
10. Naraynsingh V, Raju GC. Familial multiple fibroadenomas of the breast. Postgrad Med J 1985; 61: 439–440.
11. Morris JA, Kelly JF. Multiple bilateral breast adenomata in identical Negro twins. Histopathol 1982; 6: 539–547.
12. Cheng FCY, Tsang PH, Shum JDP, Ong GB. Maffucci's syndrome with fibroadenomas of the breasts. J Roy Coll Surg, Edinb 1981; 26: 181–183.
13. Carney JA, Toorkey BC. Myxoid fibroadenoma and allied conditions (myxomatosis) of the breast. A heritable disorder with special associations including cardiac and cutaneous myxomas. Am J Surg Pathol 1991; 15: 713–721.
14. Mies C, Rosen PP. Juvenile fibroadenoma with atypical epithelial hyperplasia. Am J Surg Pathol 1987; 11: 184–190.
15. Page DL, Rogers LW. Combined histologic and cytologic criteria for the diagnosis of mammary atypical hyperplasia. Hum Pathol 1992; 23: 1095–1097.
16. Fechner RE. Fibroadenoma and related conditions. In: Page DL, Anderson TW, eds. Diagnostic histopathology of the breast. Edinburgh: Churchill Livingstone, 1987; 72–85.
17. Azzopardi JG. Fibroadenoma. In: Azzopardi JG, ed. Problems in breast pathology. London: WB Saunders, 1979; 39–56.
18. Tavassoli FA. Biphasic tumors. In: Tavassoli FA, ed. Pathology of the breast. Norwalk: Appleton and Lange, 1992; 425–481.
19. Spagnolo DV, Shilkin KB. Breast neoplasms containing bone and cartilage. Virchows Arch (A) Pathol Anat 1983; 400: 287–295.
20. Goodman ZD, Taxy JB. Fibroadenomas of the breast with prominent smooth muscle. Am J Surg Pathol 1981; 5: 99–101.
21. Cooper A. Anatomy and diseases of the breast. In: Diseases of the breast. Lea and Blanchard, 1845; 39.
22. World Health Organization. International histological classification of tumours. Histologic types of breast tumours. Geneva: World Health Organization, 1981.
23. Sloane JP. Biopsy pathology of the breast. London: Chapman and Hall, 1987.
24. Carter D. Interpretation of breast biopsies. 2nd ed. New York: Raven, 1990.
25. Smith BL. Fibroadenomas. In: Harris JT, Hellman S, Henderson IC et al, eds. Breast diseases. Philadelphia: Lippincott, 1991; 34–37.
26. Symmers W St C. The breasts. In: Symmers W St C, ed. Systemic pathology. 3rd ed, vol 4. Edinburgh: Churchill Livingstone, 1978; 1759–1861.
27. Hanson CA, Snover DC, Dehner LP. Fibroadenomatosis (fibroadenomatoid mastopathy): a benign breast lesion with composite pathologic features. Pathol 1987; 19: 393–396.
28. Demetrakopoulos NJ. Three dimensional reconstruction of a human mammary fibroadenoma. Quart Bull Northwest Univ Med Sch 1958; 32: 221–227.
29. Orcel L, Douvin D. Contribution à l'étude histogénétique des fibro-adénomes mammaires. Ann Anat Pathol Paris 1973; 18: 255–276.
30. Pesce C, Colacino R. Morphometry of the breast fibroadenoma. Pathol Res Pract 1986; 181: 718–720.
31. Noguchi S, Motomura K, Inaji H et al. Clonal analysis of fibroadenoma and phyllodes tumor of the breast by means of polymerase chain reaction. Cancer Res 1993; 58: 4071–4074.
32. Martin PM, Kuttenn F, Serment H, Mauvais-Jarvis P. Progesterone receptors in breast fibroadenomas. J Steroid Biochem 1979; 11: 1295–1298.
33. Sitruk-Ware R, Sterkers N, Mauvais-Jarvis P. Benign breast disease I: Hormonal investigation. Obstet Gynecol 1979; 53: 457–460.
34. Wargotz ES, Norris HJ, Austin RM et al. Fibromatosis of the breast. A clinical and pathologic study of 28 cases. Am J Surg Pathol 1987; 11: 38–45.
35. Rosen PP, Ernsberger D. Mammary fibromatosis. A benign spindle cell tumor with significant risk for local recurrence. Cancer 1989; 63: 1363–1369.
36. Wilkinson S, Anderson TJ, Rifkind E et al. Fibroadenoma of the breast: a follow-up of conservative management. Brit J Surg 1989; 76: 390–391.
37. Sainsbury JRC, Nicholson S, Needham GK et al. Natural history of the benign breast lump. Brit J Surg 1988; 75: 1080–1082.
38. Cant PJ, Madden MV, Close PM et al. Case for conservative management of selected fibroadenomas of the breast. Brit J Surg 1987; 74: 857–859.
39. Ellis IO, Galea MH, Locker A et al. Early experience in breast cancer screening: Emphasis on development of protocols for triple assessment. Breast 1993; 2: 148–153.
40. Galea MH, Dixon AR, Pye G et al. Non-operative management of discrete breast lumps in women over 35 years of age. The Breast 1992; 1: 164 (Abstract).
41. Van Bogaert L, Gilbert M. Reliability of the cyto-radio-clinical triplet in breast pathology diagnosis. Acta Cytol 1977; 21: 60–62.
42. Hermansen C, Poulsen H, Jensen J et al. Diagnostic

reliability of combined physical examination, mammography and fine needle puncture ('triple-test') in breast tumors. A prospective study. Cancer 1987; 60: 1866–1871.

43. Wilkinson L, Green WO Jr. Infarction of breast lesions during pregnancy and lactation. Cancer 1964; 17: 1567–1572.

44. Majmudar B, Rosales-Quintana S. Infarction of breast fibroadenomas during pregnancy. J Am Med Assoc 1975; 231: 963–964.

45. Pambakian H, Tighe JR. Mammary infarction. Brit J Surg 1971; 58: 601–602.

46. Buzanowski-Konakry K, Harrison EG Jr, Payne WS. Lobular carcinoma arising in fibroadenoma of the breast. Cancer 1975; 35: 450–456.

47. Yoshida Y, Takaoka M, Fukumoto M. Carcinoma arising in fibroadenoma: case report and review of the world literature. J Surg Oncol 1985; 29: 132–140.

48. Diaz NM, Palmer JO, McDivitt RW. Carcinoma arising within fibroadenomas of the breast. Am J Clin Pathol 1991; 95: 614–622.

49. Ashikari R, Farrow JH, O'Hara J. Fibroadenomas in the breasts of juveniles. Surg Obstet Gynec 1971; 132: 259–262.

50. Oberman HA. Breast lesions in the adolescent female. Ann Pathol 1979; 14: 175–201.

51. Fekete P, Petrek J, Majmudar B et al. Fibroadenomas with stromal cellularity. Arch Pathol Lab Med 1987; 111: 427–432.

52. Pike AM, Oberman HA. Juvenile (cellular) adenofibromas. A clinicopathologic study. Am J Surg Pathol 1985; 9: 2891–2905.

53. Jordal K, Sorensen B. Giant fibroadenomas of the breast. Report of two cases, one treated with mammoplasty. Acta Chir Scand 1961; 122: 147–151.

54. Persaud V, Talerman A, Jordan RP. Pure adenoma of the breast. Arch Pathol Lab Med 1968; 86: 481–483.

55. Hertel BG, Zaloudek C, Kempson RL. Breast adenomas. Cancer 1976; 37: 2891–2905.

56. Moross T, Lang AP, Mahoney L. Tubular adenoma of the breast. Arch Pathol Lab Med 1983; 107: 84–86.

57. O'Hara MF, Page DL. Adenomas of the breast and ectopic breast under lactational influences. Hum Pathol 1985; 16: 707–712.

58. James K, Bridger J, Anthony PP. Breast tumour of pregnancy ('lactating adenoma'). J Pathol 1988; 156: 37–44.

59. Slavin JL, Billson VR, Ostor AG. Nodular breast lesions during pregnancy and lactation. Histopathol 1993; 22: 481–485.

60. Arrigoni MG, Dockerty MB, Judd ES. The identification and treatment of mammary hamartoma. Surg Gynecol Obstet 1971; 132: 259–262.

61. Hessler C, Schnyder P, Ozzello L. Hamartoma of the breast: diagnostic observations of 16 cases. Radiol 1979; 126: 95–98.

62. Linell F, Ostberg G, Sodersstrom J et al. Breast hamartomas. An important entity in mammary pathology. Virchows Arch (A) Pathol Anat 1979; 383: 253–264.

63. Jones MW, Norris HJ, Wargotz ES. Hamartomas of the breast. Surg Gynecol Obstet 1991; 173: 54–56.

64. Fisher C, Hanby AM, Robinson L, Millis RR. Mammary hamartoma — a review of 35 cases. Histopathol 1992; 20: 99–106.

65. Prym P. Pseudoadenome, adenome und mastome der weiblichen brastdrüse. Beitr Pathol Anat 1928; 81: 1–44.

66. Spalding JE. Adenolipoma and lipoma of the breast. Guys Hosp Rep 1945; 94: 80–84.

67. Dyreborg U, Starklint H. Adenolipoma mammae. Acta Radiol 1975; 16: 362–366.

68. Mendiola H, Henrik-Nielsen R, Dyreborg U et al. Lobular carcinoma in situ occurring in adenolipoma of the breast. Report of a case. Acta Radiol Diagnosis 1982; 23: 503–505.

69. Kersschot E, Dochez C, Beelaerts W. Fibroadenolipoma (hamartoma) of the breast: a case report. J Belge Radiol 1984; 67: 133–134.

70. Crothers JG, Butler NF, Fortt RW. Fibroadenolipoma of the breast. Brit J Radiol 1985; 58: 191–202.

71. Davies JD, Riddell RH. Muscular hamartoma of the breast. J Pathol 1971; 111: 209–211.

72. Bussolati G, Ghiringhello B, Papotti M. Subareolar muscular hamartoma of the breast. Appl Pathol 1984; 2: 94–95.

73. Hunkatroon M, Lin F. Muscular hamartoma of the breast. An electron microscopic study. Virchows Arch (A) Pathol Anat 1984; 403: 307–312.

74. Coyne J, Hobbs FM, Boggis C, Harland R. Lobular carcinoma in a mammary hamartoma. J Clin Pathol 1992; 45: 936–937.

75. Fiks A. Cystosarcoma phyllodes of the mammary gland — Müllers tumor. Virchows Arch (A) Pathol Anat 1981; 392: 1–6.

76. Müller J. Uber den feineren Bau und die Formen der krankhaften Geshwulst. Berlin: Reimer, 1838; 54–60.

77. Dyer NH, Bridger JE, Taylor RS. Cystosarcoma phyllodes. Brit J Surg 1966; 53: 450–455.

78. Kessinger A, Foley JF, Lemon HM, Miller DM. Metastatic cystosarcoma phyllodes: a case report and review of the literature. J Surg Oncol 1972; 4: 131–147.

79. Keelan PA, Myers JL, Wold LE et al. Phyllodes tumor: clinicopathologic review of 60 patients and flow cytometric analysis in 30 patients. Hum Pathol 1992; 23: 1048–1054.

80. Moffat CJC, Pinder SE, Dixon AR et al. Phyllodes tumours of the breast: a clinicopathological review of 32 cases. Histopathol 1995; 27: 205–218.

81. Haagensen CD. Cystosarcoma phyllodes. In: Haagensen CD, ed. Diseases of the breast. Philadelphia: Saunders, 1986b; 284–312.

82. Looi L–M. Personal communication. 1994.

83. Pietruska M, Barnes L. Cystosarcoma phyllodes. A clinico-pathologic analysis of 42 cases. Cancer 1978; 41: 1974–1983.

84. Hawkins RE, Schofield JB, Fisher C et al. The clinical and histologic criteria that predict metastases from cystosarcoma phyllodes. Cancer 1992; 69: 141–147.

85. Norris HJ, Taylor HB. Relationship of histologic features to behaviour of cystosarcoma phyllodes. Analysis of ninety four cases. Cancer 1967; 20: 2090–2099.

86. Qizilbash AH. Cystosarcoma phyllodes with liposarcomatous stroma. Am J Clin Pathol 1976; 65: 321–327.

87. Cohn-Cedermark G, Rutquist LE, Rosendahl O et al. Prognostic factors in cystosarcoma phyllodes. A clinicopathologic study of 77 patients. Cancer 1991; 68: 2017–2022.

88. Mentzel T, Kosmehl H, Katenkamp D. Metastasizing phyllodes tumour with malignant fibrous histiocytoma-like areas. Histopathol 1991; 19: 557–560.

89. Hajdu SI, Espinosa MH, Robbins GF. Recurrent cystosarcoma phyllodes. A clinicopathologic study of 32 cases. Cancer 1976; 38: 1402–1406.

90. Hart WR, Bauer RC, Oberman HA. Cystosarcoma phyllodes. A clinicopathologic study of twenty six hypercellular periductal stromal tumours of the breast. Am J Clin Pathol 1978; 70: 211–216.

91. Ward RM, Evans HL. Cystosarcoma phyllodes. A clinicopathologic study of 26 cases. Cancer 1986; 58: 2282–2289.

92. Murad TM, Hines JR, Beal J et al. Histopathological and clinical correlations of cystosarcoma phyllodes. Arch Pathol Lab Med 1988; 112: 752–756.

93. El-Naggar A, Ro JY, McLemore D, Garnsy L. DNA content and proliferative activity of cystosarcoma phyllodes of the breast. Am J Clin Pathol 1990; 93: 480–485.

94. Layfield LJ, Hart J, Neuwirth H et al. Relation between DNA ploidy and the clinical behavior of phyllodes tumors. Cancer 1989; 64: 1486–1489.

95. Palko MJ, Wang SE, Shackney SE et al. Flow cytometric S fraction as a predictor of clinical outcome in cystosarcoma phyllodes. Arch Pathol Lab Med 1990; 114: 949–952.

96. Noguchi S, Yokouchi H, Aihara T et al. Progression of fibroadenoma to phyllodes tumor demonstrated by clonal analysis. Cancer 1995; 76: 1779–1785.

97. McDivitt RW, Urban JA, Farrow JH. Cystosarcoma phyllodes. Johns Hopk Med J 1967; 120: 33–45.

98. Elston CW, Ellis IO. Pathological prognostic factors in breast cancer. I. The value of histological grade in breast cancer: experience from a large study with long-term follow-up. Histopathol 1991; 19: 403–410.

99. Johnson RL. Sarcomas of the breast. In: Page DL, Anderson TJ, eds. Diagnostic histopathology of the breast. Edinburgh: Churchill Livingstone, 1987.

100. Rosen PP, Urban JA. Coexistent mammary carcinoma and cystosarcoma phyllodes. Breast 1975; 1: 9–15.

101. Azzopardi JG. Sarcomas of the breast. In: Azzopardi JG, ed. Problems in breast pathology. Philadelphia: Saunders, 1979; 346–378.

102. Knudsen PJT, Ostergaard J. Cystosarcoma phylloides with lobular and ductal carcinoma in situ. Arch Pathol Lab Med 1987; 111: 873–875.

103. Harris M, Persaud V. Cystosarcoma of the breast. J Pathol 1974; 112: 99–104.

104. Grove A, Kristensen LD. Intraductal carcinoma within a phyllodes tumor of the breast: a case report. Tumori 1986; 72: 187–190.

105. Cornog JL, Mobini J, Steiger E et al. Squamous carcinoma of the breast. Am J Clin Pathol 1971; 55: 410–417.

106. Leong AS-Y, Meredith DJ. Tubular carcinoma developing within a recurring cystosarcoma phyllodes of the breast. Cancer 1980; 46: 1863–1867.

107. Hines JR, Murad TM, Beal JM. Prognostic indication in cystosarcoma phyllodes. Am J Surg 1987; 153: 276–280.

108. Salvadori B, Cusumano F, del-Bo R et al. Surgical treatment of phyllodes tumors of the breast. Cancer 1989; 63: 2532–2536.

109. Treves N, Sunderland DA. Cystosarcoma phyllodes of the breast: a malignant and a benign tumor. A clinico-pathologic study of seventy seven cases. Cancer 1951; 4: 1286–1332.

Inflammatory conditions

INTRODUCTION

In this chapter inflammatory conditions which affect the breast will be considered. Some of these lesions are clearly the result of a response to a local insult such as infection, in others the processes in the breast reflect a local manifestation of systemic disease and in others still the etiology is not established. These lesions are important not only in terms of local symptoms and discomfort, but also because many may exhibit clinical features of malignancy.

DUCT ECTASIA

This is a distinctive lesion involving the major, predominantly subareolar, ducts. A number of terms have been proposed, including 'varicocele tumor of the breast',[1–4] reflecting the clinical and various morphological features of the condition. The term 'duct ectasia' was introduced in 1951 by Haagensen[5] and is now the one most widely employed. The condition of recurrent periareolar abscesses and fistulae is related to duct ectasia in many cases. However as there appear to be at least two separate pathogenic mechanisms for this entity it is discussed separately in the next section.

CLINICAL FEATURES

Mild forms of the condition are asymptomatic and may form part of the spectrum of aberrant involution (ANDI).[6] Clinically evident disease is most common in peri- or postmenopausal women. Presentation varies but a serous, bloody or pus-like nipple discharge may be seen in about 25% of women and may be associated with an underlying palpable mass. Local pain is also common. Episodic acute inflammatory changes may occur and usually subside without treatment within a week or two. With disease progression, fibrotic shortening and thickening of the duct wall occurs and may result in nipple retraction.[4,7]

Furthermore, the acute inflammatory episodes may result in the formation of periareolar abscesses and fistulae or sinuses.[8] Some of these features, particularly nipple retraction associated with an underlying mass, may be mistaken clinically for carcinoma. Characteristic mammographic appearances of dilated subareolar ducts and annular or tubular calcifications are described, but these may be misinterpreted or absent.[9]

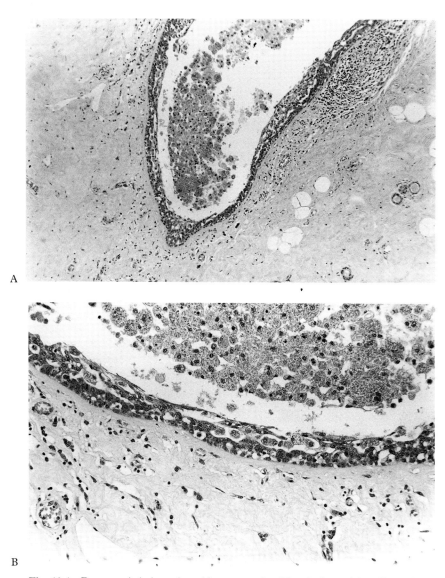

A

B

Fig. 10.1 Duct ectasia in its early and late stages. A mild early form with a dilated duct containing amorphous debris (A) and early active inflammation involving the duct lining epithelium (B). Hematoxylin–eosin, A × 57; B × 400.

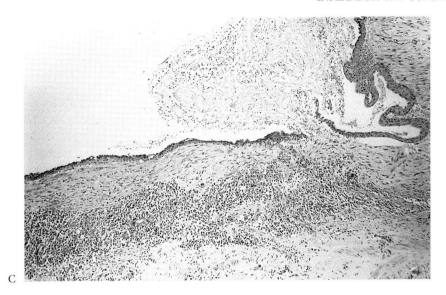

C

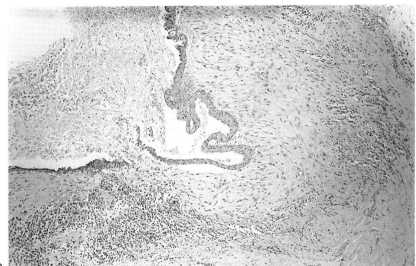

D

Fig. 10.1 Duct ectasia in its early and late stages. In established duct ectasia the inflammatory process extends to involve the duct wall (C) and periductal tissues with associated fibrosis (D). Hematoxylin–eosin, C × 57; D × 57.

MACROSCOPIC FEATURES

As stated above, the disease affects the larger, predominantly subareolar, ducts. Occasionally more peripheral ducts may be affected. Usually, it is confined to a segment which contains palpable dilated ducts filled with pultaceous material resembling comedo-type ductal carcinoma in situ.

MICROSCOPIC FEATURES

Characteristically, the dilated ducts contain amorphous debris, often foamy macrophages and occasionally crystalline structures (Fig. 10.1A). The duct lining epithelium, which may contain interspersed inflammatory cells and foamy macrophages (Fig. 10.1B) may appear ragged in the earlier stages before eventually becoming attenuated. The duct wall and periductal stroma also contain an inflammatory cell infiltrate (Fig. 10.1C) including prominent plasma cells and foamy macrophages, the latter often containing brown ceroid pigment.[10] The infiltrate may be intense and granulomatous with foreign body type giant cells. Alternatively, the plasma cell infiltrate may be sufficiently dense that the term 'plasma cell mastitis' has been applied to the condition.[11] As the disease progresses, fibrosis and reparative changes replace the inflammatory reaction and periductal fibrosis becomes prominent (Fig. 10.1D). Azzopardi has also drawn attention to the formation of eccentric fibrous cushions which may bulge into the duct lumen instead of the more usual concentric periduct fibrosis.[4] Occasionally, fibrous obliteration of the ducts may occur, leaving irregular masses of fibrous and elastic tissue with varying amounts of inflammation.[12] This appearance resulted in the term 'mastitis obliterans' applied by some authors.[2] Regenerating epithelium can produce a garland effect of epithelial lined tubules surrounding the fibrous tissue occupying the original lumen or, more commonly, can produce recanalization of the fibrous plug. Intraluminal mural and periductal calcification may occur.

PATHOGENESIS

Both the pathogenesis and the etiology of duct ectasia remain unknown. Earlier workers regarded duct dilatation as the primary event with periductal inflammation following leakage of duct contents.[3,5] More recently periductal inflammation, which is seen more commonly in younger women, has been considered to be the initial event, proceeding by destruction of elastic tissue, to duct ectasia and periductal fibrosis.[12–14] It has also recently been identified that these initial stages may be precipitated by smoking.[15]

Pregnancy and lactation have also been cited as potential etiological factors, possibly due to mechanical damage to the major ducts. However the disease can occur in nulliparous women[16] and has been described in males[17–19] and in children.[19] Furthermore, in a study of 108 patients with duct ectasia, Dixon et al found no differences in parity or breast feeding in these patients when compared

with age-matched controls suggesting that neither is an important etiological factor.[14]

Haagenesen suggested age-related involutional changes as an etiological factor. However, the rare reports of its occurrence in children[19] argues against this being so in all cases.[20] On the other hand, milder forms of this condition are asymptomatic and autopsy studies indicate they are common, occurring in 25% of clinically normal breasts,[21] leading to the suggestion that such cases form part of the spectrum of aberrant involution (ANDI).[6]

Other proposed etiological factors include hyperprolactinemia[22,23] and congenital inverted nipples.[7]

The role of bacterial infection in the pathogenesis of duct ectasia remains unresolved. While a variety of bacteria including anaerobes have been isolated from non-lactational abscesses and fistulae (see below)[24,25] several workers have been unable to demonstrate bacterial infection in uncomplicated or early lesions of duct ectasia,[26,27] suggesting infection is a secondary and possibly exacerbating factor.

DIFFERENTIAL DIAGNOSIS

The clinical and pathological features of duct ectasia are distinctive and there is little that enters the differential diagnosis. Despite this it has previously been included as part of the spectrum of fibrocystic change. Ectatic ducts are distinguished from cysts by their usual central location, linear configuration, inspissated luminal contents and presence of elastic tissue in the wall. Cysts, on the other hand, are usually round or oval, have empty lumens or contain homogeneous pale material, lack elastic tissue in their wall and often show apocrine metaplasia.

MANAGEMENT AND PROGNOSIS

There is little evidence that antibiotics can provide long-term benefit and symptomatic disease may require excision of the affected segment. Duct ectasia is not associated with any increased cancer risk. Its more frequent occurrence in older women, the age group more likely to have a carcinoma, together with the observation that breasts with duct ectasia tend to be more radiolucent, thereby aiding the mammographic detection of carcinoma, has led to the false impression of a relationship between the two diseases.[28]

MASTITIS

This broad term covers a range of inflammatory lesions of the breast, including some with an infectious etiology and other well-defined entities in which the etiology is unknown.

ACUTE MASTITIS

Cracks in the skin of the nipple or stasis of milk in lactating women may allow direct or retrograde ductal spread of bacteria (commonly *Staphylococcus aureus* or *Streptococcus pyogenes*) and development of localized acute inflammation of the breast. Haagensen has suggested that these skin cracks are the result of a change to an alkaline pH and that the problem may be alleviated by a slightly acidic topical application.[29] Minor inflammation usually resolves. However, occasionally, abscess formation may supervene and may require surgical drainage. Attention to the clinical setting should prevent confusion with other diseases presenting as an abscess-like lesion such as duct ectasia and so-called 'inflammatory carcinoma'.

Breast abscesses, commonly associated with *Staphylococcus aureus* infection, can also occur in neonates and often present in the second or third week of life.[30] The pathogenesis of these abscesses is not clear; physiological breast enlargement and breast manipulation to express colostrum, commonly regarded as etiological factors, were not identified as such in Rudoy and Nelson's review of 39 cases,[30] although they admit that their records were incomplete in many cases. These abscesses are usually treated by antibiotics and surgical drainage.

PERIAREOLAR ABSCESS

Sub- and periareolar abscesses may form part of a separate condition which is not confined to lactating women. Although most common in women of reproductive age, it is found in postmenopausal women and has also been described in men.[31] These abscesses are most commonly associated with duct ectasia (see above) and are now much more common than those occurring in the puerperium. In a retrospective review of women presenting with breast abscesses in Sheffield, UK during a 10 year period (1976–1985) Scholefield et al found only 8.5% of all abscesses occurred in the puerperium, with only 3% occurring in women who were lactating at the time of presentation.[32] Symptoms may persist for several years and multiple recurrences are common.[31] The disease may be bilateral and often associated with congenital or acquired nipple retraction.[24,31] Fistula formation between ducts and skin is common. Histologically, the abscesses may be associated with squamous metaplasia of the lactiferous ducts and plugging by keratin debris. These cases appear to form a distinct subgroup in which squamous metaplasia is probably congenital and associated with an inverted nipple in many cases.[31] Duct ectasia, as discussed above, is strongly implicated in the pathogenesis.[8,32–34] In contrast to abscesses occurring during lactation, a wide variety of bacteria have been isolated from these suppurative lesions, including *Staphylococcus*, *Streptococcus*, *Proteus* and *Bacteroides*; they are often mixed infections which are predominantly anaerobic.[24,25,32,35] Treatment is by drainage and surgical excision of the affected area which may be extensive.

GRANULOMATOUS INFLAMMATIONS OF INFECTIVE ETIOLOGY

Although very rare in most Western countries, mammary tuberculosis continues to be reported[36–38] and recent reports include a case occurring as a presenting manifestation of AIDS.[39] Infection is believed to follow either hematogenous spread from an active or occult focus elsewhere or retrograde lymphatic spread from involved axillary lymph nodes. Over a third of the 28 cases reported by Gottschalk et al occurred in pregnant or lactating women.[36] The lesions may present as a mass or as recurrent abscesses with ulceration and sinus formation and may be mistaken clinically for carcinoma. Rarely the two conditions may coexist.[40]

Histologically, typical caseating granulomas are seen which destroy breast parenchyma. The axillary lymph nodes often also contain granulomata. Caseous lymphadenitis is rare and the presence of necrotizing granulomas in axillary or intra-mammary lymph nodes is generally due to a non-tuberculous, extra-mammary cause such as cat-scratch disease.[41,42] Ideally, both histological identification of acid, alcohol-fast bacilli and isolation of the organism are required for diagnosis. However, bacilli were seen in only two of the 28 cases in the Gottschalk et al series. Diagnostic criteria vary. Symmers[43] emphasizes the need for isolation of the organism to confirm the diagnosis as a number of other infections (e.g. syphilis, cryptococcus), infestations (e.g. Hydatid cyst, Cysticercosis) and iatrogenic causes (e.g. paraffin injection) may result in similar features, whereas other authors are less stringent in their requirements and place more reliance on histological features, even in the absence of identification of acid alcohol fast bacilli in the sections.[38]

Fungal infections of the breast are rare and reported cases include cryptococcosis,[44,45] histoplasmosis,[45,46] blastomycosis[47] and coccidioidomycosis.[48] They may be asymptomatic and detected mammographically or present as a mass, cyst or abscess. Many cause necrotizing granulomatous inflammation resembling tuberculous mastitis. Actinomyces infection is also very rare and usually spreads into the breast from a deep-seated infection of the lung or chest wall. Its manifestations are similar to those in other parts of the body.[41,49] Other rare infections reported in the breast include syphilis, which results in an ulcerating gummatous mastitis[50,51] and filiariasis.[52] Twenty cases of parasitic, mycotic and other rare infections from the files of the Armed Forces Institute of Pathology and interpreted over a 40 year period, have been reviewed by Tavassoli.[53] They include filiariasis, which was the most common (12 cases), leprosy, histoplasmosis, syphilis, cat-scratch disease, molluscum contagiosum and schistosomiasis.

Unusual infections have also been reported in association with prosthetic implants. Symmers reported a case of infection by a species of *Rhizopus* following implantation of a prosthesis[41] and more recently a case of *Mycobacterium fortuitum* infection presenting as recurrent abscesses one month after augmentation mammoplasty has been reported.[54]

Continued recognition of such rare infections in the breast requires a high level of suspicion supplemented by special stains for fungi and other microorganisms where necessary.

EOSINOPHILIC MASTITIS

Intense tissue eosinophilia is rare in the breast. It has been described in three situations. Firstly, in association with parasitic infection which should be excluded in all cases. Secondly, a form of inflammatory infiltrate consisting predominantly of eosinophils and centered on ducts and lobules may occur in the absence of any systemic manifestations and is probably a localized response to leakage of duct contents. Finally, a case has been described in which bilateral eosinophilic mastitis was the presenting manifestation of the hypereosinophilic syndrome.[55]

IDIOPATHIC GRANULOMATOUS MASTITIS

This term 'idiopathic' is employed to contrast this well-defined condition of unknown etiology with other rare specific granulomatous conditions of the breast such as tuberculosis, sarcoidosis and Wegener's granulomatosis (see p. 197). Kessler and Wolloch described five cases in 1972[56] and several further reports have been described since.[57–61]

CLINICAL FEATURES

Granulomatous mastitis generally occurs in women of reproductive age and has been associated with recent pregnancy although Going et al describe two cases in which the last pregnancy was 15 years prior to presentation.[61] Clinically, despite the relatively young age group affected, carcinoma may be suspected due to its presentation as a palpable mass which is often but not always tender and which may be associated with axillary lymphadenopathy. The disease may be bilateral.

MACROSCOPIC FEATURES

The masses are generally ill-defined and in size range from 0.5 to 8 cm.[61] There are no characteristic gross features, but the tissue cut surface usually has a variable character and may appear fibrous, show features of fat necrosis with yellow areas or show evidence of microabscess formation with visible flecks of inflammatory exudate.

MICROSCOPIC FEATURES

Characteristically, a granulomatous inflammatory cell infiltrate including epithelioid histiocytes, occasional Langhans-type giant cells, lymphocytes, plasma cells and neutrophil polymorphs is centered on and distorts lobules. Extension into surrounding tissue with microabscess formation may occur in more advanced disease (Figs 10.2, 10.3). Specific etiological features are absent. Apart from within the microabscesses, no necrosis or caseation is seen and neither foreign material nor infective agents should be identifiable. Vasculitis has not been described and if found should suggest an alternative diagnosis.

PATHOGENESIS

Both pathogenesis and etiology are unknown although a number of observations have been made. For example, an association with recent pregnancy and hyperprolactinemia has been noted.[59–62] These are not absolute requirements for the development of the condition and the most recent pregnancy may have been several years previously.[61] An infective etiology is unlikely, given that organisms have never been identified either histologically or following culture. However, such an etiology factor cannot yet be totally dismissed. Finally, the possibility of an immune etiology was suggested by Kessler and Wolloch because of the morphological resemblance to granulomatous orchitis.[56] More recently, Axelsen and Reasbeck have described a case showing intense mononuclear cell infiltration of ductular epithelium associated with apoptotic bodies suggesting a role for cell mediated destruction of mammary epithelium.[63] Immunological abnormalities were not identified in these patients to confirm this.

A plausible unifying hypothesis has been offered by Fletcher and colleagues. They suggest that the granulomatous response is a reaction to ductular epithelial damage of any sort, whether infective, chemical, traumatic or immunologically mediated, which allows leakage of luminal contents into the lobular connective tissue.[59]

DIFFERENTIAL DIAGNOSIS

This diagnosis is essentially one of exclusion. An infective etiology should always be considered and fresh tissue obtained for culture wherever possible. For the same reason, special stains for mycobacteria and fungi should always be performed. Other differential diagnoses to be considered include sarcoidosis and Wegener's granulomatosis and appropriate clinical information should be sought.

MANAGEMENT AND PROGNOSIS

Response to high dose steroid treatment has been described[59,64] but requires further evaluation. Currently, refractory cases require surgical excision. There is, however, a tendency for recurrence postsurgery and postoperative wound infection appears to be a particular problem.[57–59]

SARCOIDOSIS

Sarcoidosis rarely involves the breast and when it does so is usually associated with extra-mammary manifestations, thereby producing little diagnostic difficulty.[65,66] Indeed, in some of the earlier reports, confirmatory biopsy evidence of breast involvement was not obtained.[67–69] However, cases

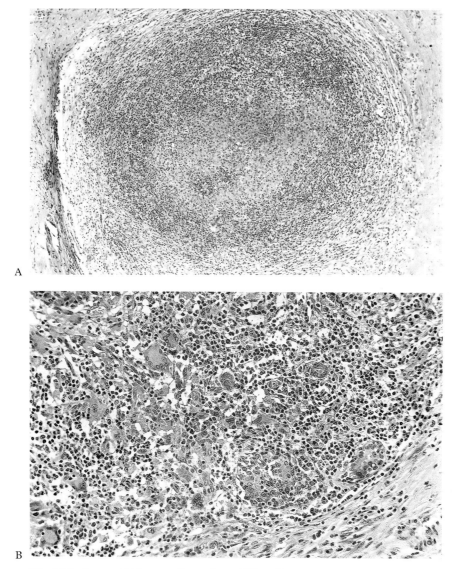

Fig. 10.2   Low and high power illustrations of idiopathic granulomatous mastitis showing the lobulocentric nature of the inflammatory process (A) and the cellular constituents of the granulomatous inflammatory infiltrate. Hematoxylin–eosin, A × 57; B × 185.

are reported in which the disease has presented in the breast[70–72] although the diagnosis does not appear to have been substantiated clinically in all reported cases.[71,73]

The breast lesions present as single, multiple or bilateral nodules and may simulate carcinoma. The histological features are similar to those found in other sites, namely, non-caseating epithelioid granulomata with multinucleate giant cells and occasional central fibrinoid hyalinization which are found in both the lobules and interlobular stroma. The diagnosis requires both exclusion of other causes of a granulomatous mastitis and confirmatory clinical evidence of sarcoidosis. If such confirmatory evidence is not found then an alternative diagnosis such as idiopathic granulomatous mastitis should be considered. It is also worth noting that sarcoid-like

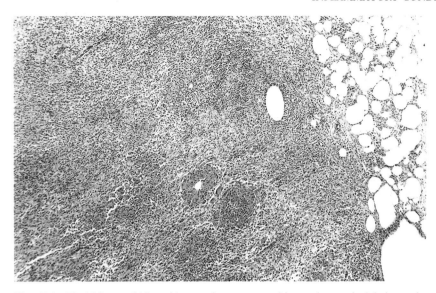

Fig. 10.3   Florid forms of idiopathic granulomatous mastitis may loosen the lobulocentric arrangement of inflammation and be associated with abscess formation. Hematoxylin–eosin × 57.

epithelioid granulomata may be seen in axillary lymph nodes in association with breast carcinoma and may be mistaken as a manifestation of sarcoidosis.[41]

LYMPHOCYTIC MASTOPATHY

This entity has been recognized under a variety of terms including fibrous mastopathy,[74] fibrous disease of the breast[75] and, more recently, sclerosing lymphocytic lobulitis[76] and lymphocytic mastopathy,[76–79] all reflecting the morphological features. Another recognized designation, diabetic mastopathy,[80,81] indicates its association with diabetes mellitus. Despite reluctance to accept some of the earlier descriptions of predominantly sclerotic lesions as truly pathological rather than an exaggerated involutional process, lymphocytic mastopathy is now emerging as a distinct clinico-pathological entity in which there is a strong association with autoimmune disease.

CLINICAL FEATURES

This condition affects predominantly young and middle aged women but overall has a wide age range of 19 to 72 years. It presents as a firm, ill-defined, palpable mass which is usually painless but may be tender. In some cases the masses are bilateral and the disease has been described in men.[81] There may be a personal or family history of autoimmune disease, particularly diabetes mellitus, as discussed in the section on pathogenesis.

MACROSCOPIC FEATURES

Resected mass lesions consist of ill-defined firm rubbery grey-white tissue reflecting the fibrosis but otherwise unremarkable. Reported cases range from 0.8 to 6 cm in size.

MICROSCOPIC FEATURES

Varying degrees of perivascular and lobulocentric lymphocytic infiltration and stromal fibrosis occur with obliteration of ducts and lobules (Fig. 10.4). Although endothelial cell swelling is described, there is no true vasculitis. There is an apparent morphological progression from an initial stage in which there is a dense lobular lymphoid infiltrate (Fig. 10.4) followed by increasing lobular sclerosis and atrophy accompanied by reduction of the lymphoid infiltrate (Fig. 10.5). The infiltrate is predominantly B-cell, polyclonal and may include

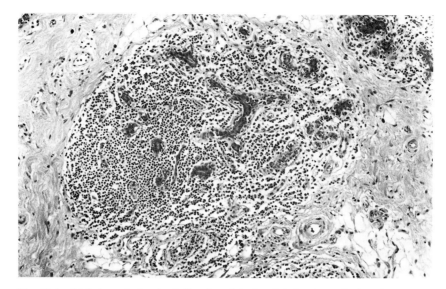

Fig. 10.4   A lobular unit showing infiltration of the intralobular stroma by lymphocytes with little extension into the surrounding tissue, typical of lymphocytic mastopathy. Hematoxylin–eosin × 185.

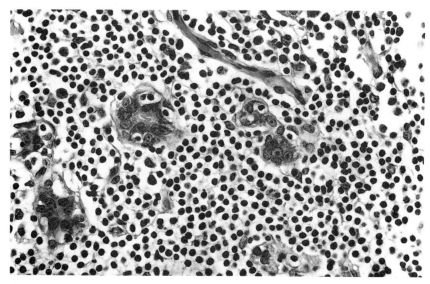

Fig. 10.5   The lymphoid cell infiltrate in lymphocytic mastopathy is composed of small mature lymphocytes. Note that there is some infiltration of the epithelial acini. Hematoxylin–eosin × 400.

follicles with germinal centers. Intra-epithelial lymphocytes are typically prominent and may form lymphoepithelial lesions. Lammie et al[76] describe a case showing epithelial destruction associated with a dense lymphohistiocytic infiltrate containing giant cells. Large epithelioid stromal cells have been noted by some and may be dispersed as isolated cells or in clusters in the sclerotic stroma.[81,82] They may be mistaken for infiltrating carcinoma, but show negative immunohistochemical staining for cytokeratins and have been found to contain actin, favoring a myofibroblastic origin.

PATHOGENESIS

Well-documented associations with diabetes mellitus, thyroiditis and arthropathy[75,77,80,81] and some similarity between the histological features of lymphocytic mastopathy and those of pancreatic 'insulitis', Sjögren's syndrome and Hashimoto's thyroiditis suggest an autoimmune pathogenesis. This has been investigated further by Lammie et al.[76] Three of the 13 women in their series had type 1 diabetes mellitus and one had Hashimoto's disease diagnosed 5 months after presenting with bilateral lymphocytic mastopathy. These investigators were able to confirm previous findings of increased HLA-DR antigen expression in involved lobular epithelium[77] and an association with HLA-DR 3 or 4 status,[75] itself associated with autoimmune disease. Furthermore, autoantibodies were identified in four of seven patients investigated; in two of the diabetic women, a woman subsequently identified as having Hashimoto's disease and a fourth woman not known to be suffering from an autoimmune disease in whom smooth muscle antibodies were found. These cases demonstrate that although the pathogenesis of lymphocytic mastopathy is far from certain, autoimmunity appears to be strongly implicated.

DIFFERENTIAL DIAGNOSIS

A number of breast lesions may be associated with marked lymphocytic infiltration and enter the differential diagnosis. In duct ectasia the infiltrate is periductal rather than lobulocentric and the infiltrate is predominantly T-cell rather than B cell.[83] Dense lymphoid infiltrates may also accompany carcinoma but again, these tend to be periductal and to be predominantly T-cell.[83] However, lobular carcinoma in situ may be associated with an intense lymphocytic mastopathy-like infiltrate and a recent case report describes lymphocytic mastopathy in association with invasive lobular carcinoma.[84] For these reasons, careful attention should be given to the epithelial elements before interpreting a lobulocentric lymphocytic infiltrate as lymphocytic mastopathy.

MANAGEMENT AND PROGNOSIS

Palpable lumps are often resected but recurrences, often at different sites, are not uncommon. The morphological similarities with Hashimoto's thyroiditis and Sjögren's syndrome and the increased incidence of lymphoma in these conditions, raises the possibility that lymphocytic mastopathy might precede the development of mammary lymphoma of MALT type. A recent study from Japan supports this assertion.[79] The authors examined 19 cases of primary non-Hodgkin's lymphoma of the breast and in 11 of these, found histological evidence of lymphocytic mastopathy. Half of these lymphomas showed features of MALT type. Interestingly, none of their patients had any clinical history of autoimmune disease. The significance of their findings in terms of follow-up and prognosis of women presenting with lymphocytic mastopathy has yet to be evaluated. It should be noted that this Japanese series of breast lymphoma appears to be different from two European series[85,86] and a more recent case report[87] in which lymphomas of predominantly high-grade B-cell type without specific features of MALT lymphoma occurring in older women were associated with perilobular lymphoid infiltrates in which there is a predominance of T-cells, and not typical of lymphocytic mastopathy.

PLASMA CELL GRANULOMA

A single case of plasma cell granuloma or inflammatory pseudotumor has been reported[88] in a 29-year-old woman who presented with a 3.5 cm tender, mobile breast mass of one year's duration. As in similar lesions described elsewhere, histological examination revealed a prominent plasma cell infiltrate in a hyalinized fibrous stroma with scattered lymphocytes and fibroblasts. No recurrence was recorded 30 months after surgical excision.

VASCULITIDES

Wegener's granulomatosis,[89–93] gaint cell arteritis[94–98] and polyarteritis nodosa[99] have all, rarely, been described in the breast. The average age at presentation of the reported cases is in the mid forties for Wegener's granulomatosis and in the mid sixties for giant cell arteritis and polyarteritis nodosa. In each condition the disease may present as a breast mass which may be tender and bilateral. The size of the reported lesions ranges from 1 to 8 cm with an average of 3 cm and nipple retraction and skin tethering have been described. Often the clinical impression is of malignancy. Whereas systemic involvement is invariable in Wegener's granulomatosis, giant cell arteritis and polyarteritis nodosa can remain localized to the breast and such localized disease appears to have an excellent prognosis based on the limited follow-up information available.

RHEUMATOID NODULE

A single case of rheumatoid nodule has been reported[100] in a woman with a 12-year history of rheumatoid arthritis who presented with a breast lump associated with pain and nipple discharge. The histological features were typical of rheumatoid nodules occurring elsewhere.

FAT NECROSIS

While commonly seen in association with duct ectasia and in the region of a recent biopsy site or following irradiation, isolated fat necrosis presenting as a clinically detectable mass is an unusual but well recognized clinical entity, accounting for approximately one in 200 resected lesions in one series.[101] Most cases are believed to result from local trauma, although such a history is only obtained in a minority of patients and local ischemia may be a factor in some cases. Mammographically, fat necrosis may show a characteristic benign ring-like calcification[102] representing calcification of a lipid cyst wall. However, the mammographic appearances may mimic almost any other type of pathology.[103] The associated inflammation and subsequent scarring may result in pain, tenderness and fixation to the overlying skin and can clinically mimic both abscess and carcinoma.

Most lesions are small, with an average size of less than 2 cm, firm and fixed to adjacent tissues. Slicing reveals a rounded outline with an indurated appearance often with hemorrhage in early lesions and oily, cystic areas in older ones. Eventually, the area may be replaced by a fibrous scar or transform into a thick walled cyst which may become calcified.

The histological appearances are well described. Foamy macrophages accumulate around the periphery of early lesions and foreign body-type giant cells surround fat globules (Fig. 10.6). Hemosiderin indicating previous hemorrhage may be seen. As the lesion ages, fibrosis becomes more prominent and dystrophic calcification may occur.

COUMARIN (WARFARIN) NECROSIS

Tissue necrosis is a rare but well-recognized complication of treatment with coumarin anticoagulants such as warfarin. The necrosis has a tendency to involve the breasts;[104,105] bilateral involvement has been reported.[106] The pathophysiology of the condition appears to involve an imbalance between circulating clotting and anticoagulant factors, with initiation of the coumarin therapy reducing the anticoagulant, protein C, levels before the levels of the clotting factors prothrombin, Factor IX and Factor X fall, thereby inducing a hypercoaguable state.[107]

Clinically, several days after initiation of the anticoagulant, local pain, swelling and echymoses appear, to be followed by blistering, ulceration and necrosis. Histologically, viable areas are interspersed with foci of hemorrhage and necrosis associated with thrombosis of small veins and arteries and a variable inflammatory cell infiltrate. Although spontaneous healing may occur following conservative treatment and discontinuation of the anticoagulant,[108] the majority of cases have required mastectomy.

TISSUE REACTION TO BREAST IMPLANTS

There is much controversy regarding the systemic effects associated with silicone implants, but the

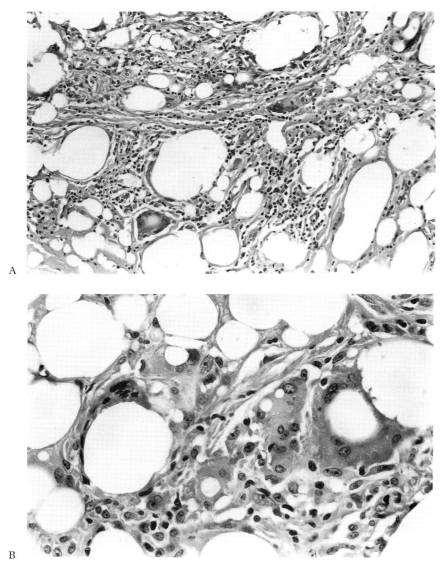

Fig. 10.6A,B Traumatic fat necrosis is typified by florid infiltration of adipose tissue by macrophages and multinucleate giant cells. A lake of released lipid can also be seen in this example. Hematoxylin–eosin, A × 185; B × 400.

local effects are well described. The majority of implants are composed of silicone gel surrounded by a capsule composed of silicone elastomer. A fibrous capsule develops around the prosthesis and in some cases contraction of this capsule is sufficient to require either capsulotomy or removal of the prosthesis and periprosthetic tissue. Histological examination of such specimens confirms the presence of fibrous scarring and capsule formation. Several recent studies have identified

a cellular lining at the implant-tissue interface composed of cells with histological, immunohistochemical and ultrastructural features of synovial cells.[109–113] Within the fibrous capsule itself, relatively large fragments of foreign material may be seen (Fig. 10.7) representing either silicone elastomer or birefringent talc granules. These elicit a typical foreign body granulomatous response. With time a dense fibrous capsule may be formed which can undergo focal microcalcifi-

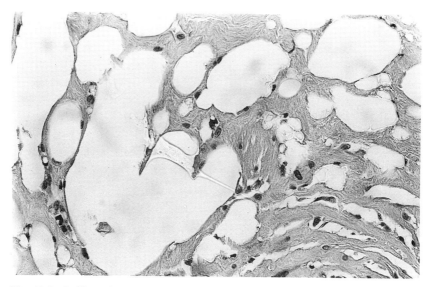

Fig. 10.7 A silicone implant capsulotomy specimen composed of collagenous fibrous tissue containing deposits of silicone gel. Hematoxylin–eosin × 185.

cation (Fig. 10.8). Peripheral to this is a zone of vacuoles and foamy macrophages filled with finely dispersed non-birefringent, silicone gel, much of which may have dissolved during processing.

Some modifications to this appearance may be seen with different types of implant. For example, Kasper has described a reaction to a saline implant surrounded by silicone elastomer; fibrous scarring and foreign body reaction to silicone elas-

tomer were seen as above but the peripheral zone of vacuolation and foamy macrophages were, not surprisingly, absent.[113] Capsules associated with polyurethane-covered implants contained non-polarizing or partially polarizing geometrical crystals associated with a prominent foreign body tissue response.[113]

The foregoing descriptions refer to tissue responses associated with intact implants. Should

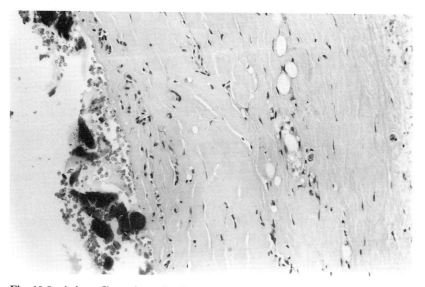

Fig. 10.8 A dense fibrous breast implant capsule showing focal calcification. Hematoxylin–eosin × 125.

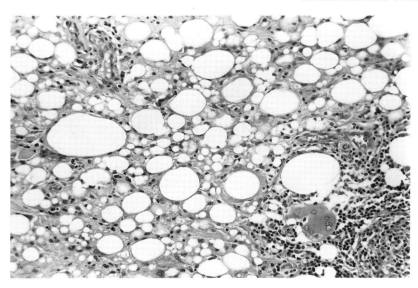

Fig. 10.9 Rupture of a silicone implant results in a florid foreign body type giant cell reaction resembling fat necrosis. Hematoxylin–eosin × 185.

a silicone gel implant rupture, then large tumor-like silicone granulomas form, composed of lake-like accumulations of liquid silicone surrounded by sheets of foamy macrophages and foreign body macrophages (Fig. 10.9). Clinically, these may be confused with carcinomas and may be sited some distance from the implant as a result of the tendency for liquid silicone to migrate through tissue.

The development of silicone granulomas following implant rupture is the result of a normal foreign body inflammatory reaction. However, the fibrous scarring and tissue reactions associated with intact prostheses are less easy to explain. Silicone gel is known to migrate or 'bleed' from an intact bag-gel implant into periprosthetic tissue[114–116] and there is evidence to suggest that the extent of the tissue reaction is related to the amount of this silicone bleed.[117,118] It has been postulated[117] that silicone gel enters the soft tissue surrounding the implant where it is ingested by macrophages, resulting in the release of a variety of cytokines trophic for fibroblasts and myofibroblasts among other cells which in turn are responsible for collagen synthesis and capsular contracture.

The pathogenesis of the synovial-like metaplasia lining the fibrous capsules remains unknown but similar changes have been described at other sites surrounding orthopedic prostheses, in skin following surgical procedures and in subcutaneous tissue following injection of air or oily fluids,[109] suggesting it represents a fundamental biological phenomenon rather than a specific response to silicone implants.

REFERENCES

1. Bloodgood JC. The clinical picture of dilated ducts beneath the nipple-The varicocoele tumour of the breast. Surg Gynaecol Obstet 1923; 36: 486–495.
2. Payne RL, Straus AF, Glasser RE. Mastitis obliterans. Surgery 1943; 14: 719–727.
3. Tice GE, Dockerty MB, Harrington SW. Comedomastitis. A clinical and pathological study of data in 172 cases. Surg Gynecol Obstet 1948; 51: 350–355.
4. Azzopardi JG. Cystic disease and duct ectasia. In: Problems in Breast Pathology. Philadelphia: W B Saunders, 1979; pp. 72–87.
5. Haagensen CD. Mammary duct ectasia — a disease that may simulate carcinoma. Cancer 1951; 4: 749–761.
6. Hughes LE, Mansel RE, Webster DJT. Aberrations of normal development and involution (ANDI): A new perspective on pathogenesis and nomenclature of benign breast disorders. Lancet 1987; ii: 1316–1319.

7. Rees BI, Gravelle H, Hughes LE. Nipple retraction in duct ectasia. Br J Surg 1977; 64: 577–580.
8. Abramson DJ. Mammary duct ectasia, mammillary fistula and subareolar abscess. Ann Surg 1969; 169: 217–226.
9. Millis RR. Mammography. In: Azzopardi JG, ed. Problems in Breast Pathology. Philadelphia: WB Saunders, 1979; pp. 437–459.
10. Davies JD. Pigmented periductal cells (ochrocytes) in mammary dysplasia: Their nature and significance. J Pathol 1974; 114: 205–216.
11. Haagensen CD. In: Diseases of the Breast. 3rd ed. Philadelphia: W B Saunders, 1986; p. 362.
12. Davies JD. Inflammatory damage to ducts in mammary dysplasia: A cause of duct obliteration. J Pathol 1975; 117: 47–54.
13. Bonser GM, Dossett JA, Jull JW. Human and Experimental Breast Cancer. London: Pitman Medical, 1961.
14. Dixon JM, Anderson TJ, Lumsden AB, Elton RA, Roberts MM, Forrest APM. Mammary duct ectasia. Br J Surg 1983; 70: 601–603.
15. Bundred NJ, Dover MS, Aluwihare N, Faragher EB, Morrison JM. Smoking and periductal mastitis. Br Med J 1993; 307: 772–773.
16. Walker JC, Sandison AT. Mammary duct ectasia. A clinical study. Br J Surg 1964; 512: 350–355.
17. Tedeschi LG, McCarthy PE. Involutional mammary duct ectasia and periductal mastitis in a male. Hum Pathol 1974; 5: 532–536.
18. Ashworth MT, Corcoran GD, Haqqani MT. Periductal mastitis and mammary duct ectasia in a male. Postgrad Med J 1985; 61: 621–623.
19. Stringel G, Perelman A, Jimenez C. Infantile mammary duct ectasia: a cause of bloody nipple discharge. J Pediat Surg 1986; 21: 671–674.
20. Haagensen CD. In: Diseases of the Breast. 3rd ed. Philadelphia: WB Saunders, 1986; pp. 357–368.
21. Frantz VK, Pickren JW, Melcher GW, Auchincloss H. Incidence of cystic disease in so-called 'normal breasts'. A study based on 225 postmortem examinations. Cancer 1951; 4: 762–783.
22. Peters F, Schuth W. Hyperprolactinemia and nonpuerperal mastitis (duct ectasia). JAMA 1989; 261: 1618–1620.
23. Shousha S, Backhouse CM, Dawson PM, Alaghband-Zadeh J, Burn I. Mammary duct ectasia and pituitary adenomas. Am J Surg Pathol 1988; 12: 130–133.
24. Leach RD, Eyken SJ, Phillips I et al. Anaerobic subareolar breast abscess. Lancet 1979; 1: 35–37.
25. Walker AP, Edmiston CE, Krepel CJ et al. A prospective study of microflora of non-puerperal breast abscess. Arch Surg 1988; 123: 908–911.
26. Aitken RJ, Hood J, Going JJ, Miles RS, Forrest AP. Bacteriology of mammary duct ectasia. Br J Surg 1988; 75: 1040–1041.
27. Hughes LE. Non-lactational inflammation and duct ectasia. Br Med Bull 1991; 47: 272–283.
28. Young GB. Mammography in carcinoma of the breast. J Roy Coll Surg Edin 1968; 13: 12–33.
29. Haagensen CD. In: Diseases of the Breast. 3rd ed. Philadelphia: W B Saunders, 1986; pp. 384–393.
30. Rudoy RC, Nelson JD. Breast abscesses during the neonatal period. A review. Am J Dis Child 1975; 129: 1031–1034.
31. Habif D, Perzin K, Lattes R. Subareolar abscess associated with squamous metaplasia. Am J Surg 1970; 119: 523–526.
32. Scholefield JH, Duncan JL, Rogers K. Review of a hospital experience of breast abscesses. Br J Surg 1987; 74: 469–470.
33. Sandison AT, Walker JC. Inflammatory mastitis, mammary duct ectasia and mammillary fistula. Br J Surg 1962; 50: 57–64.
34. Bundred NJ, Dixon JM, Chetty U, Forrest AP. Mammillary fistula. Br J Surg 1987; 74: 466–468.
35. Edmiston C Jr, Walker AP, Krepel CJ, Gohr C. The nonpuerperal breast infection: aerobic and anaerobic microbial recovery from acute and chronic disease. J Infect Dis 1990; 162: 695–699.
36. Gottschalk FAB, Decker GAG, Schmaman A. Tuberculosis of the breast. S Afr J Surg 1976; 14: 19–22.
37. Apps MC, Harrison NK, Blauth CI. Tuberculosis of the breast. Br Med J 1984; 288: 1874–1875.
38. Sharma PK, Babel AL, Yadav SS. Tuberculosis of breast (study of 7 cases). J Postgrad Med 1991; 37: 24–26.
39. Hartstein M, Leaf HL. Tuberculosis of the breast as a presenting manifestation of AIDS. Clin Infect Dis 1992; 15: 692–693.
40. Miller RE, Salomon PF, West JP. The coexistence of carcinoma and tuberculosis of the breast and axillary lymph nodes. Am J Surg 1982; 121: 338–340.
41. Symmers WSC. The Breasts. In: Symmers WSC, ed. Systemic Pathology. Edinburgh: Churchill Livingstone, 1978; vol. 4, pp. 1759–1861.
42. Lefkowitz M, Wear DJ. Cat-scratch disease masquerading as a solitary tumour of the breast. Arch Pathol Lab Med 1989; 113: 473–475.
43. Symmers WSC, McKeown KC. Tuberculosis of the breast. Br Med J 1989; 289: 48–49.
44. Symmers WSJ. Deep-seated fungal infections currently seen in histopathologic service of a medical school laboratory in Britain. Am J Clin Pathol 1966; 46: 515–537.
45. Salfelder K, Schwarz J. Mycotic 'pseudotumour' of the breast: Report of four cases. Arch Surg 1975; 110: 751–754.
46. Osborne BM. Granulomatous mastitis caused by Histoplasma and mimicking inflammatory breast carcinoma. Hum Pathol 1989; 20: 47–52.
47. Azzopardi JG. Miscellaneous entities. In: Problems in Breast Pathology. London: WB Saunders, 1979; p. 400.
48. Bocian JJ, Fahmy RN, Michas CA. A rare case of 'coccidioidoma' of the breast. Arch Pathol Lab Med (United States) 1991; 115: 1064–1067.
49. Jain BK, Sehgal VN, Jagdish S, Ratnakar C, Smile SR. Primary actinomycosis of the breast: a clinical review and a case report. J Dermatol 1994; 21: 497–500.
50. Whitaker HT, Moore RM. Gumma of the breast. Surg Gynecol Obstet 1954; 98: 473.
51. Yuehan C, Qun X. Filiarial granuloma of the female breast: A histopathological study of 131 cases. Am J Trop Med Hyg 1981; 30: 1206–1210.
52. MacDougall LT, Magoon CC, Fritsche TR. Dirofilaria repens manifesting as a breast nodule. Diagnostic problems and epidemiologic considerations. Am J Clin Pathol 1992; 97: 625–630.

53. Tavassoli FA. Miscellaneous lesions. In: Pathology of the Breast. Appleton and Lange, 1992; pp. 621–622.

54. Juang YC, Wang LS, Chen CH, Lin CY. Mycobacterium fortuitum mastitis following augmentation mammaplasty: report of a case. Taiwan I Hsueh Hui Tsa Chih 1989; 88: 278–281.

55. Thompson AB, Barron MM, Lapp NL. The hypereosinophilic syndrome presenting with eosinophilic mastitis. Arch Intern Med 1985; 145: 564–565.

56. Kessler E, Wooloch Y. Granulomatous mastitis; a lesion clinically simulating carcinoma. Am J Clin Pathol 1972; 58: 642–646.

57. Koelmeyer TD, MacCormick DEM. Granulomatous mastitis. Aust NZ J Surg 1976; 46: 173–176.

58. Brown LK, Tang PHL. Post-lactational tumoral granulomatous mastitis: a localised immune phenomenon. Am J Surg 1979; 138: 326–329.

59. Fletcher A, Magrath IM, Riddel RH, Talbot IC. Granulomatous mastitis: A report of seven cases. J Clin Pathol 1982; 35: 941–945.

60. Davies JD, Burton PA. Post-partum lobular granulomatous mastitis. J Clin Pathol 1983; 36: 363.

61. Going JJ, Anderson TJ, Wilkinson S, Chetty U. Granulomatous lobular mastitis. J Clin Pathol 1987; 40: 535–540.

62. Rowe PH. Granulomatous mastitis associated with a pituitary prolactinoma. Br J Clin Pract 1984; 38: 32–34.

63. Axelsen RA, Reasbeck P. Granulomatous lobular mastitis: report of a case with previously undescribed histopathological abnormalities. Pathology 1988; 20: 383–389.

64. DeHertogh DA, Rossof AH, Harris AA, Economou SG. Prednisone management of granulomatous mastitis. N Eng J Med 1980; 303: 799–800.

65. Scadding JG. Sarcoidosis. In: London: Eyre and Spottiswoode, 1967; p. 335.

66. Ross MJ, Merino MJ. Sarcoidosis of the breast. Hum Pathol 1985; 16: 185–187.

67. Strandberg J. Contribution a la question de la clinique et de la pathologenie de la sarcoide de Boeck. Acta Derm Venereol 1921; 2: 253–257.

68. Reisner D. Boeck's sarcoid and systemic sarcoidosis: a study of 35 cases. Am Rev Tuberc 1944; 437: 462.

69. Longcope T, Freiman DG. A study of sarcoidosis. Medicine 1952; 31: 1–121.

70. Stallard HB, Tait CB. Boeck's sarcoidosis: a case record. Lancet 1939; 1: 440–442.

71. Fitzgibbons PL, Smiley DF, Kern WH. Sarcoidosis presenting initially as a breast mass: report of two cases. Hum Pathol 1985; 16: 851–852.

72. Banik S, Bishop PW, Ormerod LP. Sarcoidosis of the breast. J Clin Pathol 1986; 39: 446–448.

73. Rigden B. Sarcoid lesion in breast after probable sarcoidosis in lung. Br Med J 1978; 2: 1533–1534.

74. Minkowitz S, Hedayati H, Hiller S, Gardner B. Fibrous mastopathy: A clinical histopathologic study. Cancer 1973; 32: 913–916.

75. Soler NG, Khardori R. Fibrous disease of the breast, thyroiditis and cheiroarthropathy in type I diabetes mellitus. Lancet 1984; 1: 193–194.

76. Lammie GA, Bobrow LG, Staunton MD, Levison DA, Page G, Millis RR. Sclerosing lymphocytic lobulitis of the breast-evidence for an autoimmune pathogenesis. Histopathology 1991; 19: 13–20.

77. Schwartz IS, Strauchen JA. Lymphocytic mastopathy. An autoimmune disease of the breast? Am J Clin Path 1990; 93: 725–730.

78. Mills SE. Lymphocytic mastopathy, a 'new' autoimmune disease? Am J Clin Pathol 1990; 93: 834–835.

79. Aozasa K, Ohsawa M, Saeki K, Horiuchi K, Kawano K, Taguchi T. Malignant lymphoma of the breast. Immunologic type and association with lymphocytic mastopathy. Am J Clin Pathol 1992; 97: 699–704.

80. Byrd B Jr, Hartmann WH, Graham LS, Hogle HH. Mastopathy in insulin-dependent diabetics. Ann Surg 1987; 205: 529–532.

81. Tomaszewski JE, Brook JSJ, Hicks D, Livolsi VA. Diabetic mastopathy: A distinctive clinicopathologic entity. Hum Pathol 1992; 23: 780–786.

82. Ashton MA, Lefkowitz M, Tavassoli FA. Epithelioid stromal cells in lymphocytic mastitis — a source of confusion with invasive carcinoma. Mod Pathol 1994; 7: 49–54.

83. Giorno R. Mononuclear cells in malignant and benign human breast tissue. Arch Pathol Lab Med 1983; 107: 415–417.

84. Chetty R, Butler AE. Lymphocytic mastopathy associated with infiltrating lobular breast carcinoma. J Clin Pathol 1993; 46: 376–377.

85. Bobrow LG, Richards MA, Happerfield LC et al. Breast lymphomas: a clinicopathological review. Hum Pathol 1993; 24: 274–278.

86. Hansen TG, Ottesen GL, Pedersen NT, Anderson JA. Primary non-Hodgkin's lymphoma of the breast (PLB): a clinicopathological study of seven cases. APMIS 1992; 100: 1089–1096.

87. Rooney N, Snead D, Goodman S, Webb AJ. Primary breast lymphoma with skin involvement arising in lymphocytic lobulitis. Histopathology 1994; 24: 81–84.

88. Pettinato G, Manivel JC, Insabato L, De Chiara A, Petrella G. Plasma cell granuloma (inflammatory pseudotumor) of the breast. Am J Clin Pathol 1988; 90: 627–632.

89. Elsner B, Harper FB. Disseminated Wegener's granulomatosis with breast involvement. Arch Pathol 1969; 87: 544–547.

90. Pambakian H, Tighe JR. Breast involvement in Wegener's granulomatosis. J Clin Pathol 1971; 24: 343–347.

91. Oimoni M, Suehiro I, Mizuno N, Baba S, Okada S, Kanazawa Y. Wegener's granulomatosis with intracerebral granuloma and mammary manifestation. Arch Intern Med 1980; 140: 853–854.

92. Deininger HZ. Wegener's granulomatosis of the breast. Radiology 1985; 154: 59–60.

93. Jordan JM, Rowe WT, Allen NB. Wegener's granulomatosis involving the breast. Report of three cases and review of the literature. Am J Med 1987; 83: 159–164.

94. Potter BT, Housley E, Thomson D. Giant-cell arteritis mimicking carcinoma of the breast. Br Med J 1981; 282: 1665–1666.

95. Thaell SF, Saue GL. Giant cell arteritis involving the breasts. J Rheumatol 1983; 10: 329–331.

96. Nirodi NS, Stirling WJI, White MFI. Giant cell arteritis presenting as a breast lump. Br J Clin Pract 1985; 39: 84–86.

97. Stephenson TJ, Underwood JCE. Giant cell arteritis: An unusual cause of palpable masses in the breast. Br J Surg 1986; 73: 105.

98. McKendry RJR, Guindi M, Hill DP. Giant cell arteritis (temporal arteritis) affecting the breast: report of two cases and review of published reports. Ann Rheum Dis 1990; 49: 1001–1004.

99. Ng WF, Chow LTC, Lam PWY. Localized polyarteritis of the breast — report of two cases and a review of the literature. Histopathology 1993; 23: 535–539.

100. Cooper NE. Rheumatoid nodule in the breast. Histopathology 1991; 19: 193–194.

101. Meyer JE, Silverman P, Gandbhir L. Fat necrosis of the breast. Arch Surg 1978; 113: 801–805.

102. Orson LW, Cigtay OS. Fat necrosis of the breast: Characteristic xeromammographic appearance. Radiology 1983; 146: 35–38.

103. Roebuck EJ. Clinical Radiology of the Breast. Oxford: Heinemann Medical Books, 1990.

104. Nudelman HL, Kempson RL. Necrosis of the breast: A rare complication of anticoagulant therapy. Am J Surg 1966; 111: 728–733.

105. Manstein CH, Steerman PH, Goldstein J. Sodium warfarin-induced gangrene of the breast. Ann Plast Surg 1985; 15: 161–162.

106. Lopez Valle CA, Herbert G. Warfarin-induced complete bilateral breast necrosis. Br J Plast Surg 1992; 45: 606–609.

107. Clouse LH, Comp PC. The regulation of haemostasis: The protein C system. N Engl J Med 1986; 314: 1298–1304.

108. Mason JR. Haemorrhage induced breast gangrene. Br J Surg 1970; 57: 700–702.

109. Chase DR, Oberg KC, Chase RL, Marlott RL, Weeks DA. Pseudoepithelialization of breast implant capsules. Int J Surg Pathol 1994; 1: 151–154.

110. Raso DS, Crymes LW, Metcalf JS. Histological assessment of fifty breast capsules from smooth and textured augmentation and reconstruction mammoplast prostheses with emphasis on the role of synovial metaplasia. Mod Pathol 1994; 7: 310–316.

111. del Rosario AD, Bui HY, Singh J, Petrocine S, Sheehan C, Ross JS. The synovial metaplasia of breast implant capsules: a light and electron microscopic study (Abstract). Lab Invest 1994; 70: 14A.

112. Hameed M, Erlanson R, Rosen PP. Capsular synovial metaplasia around mammary implants, similar to detritic synovitis: a morphologic and immunohistochemical study of 15 cases (Abstract). Lab Invest 1994; 70: 16A.

113. Kasper CS. Histologic features of breast capsules reflect surface configuration and composition of silicone bag implants. Am J Clin Pathol 1994; 102: 655–659.

114. Barker DE, Retsky MI, Schultz S. 'Bleeding' of silicone from bag-gel implants and its clinical relation to fibrous capsule reaction. Plas Reconstr Surg 1978; 61: 836–841.

115. Bergman RB, van der Ende AE. Exudation of silicone through the envelope of gel-filled breast prostheses. An in vitro study. Br J Plast Surg 1979; 32: 31–34.

116. Baker JL, LeVier RR, Spielvogel DE. Positive identification of silicone in human mammary capsular tissue. Plast Reconstr Surg 1982; 69: 56.

117. Schnitt SJ. Tissue reactions to mammary implants: A capsule summary. Adv Anat Pathol 1994; 2: 24–27.

118. Thomsen JL, Chrissensen L, Nielsen M et al. Histologic changes and silicone concentrations in human breast tissue surrounding silicone breast prostheses. Plast Reconstr Surg 1990; 91: 38–41.

11

I. O. Ellis, C. W. Elston, H. Goulding and S. E. Pinder

Miscellaneous benign lesions

INTRODUCTION

This chapter describes benign neoplastic and non-neoplastic entities not covered elsewhere in this volume. Thus, a range of stromal alterations will be considered; some may occur in association with carcinoma and the prognostic implications are discussed in Chapter 18. The locally aggressive fibromatosis is described here together with benign connective tissue neoplasms which are not specific to the breast. In addition benign tumors of salivary gland and sweat gland type, most frequently occurring in a sub-areolar location, are described.

NON-NEOPLASTIC LESIONS

STROMAL ALTERATIONS

Amyloid

Amyloid deposits may rarely occur in the breast either as a localized tumor or as a manifestation of systemic amyloidosis. The first reported case of a localized amyloid tumor in the breast was by Fernandez and Hernandez in 1973[1] in a 62-year-old woman who presented with a 3 cm firm mobile mass which was suspicious of carcinoma on mammography due to the presence of calcification and radiating spicules. Several cases have been reported since[2,3,4] including women with bilateral breast involvement.[5,6] Most have occurred in elderly women and, as for the first case, carcinoma was often suspected clinically.

Breast involvement in systemic amyloidosis is also described, complicating rheumatoid arthritis[7] and plasma cell dyscrasias.[8,9] Again, these women are usually elderly and bilateral involvement may occur. Following a review of 27 cases of primary amyloidosis, O'Connor et al identified breast involvement in five, suggesting that this may be more common than previously recognized.[9]

Macroscopically, the amyloid deposits appear as indurated areas often with a waxy cut surface. They present as discrete nodules a few centimeters across or as massive diffuse infiltrates.

Microscopically, the homogeneous, eosinophilic amyloid can be confirmed as such using standard techniques such as Congo red staining, immunohistochemical staining for light chains (primary amyloid) or amyloid-P-component and electron microscopy if necessary. It is deposited both in the stroma and in the walls of vessels and ducts and is associated with an inflammatory cell infiltrate including foreign body-type giant cells.

Santini et al have reported an unusual 'tubular' amyloid deposition in association with breast carcinoma, confirming their light microscopical impression with electron microscopy.[10] A granulomatous inflammatory response was also present in this case. The differential diagnosis of tumor associated amyloid is massive stromal elastosis which may accompany some carcinomas and in this respect, Azzopardi did not accept the case of Patil et al[11] as tumor associated amyloid but interpreted the features as elastosis.[12]

Stromal giant cells

Stromal giant cells are well documented in association with breast carcinoma and are described further in Chapter 18. Stromal giant cells are also described as an incidental finding independent of breast carcinoma, mostly in women of between 40 and 50 years old.[13] These are believed to be similar to those occurring in the lower female genital tract, bladder, prostate, urethra and in nasal polyps[14] and ultrastructural examination has shown them to be fibroblast-derived.[14,15] On light microscopy, they are seen to possess a variable number of nuclei which may display a florette arrangement and have scanty cytoplasm (Fig. 11.1). Hormonal factors may be involved in their pathogenesis and it is of interest in this respect that they have been described in adolescent gynecomastia.[15] Alternatively, they may represent a reactive or degenerative stromal response.

Stromal metachromasia

This refers to an alteration in the staining properties of the breast stroma and is commonly seen at the infiltrating edge of invasive breast carcinomas.[16] It reflects increased separation of the connective tissue strands by spaces that may become filled with a fibrillary metachromatic substance and is thought to be the result of mast cell degranulation with release of heparin and other substances.[16] Sandstad and Hartveid also described metachromatic stromal staining adjacent to ducts containing in situ carcinoma and separate from the metachromatic stroma associated with invasive tumor.[17] Furthermore, they noted that stromal metachromasia in this situation was associated with destruction of the duct wall and postulated that factors involved in the disruption of the duct wall necessary for subsequent invasion may originate in the stroma rather than directly from the tumor cells as had been accepted previously. They further suggested that the presence of metachromasia adjacent to a duct containing in situ carcinoma may be an indicator of 'incipient invasion'.

Stromal elastosis

Elastosis may be defined as the presence of focal deposits of elastic tissue in abnormal amounts or locations. It is a common stromal alteration and is described both in otherwise normal breasts and in association with benign and malignant lesions. In the normal mature breast, elastic fibres are found as a fibrillary cuff surrounding ducts, as occasional strands in the interlobular stroma and in the walls of arteries and veins; the intralobular stroma is devoid of elastin. Azzopardi and Laurini reported loss of periductal elastin accompanying premenopausal involution with no further increase occurring after the menopause.[18] Others, however, have found no correlation with age.[19,20] Many of these studies have investigated elastin deposition in material from patients with breast carcinoma. In contrast, Farahmand and Cowan studied tissue from 140 women with clinically

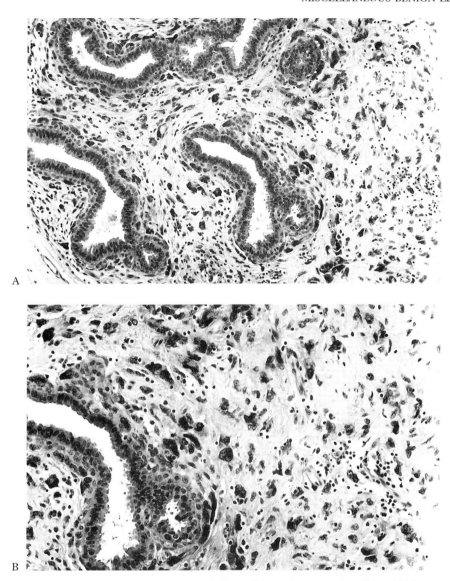

Fig. 11.1 An example of benign stromal giant cell formation seen at low (A) and high (B) magnification.

normal breasts ranging in age from 19 to 101 years.[21] These authors found elastosis to increase with age, being present in nearly half of all women over the age of 50 years with no breast disease. Periductal elastosis was found to increase with age until about 50 years and was thought to reflect parity, a finding previously reported by Davies.[22] They concluded that while periductal elastosis may be associated with cancer, it is not of itself a cause for concern. This is in contrast to marked perivascular elastosis which is uncommon at

any age and is more likely to indicate associated malignancy.[23]

Elastosis may be a prominent component of benign lesions, particularly radial scars/complex sclerosing lesions (Ch. 7)[22,24] and periductal elastosis has been described in the male breast in association with gynecomastia and neoplastic lesions.[25]

As stated above, elastosis is commonly seen in association with breast carcinoma and may be visible macroscopically as pale yellow streaks.

Microscopically, it may be found in all three locations described above, (periductal, perivascular and stromal), although many studies have concentrated on the often prominent periductal component. Ultrastructural studies suggest that the elastic fibers are synthesized by stromal fibroblasts,[26,27] possibly in response to some tumor-derived cytokine,[18] although some believe the neoplastic cells may play a more direct role in their synthesis.[28]

Histologically, elastosis may be demonstrated by the use of a standard stain for elastin such as the Verhoeff method. On routinely hematoxylin and eosin stained sections it appears as homogeneous pink material (Fig. 11.2) which has in the past been confused with amyloid[27,11] particularly in view of the affinity of amyloid stains such as Congo red for elastic fibers. The prognostic implications of tumor-associated elastosis are discussed in Chapter 18.

Stromal metaplasias

Metaplastic stromal changes are rare, but have been described in association with the biphasic lesions of fibroadenoma and phyllodes tumor. Thus, smooth muscle has been described, not only as a component of hamartoma[29] (see Ch. 9), but also as a stromal change in fibroadenomas[30]

and phyllodes tumors[31] usually affecting only a small proportion of the stroma and ascribed to a metaplastic process.[32] Osseous and cartilagenous metaplasia are also described in a number of benign and malignant breast lesions,[33,34] most frequently in phyllodes tumors and associated with sarcomatous features.[35] Similarly, rhabdomyosarcomatous and liposarcomatous elements have each been described in phyllodes tumors,[35,36] and are attributed to a metaplastic process (see also Chs 9 and 19).

Pseudoangiomatous hyperplasia

This distinctive stromal alteration was first described in nine women by Vuitch et al. in 1986.[37] These authors stressed the importance of recognition of this entity to prevent confusion with angiosarcoma, a point emphasized subsequently by Ibrahim et al.[38]

The original description[37] of this entity referred to cases presenting as palpable masses in premenopausal women aged between 22 and 52 years. However, in addition to two further cases presenting as mass lesions in premenopausal women, Ibrahim et al. found microscopic pseudoangiomatous hyperplasia, often multifocal, in 23% of 200 consecutive breast biopsy or mastectomy specimens, often in association with proliferative

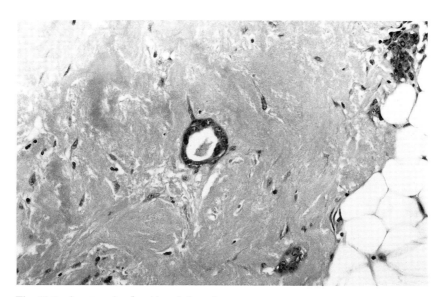

Fig. 11.2 An example of periductal elastosis.

fibrocystic changes. These were predominantly from young women but the ages ranged from 17 to 76 years and two of the cases were described in men and associated with gynecomastia.[38] Pseudo-angiomatous hyperplasia has also presented as a rapidly growing palpable mass associated with axillary gynecomastia in an immunosuppressed man.[39]

Palpable lesions generally present as a discrete, painless breast lump, often several centimeters in diameter. Fine needle aspiration is often unsuc-cessful. The lumps have been present for several weeks or months, but one of the women reported by Ibrahim et al. presented with gradual enlarge-ment of the right breast over a period of 2 years. This case was also unusual in being associated with a clinical appearance of peau-d'orange,[38] thereby heightening the suspicion of malignancy. Indeed this woman and one of the women in the original series underwent mastectomy following a false diagnosis of malignancy.

Grossly, the palpable lumps have a firm,

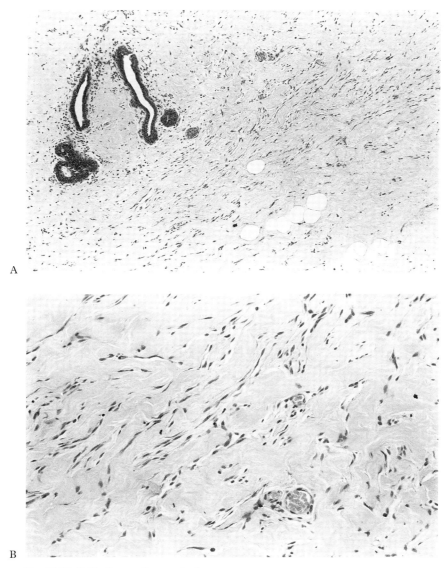

Fig. 11.3A & B   See caption overleaf.

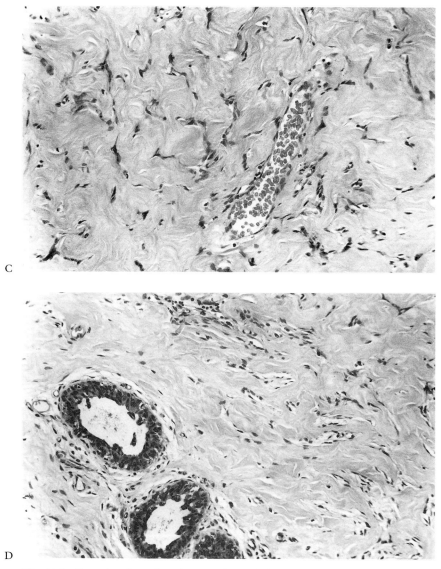

C

D

Fig. 11.3 Examples of pseudoangiomatous hyperplasia seen at low (A) and high (B,C,D,E) magnification. Note the resemblance to a microvascular stromal network but true capillaries are clearly distinguished (B,C). There is often a gynecomastia-like change affecting the parenchymal elements (A,D).

rubbery consistency. The size ranges from 1 to 7 cm. They are often well-circumscribed with a smooth external surface and a pale grey or tan cut surface without significant hemorrhage.

Microscopically, both the palpable and the microscopic lesions are characterized by a complex pattern of anastomozing empty spaces both within and between breast lobules resembling a vascular proliferation and readily appreciated at low power (Fig. 11.3a). Often the spaces are arranged concentrically immediately around the lobules. On examination at higher magnification (Fig. 11.3b), some of the spaces are seen to be lined by uniform spindle cells which are also present within the intervening, densely collagenous, stroma. Pleomorphism and mitotic activity are not features. Despite the superficial resemblance to a vascular proliferation, the spaces are empty or contain only occasional red blood cells and no basement membrane material is identified using a PAS stain. The spaces are also identified in frozen sections and do not therefore represent an artefact associated with formalin fixation or paraffin processing. The spindle cells fail to show positive immunohistochemical staining for vascular endothelial markers and no ultrastructural features to suggest an endothelial cell origin have been identified. Instead, these cells have the immunohistochemical and ultrastructural features of fibroblasts. The process tends to surround and intermingle with existing ductal and lobular structures and there may be associated epithelial hyperplasia.

It has been suggested that pseudoangiomatous hyperplasia represents a localized form of stromal overgrowth resulting from an exaggerated response to progesterone in estrogen primed tissue[37] and this is supported by the description of progesterone receptor positivity in the five cases examined immunohistochemically by Anderson et al.[40]

The most important differential diagnosis is from an angiosarcoma. Unlike angiosarcoma, however, the palpable lesions of pseudoangiomatous hyperplasia are relatively well-circumscribed, often resembling a fibroadenoma. Furthermore, as noted above, microscopic examination will fail to support a vascular origin and fail to reveal any pleomorphism, mitotic activity or necrosis. Finally, there is no destruction of epithelial elements even when the process is involving the lobules.

As referred to above, pseudoangiomatous hyperplasia is believed to represent an exaggerated physiological response and is not currently thought to be associated with any increased risk of subsequent development of carcinoma. However, two of the cases in the original series of Vuitch et al developed local recurrences requiring further excision. There was no change in the microscopical appearances in these recurrences and the authors suggested that the recurrences followed incomplete initial excision. They recommended treatment by complete local excision with short-term clinical follow-up (3 years).

COLLAGENOUS SPHERULOSIS

This is an incidental microscopical finding first described in association with benign proliferative processes such as sclerosing adenosis, radial scar and intraduct papillomas by Clement, Young and Azzopardi in 1987[41] and subsequently described by several others.[42,43] Its importance lies partly in the possible diagnostic confusion which can arise between this entity and malignancy, particularly adenoid cystic carcinoma and the rare intraduct carcinoma with signet ring cells; diagnostic confusion which has also been described in cytological preparations.[44,45]

Collagenous spherulosis is a rare finding adjacent to benign proliferative lesions in pre- and perimenopausal woman. In the original series of 15 cases, it was identified as an incidental, microscopic, asymptomatic finding and any palpable masses present were attributed to the accompanying pathology. However, one of the three cases described by Grignon et al. presented with a mass which was found to be composed predominantly of expanded lobules involved by collagenous spherulosis that were considered responsible for the palpable abnormality.[43]

There are no distinctive gross features as, apart from the case described by Grignon et al,[43] this entity represents an incidental microscopic finding. The lesions may be uni- or multi-focal and consist of aggregates of well-circumscribed eosinophilic spherules 20–100 μm in diameter, partially or completely filling the lumina of ductules, distended acini or both (Fig. 11.4). The spherules have a hyaline or fibrillar structure, are collagen-rich and may contain variable amounts of acidic mucin, elastin and PAS-positive material. Immunohistochemistry has identified the presence of basement membrane components laminin and type IV collagen which are believed to be produced by the flattened layer of myoepithelial cells seen immediately adjacent to the spherules. These may be more readily appreciated using immunohistochemical stains for S100 or actin. The spherules are usually found in association with proliferative processes and have been described in association with papillomas, radial scars and sclerosing adenosis. More recently, they have been reported in association with atypical hyperplasia.[46]

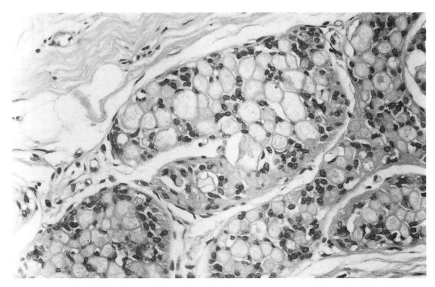

Fig. 11.4   In collagenous spherulosis the lobule contains numerous hyaline spherules replacing the normal acinar glandular structures.

The distinctive spherules have been shown to possess an ultrastructure similar to that of basement membrane.[43,42] They are believed to result from a proliferation of epithelial and myoepithelial cells, the latter being responsible for the production of the basement membrane material.

The two main differential diagnoses to be considered are adenoid cystic carcinoma and intraduct signet ring carcinoma. The hyaline spherules are similar in appearance in both collagenous spherulosis and adenoid cystic carcinoma and mistaken diagnoses have been described.[41,44] However, in most reported instances collagenous spherulosis has been an incidental microscopic finding whereas adenoid cystic carcinoma is almost always a palpable mass. Furthermore, unlike adenoid cystic carcinoma, collagenous spherulosis does not exhibit invasion and while both conditions are associated with the production of both Alcian blue and PAS-positive staining material, in adenoid cystic carcinoma the staining reactions are distinct, with PAS-positive material within the duct-like spaces and Alcian blue positive material within the pseudocysts in contrast to the highly variable pattern of staining in collagenous spherulosis in which there is often dual positivity for both stains within any given spherule. Finally, in contrast to the material within the

spaces of adenoid cystic carcinoma, the spherules of collagenous spherulosis often have a distinct fibrillar structure and a high collagen content which may be appreciated using a collagen stain such as a Masson trichrome.

The other main differential diagnosis is the rare intraduct carcinoma containing signet ring cells.[47] Again the lack of collagen in the signet ring cell vacuoles, together with the intracellular position of these and their clear association with malignant nuclei are important differential features.

Collagenous spherulosis of itself has no sinister prognostic implications and any treatment is directed at the associated pathology.

NEOPLASTIC

BENIGN SALIVARY AND SWEAT GLAND-LIKE LESIONS

Introduction

Tumors of the skin appendages may present as apparent masses of the breast or nipple. The reader is referred to specialist dermatopathology text books for the histopathological features of these lesions, which will not be covered in detail here. It is, however, noteworthy that occasional lesions with the histological features of sweat gland tumors have been described deep within the breast parenchyma and not apparently derived from these structures within dermis. Given the embryological relationship between breast and sweat glands this is perhaps not surprising. Panico et al, for example, described an eccrine spiradenoma deep within the breast which showed hormone receptor positivity and was apparently derived from the breast epithelium.[48] This tumor showed an aggressive behavior with three local recurrences seen within 30 months of diagnosis.

Benign tumors of the skin appendages must be distinguished not only from malignant tumors of the sweat glands of the breast, such as malignant eccrine acrospiroma[49] and carcinosarcoma arising in an eccrine spiradenoma,[50] but more particularly from primary breast neoplasms. This may be especially difficult on cytological preparations; Kumar et al for example reported the misdiagnosis of a clear cell hidradenoma[51] as a breast carcinoma.

Pleomorphic adenoma

Clinical features

Pleomorphic adenomas of the breast are uncommon tumors and there is still some debate as to whether this lesion represents a true distinct entity or a variant of either ductal adenoma or intraduct papilloma showing cartilagenous metaplasia of the stromal elements. They occur in patients from the 4th to the 9th decades of life with a median of 65 years of age and present as discrete palpable masses, often periareolar in situation or as suspicious mass lesions on mammography.[52,53,54]. Occasionally patients may present with a nipple discharge[53].

Macroscopic and microscopic appearances

Pleomorphic adenomas of the breast are single or multifocal and usually measure between 1 and 4 cm in diameter. They have a well-circumscribed, sometimes lobulated appearance with a white/grey or yellow homogeneous rubbery cut surface.

Microscopically these tumors resemble their analogues in salivary glands. By definition pleomorphic adenomas are composed of a minimum of three elements: epithelial cells, myoepithelial cells and chondromyoid tissue (Fig. 11.5). A transition between these components may be seen. The epithelium may form tubular or acinar structures arranged in islands or trabeculae; significant numbers of mitoses are not seen and minimal cellular atypia is identified. The myo-

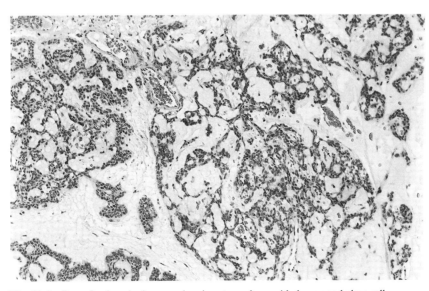

Fig. 11.5 Part of a ductal adenoma showing stromal myxoid change and clear cell alteration of myoepithelial cells giving an appearance resembling pleomorphic adenoma of salivary glands.

epithelial component often adjoins the chondro-myxoid areas and may dominate areas of the tumor. The epithelial component of a pleomorphic adenoma can be distinguished immuno-histochemically using low molecular weight cytokeratin antibodies and the myoepithelial component using S100 or anti-smooth muscle actin antibodies, although this latter portion of the tumor may also focally express cytokeratin markers. The chondromyxoid stromal tissue may contain areas of well-formed hyaline cartilage. Focal calcification may be present and bone formation is also found in up to 50% of cases.[33,55]

Pleomorphic adenomas are generally circumscribed and may have a collagen rich fibrous pseudocapsule. On occasions there is evidence of an origin from an underlying papilloma, with a residual surrounding luminal space identifiable. Other coincidental but coexisting histological features may be noted, such as epithelial hyperplasia, sclerosing adenosis, cystic change or apocrine metaplasia.

Differential diagnosis

Cartilage formation may be present in a variety of other breast tumors including fibroadenoma and hamartoma, intraduct papilloma and ductal adenoma; it may also be seen in some malignant tumors including phyllodes tumor and metaplastic carcinoma. Indeed pleomorphic adenomas may be indistinguishable from a complex intraduct papilloma or ductal adenoma and there is no real merit in attempting to differentiate between these conditions. The diagnosis of pleomorphic adenoma, however, rests on the purity of its histology and coexistence of bland epithelial tissue with myoepithelial proliferation and chondromyxoid stroma.

Prognosis and treatment

Diaz et al described a series of ten patients with pleomorphic adenomas of the breast and found with approximately 5 years median follow-up none had developed metastatic disease, indeed malignant transformation is exceedingly rare. However these lesions also arise in dogs and in these animals more commonly show malignant behavior. In the series of Diaz et al, one patient suffered local recurrence, although this is also very unusual.[53,56] Simple excision with a narrow circumferential margin of uninvolved tissue is sufficient treatment for these lesions although review of the literature demonstrates mistaken diagnosis has frequently led to inappropriate mastectomy.[56,57]

Syringomatous adenoma

Introduction

Syringomatous adenoma of the nipple[58] is a relatively rare benign tumor which has histological features similar to those of eccrine syringoma. The origin of the neoplasm is, however, unclear; some authors suggest that syringomatous adenomas may arise from breast parenchyma and that there is no evidence of transition from overlying skin or nipple epidermis.[59] Others suggest that occasional connections to the overlying skin may be identified[60] and propose that these tumors are truly of skin adnexal origin.[61] The major significance of this lesion, however, lies primarily in its correct recognition as a distinctive benign neoplasm which should not be mistaken for a malignant tumor.

Clinical

Clinically syringomatous adenomas most frequently present as firm well-defined masses or plaques in the nipple. These tumors have been reported in women of all ages and also very rarely in men.[58]

Macroscopic and microscopic appearances

Syringomatous adenomas range in size from 1 to 3 cm.[61] Macroscopically they are poorly-defined pale masses with small cystic areas sometimes visible on the cut surface.

Histologically a proliferation of angulated, round or comma-shaped, solid and tubular islands of epithelium are identified infiltrating the fibrous stroma of the nipple. This stroma may be histological unremarkable or may show edema or more cellular desmoplastic reactive changes.[62] The epithelial elements may also extend into the smooth muscle of the nipple.

The tubular structures are formed of glandular epithelium with foci of squamous metaplasia; keratinising squamous cysts may also be seen (Fig. 11.6). The tubules may be small and inconspicuous and may be overlooked on low-power examination. A dual cell population may be seen, including scattered clear cells but a consistent distinct basal myoepithelial layer is not typically evident. In some cases usual epithelial hyperplasia may occur within the larger duct-like tubules of the lesion and this is also frequently seen in the surrounding breast parenchyma.[59] Ward et al described two cases of 'syringomatous tumor of the nipple' and noted that mitotic figures were sparse. In addition, however, both these[60] and other authors[62] have reported perineural invasion by these tumors; a feature which should not be over-interpreted as indicative of malignancy.

Differential diagnosis

Syringomatous adenomas of the nipple may be

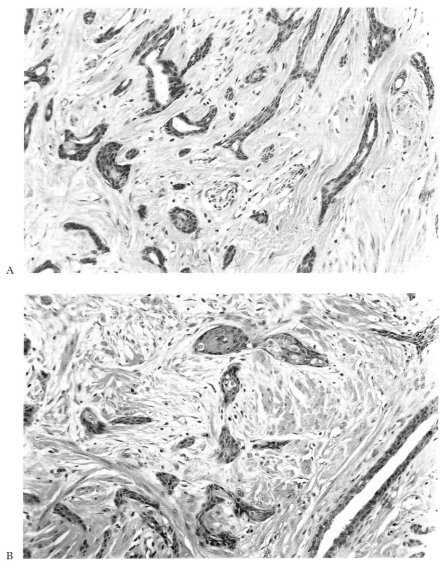

Fig. 11.6   See caption overleaf.

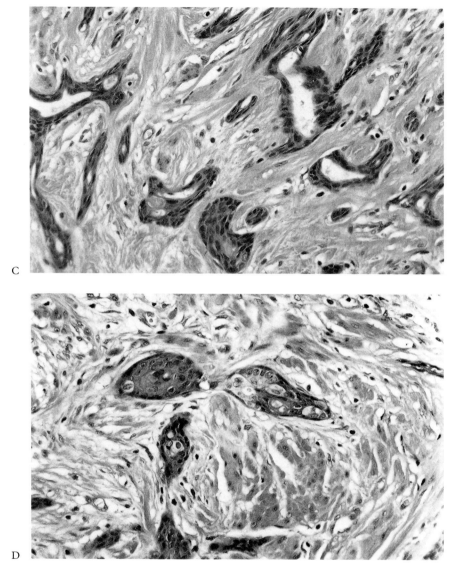

Fig. 11.6   A syringomatous adenoma arising in the nipple and composed of angulated nests of cells infiltrating collagenous stroma (A, B). These nests may show lumen formation (C) or rudimentary squamous pearl formation (D). An epithelial/myoepithelial bilayer is usually not apparent.

misdiagnosed as tubular carcinoma or nipple adenoma.[62,63] The tubules of tubular carcinomas lack the dual cell population which is present in syringomatous adenomas. In addition the tubules in the former lesion area are often larger and lack the squamous differentiation seen in syringomatous adenoma.

Nipple adenomas form well-defined lesions which displace rather than infiltrate the stroma of the nipple. Indeed the epithelial proliferation is more often hyperplastic in the former lesion with less stroma seen between the epithelial islands than in syringomatous adenomas where the stroma is abundant. Squamous metaplasia may be seen in nipple adenomas, but only in the superficial portions of the lesion and is not present in the deep parts of these tumours as in syringomatous adenomas where squamous metaplasia is often prominent throughout.

Prognosis and treatment

Although these tumors have an infiltrative margin and may be histologically and clinically worrying, metastatic disease has not been reported. If incompletely excised they may recur locally and adequate treatment may require nipple resection,[58,62] but more aggressive surgery than this does not appear to be warranted.

FIBROMATOSIS

Fibromatosis may be defined as an infiltrating, fibroblastic and myofibroblastic proliferation which is locally aggressive, recurring if incompletely excised, but does not metastasize. It has been described in many different anatomical locations, most commonly in the abdominal wall ('abdominal desmoid'). Occurrence in the breast, probably in this case following spread from a lesion arising in the chest wall, was first described in 1923[64] and since then occurrence at this site, either primarily or following spread from the chest wall, has been the subject of several case reports and three

more recent series.[65,66,67] Importantly, when occurring in the breast it may be mistaken clinically, radiologically and occasionally histologically for malignancy.

Clinical features

The age range in reported cases is from 14 to 80 years. Initial presentation is with a firm to hard, usually discrete but occasionally ill-defined, nontender, mass. Skin tethering is not uncommon and nipple retraction has been reported. The lesion is usually unilateral although bilaterality has been reported.[66,68] Mammography may show no distinctive features or may show a stellate lesion, adding to the suspicion of malignancy[65,67,69] and dense calcification on mammography has been reported in a 70-year-old woman subsequently shown to have an ossifying fibromatosis.[70]

Macroscopic features

The size of the lesion is variable, with a range of 0.7 cm to 10 cm reported. The poorly circumscribed, infiltrative nature of the process is readily appreciated macroscopically and the margins difficult to discern. The cut surface is grey-white and appears fibrous with few distinguishing features. Often the lesion appears less impressive

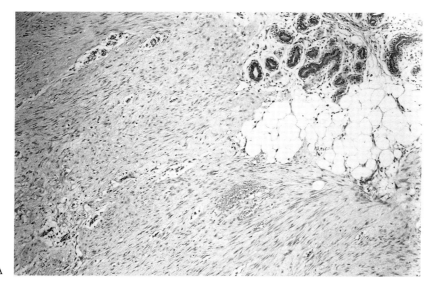

Fig. 11.7A See caption overleaf.

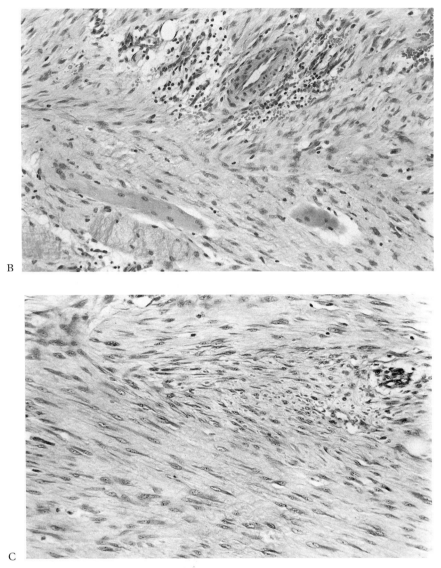

Fig. 11.7B & C   An example of fibromatosis showing infiltration of breast tissue (A) and underlying muscle (B) by a population of uniform bland spindle cells (C).

than the amount of skin tethering and retraction associated with it.

Microscopic features

The majority of these lesions are composed of a uniform population of spindle cells arranged in interlacing bundles and fascicles and surrounding and entrapping parenchymal elements (Fig. 11.7). The cellularity varies throughout the lesion; often being greater at the periphery. Stromal collagen is also variable. Some lesions are predominantly collagenous, with prominent hyalinization, often with a keloid-like appearance. More often cellular and collagenous area intermingle within the same lesion. Myxoid areas and calcification are described[66] and ossification has been reported.[70] The margins are largely infiltrative, with finger-like projections extending into adjacent stroma, although a more lobulated margin may be seen focally. A patchy lymphoid infiltrate is often seen and tends to be more dense at the periphery

(Fig. 11.8). Follicles with germinal centers may be seen. Other inflammatory cells are inconspicuous or absent unless there has been previous surgery.

The spindle cells usually show at most mild nuclear pleomorphism although areas containing large atypical, often multinucleated, fibroblasts have been described.[66,67] Importantly, mitotic figures are infrequent. Wargotz et al identified a maximum rate of three per 10 high power fields (field area 0.153 mm²) in one of their 28 cases.

Three other lesions which also showed mild cellular atypia had a rate of one per 10 high power fields.[67] Necrobiosis is described, but necrosis should not be identified.

The entrapped ductal and lobular elements may be distorted such that their nuclei appear abnormal and mild epithelial hyperplasia is frequently described (Fig. 11.8).

Ultrastructural examination of the spindle cells has identified two cell types: fibroblasts and myofibroblasts; the former containing numerous

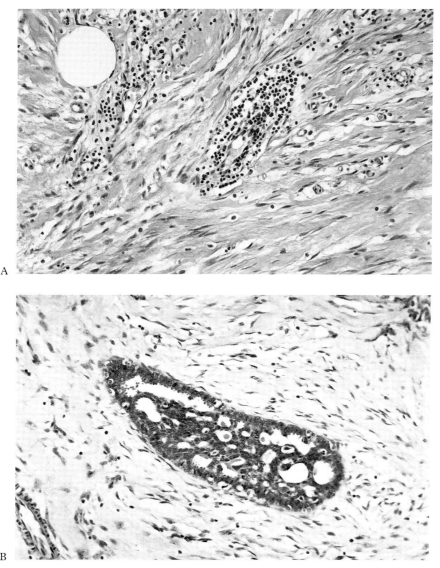

Fig. 11.8 Fibromatoses may have accompanying features of a perivascular lymphocytic infiltrate (A) and gynecomastia-like changes of entrapped glandular structures (B).

dilated stacks of rough endoplasmic reticulum and the latter cytoplasmic bundles of fine filaments with dense bodies.[71,72] The contractile nature of these cells is probably responsible for the skin retraction that is so often an associated feature.

Pathogenesis

The etiology and pathogenesis of fibromatosis is unknown although genetic, physical and hormonal factors have been implicated. Rarely, breast fibromatosis may occur in association with a familial syndrome such as Gardner's syndrome[68,73] or familial multicentric fibromatosis[74] and bilateral involvement is described.[68] However, although a familial syndrome should be considered, the vast majority of fibromatoses presenting in the breast are not associated with such syndromes.

A history of trauma is obtained in some cases and has been implicated in pathogenesis. Similarly, there are reported cases of its occurrence in association with breast implants;[66,75] an association which may be coincidental or related to surgical trauma or inflammation. It is possible that trauma may play an etiological role in most cases but has been forgotten by the time the patient presents.

The role of hormones in the pathogenesis of mammary fibromatosis has been considered in view of the significant positive association between abdominal fibromatosis and pregnancy and the reported regression with tamoxifen therapy.[76] However, an association with pregnancy is not identified in breast fibromatosis which has been observed in nulliparous women. The presence of estrogen and progesterone receptors has been identified using biochemical methods in fibromatoses,[77] including a case in the breast.[78] However, more recently, Rasbridge et al. investigated estrogen and progesterone expression in six cases of breast fibromatosis using both biochemical and immunohistochemical methods and were unable to identify significant expression. Similarly, one of the cases in Rosen and Ernsbergers' series underwent estrogen and progesterone receptor analysis and was also found to be negative.[66] Thus, while there is some evidence for the role of hereditary factors, trauma and hormonal fac-

tors, the pathogenesis of mammary fibromatosis remains unknown. A combination of factors may be involved.

Differential diagnosis

Fibromatosis must be differentiated from malignant lesions capable of metastasis on the one hand, and from benign lesions lacking the potential for recurrence on the other. An important differential diagnosis is spindle cell metaplastic carcinoma (see Ch. 15). This is not usually a problem due to the prominent carcinomatous element in most cases of metaplastic carcinoma but rarely, the entrapped ductal elements in fibromatosis may be a source of confusion, particularly if showing hyperplasia. Helpful features are the usual lack of pleomorphism and presence of keloid-like foci and lymphoid aggregates in fibromatosis compared with the highly cellular and pleomorphic spindle cell component in metaplastic carcinoma.

Fibromatosis must also be distinguished from high grade fibrosarcoma (see Ch. 19). This is determined on the basis of cellularity, pleomorphism, necrosis and importantly, mitotic activity. The finding of a mitotic rate of three per 10 high power fields by Wargotz et al.[67] is unusual. Most reported cases have no or less than one mitotic figure per 10 high power fields in contrast to fibrosarcoma.

Malignant fibrous histiocytoma (see Ch. 19) may also enter the differential diagnosis. However, although fibromatosis may contain storiform areas, these are not usually prominent. Furthermore, the pleomorphism, necrosis and mitotic activity of malignant fibrous histiocytoma are lacking in fibromatosis.

Benign processes included in the differential diagnosis of fibromatosis include scars associated with healed fat necrosis and surgery. Although occasionally seen in fibromatosis, calcification is more likely to be associated with fat necrosis and even when largely replaced by fibrous tissue, areas of previous fat necrosis often still contain cystic cavities (see Ch. 10). The recognition of post-surgical scarring is aided by both the history and the presence of small stitch granulomata and hemosiderin. However, particular problems may be encountered when assessing the possibility of recurrence following previous surgery. In this situation, the extent of the lesion may be of use.

Nodular fasciitis can be difficult to separate from fibromatosis. However, in contrast to the focal lymphoid infiltrates, often located in the periphery of the lesion in fibromatosis, in nodular fasciitis, the inflammatory infiltrate is more heterogeneous and tends to be dispersed throughout the lesion. Furthermore, nodular fasciitis tends to be more circumscribed, has a higher mitotic activity, an increased mucoid matrix and tends to bear a greater similarity to granulation tissue.

Prognosis and treatment

One of the most important features of this entity is its propensity for recurrence. Recurrence rates in the three series reported are 23%[65], 21%[67] and 27%.[66] In some cases multiple recurrences have occurred. When recurrences have occurred they have generally, but not always, done so within three years of the initial diagnosis. The risk of recurrence does not appear to be associated with size, nuclear atypia or mitotic activity but most closely correlates with adequacy of excision, the vast majority of recurrences associated with inadequate initial excision. Recurrences have the same histological appearance as the initial lesion with no evidence for progressive development of atypia or increased mitotic activity.

Not all patients with documented incomplete excision will develop recurrence. Gump et al. described two patients who had no recurrence despite the presence of fibromatosis at the surgical margin. It is not clear how long these two particular women had been followed up, but the minimum length of follow up for the series as a whole was 2 years[65] and may therefore have been inadequate in these two cases. These authors also described a third woman who had incomplete excision of a first recurrence followed by a second recurrence which was deemed inoperable. Her lesion showed no clinical change over the next 5 years or so then underwent remarkable regression.

Despite these rare exceptions, adequacy of excision is considered to be of paramount importance in the prevention of recurrence and wide local excision is recommended. As recurrences deep within the breast or close to the chest wall are notoriously difficult to control, immediate re-excision of the biopsy site is recommended following incomplete excision at these sites. For more superficial or subareolar lesions close follow-up may be preferable to early re-excision.[66]

Although the use of tamoxifen therapy has reportedly induced remission in fibromatoses at other sites,[76,79] this has not been shown in the breast.

MYOFIBROBLASTOMA

The largest series of myofibroblastomas was described in 1987 by Wargotz et al. who identified 16 cases of this rare neoplasm in the files of the Armed Forces Institute of Pathology.[80] Eleven of these occurred in males and it was originally believed that this neoplasm showed a male preponderance; this lesion is thus described in Chapter 21. Recent reports, however, have included more female patients raising doubts about this male predominance.[81,82]

LIPOMA, ANGIOLIPOMA AND CHONDROLIPOMA

Several tumors containing mature adipose tissue have been described in the breast and three are considered here.

As lipomata are so common elsewhere in the body, it is not surprising that they are also frequently found in the breast.[83,84] They tend to present in middle-age or older women although may have been there for many years as they produce no symptoms and grow only slowly. In Haagensen's series of 186 patients presenting with lipomata over a 20 year period, the mean age was 45 years with fewer than 3% occurring in women less than 25 years.[84] They occur as soft, mobile masses, the vast majority of which are solitary.

Macroscopically, lipomas of the breast are usually less than 5 cm in diameter although several of more than 10 cm in diameter have been described.[84] They may be difficult to distinguish from normal breast adipose tissue unless their thin capsule is identified by close inspection. Microscopically, their appearance is typical of lipomas occurring elsewhere, consisting of mature adipocytes and surrounded by a delicate capsule.

Angiolipomas are also described in the breast[85, 86,87] and may be multiple.[87,85] Otherwise they resemble lipomas clinically, being more common in older women and, unlike angiolipomata occurring elsewhere, are usually painless. Like lipomas, they are encapsulated, but may contain focal grey or pink areas. Microscopically, multiple, interconnected small vessels are seen within mature adipose tissue. Typically, microthrombi are found within these small vessels. The degree of vascularity is variable but is often most impressive in the subcapsular area and the most cellular lesions have been termed cellular angiolipomas.[88] One such lesion has been described in the breast of a 64-year-old woman[89] and contained highly cellular spindle cell areas forming vascular spaces admixed with areas of mature adipose tissue. The degree of cellularity may give rise to confusion with Kaposi's sarcoma or angiosarcoma and important distinguishing features include the circumscription and encapsulation, presence of intravascular thrombi and lack of cytological atypia, mitotic activity and necrosis in cellular angiolipomas.

Chondrolipomas have been reported in the female breast.[90–93] All presented as firm mobile masses in women aged between 39 and 68 years. Pathologically they were all well-circumscribed and consisted of an admixture of mature adipose tissue, cartilage, fibrous tissue and benign breast parenchymal tissue. It is uncertain whether the parenchymal elements represent entrapped tissue or form part of the lesion. Similarly the histogenesis of these lesions is uncertain, but they may represent hamartomas showing chondroid metaplasia. The differential diagnosis includes other rare benign and malignant breast lesions which have been reported as showing chondroid metaplasia,[34,33] the more important being the malignant lesions which more commonly show this feature but which are usually readily identified as malignant.

The pathogenesis of these entities is uncertain, some may represent neoplastic processes but, particularly for those containing more than one mesenchymal element an alternative, hamartomatous origin may be considered (see Ch. 9).

GRANULAR CELL TUMOR

Granular cell tumor can occur at a variety of sites with around 6 to 8% occurring in the breast.[94] One of the earliest descriptions of the tumor at this site was provided by Haagensen and Stout who reported five cases[95] and there have been many others recorded since.[94,96–99] The importance of its occurrence in the breast lies in the possible clinical confusion with malignancy which results from its firm fibrous texture and possible fixation to skin and fascia. Suspicion may be strengthened by mammographic findings of a stellate or spiculate lesion[99,100] and there are reports of these tumors being mistaken for malignancy on frozen section.[101]

Clinical features

The average age at presentation is around 30 years but with a wide range from the mid teens to the eighties.[94] Palpable lesions may give a clinical impression of a fibroadenoma, or importantly, carcinoma if fixed or associated with skin retraction. The mammographic appearances vary from discrete rounded nodules to suspicious stellate or spiculate lesions and an impalpable lesion presenting at mammography for breast screening has been described.[99]

Macroscopic features

Macroscopically, these tumors may continue to mimic breast carcinoma due to their hard, fibrous constituency and infiltrative margins, although most are more circumscribed and have a more uniform pale gray cut surface than carcinomas. Most are less than 2 cm in diameter although larger tumors have been described.[94]

Microscopic features

Typically, granular cell tumor is composed of large round or polygonal cells with abundant coarsely granular eosinophilic cytoplasm and small, central vesicular nuclei (Fig. 11.9). The margins may be expansile or infiltrative. Occasionally, small areas showing mild to moderate nuclear pleomorphism but lacking mitotic activity may be found. The

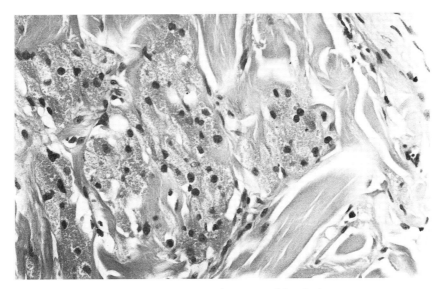

Fig. 11.9   A granular cell tumour involving the stroma of the nipple.

cells may be arranged in solid sheets or in islands and trabeculae divided by fibrous connective tissue and there may be marked desmoplasia in older lesions. The granular cells frequently encompass small nerves; a histogenetically significant feature.

The granules show weak PAS-diastase resistant positivity and expression of S-100 protein is well established and an important indicator of both histogenesis and diagnosis.[102,103] Expression of carcinoembryonic antigen has also been described.[104,103] The ultrastructural features have been described by Demay and Kay among others.[94] The granules correspond to lysosomal bodies containing cellular debris including myelin-like figures. The tumor cells are surrounded by a complete basal lamina and may possess long, fine cytoplasmic extensions with an incomplete basal lamina similar to those seen in Schwannomas.

Pathogenesis

Since the initial description of a granular cell tumor of the tongue in 1926[105] there has been some debate as to its histogenesis with various authors suggesting an origin from mesenchymal cells, fibroblasts, histiocytes and striated muscle cells. More recently, a Schwann cell origin has been accepted, supported by the immunohistochemical and ultrastructural findings (see above).

These tumors are more common in women than men at all sites but particularly in the breast; in one of the larger series of 12 tumors only one was in a male.[94] This suggests a hormonal influence, although neither estrogen nor progesterone receptors were identified in the four cases studied by Ingram et al.[106]

Differential diagnosis

The most important differential diagnosis is from breast carcinoma. This is primarily a clinical and radiological problem but granular cell tumor has been mistaken for carcinoma on frozen section.[101, 96,107] Important pointers to the correct diagnosis are the granular cytoplasm, paucity of mitotic activity and absence of malignant nuclear features. If there is any doubt as to the correct diagnosis an S-100 immunostain is recommended.

Malignant granular cell tumors are rare at any site but have been reported in the breast,[108,109] including one case in a male.[110] Clinically they are more likely to be larger tumors and there may be a history of recent increase in size. Increased mitotic activity may be an indicator of malignancy and Enzinger regards more than two mitotic figures in 10 high power fields suspicious although does not state the field area.[111] In general, malignant granular cell tumors are more cellular and display more nuclear pleomorphism. Necrosis may also be a feature.

Prognosis and management

As the vast majority of these uncommon tumors are benign, local excision is adequate treatment. Chemotherapy or radiotherapy appear to have little place in the management of malignant granular cell tumour and wide local excision is the treatment of choice for malignant lesions.

NEUROFIBROMA AND NEURILEMMOMA

These benign peripheral nerve sheath tumours have only rarely been reported in the breast[112–116] although many probably go unreported.[87] Their gross and microscopical features are the same as those occurring at other sites and they require only local excision as treatment.

LEIOMYOMA

Benign pure smooth muscle tumors of the breast may be considered in two groups; those occurring in the periareolar region and the much rarer tumors occurring within the breast parenchyma. The histogenesis of the latter is uncertain, but an origin from blood vessel walls or from displaced areolar muscle have been proposed. The age range for reported cases of these rare deep leiomyomas is from 34[117] to 69[118] years. The patients present with a mobile mass which may have been present for years and which may be associated with pain and tenderness. The largest described is 13.8 cm[119] and the smallest 0.5 cm.[120] Macroscopically they appear as pale gray or pink circumscribed, firm masses with a whorled cut surface. Microscopically, they consist of interlacing fascicles of smooth muscle cells without atypia and with minimal mitotic activity (see below). Immunohistochemical staining for desmin or smooth muscle actin and lack of immunostaining for S-100 or cytokeratin will confirm the cell type. A recent report of an epithelioid leiomyoma in a 42-year-old woman was described as containing granular cells,[121] a feature previously reported in uterine leiomyomas [122] and corresponding to numerous lysosomes on ultrastructural examination.

Smooth muscle has been described in a number of benign breast lesions which may therefore enter the differential diagnosis; smooth muscle may be a component of fibroadenomas,[30] hamartomas[29] and phyllodes tumors.[31] In each of these cases, the presence of other elements apart from smooth muscle precludes a diagnosis of leiomyoma. Myoepitheliomas may also be confused with leiomyomas. However, although both show positive immunostaining for actin, myoepithelial lesions will also show positive staining for S-100 and focal positivity for cytokeratin (see Ch. 16).

The most important differential diagnosis is leiomyosarcoma. Benign smooth muscle tumors should not show any necrosis or atypia and mitotic activity is minimal, although opinions differ slightly as to how much activity is acceptable. Chen et al suggested that three or more mitotic figures in 10 high power fields indicates malignancy[123] whereas Nielsen proposed that tumors which recur or have two or more mitotic figures in 10 high power fields should be considered leiomyosarcomas although accepted that this was somewhat arbitrary.[124] Neither author stated the field size and problems with both performance and interpretation of mitotic figure counting should be borne in mind when attempting to predict the behavior of any smooth muscle tumor. Some may have to be considered of uncertain malignant potential, requiring long term follow-up (see also Ch. 19).

BENIGN VASCULAR LESIONS

In this section benign vascular lesions occurring in the breast, excluding those arising from overlying skin, will be discussed. The importance of these lesions lies in the differential diagnosis of angiosarcoma and it should be remembered that the majority of vascular lesions arising in the breast (in contrast to the overlying skin) are, in fact, malignant. Thus, in all vascular lesions, a careful search for cytological atypia should be undertaken. The entities considered here are: hemangiomas, which may be subdivided into microscopic, palpable and atypical types, angiomatosis and hemangiopericytoma. Angiolipoma is discussed in a preceding section and malignant vascular tumors in Chapter 19.

Microscopic hemangiomas

The majority of hemangiomas in the breast parenchyma are impalpable, incidental findings in breast tissue removed for other reasons. Most are found in a perilobular location with occasional periductal hemangiomas. Rosen and Ridolfi reviewed tissue from 555 female mastectomy specimens performed for carcinoma; at least two blocks of uninvolved breast parenchyma and a block of nipple was available on each. They identified perilobular hemangiomas in seven (1.2%) with multiple hemangiomas in two specimens.[125] In contrast, in a forensic autopsy series of 210 consecutive female subjects performed at the Melbourne City Morgue, Lesueur and colleagues identified 32 microscopic hemangiomas in 23 cases (11%).[126] These workers examined at least 10 blocks from each breast and this figure is therefore probably nearer the true incidence, at least for this population. The mean age in this study was 51.5 years and in Rosen and Ridolfi's study, 56 years. Cases are also recorded in males with gynecomastia.[127,128]

These lesions are a few millimeters in diameter (0.3 to 3.6 mm in Lesueur's study) and are not visible macroscopically. Despite their name, they may be found in perilobular, intralobular, periductal or other stromal sites in the breast. Microscopically, they consist of an ill-defined meshwork of small, thin-walled, vascular channels lined by a single layer of endothelium similar to those in a cavernous hemangioma (Fig. 11.10). They may contain erythrocytes or proteinaceous fluid. The endothelial cells should not show any cytological atypia.

Palpable hemangiomas

Excluding those occurring in overlying skin, palpable benign hemangiomas of the breast are rare. Most have been reported in females although hemangiomas in males are recorded.[129,128] The age range is wide, with reports of their occurrence in children[130] and in women up to 85 years.[128] As for hemangiomas at other sites, they may be subdivided on the basis of their microscopic appearances into cavernous, capillary, venous, arteriovenous and juvenile. All have well-defined margins. Cavernous hemangiomas are composed of ectatic thin-walled, blood-filled vessels whereas capillary hemangiomas are composed of small, capillary-sized vessels. The vascular channels of venous and

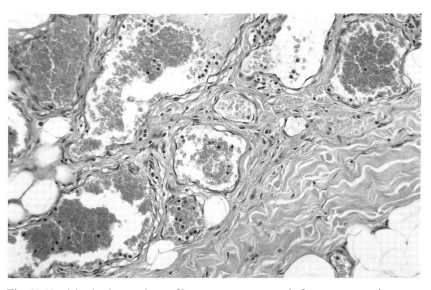

Fig. 11.10 A benign hemangioma of breast stroma composed of cavernous vascular channels.

arteriovenous hemangiomas are thick walled and muscular, with elastin in the arterial component. The vascular channels in all these subtypes are lined by flattened endothelial cells. This is in contrast to the juvenile subtype, in which some of the vessels are lined by plump endothelial cells and mitotic activity may be seen. This subtype probably represents an immature capillary hemangioma.

As stated in the introduction to this section, the important differential diagnosis of a vascular lesion is angiosarcoma. Azzopardi has emphasized that whereas a benign lesion is unlikely to be mistaken for malignancy, angiosarcoma may be misdiagnosed as benign.[131] Thus, palpable vascular lesions in particular should be thoroughly sampled to search for features of malignancy which include ill-defined, infiltrative margins, irregularity of vessel caliber, anastomozing vessels and endothelial atypia (see also Ch. 19). Occasionally, otherwise benign vascular lesions may display some of these features; these have been termed atypical hemangiomas and are discussed below.

Atypical hemangioma

In 1985, Josefcyk and Rosen described a further subset of 13 vascular tumors of the breast which exhibited characteristics raising the question of, but not qualifying for, a diagnosis of low grade angiosarcoma[132] and which they termed atypical hemangiomas. Subsequently, Hoda and colleagues have described a series of 18 such lesions[133] occurring in women aged between 19 and 82 years. They are characterized by small size (less than 2 cm) relative circumscription, broadly anastomozing vascular channels and endothelial hyperplasia. Destructive invasion, solid areas, hemorrhage and necrosis, except that associated with a needling procedure, are notably absent. Follow-up (1 to 140 months) of the 18 patients in Hoda's series, 11 of which were detected mammographically, has indicated a benign behavior with no recurrences recorded and the authors recommend complete excision alone as treatment.

Angiomatosis

This is a very rare benign vascular entity which can be extremely difficult to differentiate from angiosarcoma. The few cases reported in the breast have affected predominantly young women, but with an age range extending from birth[134] to 61 years[128] and it has been described in a male.[128] Presentation is with a breast mass which is generally several centimeters in diameter. The largest documented case measured 22 cm; this case being of further interest in that the tumor recurred and underwent massive enlargement during pregnancy, raising the possibility of hormone dependence. However, estrogen and progesterone receptor analyses were negative.[135]

Macroscopically, the resected specimens may not appear obviously vascular.[134] Two of the cases described have been cystic.[135,128] Microscopically, there is a network of anastomozing vascular channels which may appear empty or contain blood or lymph and which diffusely infiltrate the breast tissue without conspicuous intralobular growth.

The infiltrative nature of this process can render its distinction from well differentiated angiosarcoma extremely difficult. However, endothelial atypia and disruption of lobules are not a feature of angiomatosis and should be carefully sought before the diagnosis is made. In view of the difficulty of excluding well differentiated angiosarcoma on the basis of a small biopsy specimen, these lesions should be completely excised. Furthermore, as there is a tendency for these lesions to undergo local recurrence, wide local excision is the treatment of choice and long term follow up recommended.

Hemangiopericytoma

This rare soft tissue tumor, whose clinical behaviour can be difficult to predict, has been reported in the breast[136,137,138,128] in patients ranging from 5 to 67 years including a young boy.[137] The tumors are usually a few centimeters in diameter although lesions of 19 and 20 cm are described.[136,139] Macroscopically, they are pale grey to pink and may contain myxoid or cystic areas. Microscopically, these cellular tumors are composed of closely packed spindle cells surrounding ramifying vascular spaces which have a characteristic branching, stag-horn shape. The vascularity is emphasized by a reticulin stain. Immunohistochemical staining for vimentin and actin is positive in the spindle cells whereas the endothelial cells will show positive immunostaining for Factor VIII. The cases occurring in the breast appear to have a benign clinical course, being reported as showing no recurrence after local resection and follow-up periods ranging from 0.5 to 23 years. At other sites, a mitotic rate of four or more per 10 high power fields is taken to indicate an increased capability for recurrence and metastasis, as are the presence of increased cellularity, cytological atypia and foci of hemorrhage or necrosis.[111] Until more is known of the behavior of this rare tumor at this site, it is advisable to ensure complete excision of these tumors and long-term follow-up.

RARE TUMORS

There are case reports of unusual lesions arising in the breast which are of interest for a variety of reasons; they may mammographically or clinically resemble invasive carcinoma, may have histological features similar to more common or malignant entities and therefore need to be correctly interpreted, or simply be very rare, previously undescribed, exotica. Some of these lesions are well described at other, usually soft tissue sites, including nodular fasciitis,[140] leiomyoma,[118] chondrolipoma,[93] myxoma.[141] Others are more unusual; fibroma with cartilagenous differentiation,[34] choristoma showing a mixture of mesenchymal elements,[142] benign spindle cell tumor of Toker et al.,[143-145] ochronosis,[146] smooth muscle cell metaplasia.[147]

REFERENCES

1. Fernandez BB, Hernandez FJ. Amyloid tumour of the breast. Arch Pathol 1973; 95: 102–105.
2. Lipper S, Kahn LB. Amyloid tumour. A Clinicopathologic study of four cases. Am J Surg Pathol 1978; 2: 141–145.
3. McMahon RFT, Waldron D, Given HF, Connolly CE. Localised amyloid tumour of the breast — a case report. Ir J Med Sci 1984; 159: 323–324.
4. Lew W, Seymour A. Primary amyloid tumour of the breast. Case reports and literature review. Acta Cytol 1985; 29: 7–11.
5. Cheung PS, Yan KW, Alagaratnam TT, Collins RJ. Bilateral amyloid tumour of the breast. Aust NZ J Surg 1986; 56: 375–377.
6. Silverman JF, Dabbs DJ, Norris HT, Pories WJ, Legier J, Kay S. Localized primary (AL) amyloid tumour of the breast. Am J Surg Pathol 1986; 10: 539–545.
7. Sadaghee SA, Moore SW. Rheumatoid arthritis, bilateral amyloid tumours of the breast and multiple cutaneous amyloid nodules. Am J Clin Pathol 1984; 62: 472–476.
8. Hardy TJ, Myerowitz RL, Bender BL. Diffuse parenchymal amyloidosis of lungs and breast: Its association with diffuse plasmacytosis and k chain gammopathy. Arch Pathol Lab Med 1979; 103: 583–585.
9. O'Conner CR, Rubinow A, Cohen AS. Primary (AL) amyloidosis as a cause of breast masses. Am J Med 1984; 77: 981–986.
10. Santini D, Pasquinelli G, Alberghini M, Martinelli GN, Taffurelli M. Invasive breast carcinoma with granulomatous response and deposition of unusual amyloid. J Clin Pathol 1992; 45: 885–888.
11. Patil SD, Joshi B, Datar KG. Amyloid deposit in the carcinoma of breast. Indian J Cancer 1970; 7: 60–62.
12. Azzopardi JG. Miscellaneous entities. In: Problems in Breast Pathology. London: WB Saunders, 1979; pp.395–406.
13. Rosen PP. Multinucleated mammary stromal giant

cells: a benign lesion that simulates invasive carcinoma. Cancer 1979; 44: 1305–1308.
14. Abdul-Karim FW, Cohen RE. Atypical stromal cells of the lower female genital tract. Histopathology 1990; 17: 249–253.
15. Campbell AP. Multinucleated stromal giant cells in adolescent gynaecomastia. J Clin Path 1992; 45: 443–444.
16. Hartveit F. Mast cells and metachromasia in human breast cancer: their occurrence, significance and consequence: a preliminary report. J Pathol 1981; 134: 7–11.
17. Sandstad E, Hartveit F. Stromal metachromasia: a marker for incipient invasion in ductal carcinoma of the breast. Histopathology 1987; 11: 73–80.
18. Azzopardi JG, Laurini RN. Elastosis in breast cancer. Cancer 1974; 33: 174–183.
19. Humeniuk V, Forrest APM, Hawkins RA, Prescott R. Elastosis and primary breast cancer. Cancer 1983; 52: 1448–1452.
20. Glaubitz LC, Bowen LH, Cox ED. Elastosis in human breast cancer. Correlation with sex steroid receptors and comparison with clinical outcome. Arch Pathol Lab Med 1984; 108: 27–30.
21. Farahmand S, Cowan DF. Elastosis in the normal ageing breast. Arch Pathol Lab Med 1991; 115: 1241–1246.
22. Davies JD. Hyperelastosis, obliteration and fibrous plaques in major ducts of the human breast. J Pathol 1973; 110: 13–26.
23. Bogomoletz WV. Elastosis in breast cancer. Pathol Annu 1986; 21: 347–366.
24. Tremblay G, Buell RH, Seemayer TA. Elastosis in benign sclerosing ductal proliferations of the female breast. Am J Surg Pathol 1977; 1: 1155–1158.
25. Raju GC, Lee Y-S. Elastosis in the male breast. Histopathology 1988; 12: 203–209.
26. Fisher ER, Gregorio RM, Fisher B. The pathology of invasive breast cancer. A syllabus derived from findings

of the National Surgical Adjuvant Breast Project (No. 4). Cancer 1975; 36: 1–85.

27. Schiodt T, Jensen H, Nielsen M, Ranlov P. On the nature of amyloid-like duct wall changes in carcinoma of the breast. Acta Pathol Microbiol Scand (A) 1972; 80(Suppl. 233): 151–157.

28. Ghosh L, Ghosh BC, Das Gupta TK. Ultrastructural study of stroma in human mammary carcinoma. Am J Surg 1980; 139: 229–232.

29. Davies JD, Riddell RH. Muscular hamartomas of the breast. J Pathol 1973; 111: 209–211.

30. Mackenzie DH. A fibroadenoma of the breast with smooth muscle. J Pathol Bacteriol 1968; 96: 231–232.

31. Norris HJ, Taylor HB. Relationship of histological features to behaviour of cystosarcoma phylloides. Cancer 1967; 20: 1090–1099.

32. Eusebi V, Cusolo A, Fedeli F. Benign smooth muscle metaplasia in the breast. Tumori 1980; 66: 643–653.

33. Smith BG, Taylor HB. The occurrence of bone and cartilage in mammary tumours. Am J Clin Pathol 1969; 51: 610–618.

34. Lawler RG. Cartilagenous metaplasia in a breast tumour. J Pathol 1969; 97: 385–387.

35. Pietruszka M, Barnes L. Cystosarcoma phyllodes. A clinicopathologic analysis of 42 cases. Cancer 1978; 41: 1974–1983.

36. Qizilbash AH. Cystosarcoma phyllodes with liposarcomatous stroma. Am J Clin Pathol 1976; 65: 321–327.

37. Vuitch MF, Rosen PP, Erlandsen RA. Pseudoangiomatous hyperplasia of mammary stroma. Hum Pathol 1986; 17: 185–191.

38. Ibrahim RE, Sciotto CG, Weidner N. Pseudoangiomatous hyperplasia of mammary stroma. Cancer 1989; 63: 1154–1160.

39. Seidman JD, Borkowski A, Aisner SC, Sun CS. Rapid growth of pseudoangiomatous hyperplasia of mammary stroma in axillary gynecomastia in an immunosuppressed patient. Arch Pathol Lab Med 1993; 117: 736–738.

40. Anderson C, Ricci A, Pedersen CA, Cartun RW. Immunocytochemical analysis of estrogen and progesterone receptors in benign stromal lesions of the breast. Evidence for hormonal etiology in pseudoangiomatous hyperplasia of mammary stroma. Am J Surg Pathol 1991; 15: 145–149.

41. Clement PB, Ypung RH, Azzopardi JG. Collagenous spherulosis of the breast. Am J Surg Pathol 1987; 11: 411–417.

42. Wells CA, Wells CW, Yeomans P, Vina M, Jordan S, d'Ardenne AJ. Spherical connective tissue inclusions in epithelial hyperplasia of the breast ('collagenous spherulosis'). J Clin Pathol 1990; 43: 905–908.

43. Grignon DJ, Ro JY, Mackay BN, Ordonez NG, Ayala AG. Collagenous spherulosis of the breast. Immunohistochemical and ultrastructural studies. Am J Clin Pathol 1989; 91: 386–392.

44. Tyler X, Coghill SB. Fine needle aspiration cytology of collagenous spherulosis of the breast. Cytopathology 1991; 2: 159–162.

45. Highland KE, Finley JL, Neill JS, Silverman JF. Collagenous spherulosis. Report of a case with diagnosis by fine needle aspiration biopsy with immunocytochemical and ultrastructural observations. Acta Cytol 1993; 37: 3–9.

46. Guarino M, Tricomi P, Cristofori E. Collagenous spherulosis of the breast with atypical hyperplasia. Pathologica 1993; 85: 123–127.

47. Fisher ER, Brown R. Intraductal signet ring carcinoma. A hitherto undescribed form of intraductal carcinoma of the breast. Cancer 1985; 55: 2533–2537.

48. Panico L, Dantonio A, Chiacchio R, Delrio P, Petrella G, Pettinato G. An unusual, recurring breast tumor with features of eccrine spiradenoma: A case report. Am J Clin Pathol 1996; 106: 665–669.

49. Cyrlak D, Barr RJ, Wile AG. Malignant eccrine acrospiroma of the breast. Internat J Dermatol 1995; 34: 271–273.

50. Saboorian MH, Kenny M, Ashfaq R, Albores Saavedra J. Carcinosarcoma arising in eccrine spiradenoma of the breast: Report of a case and review of the literature. Arch Pathol Lab Med 1996; 120: 501–504.

51. Kumar N, Verma K. Clear cell hidradenoma simulating breast carcinoma: A diagnostic pitfall in fine-needle aspiration of breast. Diagn Cytopathol 1996; 15: 70–72.

52. Narita T, Matsuda K. Pleomorphic adenoma of the breast: Case report and review of the literature. Pathol Internat 1995; 45: 441–447.

53. Diaz NM, McDivitt RW, Wick MR. Pleomorphic adenoma of the breast: A clinicopathologic and immunohistochemical study of 10 cases. Hum Pathol 1991; 22: 1206–1214.

54. Moran CA, Suster S, Carter D. Benign mixed tumors (pleomorphic adenomas) of the breast. Am J Surg Pathol 1990; 14: 913–921.

55. Walt JVD, Rohlova B. Pleomorphic adenoma of the human breast. A report of a benign tumour closely mimicking a carcinoma clinically. Clin Oncol 1982; 8: 361–365.

56. Soreide JA, Anda O, Eriksen L, Holter J, Kjellevold KH. Pleomorphic adenoma of the human breast with local recurrence. Cancer 1988; 61: 997–1001.

57. Chen KTK. Pleomorphic adenoma of the breast. Am J Clin Pathol 1990; 93: 792–794.

58. Rosen PP. Syringomatous adenoma of the nipple. Am J Surg Pathol 1983; 7: 739–745.

59. Suster S, Moran CA, Hurt MA. Syringomatous squamous tumors of the breast. Cancer 1991; 67: 2350–2355.

60. Ward BE, Cooper PH, Subramony C. Syringomatous tumor of the nipple. Am J Clin Pathol 1989; 92: 692–696.

61. Tavassoli FA. Diseases of the nipple. In: Tavassoli FA, ed. Pathology of the Breast. Connecticut: Appleton and Lange, 1992; pp. 583–589.

62. Jones MW, Norris HJ, Snyder RC. Infiltrating syringomatous adenoma of the nipple. A clinical and pathological study of 11 cases. Am J Surg Pathol 1989; 13: 197–201.

63. Slaughter MS, Pomerantz RA, Murad T, Hines JR. Infiltrating syringomatous adenoma of the nipple. Surgery 1992; 111: 711–713.

64. Nichols RW. Desmoid tumours; a report of 31 cases. Arch Surg 1923; 7: 227–236.

65. Gump FE, Sternschein MJ, Wolff M. Fibromatosis of the breast. Surg Gynecol Obstet 1981; 153: 57–60.

66. Rosen PP, Ernsberger D. Mammary fibromatosis. A benign spindle-cell tumour with significant risk for local recurrence. Cancer 1989; 63: 1363–1369.

67. Wargotz ES, Norris HJ, Austin RM, Enzinger FM. Fibromatosis of the breast. A clinical and pathological study of 28 cases. Am J Surg Pathol 1987; 11: 38–45.

68. Haggitt RC, Booth JL. Bilateral fibromatosis of the breast in Gardner's syndrome. Cancer 1970; 25: 161–166.

69. Kalisher L, Long JA, Peyster RG. Extra-abdominal desmoid of the axillary tail mimicking breast carcinoma. Am J Roentgen 1976; 126: 903–906.

70. Mayers MM, Evans P, MacVicar D. Case report: Ossifying fibromatosis of the breast. Clin Radiol 1994; 49: 211–212.

71. Hanna WM, Jambrosik J, Fish E. Aggressive fibromatosis of the breast. Arch Pathol Lab Med 1985; 109: 260–262.

72. El-Naggar A, Abdul-Karim FW, Marshalleck JJ, Sorensen K. Fine needle aspiration of fibromatosis of the breast. Diagn Cytopathol 1987; 3: 320–322.

73. Simpson RD, Harrison EG, Mayo CW. Mesenteric fibromatosis in familial polyposis: a variant of Gardner's syndrome. Cancer 1964; 12: 526–534.

74. Zayid I, Dihmis C. Familial multicentric fibromatosis-desmoids. Cancer 1969; 24: 786–795.

75. Jewett STJ, Mead JH. Extra-abdominal desmoid arising from a capsule around a silicone breast implant. Plast Reconstr Surg 1979; 63: 577–579.

76. Kinzbrunner B, Ritter S, Domingo J, Rosenthal J. Remission of rapidly growing desmoid tumours after tamoxifen therapy. Cancer 1983; 52: 2201–2204.

77. Hayry P, Reitamo JJ, Bikho R. The desmoid tumour III. A biochemical and genetic analysis. Am J Clin Pathol 1982; 77: 681–685.

78. Pierce VE, Rives DA, Sisley JF, Allsbrook WC. Estradiol and progesterone receptors in a case of fibromatosis of the breast. Arch Pathol Lab Med 1987; 11: 870–872.

79. Waddell WR, Gerner R, Reich MP. Nonsteroid anti-inflammatory drugs and tamoxifen for desmoid tumours and carcinoma of the stomach. J Surg Oncol 1983; 22: 197–211.

80. Wargotz ES, Weiss SW, Norris HJ. Myofibroblastoma of the breast. Sixteen cases of a distinctive benign mesenchymal tumour. Am J Surg Pathol 1987; 11: 493–502.

81. Julien M, Trojani M, Coindre JM. Myofibroblastoma du sein. Etude de 8 cas. Ann Pathol 1994; 14: 143–147.

82. Lee AHS, Sworn MJ, Theaker JM, Fletcher CDM. Myofibroblastoma of the breast: an immunohistochemical study. Histopathol 1993; 22: 75–78.

83. Spalding JE. Adenolipoma and lipoma of the breast. Guys Hosp Rep 1945; 94: 80–84.

84. Haagensen CD. Diseases of the Breast. (3rd ed.) WB Saunders, 1986; pp. 333–335.

85. Brown RW, Bhathal PS, Scott PR. Multiple bilateral angiolipomas of the breast. Aust NZ J Surg 1982; 52: 614–616.

86. Franzini M, Castigluini G, Martinelli R. Angiolipoma of the breast. Pathologica 1981; 73: 823–826.

87. Tavassoli FA. Mesenchymal Lesions. In: Tavassoli FA, ed. Pathology of the Breast. Connecticut: Appleton and Lange, 1992; pp. 517–563.

88. Hunt SJ, Santa Cruz DJ, Barr RJ. Cellular angiolipoma. Am J Surg Pathol 1990; 14: 75–81.

89. Yu GH, Fishman SJ, Brooks JSJ. Cellular angiolipoma of the breast. Mod Pathol 1993; 6: 497–499.

90. Kaplan L, Walts AE. Benign chondrolipomatous tumour of the human female breast. Arch Pathol Lab Med 1977; 101: 149–151.

91. Dharkar DD, Kraft JR. Benign chondrolipomatous tumour of the breast. Postgrad Med J 1981; 57: 129–131.

92. Lugo M, Reyes JM, Putong PB. Benign chondrolipomatous tumours of the breast (letter). Arch Pathol Lab Med 1982; 106: 691–692.

93. Marsh WL, Lucas JG, Olsen J. Chondrolipoma of the breast. Arch Pathol Lab Med 1989; 113: 369–371.

94. Demay RM, Kay S. Granular cell tumour of the breast. Pathol Annu 1984; 19: 121–148.

95. Haagensen CD, Stout AT. Granular cell myoblastoma of the mammary gland. Ann Surg 1946; 124: 218–227.

96. Mulcare R. Granular cell myofibroblastoma of the breast. Ann Surg 1968; 168: 262–268.

97. Gordon AB, Fisher C, Palmer B et al. Granular cell tumours of the breast. Br J Surg Oncol 1985; 11: 269–273.

98. Strobel SL, Shah NT, Lucas JG, Tuttle SE. Granular cell tumour of the breast. A cytologic, immunohistochemical and ultrastructural study of two cases. Acta Cytol 1985; 29: 598–601.

99. Rickart MT, Sendel A, Burchett I. Case report: Granular cell tumour of the breast. Clin Radiol 1992; 45: 347–348.

100. Komoss F, Mercer L, Schmidt RA, Talerman A. Granular cell tumour of the breast mimicking carcinoma. Obstet Gynecol 1989; 73: 898–900.

101. Umansky C, Bullock WK. Granular cell myoblastoma of the breast. Ann Surg 1968; 168: 810–817.

102. Stefansson K, Wollmann RL. S-100 protein in granular cell tumours (granular cell myoblastomas). Cancer 1982; 49: 1834–1838.

103. Raju GC, O'Reilly AP. Immunohistochemical study of granular cell tumour. Pathology 1987; 19: 402–406.

104. Shousha S, Lyssiotis T. Granular cell myoblastoma: Positive staining for carcinoembryonic antigen. J Clin Pathol 1979; 32: 219–224.

105. Abrikossoff A. Über Myome, augehend von der quergestreiften willkürlichen Muskulatur. Virch Arch. (A) 1926; 260: 215–233.

106. Ingram DL, Mossler JA, Snowhite J, Leight GS, McCarty KSJ. Granular cell tumours of the breast. Steroid receptor analysis and localisation of carcinoembryonic antigen, myoglobin and S100 protein. Arch Pathol Lab Med 1984; 108: 897–901.

107. Azzopardi JG. Granular-cell 'myoblastoma'. In: Bennington JL, ed. Problems in Breast Pathology. London: W B Saunders, 1979; pp. 398–399.

108. Crawford ES, deBakey ME. Granular cell myoblastoma: Two unusual cases. Cancer 1953; 6: 786–789.

109. Chetty R, Kalan MR. Malignant granular cell tumour of the breast. J Surg Oncol 1992; 49: 135–137.

110. Khansur T, Balducci L, Tavassoli M. Granular cell tumour. Clinical spectrum of the benign and malignant entity. Cancer 1987; 60: 220–222.

111. Enzinger FM, Weiss SW. Soft Tissue Tumours. (second ed.) St Louis: CV Mosby 1988: 757–768.

112. Collins R, Gau G. Neurilemoma presenting as a lump in the breast. Br J Surg 1973; 60: 242–243.

113. Majmudar B. Neurilemoma presenting as a lump in the breast. South Med J 1976; 69: 463–464.

114. Van der Walt JD, Reid HAS, Shaw JHF. Neurilemoma appearing as a lump in the breast (letter). Arch Pathol Lab Med 1982; 106: 539–540.

115. Fisher PE, Estabrook A, Cohen MB. Fine needle aspiration biopsy of intramammary neurilemoma. Acta Cytol 1990; 34: 35–37.

116. Bernardello F, Caneva A, Bresaola E et al. Breast solitary schwannoma: fine needle aspiration biopsy and immunocytochemical analysis. Diagn Cytopathol 1994; 10: 221–223.

117. Schauder H. Über leiomyome der brustdruse. Arch Pathol 1927; 14: 794–798.

118. Diaz-Arias AA, Hurt MA, Loy TS, Seeger RM, Bickel JT. Leiomyoma of the breast. Hum Pathol 1989; 20: 396–399.

119. Lebowich RJ, Lenz G. Primary fibromyoma of the breast. Am J Cancer 1940; 38: 73–75.

120. Libcke JH. Leiomyoma of the breast. J Pathol 1969; 98: 89–91.

121. Roncaroli F, Rossi R, Severi B, Martinelli GN, Eusebi V. Epithelioid leiomyoma of the breast wih granular cell change: A case report. Hum Pathol 1993; 24: 1260–1263.

122. Shimokama T, Watanabe T. Leiomyoma exhibiting a marked granular change: Granular cell leiomyoma versus granular cell Schwannoma. Hum Pathol 1992; 23: 327–331.

123. Chen KTK, Kuo TT, Hoffman KD. Leiomyosarcoma of the breast. Cancer 1981; 47: 1883–1886.

124. Nielsen BB. Leiomyosarcoma of the breast with late dissemination. Virchows Archiv (Pathol Anat) 1984; 403: 241–245.

125. Rosen PP, Ridolfi RL. The perilobular haemangioma. A benign microscopic vascular lesion of the breast. Am J Clin Pathol 1977; 68: 21–23.

126. Lesueur GC, Brown RW, Bhathal PS. Incidence of perilobular hemangioma in the female breast. Arch Pathol Lab Med 1983; 107: 308–310.

127. Scwartz IS, Marchevsky A. Haemangioma of male breast (letter). Am J Surg Pathol 1987; 11: 739.

128. Tavassoli FA. Vascular lesions. In: Tavassoli FA, ed. Pathology of the Breast. Connecticut: Appleton and Lange, 1992; pp. 483–516.

129. Shousha S, Theodorou NA, Bull TB. Cavernous haemangioma of breast in a man with contralateral gynaecomastia and a family history of breast carcinoma. Histopathology 1988; 13: 221–223.

130. Nagar H, Marmor S, Hammer B. Haemangiomas of the breast in children. Eur J Surg 1992; 158: 503–505.

131. Azzopardi JG. Breast Sarcomas. In: Bennington JL, ed. Problems in Breast Pathology. London: WB Saunders, 1979; pp. 346–378.

132. Jozefcyk MA, Rosen PP. Vascular tumours of the breast II: perilobular hemangiomas and hemangiomas. Am J Surg Pathol 1985; 9: 491–503.

133. Hoda SA, Cranor ML, Rosen PP. Hemangiomas of the breast with atypical histological features. Further analysis of histological subtypes cofirming their benign character. Am J Surg Pathol 1992; 16: 553–560.

134. Rosen PP. Vascular tumours of the breast III. Angiomatosis. Am J Surg Pathol 1985; 9: 652–658.

135. Morrow M, Berger D, Thelmo W. Diffuse cystic angiomatosis of the breast. Cancer 1988; 62: 2392–2396.

136. Arias-Stella JJ, Rosen PP. Haemangiopericytoma of the breast. Mod Pathol 1988; 1: 98–103.

137. Kaufman SL, Stout AP. Hemangiopericytoma in children. Cancer 1960; 13: 695–710.

138. Mittal KR, Gerald W, True LD. Hemangiopericytoma of breast: Report of a case with ultrastructural and immunohistochemical findings. Hum Pathol 1986; 17: 1181–1183.

139. Callery CD, Rosen PP, Kinne DW. Sarcoma of the breast. Ann Surg 1985; 201: 527.

140. Page DL, Anderson TJ. Diagnostic Histopathology of the Breast. Edinburgh: Churchill Livingstone, 1987; p. 352.

141. Chan YF, Yeung HY, Ma L. Myxoma of the breast:report of a case and ultrastructural study. Pathology 1986; 18: 153–157.

142. Metcalf JS, Ellis B. Choristoma of the breast. Hum Pathol 1985; 16: 739–740.

143. Toker C, Tang CK, Whitely JF, Berkheiser Sw, Rachman R. Benign spindle cell breast tumour. Cancer 1981; 48: 1615–1622.

144. Böger A. Benign spindle cell tumour of male breast. Pathol Res Pract 1984; 178: 395–398.

145. Chan K, Ghadially FN, Alagaratnam TT. Benign spindle cell tumour of breast — a varient of spindle cell lipoma or fibroma of breast? Pathology 1984; 16: 331–337.

146. Lefer LG, Rosier RP. Ochronosis of the breast. Am J Clin Pathol 1979; 71: 349–352.

147. Eusebi V, Cunsolo A, Fedeli F, Severi B, Scarini P. Benign smooth muscle metaplasia in the breast. Tumori 1980; 66: 643–653.

12

R. W. Blamey

Clinical aspects of benign breast lesions

INTRODUCTION

From the foregoing chapters it is apparent that benign breast conditions make up a heterogeneous collection presenting a variety of management problems. One group is those which are recognized as lesions associated with a higher risk of developing breast cancer. The management of these is best discussed alongside that of breast carcinoma (see Ch. 22).

In this chapter benign conditions will be considered which have no association with breast cancer. The reason why the phrase benign 'disease' should be avoided, is that the majority do not produce dis-ease (discomfort or a dangerous condition). They may be considered according to their mode of presentation: lumps, nipple discharge, inflammatory lesions and discomfort (mastalgia).

BENIGN BREAST LUMPS

Benign breast lumps do not constitute a disease in their own right, since if there was no breast cancer the presence of a breast lump would not cause concern. The commonest lumps are cysts (which are part of the involutional process of fibrocystic change) and fibroadenomas (which are developmental abnormalities). They have a very different age distribution (Fig. 12.1).

FIBROCYSTIC CHANGE

Fibrocystic change gives two clinical problems —

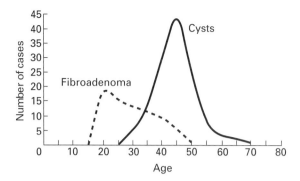

Fig. 12.1 Age distribution of cysts and fibroadenomata presenting in the GP referral clinic.

a lumpy area with an ill-defined edge or a discrete lump formed by a cyst.

A clinically lumpy area

This is a common presentation. Since the clinical judgment between lumpiness within the normal range and the presence of a true but indefinite lump is blurred, they may present a diagnostic problem. A clinically lumpy area on histology shows the normal involutional change associated with the age of the patient, fibrosis with some microcyst formation. The diagnostic problem is that occasionally, in retrospect, carcinoma in situ may be seen to have presented as a lumpy area; the difficulty is that very many women have asymmetric lumpy areas in the breast at some time during their 30s and 40s, and full investigation of all such patients is not a practical proposition.

Until comparatively recently, biopsy of a lumpy area clinically mimicking a lump was a frequent operative procedure. With careful triple assessment (Ch. 2) the problem is now usually resolved without operation.

The examining surgeon has to stick firmly to the principles of clinical examination, the most important of which is to decide whether or not a true lump is present. If it is thought that there is a generally lumpy area then a subjective decision has to be made which is difficult to describe; four examples will be given:

1. On careful palpation it may be clear that the patient is simply feeling the edge of the breast disc; the diagnosis is made by creeping the fingers towards the edge feeling only skin and subcutaneous fat and then easing across the relatively sudden edge of the breast tissue. No further investigation is then required.

2. Palpation reveals an area approximately 4 cm in diameter in the axillary tail, which the examiner initially thinks may be a true lump; palpation of the contralateral breast shows a very similar area. No further investigation is required.

3. The breasts are generally lumpy. They may be tender and there may be a cyclical element. No further investigation is required.

4. There is an asymmetrical lumpy area — quite prominent but with indistinct edges so that the examiner is uncertain whether or not a true lump is present. This requires ultrasound and mammographic examination and category C fine needle aspiration cytology (FNAC) or needle core biopsy (Ch. 2).

Cysts

Unless there are clear physical signs of malignancy any lump in the breast may prove to be a cyst. Clinically cysts may measure a few mm up to 10 cm in diameter. They may feel firm or soft and fluctuation cannot usually be elicited since they are too tense. The surface is usually smooth and the lump discrete; there may be associated discomfort.

Sometimes there is a clear history that a large cyst appeared overnight. This reflects the pressure within a cyst and the resistance; the analogy is the blowing up of a balloon: high pressure is needed to overcome the initial resistance, then there is a rapid expansion whilst the pressure within actually drops.

Cysts may be divided into those in which there is active secretion (high potassium content) and those where the content is extracellular fluid (diffusion cysts);[1] although the former are more likely to be multiple and recurrent, this is of no practical value. Cysts are uncommon before the age of 30 (Fig. 12.1) and some years ago were rare in women over 50. This has changed with the increasing prescription of hormone replacement therapy.

The easiest way to confirm that a lump is a cyst is to aspirate with a 23 gauge needle; however if the lump then proves to be solid, this may cause a hematoma and make further investigation more difficult. Ideally an ultrasound examination should be carried out to confirm that the lump is a cyst before needling (Ch. 2). If the cyst has presented as a clinical lump then it is aspirated completely, pressing with one hand whilst aspirating with the other. Cytological examination of the fluid is not required, but re-palpation must confirm that the lump has disappeared; if a solid lump remains then full investigation is required. Cysts found on screening mammography do not need to be aspirated.

FIBROADENOMA AND RELATED CONDITIONS

Fibroadenoma

Fibroadenomata present typically as smooth, very mobile, very well demarcated, ovoid lumps. The age distribution for their symptomatic presentation is shown in Figure 12.1; they may also be recognized at mammographic screening in women of over 50, when they are often small. They are usually 1–2 cm in diameter and once found the majority do not increase in size. Their occurrence is probably extremely common and with a pyramidal size distribution, so that only those few near the peak at 1–2 cm present clinically (Fig. 12.2).

Juvenile fibroadenoma/hamartoma

These conditions, which are similar in clinical presentation and overlap from the histological point of view, are actually seen more commonly in the post-juvenile age range, around 18–22 years

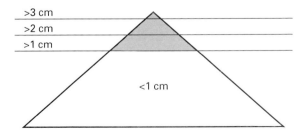

Fig. 12.2 Suggested distribution of fibroadenomata in the population. Only those at the peak of the pyramid reach the size at which they are discovered.

and occasionally up to 40. As the breast undergoes postpubertal enlargement, the woman finds that she has a large, unilateral, irregular, ill-demarcated, breast lump, occupying perhaps a quarter of the breast tissue. Needle core biopsies may show the histological appearance of a fibroadenoma or of non-specific benign breast tissue. The lump does not resolve and does not enlarge, the only problem is cosmetic; if the lesion is not distressing the patient then it may be left in situ.

If the patient decides that she would like the lump removed the surgeon may be worried at excising such a large volume of breast tissue, but the cosmetic results are quite good; the lesion is largely an overgrowth, leaving a comparatively normal residual breast volume for that patient.

Lactational nodules

We prefer to term this condition 'adenosis of pregnancy', for there is no pathological lesion. A smooth, demarcated, ovoid lump, around 4–6 cm in length (the longer axis lying horizontal), is found at around 30 weeks of pregnancy. The clinical signs are alarming, for carcinomas detected in pregnancy are often large. The rule in the Nottingham Breast Clinic is to take needle core biopsies from both poles: these show breast tissue with lactational change only. The woman is seen one month later and the biopsies are repeated.

The apparent 'lump' becomes impalpable after cessation of lactation. Interestingly we have seen the 'lump' return in the same place during a subsequent pregnancy. Presumably the clinical finding represents a tenser feel to one lobe.

Phyllodes tumor

Phyllodes tumors usually present as large lesions, around 4 cm diameter; they are seen predominantly in middle-aged or elderly patients and the average age of presentation is 45–50 years. They may be smaller and indistinguishable clinically from fibroadenomata or may be bosselated masses occupying the whole breast. The clinical differentiation from locally advanced carcinoma is that despite their often considerable size, they do not show the malignant features of skin tether nor deep fixity. The lump may be so large as to cause patchy pressure necrosis of the skin.

Impalpable phyllodes tumors of 3–4 cm may be seen on mammography at breast screening. It is consistency and not size which makes a lump feel different from the surrounding breast tissue.

Needle core histology confirms the diagnosis. Lumps thought clinically to be fibroadenomas, but which are greater than 3 cm in extent, should undergo needle core biopsy to exclude the possibility of phyllodes tumor.

The majority of phyllodes tumors are benign, but they may grow extensively locally and tend to recur after excision. A few are sarcomatous and metastasize. Histological prediction of these events is inexact (Ch. 9). Excision must be complete, with a clear margin of at least 1 cm on postoperative histological examination. As in excising a breast cancer (Ch. 22) the surface of the specimen must be painted with Indian ink so that the pathologist can recognize the margins at microscopy and the specimen must be orientated. If marginal clearance is anywhere less than 1 cm then that margin must be re-excised. Large tumors and local recurrences should be treated by mastectomy or subcutaneous mastectomy (the tumor does not invade skin). Distant metastases are sarcomatous (Ch. 22). Of 33 phyllodes tumors managed on the Nottingham Unit, 7 recurred locally (one aggressive and difficult to control) and one (a tertiary referral) behaved aggressively locally and produced lung metastases as an osteosarcoma.

EPITHELIAL HYPERPLASIA

Hyperplastic lesions may give rise to palpable lumps. Lesions which on histology show epithelial hyperplasia of usual type (Ch. 5) require no further follow-up but management in lesions showing atypia is considered in Chapter 22.

PAPILLOMA/PAPILLARY LESIONS

Single

Small single papillomas present as single duct nipple discharge (see below).

Multiple

Multiple larger papillomata are more peripheral in the breast and may present as a lump. Needle core biopsy and FNAC are interpreted only as 'papillary lesion', which means that the lump must be removed for full diagnosis, since the lump may be a papillary carcinoma or ductal carcinoma in situ (DCIS) or a papilloma with atypia, all of which are managed accordingly. If histology shows a straightforward benign papilloma without atypia, then excision biopsy alone is all that is needed.

SCLEROSING LESIONS

Sclerosing lesions are usually impalpable and found at mammographic screening. Occasionally a breast lump mimicking a fibroadenoma is found to show only sclerosing adenosis[2] and a radial scar/complex sclerosing lesion may be palpable as a diffuse lump. When a lump is diagnosed as a radial scar by needle core biopsy, subsequent open incision biopsy is recommended currently, since carcinoma and radial scar may co-exist. Likewise impalpable lesions which appear spiculate on mammography (Ch. 2) require tissue diagnosis by open surgical biopsy, even if benign tissue has been obtained by needle core biopsy (Ch. 22).

DIAGNOSIS AND MANAGEMENT OF A BENIGN LUMP

Until recently a solid breast lump was always excised for diagnosis, to ensure that it was not a cancer. With the increasing use and sensitivity and specificity for the diagnosis of cancer, of aspiration cytology in the UK over the past few years, brought about by the introduction of the breast screening program, the possibility arose to make a positive benign diagnosis. At Nottingham City Hospital criteria by which a palpable lump is diagnosed as benign without operative excision, have been set. These criteria have been modified with the increasing readoption of needle core biopsy, brought about by the introduction of guns to fire the needles.

The older the patient the more likely any solid lump may be a cancer and for this reason, the older the patient the more strict are the criteria. Those for a woman of 35 or over are: (i) that the lump must feel benign, be smooth and mobile, and measure 3 cm or less (see phyllodes tumor, below); (ii) the lump must appear benign on ultrasound and/or mammography or not image; (iii) one needle core biopsy showing features of definite lesion, e.g. a fibroadenoma, is sufficient to confirm the diagnosis. If no confirmation has been obtained from needle core then (iv) two FNACs are taken 6 weeks apart and both must show an adequate number of benign epithelial cells (Category B, see Ch. 2) and (v) as a further precaution the size is recorded (preferably by ultrasound) and the patient is reassessed 6 months from her first attendance; the lump is re-measured and a third FNAC is performed (Category C).

Many fibroadenomata occur before 25 years of age, whereas breast cancer before that age is extremely rare (only 1–2 cases per annum in the UK). Some surgeons therefore do not now excise a lump which feels like a fibroadenoma in a woman under 25 years. In the Nottingham City Hospital Breast Clinic we take one FNAC (Category C, see Ch. 2) and excision is advised only if abnormal cells are seen.

For women aged 26–35, ultrasound examination is added to clinical examination but x-ray mammography is not appropriate; a Category B FNAC is taken (see Ch. 2), and management is then as for a lump in women of over 35. Ideally one of the cytology specimens should be taken under ultrasound, to ensure that the sample is from the lump and not from the adjacent tissue.

In a study of 412 clinically benign feeling lumps in women of 35 or over we have shown that as long as the criteria are closely followed, these are safe policies[3] (Fig. 12.3). The majority of patients accept the assurance that the lump is benign and under these circumstances prefer to have it left in situ. In 26 patients who chose to undergo excision after the criteria had been satisfied, all proved to have fibroadenomas.

Asymptomatic fibroadenomas, seen at basic mammographic screening, are often diagnosed as such by the radiologist and the woman is not then recalled for assessment. If a woman is recalled and the lump is palpable it is managed as above. If it is impalpable and judged by the radiologist, after

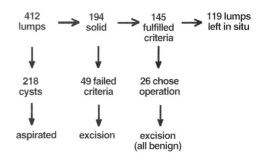

Fig. 12.3 The results in women of 35 years and over of the non-operative approach to the management of benign breast lumps.

further imaging with ultrasound and possibly extra mammographic views, to be benign, then one FNAC is taken (Category C, Ch. 2); excision is only advised if abnormal cells are present in the aspirate (C 3, Equivocal or above).

INFLAMMATORY LESIONS

Acute abscess

Acute abscess is most often a complication of pregnancy or lactation. All the features of acute abscess are present: tumor, rubor, dolor. An abscess may be treated by aspiration of pus with a 23 gauge needle followed by a course of antibiotics. If the abscess is very large or if conservative treatment fails, then incision is required.

Patients are sometimes seen in the clinic after antibiotic treatment by the general practitioner and the lesion may have resolved. To make the diagnosis the patient should be asked if it was red, hot and very tender. Alternatively the inflammation resolves but leaves a palpable lump; this is an 'antibioma', filled with sterile pus and may require incision and drainage or, if small, excision.

The only confusion in differential diagnosis in the acute stage is with so-called 'inflammatory' carcinoma. Carcinomas with overlying erythema and skin edema (Ch. 22) are not as acutely tender as an abscess but a dangerous trap is that the inflammatory appearance may resolve somewhat with antibiotic treatment; when this occurs, needle core biopsy of the residual lump should be carried out to exclude carcinoma. The patient is then watched until the acute inflammation clears completely and subsequently for complete resolution of the lump. If the lump does not resolve within 6 weeks a further needle core biopsy or incision/excision biopsy must be carried out to confirm the diagnosis.

Periareolar abscess/periductal mastitis/mammillary fistula

This group of conditions present as indefinite lumps under the areolar edge, usually somewhat tender. There may be associated nipple discharge. The lump does not generally image and FNAC shows inflammatory change with macrophages. If painful and tender, incision is indicated and is made following the areolar edge. A search for the involved duct is made, a probe passed up to the nipple and an incision made along the probe. The small, T-shaped wound is left to granulate.

Prior to incision the abscess may itself discharge at the areolar edge, giving a mammillary fistula from duct to skin (Fig. 12.4), the probe is then easy to pass and incision and granulation follow.

The condition may be recurrent or multiple around the areola and may be bilateral. It is commoner in smokers.[4] If the patient suffers several abscesses then excision of the central duct system (all the tissue beneath the areola) is undertaken. Unfortunately not even this always prevents further recurrence,[5] as chronic infection has extended to the whole duct system. A long course of ciprofloxacillin may be given.

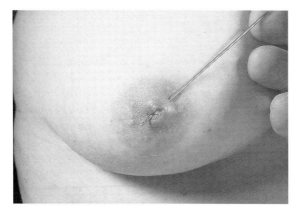

Fig. 12.4 Mammillary fistula.

TRAUMATIC FAT NECROSIS/HEMATOMA

This is the condition that may most resemble breast cancer; it particularly occurs in the elderly and there may be no history of trauma. A lump is felt which is neither smooth nor freely mobile; sometimes there is even discernible skin tether. FNAC shows inflammatory cells and macrophages and may be reported as 'suspicious'. If the condition is suspected then needle core biopsy is the best investigation; this must not be done as the primary investigation, since a previous needle aspirate itself produces the histological appearance of fat necrosis.

Traumatic fat necrosis is the one condition for which a lump which does not feel entirely benign may be left unoperated when investigations have not shown carcinoma. The diagnosis may be suspected because of a recent history of severe bruising of the breast (e.g. from seat belt injury) or from the findings on FNAC or needle core biopsy. The patient is seen again one month later and the lump should be resolving by then; she is followed until complete resolution, which is usually within 2 months.

Granulomatous conditions

Tuberculosis and sarcoidosis rarely present as breast lumps: tuberculosis usually as a chest wall mass lying under the breast.

Granulomatous mastitis gives rise to a breast lump, which since it does not feel entirely benign, is removed. It is an uncommon condition and may give rise to multiple or recurrent lumps.[6]

CONNECTIVE TISSUE LESIONS

Fibromatosis

A focus of fibromatosis may occur within the pectoral muscles or within the breast itself. The potential for local recurrence is well recognized and fibromatoses sometimes invade the thoracic cavity. Therefore the surgeon must ensure that excision is very wide, even at the expense of cosmesis. If the tumor lies in muscle then the whole of that muscle should be removed. Clearance must be deep enough and excision of the underlying chest wall may be advisable. If excision appears incomplete at histology and further surgery is not possible then adjuvant radiotherapy may be advantageous.[7] Treatment with peripheral estrogen antagonists has also been recommended.[8]

Adenoma of the nipple

Adenoma presents as a lump directly beneath and attached to the nipple; the nipple skin may be inflamed. The only treatment is to excise, which means removal of the nipple.

GALACTOCELE

Galactocele presents as a lump, 1–3 cm in diameter, in late pregnancy or lactation. Needling confirms a milk cyst. There is no need for further treatment and the condition resolves when lactation ceases.

MISCELLANEOUS SYMPTOMATIC PROBLEMS

NIPPLE DISCHARGE

The surgeon first determines from the history or examination whether there is discharge from a single or from multiple ducts.

Multiduct

Often bilateral this is a physiological upset rather than a pathological entity. No diagnostic steps are needed. If heavy enough to cause a social problem, the ducts are divided directly under the nipple; prolactin secreting adenoma is very rarely the underlying cause.

Single duct

Five percent of single duct discharges are due to DCIS.[9] If clinical examination or mammography reveals an abnormality, it is investigated and if cytological examination of the discharge (Ch. 2) shows malignant cells, then the discharging duct is explored (microdochectomy) and removed for histology. Otherwise the patient is followed with yearly mammography for 3 years or until the discharge ceases.

The common causes of single duct discharge are duct ectasia or papilloma.[9]

BREAST PAIN

Breast pain is a common presenting symptom which has no histological correlate. Clinical examination is all that is required to proceed to reassure the woman that the pain does not indicate that a breast cancer is present. However the discomfort may be bad enough to intrude into the patient's life and the woman wants treatment. Before treating the pain is classified.

The causes are:[10]

1. Localized fibromyalgia (lateral chest wall tenderness). Pain is thought to be in the breast but palpation of one or several ribs or costal cartilages (Tietze syndrome) reveals extreme tenderness. An injection of corticosteroid down to the tender rib may be helpful.

2. Cyclical. There is a clear relation to the menstrual cycle and if bad enough the patient is only free of pain in the menstrual week. Danazol (Sanofi-Winthrop) used at a dose with mild androgenic side effects (300 mg per day) for 3 months is a useful treatment. Oil of Evening Primrose may be helpful. Recalcitrant cases are treated by suppressing the ovaries using the LH/RH agonist Zoladex.

3. Referred pain from cervical spondylitis: in addition to giving referred pain to the arm, this may produce pain in the breast.

GYNECOMASTIA IN MALES (see Ch. 22)

Gynecomastia may present as a small lump, placed directly under the nipple or as a general breast enlargement ('fatty' gynecomastia). It is seen largely in two age groups: adolescents (a small lump under the nipple is a common finding at routine medical examination)[11] and men aged 50 or above. A number of the latter are on medications which cause secondary gynecomastia, the best known being anabolic steroids, estrogens, cimetidine (which disturbs gonadotrophic control) and digoxin (which binds to the estrogen receptor). There is a table of medications which have been said to be associated with gynecomastia in Chapter 21.

The diagnosis is usually clinically obvious; breast cancer in the male has a very different presentation (Ch. 21). Most cases need no treatment, although a number of adolescents ask for excision because of embarrassment.

REFERENCES

1. Miller WR, Dixon JM, Scott WN, Forrest APF. Classification of human breast cysts according to electrolytes and androgen conjugate composition. Clin Oncol 1990; 9: 227–232.
2. Caseldine J, Elston CW, Blamey RW. The presentation of sclerosing adenosis. Br J Clinical Practice 1987; 56: 56–57.
3. Galea MH, Dixon AR, Pye G et al. Non-operative management of discrete palpable breast lumps in women over 35 years of age. The Breast 1992; 1: 164 (Abstract).
4. Bundred NJ, Dover MS, Coley S, Morrison JM. Breast abscesses and cigarette smoking. Br J Surg 1992; 79: 58–59.
5. Hartley MN, Stewart J, Benson EA. Subareolar dissection for duct ectasia and peri-areolar sepsis. Br J Surg 1991; 78: 1187–1188.
6. Galea MH, Robertson JFR, Ellis IO, Elston CW, Blamey RW. Granulomatous lobular mastitis. Aust NZJ Surg 1989; 59: 547–550.
7. Kiel KD, Suit HD. Radiation therapy in the treatment of aggressive fibromatoses (Desmoid tumors). Cancer 1984; 54: 2051–2055.
8. Kinzbrunner B, Ritter S, Domingo J, Rosenthal CJ. Remission of rapidly growing desmoid tumors after tamoxifen therapy. Cancer 1983; 52: 2201–2204.
9. Locker AP, Galea MH, Ellis IO, Elston CW, Blamey RW. Microdochectomy for single-duct discharge from the nipple. Br J Surg 1988; 75: 700–701.
10. Galea MH, Blamey RW. Non-cyclical breast pain: 1-year audit of an improved classification. In: Mansel RE, ed. Benign breast disease. Carnforth: Parthenon Publishing Group, 1992; 75–80.
11. Nydick M, Bustos J, Dale JH, Rawson RW. Gynaecomastia in adolescent boys. J Am Med Ass 1961; 178: 449–457.

Classification of malignant breast disease

INTRODUCTION

As Azzopardi[1] stated in his elegant and scholarly monograph 'no classification is perfect nor is it likely that it ever will be ... All classifications depend on our knowledge of the pathology and histogenesis of the tumors being classified and, since this knowledge is far from perfect or complete, no classification can be other than a reasonable working compromise'.

It is true to say that since these words were written our understanding of the clinicopathological aspects of malignant breast lesions have improved considerably and there is consequently closer agreement throughout the world on the appropriateness of the diagnostic categories which are currently recognized. There are minor variations in the interpretation of some specific types of tumor (which will be discussed in subsequent chapters) but most authorities have based their own classifications firmly on the morphological features outlined by the World Health Organization (WHO).[2–6]

All these classifications have followed the long-established tradition of making an initial subdivision along embryological lines into neoplasms derived from epithelial and those arising from mesenchymal tissue. We have followed this same convention and in the rest of this chapter we give a brief outline of our philosophy for the characterization of the malignant tumors shown in Table 13.1.

EPITHELIAL TUMORS

For malignant epithelial neoplasms the next, and

Table 13.1   Classification of malignant breast disease

Epithelial:	Ductal carcinoma in situ	High grade
		Intermediate grade
		Low grade
		Mixed types
	Microinvasive carcinoma	
	Invasive carcinoma — usual types	Ductal NST
		Lobular
		Medullary
		Tubular
		Invasive cribriform
		Tubular mixed
		Mucinous
		Invasive papillary
		Metaplastic
		Mixed types
	Invasive carcinoma — rare types	Squamous cell
		Mucoepidermoid
		Low-grade adenosquamous
		Adenocystic
		Adenomyoepithelioma
		Malignant myoepithelioma
		Apocrine
		Primary oat cell
		(neuroendocrine)
		Clear cell (glycogen rich)
		Secretory (juvenile)
Mesenchymal:	Angiosarcoma	
	Lymphangiosarcoma (post-mastectomy angiosarcoma)	
	Fibrosarcoma and malignant Fibrohistiocytoma (MFH)	
	Liposarcoma	
	Osteogenic sarcoma	
	Leiomyosarcoma	
	Rhabdomyosarcoma	
	Chondrosarcoma	
Miscellaneous:	Malignant lymphoma	Non-Hodgkin's lymphoma
		Hodgkin's lymphoma
	Plasmacytoma	
	Leukemia	
	Metastases	

most fundamental, division is into *in situ* and *invasive* carcinoma. Whilst emphasizing the importance of this basic concept Azzopardi[1] preferred to make an initial topographical division into lobular and ductal types, despite his acceptance of the classical study of Wellings, Jensen and Marcum[7] which showed that the majority of breast carcinomas, whatever their morphological pattern, arise in common from the terminal duct lobular unit (TDLU). A number of studies in the last 10–15 years have demonstrated that this topographical concept is rather too simplistic. For example, lobular carcinoma in situ (LCIS) is now regarded by most authorities as a risk factor for

subsequent invasive carcinoma rather than an established malignant entity, and it is also recognized that some invasive carcinomas exhibit both 'lobular' and 'ductal' patterns.[8]

We have preferred, therefore, to make a complete separation between the 'in situ' lobular and ductal lesions and the former, together with atypical lobular hyperplasia, has already been covered in Chapter 6 under the title of 'lobular neoplasia'. We recognize the current controversies surrounding the classification and behavior of the different subtypes of ductal carcinoma in situ (DCIS)[9–13] but have accepted that at the present time histological pattern has relatively little influence on clinical management. DCIS is therefore considered as a single group of related entities.

Epithelial tumors are subdivided as follows into the two main categories of *in situ* and *invasive* carcinoma.

DUCTAL CARCINOMA IN SITU

The classification of DCIS is at present under scrutiny with several groups describing new systems for sub-dividing this disease. This interest in DCIS classification has been generated by the apparent increase in the incidence of DCIS following the introduction of mammography. DCIS now accounts for 15 to 20% of breast cancer cases compared with approximately 5% prior to the advent of breast cancer screening programs.[9,14–16] This increase in incidence has been coupled with an expansion of treatment options for women with breast disease. Mastectomy was the treatment of choice for symptomatic DCIS but mammography allows identification of small localized lesions which can be managed successfully by breast conservation. There are now large clinical trials in the US (NSABP B7),[17] UK (UKCCCR) and Europe (EORTC) examining the effectiveness of conservation surgery coupled with adjuvant therapies such as radiotherapy and tamoxifen. The ability of a histological classification to predict endpoints such as in situ recurrence, invasive recurrence and survival is an important supplementary question needing to be answered by these trials.

The traditional classification of DCIS is based on both architectural growth pattern and cytological features. This method is, however, poorly reproducible, with up to 30% of cases in multi-center trials requiring re-classification.[18] The lack of correlation between pathologists may partly be due to the heterogeneity of DCIS with more atypical features often seen in the central portion of the lesion.[19] A system of classification which can be used to identify aggressive disease reproducibly is required. Most recent interest has focused on grading systems based on nuclear features, coupled in some with cellular architectural arrangement.[9,20–23] The National Co-ordinating Group for Breast Screening Pathology in the United Kingdom[24] recommend a nuclear grading system derived from Holland et al[23] which classifies DCIS into high, low or intermediate nuclear grade.

Similar systems for classification of DCIS based on necrosis and to a lesser degree nuclear grade have been proposed and appear promising since an association between the subtypes of DCIS and local recurrence and disease free survival were seen in both these series.[11,13,25] It has been shown that pathologists have high concordance in the recognition of comedo DCIS[26] and separation of other forms of DCIS on the basis of presence or absence of necrosis may achieve good reproducibility.

Holland's group have shown that DCIS is virtually always a unicentric process involving a single duct system.[14,27] DCIS, when identified in its pure form, should have no risk of local recurrence or progression to systemic disease when completely excised. If adequacy of excision can be confirmed by diligent pathological examination, prognostic grading systems may become redundant. Pathologists would then need to concentrate their efforts on ensuring adequate excision rather than on histological classification.[12,28]

The thresholds of DCIS designation are also being questioned. DCIS is conventionally regarded as an obligate precursor of invasive breast cancer[29] and atypical ductal hyperplasia (ADH) as a risk factor for the development of the disease. It is, however, becoming more widely accepted that not all DCIS progresses inexorably towards invasion and the clinical significance of this disease has been questioned.[30] In addition, at least some cases of ADH are monoclonal in nature[31] and loss of heterozygosity, of the same pattern as a more advanced lesion from the same breast, has been reported in usual and atypical epithelial hyperplasia (in up to 50% of cases), although it is seen more frequently in DCIS (80% of cases).[32] These data lead some support to the theory that at least some 'borderline' epithelial proliferations may be non-obligate precursor lesions.

ADH has, by definition, morphological similarities to low grade DCIS and these entities are also alike in molecular phenotype and DNA characteristics; 36% of ADH and 38% of cribriform DCIS show DNA aneuploidy compared to 93%

of morphologically high grade DCIS.[33] Several series have described absence[34–36] or rare[37–38] expression of p53 and c-erbB-2 in ADH. Expression of these markers is also uncommon in low grade DCIS[37,39] but immunoreactivity is seen more often in high grade disease.[40–41] The atypical ductal proliferations of the breast epithelium are now widely believed to form a spectrum of disease from high grade DCIS at one end to low grade in situ disease and ADH at the other. Future classification systems for DCIS may have to take account of these emerging data on early epithelial in situ lesions.

MICROINVASIVE CARCINOMA

Microinvasive carcinoma is a relatively contentious entity, but has been retained because of the view that tiny foci (less than 1 mm) of invasive carcinoma in association with a lesion composed predominantly of DCIS (usually of high grade/comedo type) behave like DCIS rather than an established invasive carcinoma.[24] Any tumor with foci of infiltration of a larger size is classified as established invasive breast carcinoma. High grade DCIS, especially that of comedo type, frequently has an associated lymphoid infiltrate with periductal fibrosis and distortion and, particularly when 'cancerization' of lobules is present, may mimic invasive carcinoma. However, only when unequivocal invasion is seen outside the specialized lobular stroma should microinvasive carcinoma be diagnosed. Tumors showing microinvasion are rare and if any doubt exists the lesion should be classified as DCIS.

INVASIVE CARCINOMA

As indicated above most authorities have accepted the view that the great majority of invasive carcinomas of the breast originate from epithelial cells within the TDLU despite obvious differences in morphological pattern.[1,5–6,42] Although these specialist breast pathologists have proposed specific histological subclassifications of invasive carcinoma for several decades, based on the recognizable differences in pattern, histological

typing has been slow to gain acceptance until comparatively recently.[43] For example, in the last edition of this series, published as recently as 1978,[44] apart from use of the broad terms 'scirrhous' and 'medullary' (encephaloid) to describe the gross appearances and 'mucoid carcinoma' for one histological variant, all other invasive carcinomas of the breast were designated microscopically as spheroidal cell carcinoma. Even today a great many pathologists do not bother to type or grade invasive carcinoma of the breast, content with the broad designation of invasive adenocarcinoma. This position is now no longer tenable, and there are a number of reasons why morphological typing of invasive carcinomas should form a routine part of the histopathological report.

In the first place, careful large-scale studies have confirmed that some types of invasive carcinoma of the breast carry a more favorable outcome than others. These include, in particular, the special types such as tubular carcinoma, invasive cribriform carcinoma and mucinous carcinoma.[8] Secondly, the introduction of breast cancer screening has completely changed the pattern of detection of breast carcinoma, and the special types, which form only a small percentage of tumors presenting symptomatically, are found much more frequently in mammographic programs, particularly in the prevalent round.[45–47] In this respect, histological typing of invasive carcinoma forms a useful quality assurance measure for performance in breast screening programs.[24] Lastly, the therapeutic options for the treatment of patients with breast cancer are now much broader. There is an increasing trend towards breast conservation, radiotherapeutic techniques have improved and a wider range of cytotoxic and hormonal therapies is available. This, together with the increased proportion of good prognosis tumors detected through screening, means that very careful assessment is required before appropriate treatment is given to an individual patient.

There is considerable variation in the reported frequency of the morphological subtypes of invasive carcinoma of the breast (Table 13.2).[8,42,48–52] This is due to a number of factors. Although most authorities use the WHO classification[2–3] as a basis many have introduced their own modifications. This is understandable, since the last

Table 13.2 Comparison of relative percentage of main morphological types of invasive breast cancer in different published series

Type	Study						
	Rosen, 1979, USA[49]	Fisher et al, 1975, USA[48]	Wallgren et al, 1976, Sweden[50]	Linnell and Rank, 1989, Denmark[52]	Sakamoto et al, 1981, Japan[51]	Page, Anderson and Sakamoto, 1987, UK[42]	Ellis et al, 1992, UK[8]
Ductal/NST	75%	53%	66%	41%	47%	70%	49%
Lobular	10%	5%	14%	11%	2%	10%	16%
Medullary	10%	6%	6%	9%	2%	5%	3%
Tubular	1%	1%	–	10%	–	3%	2%
Tubular mixed	–	–	–	20%[d]	–	–	14%
Mucinous	2%	2%	–	3%	2%	2%	1%
Cribriform	–	–	} 9%	–	–	4%	1%
Papillary	0.5%	4%[a]		–	22%[b]	1%	<1%
Mixed pattern	–	28%	–	–	20%[c]	2%	14%

[a]Mixed papillary, cribriform and tubular.
[b]Papillo-tubular.
[c]Solid-tubular.
[d]Tubuloductal.

edition of the WHO classification was published in 1981 and some morphological subtypes, e.g. invasive cribriform carcinoma,[53] have only been fully characterized since then. In the classification used by the Japanese Mammary Cancer Society[51] infiltrating ductal carcinoma of no special type (Ductal NST) is subdivided into three categories. One of these, solid-tubular, bears close similarities to our entity of tubular mixed carcinoma[8] whilst the other, papillo-tubular, shares features with invasive cribriform carcinoma.[53] Similarly Linell and Rank[52] appear to include a high proportion of tubular and tubuloductal carcinomas because in their definition *any* tubular component qualifies a tumor to be included in these groups. This illustrates a further reason for potential discrepancy, the lack of generally accepted diagnostic criteria for many of the subtypes. The problem is compounded by the fact that a proportion of invasive carcinomas have a heterogeneous morphological pattern. This raises the question of where the distinction should be made between a tumor designated as being of pure type and one exhibiting a mixed pattern. This dilemma is illustrated perfectly by Page et al[42] who posed the question 'how should a breast cancer be classified if 80% is of no special type, 10% is of mucinous type and 10% of infiltrating lobular type?'. Their solution is to classify the tumor in the broad category of ductal NST, but record the additional features in text. This approach is reflected in the

relatively high proportion of ductal NST carcinomas (70%) in their series (Table 13.2). We do not agree with this point of view, but recognize mixed types if the particular designation provides prognostic information. However, we endorse completely their suggestion that simple rules should be established to categorize each type; for example, to label a tumor as a particular special type at least 90% of its area must be of the dominant histological pattern.

It should be understood clearly that the descriptive terms applied to these different histological types of invasive carcinoma do not imply a specific cell of origin, but rather indicate a recognizable morphological pattern. Furthermore, it is our view that the most important reason for making a distinction between these various patterns is their correlation with clinical behavior and prognosis.

In keeping with this philosophy we have attempted to keep our classification as simple as possible, at the same providing a comprehensive view of the published literature. Reference to the long-standing debate between 'lumpers' and 'splitters' is pertinent in this respect. In our comprehensive study of histological type in the Nottingham Tenovus Primary Breast Cancer Study (NTPBCS) we deliberately split the morphological patterns recognized into as many types as possible, and then carried out a correlation with prognosis. From this study we have been able to reduce the number of common or usual type subdivisions to a sensible number without losing prognostic significance (Table 13.2). These tumors are described in detail in Chapter 15. In order to provide a comprehensive account of a subject any classification must, of course, include the uncommon or rare variants. The rare carcinomas are discussed in Chapter 16 by Eusebi and Foschini.

HISTOLOGICAL GRADE

It is something of a paradox that methods for the semiquantitative assessment of the morphological differentiation of invasive breast carcinoma were first described before a full classification of histological type had been established.[54-56] As one consequence of this the evolution and refinement of these methods for histological grading took place independently and quite separately from the categorization of the histological types which we recognize today, although both can be regarded as providing information on tumor differentiation. This resulted in an informal division amongst breast pathologists into two groups, the 'typers' and the 'graders'. Even Scarff, one of the fathers of grade, recommended in the first edition of the WHO classification of breast tumors, that it should only be carried out in invasive ductal (ductal NST) carcinoma,[56] and this view has been perpetuated ever since.[5-6] Furthermore, until very recently there has been a general reluctance amongst pathologists and clinicians alike to accept the prognostic value of histological grade, largely due to perceived problems in consistency and reproducibility of the methods. We have shown conclusively that histological grade is, in fact, as powerful a prognostic factor as lymph node stage[57-58] and the consistency and reproducibility of our method has now been confirmed in several different studies.[59-61] We have also shown that histological grading can provide useful stratification of prognosis within some of the special types (e.g. infiltrating lobular, mucinous) and have concluded that both grade and type should be assessed in all cases of invasive breast carcinoma.[62] Indeed, for types such as pure tubular carcinoma grade is one of the most important defining diagnostic features; they *must* be grade 1

(well-differentiated) to qualify for that category. For all these reasons we feel that histological grade is of sufficient importance to warrant a separate account and this is provided in Chapter 17.

MESENCHYMAL TUMORS

Primary malignant mesenchymal tumors are exceedingly uncommon in the breast, and it has proved extremely difficult to obtain universal agreement on their classification. For example, as discussed previously in Chapter 3, the WHO classification[2-3] categorizes phyllodes tumor within a section entitled 'Mixed connective tissue and epithelial tumors' together with fibroadenoma and so-called carcinosarcoma. Although Tavassoli[5] and Rosen and Oberman[6] have chosen to follow this convention and place phyllodes tumors in chapters on 'Fibroepithelial lesions', both Azzopardi[1] and Page and Anderson[42] include them with 'Sarcomas of the breast'. Whilst there are arguments for regarding *malignant* phyllodes tumors as sarcomas the same is not true for the benign and borderline categories which account for the great majority of these lesions.[63] Indeed, to include phyllodes tumor with sarcomas serves to perpetuate the myth that they all behave as malignant tumors. We therefore feel that it is more logical to follow the WHO convention and phyllodes tumors are considered in Chapter 9, on 'Fibroepithelial lesions'.

Further problems are encountered with the pure sarcomas of the breast. In the WHO classification[2-3] they are placed in the section on 'Miscellaneous tumors' and this is the convention used by Rosen and Oberman.[6] However, both Azzopardi[1] and Page and Anderson[42] have opted for separate chapters on sarcomas whilst Tavassoli[5] has included non-neoplastic mesenchymal entities together with benign and malignant tumors in a very broad chapter entitled 'Mesenchymal lesions'. As far as possible we have tried to make a fundamental distinction between benign and malignant lesions in this book and to this end the benign mesenchymal tumors are included in Chapter 11, 'Miscellaneous benign lesions'.

The pure malignant mesenchymal tumors which occur in the breast appear to exhibit the same morphological characteristics as those arising elsewhere in the body. Our subclassification reflects this (Table 13.1) and uses the terminology accepted by acknowledged specialists in the field.[64–65] They are described in Chapter 19.

MISCELLANEOUS TUMORS

Because of their comparative rarity the tumors of the lymphoreticular system do not warrant a chapter on their own. They have therefore been included with the mesenchymal tumors in Chapter 19, in the same convention as in the WHO classification.[2–3] Finally, for the sake of completeness, metastases to the breast from other sites are also covered in this chapter.

SUMMARY

We commented at the beginning of this chapter that no classification is ever perfect, and we have also pointed out some minor areas of terminological and nosological disagreement. Despite these there has been remarkable progress in the last few years towards a world-wide acceptance of the basic subdivisions outlined in Table 13.1. Further modifications will, no doubt, be made in the future, but for the present time we believe that this classification provides a practical framework for the diagnostic histopathologist in routine practice.

REFERENCES

1. Azzopardi JG. Problems in breast pathology. London: WB Saunders, 1979.
2. Azzopardi JG, Chepick OF, Hartmann WH et al. The World Health Organization histological typing of breast tumors. 2nd ed. Am J Clin Pathol 1982; 78: 806–816.
3. World Health Organization. International histological classification of tumours. Histologic types of breast tumours. Geneva: World Health Organization, 1981.
4. Page DL, Anderson TJ. Diagnostic histopathology of the breast. Edinburgh: Churchill Livingstone, 1987.
5. Tavassoli FA. Pathology of the breast. Norwalk: Appleton and Lange, 1992.
6. Rosen PP, Oberman HA. Tumors of the mammary gland. Atlas of tumor pathology. Washington: Armed Forces Institute of Pathology, 1993. Third series, fascicle 7.
7. Wellings SR, Jensen HM, Marcum RG. An atlas of subgross pathology of the human breast with special reference to possible precancerous lesions. J Natl Cancer Inst 1975; 55: 231–273.
8. Ellis IO, Galea M, Broughton N et al. Pathological prognostic factors in breast cancer. II. Histological type. Relationship with survival in a large study with long-term follow-up. Histopathol 1992; 20: 479–489.
9. Lagios MD. Duct carcinoma in situ. Pathology and treatment. Surg Clin North Am 1990; 70: 853–871.
10. Holland R, Peterse JL, Millis RR et al. Ductal carcinoma in situ: a proposal for a new classification. Semin Diagn Pathol 1994; 11: 199–207.
11. Poller DN, Silverstein MJ, Galea MH et al. Ideas in pathology. Ductal carcinoma in situ of the breast: a proposal for a new simplified histological classification association between cellular proliferation and c-erbB-2 protein expression. Mod Pathol 1994; 7: 257–262.
12. Page DL, Lagios MD. Pathological analysis of the National Surgical Adjuvant Breast Project (NSABP) B-17 trial: unanswered questions remaining unanswered considering current concepts of ductal carcinoma in situ. Editorial. Cancer 1995; 75: 1223–1227.
13. Harrison M, Coyne JD, Gorey T, Dervan PA. Comparison of cytomorphological and architectural heterogeneity in mammographically-detected ductal carcinoma in situ. Histopathol 1996; 28: 445–450.
14. Faverly DR, Burgers L, Bult P, Holland R. Three dimensional imaging of mammary ductal carcinoma in situ: clinical implications. Semin Diagn Pathol 1994; 11: 193–198.
15. Rosner D, Bedwanu R, Vana J. Non invasive breast carcinoma: result of a national survey by the American College of Surgeons. Ann Surg 1980; 192: 139–147.
16. Van Dongen JA, Fentiman IS, Harris JR et al. In situ breast cancer: the EORTC consensus meeting. Lancet 1989; ii: 25–27.
17. Fisher ER, Costantino J, Fisher B et al. Pathologic findings from the National Surgical Adjuvant Breast Project (NSABP) Protocol B-17. Intraductal carcinoma (ductal carcinoma in situ). The National Surgical Adjuvant Breast and Bowel Project Collaborating Investigators. Cancer 1995; 75: 1310–1319.
18. Van Dongen JA, Holland R, Peterse JL et al. Ductal carcinoma in-situ of the breast; second EORTC consensus meeting. Eur J Cancer 1992; 28: 626–629.
19. Lennington WJ, Jensen RA, Dalton LW, Page DL. Ductal carcinoma in situ of the breast. Heterogeneity of individual lesions. Cancer 1994; 73: 118–124.
20. Lagios MD, Margolin FR, Westdahl PR et al. Mammographically detected duct carcinoma in situ. Frequency of local recurrence following tylectomy and prognostic effect of nuclear grade on local recurrence. Cancer 1989; 63: 618–624.
21. Locker AP, Horrocks C, Gilmour AS et al. Flow cytometric and histological analysis of ductal carcinoma in situ of the breast. Br J Surg 1990; 77: 564–567.
22. Bellamy CO, McDonald C, Salter DM et al. Non invasive ductal carcinoma of the breast: the relevance of histologic categorization. Hum Pathol 1993; 24: 16–23.
23. Holland R, Peterse JL, Millis RR et al. Ductal carcinoma

in situ: a proposal for a new classification. Semin Diagn Pathol 1994; 11: 167–180.

24. National Co-ordinating Group for Breast Screening Pathology. Pathology Reporting in Breast Cancer Screening. 2nd ed. NHSBSP Publications, no 3, 1995.

25. Silverstein MJ, Poller DN, Waisman JR et al. Prognostic classification of breast ductal carcinoma-in-situ. Lancet 1995; 345: 1154–1157.

26. Sloane JP, National Coordinating Group for Breast. Consistency of histopathological reporting of breast lesions detected by screening: findings of the UK National External Quality Assessment (EQA) Scheme. Eur J Cancer 1994; 30A: 1414–1419.

27. Holland R, Connelly JL, Gelman R et al. The presence of an extensive intraduct component following a limited excision correlates with prominent residual disease in the remainder of the breast. J Clin Oncol 1990; 8: 113–118.

28. Poller DN, Ellis IO. Ductal carcinoma in situ of the breast. In: Kirkham N, Lemoine NR, eds. Progress in pathology. vol 2. Edinburgh: Churchill Livingstone, 1995.

29. Frykberg ER, Bland KI. Overview of the biology and management of ductal carcinoma in situ of the breast. Cancer 1994; 74: 350–361.

30. Fisher ER, Sass R, Fisher B, Wicherham L, Paik SM. Pathologic findings from the National Surgical Adjuvant Breast Project (protocol 6). I. Intraductal carcinoma (DCIS). Cancer 1986; 57: 197–208.

31. Lakhani SR, Collins N, Stratton MR, Sloane JP. Atypical ductal hyperplasia of the breast: clonal proliferation with loss of heterozygosity on chromosomes 16q and 17p. J Clin Pathol 1995; 48: 611–615.

32. O'Connell P, Pekkel V, Fuqua S, Osborne CK, Allred DC. Molecular genetic studies of early breast cancer evolution. Br Cancer Res Treat 1994; 32: 5–12.

33. Crissman JD, Visscher DW, Kubus J. Image cytophotometric DNA analysis of atypical hyperplasias and intraductal carcinomas of the breast. Arch Pathol Lab Med 1990; 114: 1249–1253.

34. Umekita Y, Takasaki T, Yoshida H. Expression of p53 protein in benign epithelial hyperplasia, atypical ductal hyperplasia, non-invasive and invasive mammary carcinoma: an immunohistochemical study. Virchows Arch (A) Pathol Anat 1994; 424: 491–494.

35. Allred DC, O'Connell P, Fuqua SA, Osborne CK. Immunohistochemical studies of early breast cancer evolution. Br Cancer Res Treat 1994; 32: 13–18.

36. Eriksson ET, Schimmelpenning H, Aspenblad U et al. Immunohistochemical expression of the mutant p53 protein and nuclear DNA content during the transition from benign to malignant breast disease. Hum Pathol 1994; 25: 1228–1233.

37. Lodato RF, Maguire H Jr, Greene MI et al. Immunohistochemical evaluation of c-erbB-2 oncogene expression in ductal carcinoma in situ and atypical ductal hyperplasia of the breast. Mod Pathol 1990; 3: 449–454.

38. Schmitt FC, Leal C, Lopes C. p53 protein expression and nuclear DNA content in breast intraductal proliferations. J Pathol 1995; 176: 233–241.

39. Poller DN, Roberts EC, Bell JA et al. p53 protein expression in mammary ductal carcinoma in situ: relationship to immunohistochemical expression of estrogen receptor and c-erbB-2 protein. Hum Pathol 1993; 24: 463–468.

40. Bobrow LG, Happerfield LC, Gregory WM et al. The classification of ductal carcinoma in situ and its association with biological markers. Semin Diagn Pathol 1994; 11: 199–207.

41. Leal CB, Schmitt FC, Bento MJ et al. Ductal carcinoma in situ of the breast. Histologic categorization and its relationship to ploidy and immunohistochemical expression of hormone receptors, p53, and c-erbB-2 protein. Cancer 1995; 75: 2123–2131.

42. Page DL, Anderson TJ, Sakamoto G. Infiltrating carcinoma: major histological types. In: Page DL, Anderson TJ, eds. Diagnostic histopathology of the breast. London: W B Saunders, 1987; 193–235.

43. Page DL. How should we categorize breast cancer? Breast 1993; 2: 217–219.

44. Symmers W St C. The Breasts. In: Symmers W St C, ed. Systemic pathology. 2nd ed. Edinburgh: Churchill-Livingstone, 1978; 1760–1857.

45. Anderson TJ, Lamb J, Donnan P et al. Comparative pathology of breast cancer in a randomized trial of screening. Brit J Cancer 1991; 64: 108–113.

46. Ellis IO, Galea MH, Locker A et al. Early experience in breast cancer screening: Emphasis on development of protocols for triple assessment. Breast 1993; 2: 148–153.

47. Rajakariar R, Walker RA. Pathological and biological features of mammographically detected invasive breast carcinomas. Brit J Cancer 1995; 71: 150–154.

48. Fisher ER, Gregorio RM, Fisher B. The pathology of invasive breast cancer. A syllabus derived from findings of the National Surgical Adjuvant Breast Cancer Project (protocol no 4). Cancer 1975; 36: 144–156.

49. Rosen PP. The pathological classification of human mammary carcinoma: past, present and future. Ann Clin Lab Sci 1979; 9: 144–156.

50. Wallgren A, Silferswärd C, Eklund G. Prognostic factors in mammary carcinoma. Acta Radiol 1976; 15: 1–16.

51. Sakamoto G, Sugano H, Hartmann WH. Comparative pathological study of breast carcinoma among American and Japanese women. In: McGuire WL, ed. Breast cancer. Advances in research and treatment. vol 4. New York: Plenum, 1981; 211–231.

52. Linell F, Rank F. Comments on histologic classifications with reference to histogenesis and prognosis. Universitetsförlaget Dialogos, Lund, 1989.

53. Page DL, Dixon JM, Anderson TJ et al. Invasive cribriform carcinoma of the breast. Histopathol 1983; 7: 525–536.

54. Greenhough RB. Varying degrees of malignancy in cancer of the breast. J Cancer Res 1925; 9: 452–463.

55. Patey DH, Scarff RW. The position of histology in the prognosis of carcinoma of the breast. Lancet 1928; 1: 801–804.

56. Scarff RW, Torloni H. Histological typing of breast tumours. International histological classification of tumours, no 2. Geneva: 1968. (WHO).

57. Elston CW, Ellis IO. Pathological prognostic factors in breast cancer. I. The value of histological grade in breast cancer: experience from a large study with long-term follow-up. Histopathol 1991; 19: 403–410.

58. Galea MH, Blamey RW, Elston CW et al. The Nottingham Prognostic Index in primary breast cancer. Br Cancer Res Treat 1992; 22: 187–191.

59. Dalton LW, Page DL, Dupont WD. Histologic grading of breast carcinoma: a reproducibility study. Cancer 1994; 73: 2765–2770.

60. Frierson HF, Wolber RA, Berean KW et al. Interobserver reproducibility of the Nottingham modification of the Bloom and Richardson histological grading scheme for infiltrating ductal carcinoma. Am J Clin Pathol 1995; 105: 195–199.

61. Robbins P, Pinder S, de Klerk N et al. Histological grading of breast carcinomas. A study of interobserver agreement. Hum Pathol 1995; 26: 873–879.

62. Pereira H, Pinder SE, Sibbering DM et al. Pathological prognostic factors in breast cancer. IV: should you be a typer or a grader? A comparative study of two histological prognostic features in operable breast carcinoma. Histopathol 1995; 27: 219–226.

63. Moffat CJC, Pinder SE, Dixon AR et al. Phyllodes tumours of the breast: a clinicopathological review of 32 cases. Histopathol 1995; 27: 205–218.

64. Enzinger FM, Weiss SW. Soft tissue tumors. 3rd ed. St Louis: Mosby, 1995.

65. Fletcher CDM. Soft tissue tumors. In: Fletcher CDM, ed. Diagnostic histopathology of tumors. Edinburgh: Churchill Livingstone, 1995; 1043–1096.

Ductal carcinoma in situ

INTRODUCTION

The use of mammography has led to a dramatic increase in the detection of ductal carcinoma in situ (DCIS), particularly in the form of small localized lesions.[1] This apparent change in disease incidence because of easier mammographic detection has highlighted deficiencies in our understanding of DCIS. There are difficulties in determining appropriate and reproducible criteria for the distinction between DCIS and atypical ductal hyperplasia (ADH), DCIS and lobular carcinoma in situ (LCIS), and criteria for diagnosis of DCIS with micro-invasion (DCIS Mi). Some subtypes of DCIS are difficult to classify and rarer types can be difficult to recognize and diagnose. The usefulness of various pathological sub-classification systems for DCIS is disputed; similarly the question of what constitutes an adequate pathological excision margin and the value or role, if any, of molecular markers in DCIS is unclear. The question of whether DCIS is a true 'cancer' or is better regarded as a marker for patients with a high risk of subsequent invasive breast cancer[2] is unresolved. The utility of conservation surgery and the role of adjuvant therapy (e.g. radiotherapy or endocrine therapy) in clinical management of DCIS is also uncertain.

HISTORICAL BACKGROUND

The history of DCIS has been well reviewed recently by Fechner.[2] DCIS was first recognized in 1893 by Bloodgood.[3] Lewis and Geschickter[4] described comedo DCIS although they failed to distinguish invasive carcinoma from in situ carcinoma. Later, lobular 'cancerization' in DCIS was highlighted by Azzopardi.[5] Page, Dupont and co-workers described cribriform, micropapillary and other types of non-comedo DCIS as high risk factors for the development of ipsilateral invasive breast cancer.[6]

In the original study by Page and his colleagues,[6] a review of 11 760 breast biopsies performed in the period 1950 to 1968, seven of 25 (28%) women with undiagnosed DCIS (and therefore left untreated) developed invasive breast carcinoma over a period of 15 years follow-up. The tumors were always in the same breast as that previously biopsied. The American College of Pathologists has recently adopted broadly similar diagnostic criteria for DCIS (MD Lagios, personal communication 1994) based on the studies of Page[6] and those of Lagios.[7,8] In the United Kingdom (UK) The National Breast Screening Programme has also in general followed Page's criteria for diagnosis of ADH and DCIS.

Invasive adenocarcinoma of the breast frequently has intimately associated DCIS and for this reason DCIS is regarded as a precursor lesion. DCIS is considered distinct on morphological and clinical grounds from lobular carcinoma in situ (LCIS) (see Ch. 6). LCIS is now regarded as a high risk factor for the development of invasive breast cancer, but because it is frequently multifocal, pure LCIS without co-existent DCIS (see Chs 12 and 22) is generally managed differently from DCIS. At the second European Organization for Research into the Treatment of Cancer (EORTC) DCIS consensus meeting in September 1991[9] it was recognized that DCIS is heterogeneous, histologically, radiologically, and biologically,[9] but the participants agreed on the basis of the then existing evidence that DCIS was nearly always unicentric, that its detection has increased with mammographic screening, and that not all incompletely excised lesions necessarily progress to invasive carcinoma. It was also accepted that the incidence of axillary lymph node involvement by metastatic carcinoma in DCIS is very small (<1%), and that management of pure DCIS does not require routine axillary dissection.

This view that DCIS is heterogeneous and could be regarded as part of a spectrum of disease,

originally proposed by Rosai[10] and subsequently by others,[11] is supported by studies which show chromosomal aneuploidy,[12] losses of heterozygosity (LOH) or chromosomal deletions in usual type epithelial hyperplasia, ADH and DCIS,[13-23] implying that other epithelial proliferative lesions, particularly ADH, are also part of the neoplastic spectrum of breast disease. ADH and low grade DCIS may well be examples of biologically less advanced breast pre-cancer, different from intermediate and high nuclear grade DCIS. The view of DCIS as a spectrum of disease has been explored further by Lininger and Tavassoli who advocate the concept of mammary intraepithelial neoplasia (MIN).[24] They suggest that breast pre-neoplasias may be subdivided into three categories, MIN of ductal (DIN), lobular (LIN), and papillary (PIN) types. The Armed Forces Institute of Pathology (AFIP) proposal for ductal neoplasia is shown in Table 14.1.

NATURAL HISTORY

Ductal carcinoma in situ has been shown to arise within the terminal duct lobular units (TDLU) of the breast.[25-27] The adult breast comprises 20 or so developmentally derived segments which extend from the nipple area radially outwards to the pectoralis fascia. The TDLU connects anatomically via intralobular terminal ducts to extralobular terminal ducts, subareolar ducts and thence to the nipple. The current belief is that DCIS originates in the terminal ducts and acini of the breast, grows, and expands these ducts until, at a certain stage in its natural history, it develops invasive properties and penetrates the basement membrane. Autopsy based studies have demonstrated that 15% or so of young asymptomatic women may have DCIS.[28] If such studies could be extrapolated to living patients it might be argued that DCIS could almost be a 'normal' finding, similar in disease frequency to the detection of benign physiological breast conditions such as involutional change or fibrocystic change. However, critical review of these studies suggests that some cases reported as latent 'post-mortem' DCIS might not meet modern diagnostic criteria. Nevertheless these studies demonstrate that

Table 14.1   AFIP proposal for subclassification of mammary intraepithelial neoplasia (MIN), ductal type (ductal intraepithelial neoplasia)

Proposed DIN classification	Description	Current designation	Pleomorphic nuclear atypia	Necrosis
DIN 1a	IDH	IDH	–	– or +
1b	Type 1 AIDH	ADH	–*	–
	Type 2 AIDH Monolayered and minimally hyperplastic, moderately atypical cellular proliferations ('clinging carcinoma')			
1c	Low grade DCIS	DCIS, grade 1	–*	–
DIN 2	Cribriform or micropapillary DCIS with necrosis or atypia	DCIS, grade 2	– or +	+ or –
DIN 3	DCIS with significant cytologic atypia with or without necrosis	DCIS, grade 3	+++	+++/–

AIDH=atypical intraductal hyperplasia; DCIS=ductal carcinoma in situ; DIN=ductal intraepithelial neoplasia; IDH=intraductal hyperplasia; MIN=mammary intraepithelial neoplasia.
* No significant pleomorphic nuclear atypia is present, although at least a minor degree of atypia is assumed in all DCIS (as well as AIDH) proliferations.

asymptomatic microfocal atypical epithelial proliferative lesions are relatively common in Western women. Furthermore the incidence of invasive breast cancer in Western Caucasian populations is high. The lifetime risk of development of invasive breast cancer of 1 in 8 to 1 in 12 in North America or Europe is consistent with these autopsy findings.

Three-dimensional reconstruction techniques, such as the serial subgross method of Egan[25] and similar stereomicroscopic techniques, have been used by Holland and co-workers[26,27,29] and by others (JD Davies, personal communication) to map the distribution of DCIS. These studies show that the majority, if not all, cases of DCIS exist as one lesion usually in one quadrant (66%)[26] and that DCIS should, therefore, be regarded as a unifocal disease process, although as far as is known no clearly defined anatomical boundaries exist between breast segments. Clinicians use the arbitrary boundaries of quadrants which comprise 90° sectors of breast tissue originating from the nipple and extending to the pectoralis fascia. These may include the axillary tail (for the outer upper quadrant) and in each there will be a variable number of segments. This method of ascribing a disease process to a specific region means that a proportion of lesions will extend into

more than one breast quadrant[26] and that centrally located tumors cannot be easily placed in a single quadrant.

The view that DCIS is a single clonal process has been further supported recently by the observation that in 12 cases of DCIS, although apparently anatomically multifocal, all showed loss of heterozygosity at the same chromosome locus.[30] This implies that the foci of DCIS were derived from the same clone and can be regarded as part of the same neoplastic process. That clonal selection occurs in DCIS in a way as proposed by Nowell[31] suggests that some forms of DCIS can arise through clonal evolution of atypical hyperplasias and then progress to invasive cancer. This hypothesis is in part supported by recent cytogenetic (see above) and oncogene abnormalities discovered in DCIS (detailed below), as well as by microscopic evidence of heterogeneity of lesions.[32]

Since the studies of Lewis and Geshickter,[4] showing a high frequency of progression following biopsy alone of in situ 'comedo' carcinoma to invasive carcinoma, it has been unethical not to treat histologically identified DCIS. As a consequence there is relatively little knowledge of the natural history of DCIS in all its various forms. The results of this and subsequent studies detailing the incidence of invasive breast cancer

Table 14.2 Incidence of invasive breast cancer following previous biopsy showing DCIS

Reference	Year	No. patients	Subsequent cancers	
			No.	%
Lewis[4]	1938	8	6	75
Farrow[89]	1970	25	5	20
Haagensen[90]	1971	11	8	73
Millis[91]	1975	8	2	25
Rosen[92]	1980	15	8	53
Eusebi[79]	1994	80	11	14
Page[93]	1995	28	9	32
Total		175	49	28

after incisional biopsy alone are shown in Table 14.2. The later studies largely include cases originally classified as benign, but in whom the diagnosis was revised to DCIS on retrospective review conducted many years after initial presentation. Many of these studies have an over-representation of localised low grade forms of DCIS as high grade/comedo forms of DCIS are rarely misclassified by pathologists.[33] In view of this bias these series cannot be accepted as fully representative of the full spectrum of DCIS and probably reflect only the behavior of the less aggressive forms of this disease. These data do however provide convincing evidence that DCIS can progress to invasive carcinoma if incompletely excised, but that this progression is not invariable.

For these reasons it has been argued that DCIS should be regarded and managed as a unifocal high risk factor for the development of subsequent invasive breast rather than an established form of 'cancer' with metastatic potential. Certainly the 'risk factor' view of DCIS can be applied convincingly to lower nuclear grades of DCIS or cases of DCIS without comedo type necrosis[11] but these views should be balanced by the very convincing data supporting the view that DCIS is the principle precursor of invasive adenocarcinoma:

1. DCIS is present in at least 80% of invasive breast cancers.[34]
2. It has morphological similarities to invasive carcinoma.[34]
3. It shares highly abnormal molecular abnormalities such as gross DNA aneuploidy and c-erbB-2 (neu) gene amplification.[35, 36]
4. Loss of heterozygosity studies of microdissected in situ and invasive

components of the same tumor have demonstrated identical genetic abnormalities.[30]

CLASSIFICATION OF DCIS

CRITERIA FOR DIAGNOSIS AND CLASSIFICATION

Ductal carcinoma in situ can be defined as a ... 'proliferation of epithelial cells with cytological features of malignancy within parenchymal structures of the breast ... distinguished from invasive carcinoma by the absence of stromal invasion across the basement membrane'.[37] It may be categorized on (a) clinical — symptomatic, screening detected, associated with Paget's disease, location of lesion within breast; (b) radiological — radiological size, pattern of calcifications, lesion character; or on (c) pathological grounds — microscopic size of lesion, margin status, nuclear grade, nucleolar grade, architecture, cell size, grade of necrosis or the presence of associated lesions. Molecular markers can also be used in subclassification; e.g. c-erbB-2, p53, nm23, estrogen (ER) or progesterone receptor (PR) expression, pS2, bcl-2, p21ras, cyclin D1, DNA ploidy, proliferative fraction, apoptotic index, metallothionein expression, E cadherin expression, or argyrophilic nucleolar organizer region index. In practice the optimum combination for patient management is not entirely clear, but histological features are generally used as part of this process. In this section we examine the histological criteria of DCIS and its boundaries with the closely related conditions of ADH and microinvasive carcinoma.

HISTOLOGICAL CLASSIFICATION

Distinction between atypical ductal hyperplasia and DCIS (see also Ch. 5)

Atypical ductal hyperplasia (ADH) can be defined as 'a rare lesion often co-existing with fibrocystic change, a sclerosing lesion, or a papilloma'. In UK guidelines, the current definition rests on identification of ... 'some but not all of the features of ductal carcinoma in situ'.[38] This is an area of diagnosis where even expert pathologists differ; many experience difficulty in achieving consensus or acceptable diagnostic agreement.[10] These problems can often be resolved through adherence to one diagnostic protocol coupled with training and guidance. Disagreements on the definitions of these early lesions still occur, particularly in the area of distinction of ADH from low grade non-comedo types of DCIS.[33,39] If ADH and low grade non-comedo DCIS are indeed biologically different from intermediate and high nuclear grade DCIS, then the distinction of ADH from low grade DCIS may in future become irrelevant. A recent review of inter-observer agreement in the diagnosis of atypical hyperplasias, DCIS, and microinvasive breast cancer from the UK Breast Screening External Quality Assessment (EQA) scheme showed that there was greater agreement over cases of DCIS where there was a comedo growth pattern in at least part of the lesion, prominent nucleoli, and low nucleo-cytoplasmic ratio.[33]

There was little consistency in subtyping of DCIS, with the highest agreement at average level (kappa statistic=0.4) for comedo type DCIS. There was also poor agreement among participants in the diagnosis of atypical hyperplasias (highest kappa statistic=0.25) and low agreement about the diagnosis of microinvasive carcinoma (highest kappa statistic=0.30) in this study. Such findings re-emphasize the view that the reproducibility of DCIS classification and grading has limitations, particularly as 'expert' breast pathologists in this study also seemed to have similar difficulty in the classification of DCIS subtypes and in agreeing about presence or absence of microinvasive carcinoma.

Most difficulties are encountered in distinguishing ADH from low grade variants of DCIS.[33] Guidelines for distinction of ADH and DCIS are reproduced in Table 14.3. If pathologists adhere to the view[40] that when cellular changes typical of DCIS occupy two separate duct spaces this is

Table 14.3 Microscopic features of ADH compared with low grade DCIS

	ADH	Low grade DCIS
Size	Usually small and focal <2–3 mm size. Rarely over 2–3 mm unless associated with papilloma or radial scar	Rarely under 2–3 mm and may be extensive
Cellular composition	May be uniform single population but this merges with areas of usual type hyperplasia within same duct space. Spindle cells may be prominent. Myoepithelial cells always present around periphery of duct spaces	Single population of cells. Spindle shaped cells very rare. Myoepithelial cells usually present around periphery of duct spaces
Architecture	Micropapillary, cribriform, or solid	Well developed micropapillary cribriform, or solid patterns
Lumina	May be distinct and well formed ovoid or rounded spaces in cribriform type	Well formed, regular punched out lumina in cribriform type often with cells orientated towards the luminal space
Cell orientation	May be regular, even placement at least focally. Cells may be at right angles to bridges in cribriform types	Micropapillary structures with indiscernible fibrovascular cores or smooth geometric spaces and 'rigid'. Bridges in cribriform type
Nuclear spacing	May be even	Even
Epithelial tumor cell character	Small, uniform or medium sized monotonous cell populations focally	Small, uniform monotonous cell population
Nucleoli	Single and small	Single and small
Mitoses	Infrequent, abnormal forms rare	Infrequent, abnormal forms rare
Necrosis/apoptosis	Rare	May be present as small particulate debris in cribriform and/or luminal spaces
Myoepithelial cells	Present	Present, rarely attenuated in thickness
Calcification	May be present	May be present

regarded as DCIS, if only one duct space, as ADH, then the majority of cases should be readily classifiable,[39] particularly as this also implies that ADH is a small microfocal lesion. We use two simple rules of thumb: (a) not to entertain the diagnosis of ADH unless DCIS has been seriously considered in the differential diagnosis; and (b) the larger the lesion the greater the likelihood that it is DCIS.

Page and co-workers have recently used a 3 mm size cut-off in subclassification of atypia within papillomas.[41] Tavassoli and Norris have argued that the overall geometric size of the DCIS lesion is more important than the number of duct spaces involved.[42,43] Two mm in size was used as the cut-off point for the decision between ADH or DCIS in earlier published articles, a lesion less than 2 mm in overall size indicating ADH. The AFIP criteria for DCIS have now been updated.[24] The 2 mm size criterion is now invoked *only* when assessing non-necrotic atypical intraductal prolif-erations with both architectural and cytologic features similar to those of low grade DCIS. Proliferations with high grade cytology (with or without necrosis) qualify as DCIS, regardless of size or quantity of epithelial proliferation.[24] Lesions that show comedo necrosis or high nuclear grade are not classified as ADH using updated AFIP criteria. Other pathologists would also classify a lesion as DCIS if the cellular changes typical of DCIS were present in only one duct space or if comedo type necrosis was present in the duct space in question, and even if the lesion was less than 2.0 mm in size (MD Lagios, personal communication). In our view such lesions are rare and unless present at or close to the edge of a biopsy are clearly microfocal and will have been adequately excised. Until there is a clearer understanding of the pathogenesis of DCIS these tiny lesions represent an intellectual dilemma for pathologists rather than a significant clinical problem.

Staining for α-smooth muscle actin, S100 protein and cytokeratin has been suggested to be of value in aiding the discrimination of ADH and DCIS[44] and similarly antibodies directed against basal and luminal cell cytokeratins can be used to discriminate usual type epithelial hyperplasia from DCIS in many cases[45] through identification of mixed populations of cells. Basal epithelial cells have both epithelial and myoepithelial properties and can be readily demonstrated using stains for α-smooth muscle actin. In our view the use of cytokeratins currently does not appear to be of practical value for the discrimination of usual type hyperplasia, ADH or DCIS although stains for α-smooth muscle actin are useful for the assessment of the presence or absence of microinvasion or frank invasive carcinoma in many cases (see below).

Review of classification systems for DCIS

The traditional classification of DCIS was based largely on architecture; comedo or non-comedo, papillary, micropapillary, or solid (Fig. 14.1), with special types of DCIS such as clear cell, neuro-endocrine, signet-ring, and cystic hypersecretory DCIS also recognized. Current thinking is that the architectural type is probably of less impor-tance than was earlier believed and that nuclear grade, the size of the lesion, margin status and coexisting features such as the presence or absence of comedo type necrosis are of greater importance. These and additional characteristics have been used to develop new classification systems for DCIS (Tables 14.4 and 14.5). Most of these grading systems have utilized nuclear morphology or grade as the basis for histological classification. The prototype system was that of Lagios and co-workers and is now updated to subclassify DCIS into three grades.[46] A four point nuclear grading system for DCIS which also uses the presence or absence of comedo type necrosis has been advocated by Page and co-workers.[32] In the UK and elsewhere in Europe a modified system originally proposed by the European Pathologists Working Group (EPWG)[47] utilizing nuclear grade has been adopted. In addition a number of other systems have been proposed by groups in Edinburgh,[48] Nottingham,[49] Scandinavia,[50] and Van Nuys.[51,52] These recent proposals for alterna-tive classifications and grading systems for DCIS are based on the findings from non-randomized follow-up studies showing that high nuclear grade DCIS and those cases with comedo type necrosis recur earlier than cases of low nuclear grade DCIS and those without comedo type necrosis, with size and margin status as additional prognostic factors. While a recent single center study has suggest that the Van Nuys DCIS classification may be superior to other proposed classification systems[52] further confirmatory studies are awaited. Our assessment of the available evidence is that margin status is probably the single most important factor in predicting risk of local recurrence after breast conservation.[53,54] Size and pathological subtype are also important in breast conservation and can be used to formulate a DCIS

prognostic index for treatment of DCIS by breast conservation therapy.[55] We examine below the evidence for the validity of the components of these methods and present details of the classification currently used in our Unit.

Nuclear grade: Published studies of DCIS show increased local recurrence rates after excision alone in cases of higher nuclear grade or with comedo type necrosis.[7,48–51,55–60] It should also be noted that the evaluation of nuclear grade in the grading of invasive breast cancer is one of the most

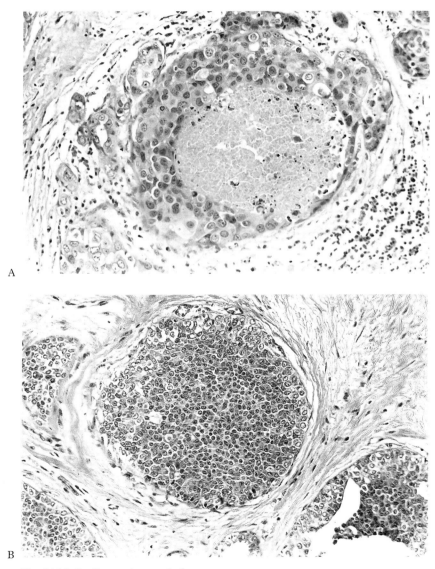

A

B

Fig. 14.1A,B See caption overleaf.

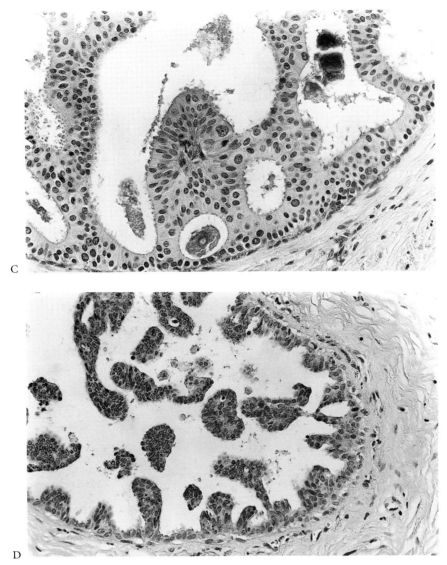

Fig. 14.1 Illustrations of the four traditional subtypes of DCIS, comedo (A), solid (B), cribriform (C) and micropapillary (D). Hematoxylin–eosin × 125.

difficult and least reproducible of the categories as compared with tubule formation and mitotic count. High nuclear grade in DCIS is also closely correlated with large cell size,[35] larger tumor size,[55,61] increased grades of intraductal necrosis,[50,55,61] increased c-erbB-2 protein expression,[55,61] higher cellular proliferation fraction, increased p53 protein expression, and absence of ER and PR expression.

Necrosis: The presence or absence of comedo type necrosis is a feature which pathologists find

easy to recognize.[33,52] This, coupled with the knowledge that most cases of DCIS showing intermediate or high nuclear grade have foci of comedo-type necrosis, together with the fact that comedo type necrosis closely correlates with coarse cast-like radiological calcifications, expression of p53, c-erbB-2, and inversely with ER and bcl-2 expression, provides a rationale for systems of DCIS classification based on necrosis.[35,49] Radiologists can identify the result of tumor necrosis mammographically (as micro-calcifica-

Table 14.4 Pathological features used in the development of new classification systems for DCIS (Table 14.5)

Size of pathological lesion (Ottensen, Van Nuys DCIS Prognostic Index)
Margin status (Van Nuys DCIS Prognostic Index)
Duct size (median or range, etc.) (none)
Nuclear grade (Edinburgh, EPWG, Lagios, Ottensen, Page, Van Nuys DCIS Class)
Nucleolar grade (implied in Edinburgh, EPWG, Lagios, Page)
Cell size (implied in EPWG, Lagios, Ottensen, Page, Van Nuys Class)
Architecture (comedo, cribriform, micropapillary, solid) (Edinburgh, EPWG, Ottensen)
Necrosis or grade of necrosis (Lagios, Nottingham, Ottensen, Page)
Pattern of microscopic calcifications (coarse, fine, psammoma body like) (EPWG, Page)
Homogeneity or heterogeneity of nuclear grade/cell size throughout lesion (Page)
Presence of co-existent AIDH (Page)
Three-dimensional studies of DCIS distribution (EPWG)
c-erbB-2 (Lagios, Nottingham, EPWG)
p53 (EPWG, Nottingham)
ER (EPWG)
PR (EPWG)
DNA ploidy (image analysis or flow cytometry) (Nottingham)
Proliferation fraction (flow cytometry or Ki67/MIB1) (EPWG, Nottingham)
Angiogenesis (none)
Tumor forming or asymptomatic (Ottensen)

Table 14.5 Classification and grading systems for DCIS

Edinburgh[48]

Main findings:

Micropapillary DCIS (also including some cases with comedo necrosis) more likely to be multiquadrantic. Non-micropapillary cases more likely to be uniquadrantic. Comedo DCIS more likely to be asymptomatic than non-comedo DCIS. High grade DCIS more likely to be incompletely excised than other patterns of DCIS. Invasive recurrence only followed high grade DCIS, in particular comedo DCIS. Necrosis, lymphoplasmacytic infiltration, periductal sclerosis not found to be of value.

European Pathologists' Working Group (EPWG)[47]

Main findings:

Development of new system of classification; clear association with molecular markers; no retrospective or prospective evaluation of validity yet performed.

Poorly differentiated, very pleomorphic nuclei with variation in size, irregular nuclear outlines, and spacing. Chromatin coarse and clumped, nucleoli prominent, mitoses often present, polarization of cells absent or minimal, central necrosis usually present, often prominent, individual cell necrosis usually present, growth pattern solid, clinging, or pseudomicropapillary or cribriform, calcifications amorphous.

Intermediately differentiated, mildly pleomorphic cells, some variation in size, outline and spacing, chromatin fine to coarse, nucleoli visible, mitoses occasionally present, polarization of cells present, central necrosis variable, individual cell necrosis may be focally present, growth pattern variable, calcifications amorphous or laminated.

Well differentiated, monomorphic cells, uniform in size, regular nuclear outline and spacing with uniform fine chromatin, insignificant nucleoli, rare mitoses. Architectural differentiation (polarization) marked, central necrosis absent or minimal, individual cell necrosis absent, growth clinging, micropapillary, cribriform or rarely solid, calcifications psammoma-like or rarely amorphous.

Nottingham[49]

Main findings:

Development of new system of classification; retrospective clinical evaluation in large series of DCIS has confirmed validity of proposal.

Pure comedo, central lumina containing necrotic debris surrounded by large pleomorphic cells in solid masses.

DCIS with necrosis, central lumina containing necrotic debris, cribriform (non-pure comedo), micropapillary, or variable architectural pattern.

DCIS without necrosis, no evidence of intraluminal necrosis, occasional apoptotic desquamated cells or mucus ignored.

Table 14.5 (*contd*)

Ottensen et al[50]

112 cases treated by excision alone, the majority (93%) were symptomatic or presented as incidental findings; only 7% detected via mammography alone. The growth pattern of DCIS (microfocal, diffuse, or tumor forming), size of lesions, the architecture (solid, clinging, cribriform and papillary), nuclear grade, presence of comedo type necrosis, and histological subtype were assessed. A strong relationship was found with growth pattern (microfocal, diffuse, or tumor forming), increased nuclear size and comedo type necrosis. Increased frequency of recurrence of DCIS was associated with larger sized lesions, high or intermediate nuclear grade, and comedo type necrosis.

Lagios[7]

High grade	Nuclear diameter greater than two red blood cells, nuclear chromatin vesicular, with one or more nucleoli, two or more mitoses per 10 hpf. +++ necrosis.
Intermediate grade	Nuclear diameter 1–2 red blood cells, coarse chromatin, infrequent nucleoli, 1–2 mitoses per 10 hpf, + necrosis.
Low grade	Nuclear diameter 1–1.5 red blood cells, diffuse chromatin, nucleoli not apparent, less than 1 mitosis per 10 hpf, no necrosis.

The mitotic index can be quite variable, some high grade lesions have rare mitoses, others exceed indexes of 20 or more.

Page[32]

Main findings:

Development of new system of classification, particularly with reference to lower grade spectrum of DCIS lesions based on referral practice of senior author (DL Page).

100 cases of DCIS reviewed. 17 cases of DCIS associated with ADH, 33 cases contained foci of comedo type necrosis with foci of non-comedo DCIS. No cases of comedo DCIS found to be associated with ADH. More 'advanced' patterns seen in middle of lesions with ADH peripherally. Argues that DCIS develops from a central focus and 'expands' peripherally. Used a 1–4 category system for nuclear grading of DCIS. The results of this study taken together with other studies of computerized image analysis in DCIS which show that ducts showing comedo type necrosis are larger, having a much greater cross sectional area than ducts with a solid pattern of intraductal carcinoma without comedo type necrosis explains much of the architectural heterogeneity in DCIS.

Van Nuys[51]

Main findings:

A development of the Nottingham Classification (see above). 425 consecutive patients with histologically confirmed DCIS treated at The Breast Center, Van Nuys, California, USA. 31 local recurrences in 238 patients (3.8% in group 1, 11.1% in group 2 and 26.5% in group 3, 8-year actuarial disease-free survivals 93%, 84% and 61% respectively.

Group 1 Non-high grade without necrosis. Intermediate or low nuclear grade cases without evidence of intraductal necrotic material.

Group 2 Non-high nuclear grade with necrosis. Any architectural pattern of DCIS allowed in which central lumina contain substantial amounts of necrotic neoplastic cells of duct origin. Occasional desquamated or individually apoptotic cells are ignored. Nuclear grade must be intermediate or low.

Group 3 High nuclear grade cases. High grade nuclei are defined as nuclei with a diameter greater than two red blood cells, with vesicular chromatin, and one or more nucleoli. Necrosis may be present or absent (e.g. as in high grade solid DCIS). Any architectural pattern may be present.

tion), but not the grade of DCIS nuclei.[62] There are some rarer forms of high grade DCIS, particularly large cell solid types in which necrosis is not seen, but these are often related to Paget's disease of the nipple and confined to the sub-areolar ducts. Lower grade forms of DCIS may have occasional necrotic cells within duct spaces or with duct spaces containing mucus and may be overclassified if necrosis alone is used.

Microscopic size of DCIS lesions: While this disease extent is undoubtedly of crucial importance for management of DCIS it has rarely been used in classification systems of DCIS to date.[50,55,61] The data on size and outcome, although limited, suggests that larger lesions are more difficult to excise and are thus more likely to have tumor extending closer to margins.[55]

Architecture: As mentioned above this has been the traditional means of subclassifying DCIS into comedo, cribriform, micropapillary, solid, and mixed types.[48] There has now been a general tendency away from this system towards those based on nuclear grade, necrosis, and differentiation since, if any given case of DCIS is examined critically, there are almost inevitably foci of both cribriform and micropapillary pattern or other mixtures of comedo and non-comedo types.[63] Reproducibility of grading systems for DCIS based on architecture alone is therefore likely to be poor or a high proportion of cases will be classified as mixed.

Cytonuclear grade: This is the basis for a classification of DCIS, together with cyto-architectural differentiation, as proposed by the European Pathologists Working Group (EPWG).[47] This system has biological validity based on studies showing increased proliferation fraction, c-erbB-2 and p53 expression in the more poorly differentiated subtypes compared with well differentiated DCIS.[36,64]

Cell size: This is a useful criterion. Its practical difficulty is that the cellular boundaries are often indistinct, and nuclear grade is therefore preferred.

Pattern of microscopic calcifications and mammographic appearances: Calcification in DCIS occurs within the ductal epithelium, and in debris or secretions found in the duct lumina. This may be granular, or linear. Linear, branch-ing, or casting calcifications are more commonly associated with comedo type necrosis. Granular microcalcifications can be formed by foci of dystrophic calcification in necrotic tumor cells that have not coalesced to form linear calcifications, or as calcified secretions or mucin with cribriform spaces and non-comedo DCIS. While there is an undoubted association of coarse calcifications with high and intermediate grade DCIS and fine granular calcifications with low grade DCIS,[1] these can be difficult to distinguish reliably on hematoxylin and eosin sections. Lesions without calcifications have a tendency to lower histological grades in our experience.[1]

RECOMMENDED SYSTEM FOR CLASSIFICATION OF DUCTAL CARCINOMA IN SITU

In 1996 a European Union Working Group on Breast Screening Pathology accepted these following guidelines for classification of DCIS.[65]

i. High nuclear grade DCIS

This is the easiest pattern to recognize.[33] Cells have pleomorphic, irregularly spaced, and usually large nuclei exhibiting marked variation in size,

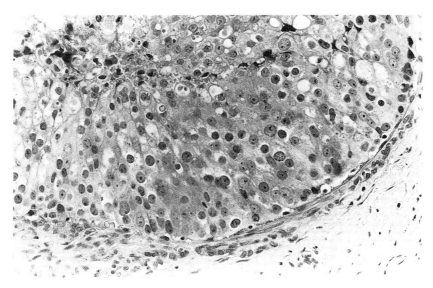

Fig. 14.2   High grade DCIS showing the very abnormal cytonuclear features. Hematoxylin–eosin × 400.

irregular nuclear contours, coarse chromatin and prominent nucleoli (Fig. 14.2). Mitoses are frequent and abnormal forms may be seen. High grade DCIS may exhibit several growth patterns; most commonly as a solid sheet of cell lining the duct and with comedo type central necrosis which frequently contains deposits of amorphous calcification. Sometimes a solid proliferation of malignant cells fills the duct without necrosis. This is relatively uncommon and may be confined to nipple ducts in cases presenting with Paget's disease. High nuclear grade DCIS may also

exhibit micropapillary and cribriform patterns which are also frequently associated with central comedo type necrosis (Fig. 14.3). Unlike low nuclear grade DCIS there is rarely any polarization of cells covering the micropapillae or lining the intercellular spaces.

ii. Intermediate nuclear grade DCIS

This type cannot be assigned easily to the high or low nuclear grade categories. The nuclei show mild to moderate pleomorphism, which is less

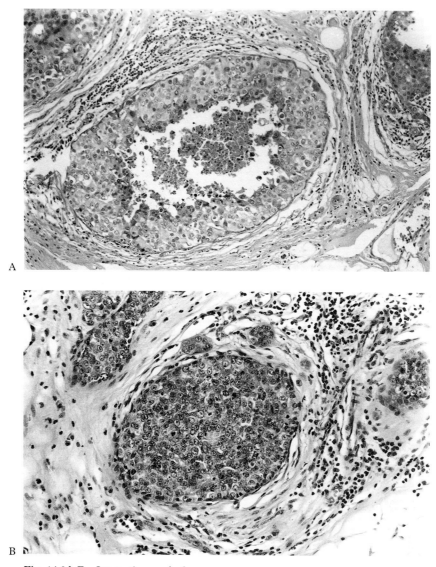

A

B

Fig. 14.3A,B See caption overleaf.

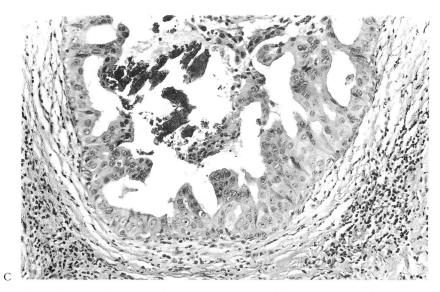

C

Fig. 14.3 Three illustrations of the growth patterns and features of high grade DCIS. Central comedo necrosis is the most frequent pattern seen (A), but solid (B) and micropapillary architecture is also found (C). Hematoxylin–eosin × 125.

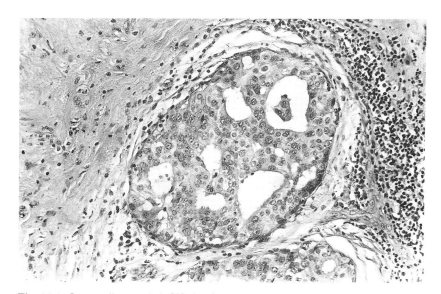

Fig. 14.4 Intermediate grade DCIS showing some cytomorphological atypia. Hematoxylin–eosin × 185.

than that seen in the large cell variety, but lacks the monotony of the small cell type (Fig. 14.4). The nuclear to cytoplasmic ratio is often high and one or two nucleoli may be identified. The growth pattern may be solid, cribriform, or micropapillary and the cells usually exhibit some degree of polarization covering papillary processes or lining inter-cellular lumina, although this is not as marked as in low grade DCIS (Fig. 14.5).

iii. Low nuclear grade DCIS

These types are composed of monomorphic, evenly spaced cells with roughly spherical, cen-

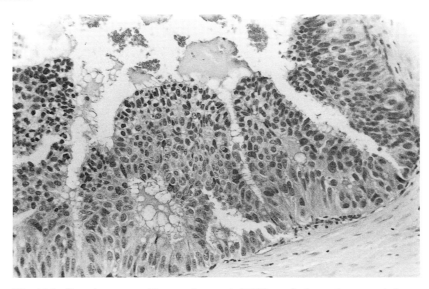

Fig. 14.5 Growth patterns of intermediate grade DCIS are similar to those seen in low grade DCIS, but lack the uniformity of structure with less distinct polarization of cells. Hematoxylin–eosin × 185.

trally-placed nuclei, and inconspicuous nucleoli. The nuclei are usually, but not invariably, small (Fig. 14.6). Mitoses are few and there is rarely individual cell necrosis. The cells are generally arranged in micropapillary and cribriform patterns which are frequently present within the same lesion, with cribriform patterns being more common. There is usually polarization of cells cover-

ing the micropapillae or lining the intercellular lumina (Fig. 14.7). Less frequently low grade DCIS has a solid pattern. When terminal duct lobular units are involved the process can be very difficult to distinguish from lobular carcinoma in situ (see also Ch. 6). Features in favor of DCIS are the slightly larger cell size, cytoplasmic basophilia, and variation in cellular arrangement and size,

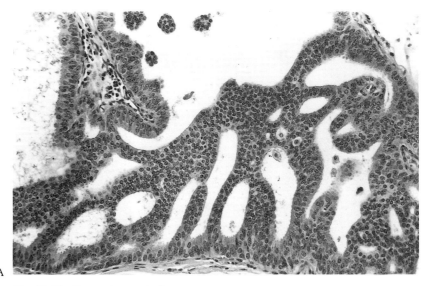

A

Fig. 14.6A See caption overleaf.

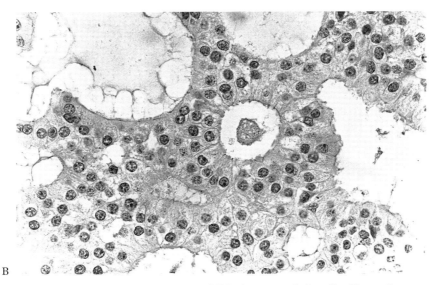

B

Fig. 14.6 Two examples of low grade DCIS both composed of small uniform cells showing little cytonuclear atypia (A and B). Note the even cellular placement and polarization of cells around the cribriform spaces (B). Hematoxylin–eosin, A × 125; B × 400.

greater cellular cohesion and lack of intracytoplasmic lumina. Occasionally there may be combinations of both processes or it may not be possible to distinguish between DCIS and LCIS and in this situation we classify the appearance as a combined lesion (Fig. 14.8).

iv. Mixed types of DCIS

A proportion of cases of DCIS exhibit features of more than one histological subtype. One of the advantages of classifying DCIS according to nuclear grade is that when there are variations

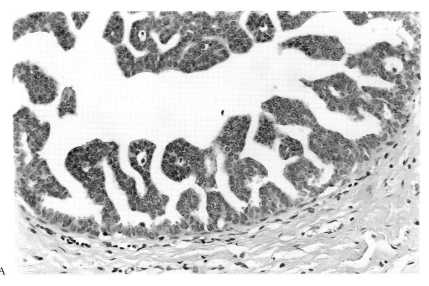

A

Fig. 14.7A See caption overleaf.

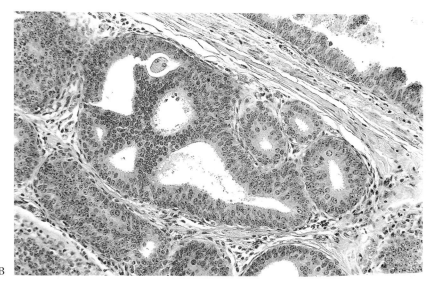

Fig. 14.7   Low grade forms of DCIS exhibit distinctive micropapillary (A) and cribriform (B) growth patterns. Hematoxylin–eosin × 125.

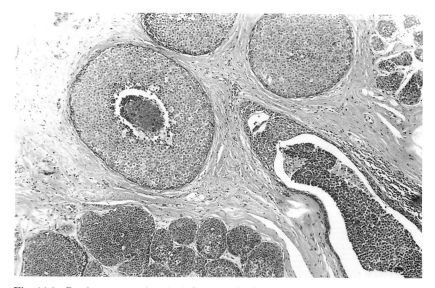

Fig. 14.8   Rarely cases can show both features of DCIS, here in the form of high grade comedo DCIS, and LCIS. Hematoxylin–eosin × 57.

in growth pattern but a dominant cell type, the lesion can be classified on the basis of nuclear grade. Foci of differing nuclear grade may be seen (Fig. 14.9), but such variation in cell type is unusual, although if present, the case should be classified according to the highest nuclear grade.

v. Microinvasive carcinoma

This is defined as a tumor in which the dominant lesion is non-invasive but in which there are one or more clearly separate foci of infiltration of non-specialized interlobular stroma, none of which measures more than 1 mm (about two high

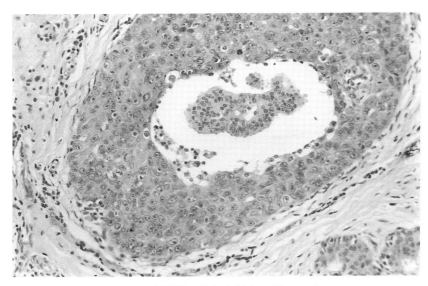

Fig. 14.9 A true mixed case of DCIS with both high and low grade components. Hematoxylin–eosin.

power fields) in diameter.[38] Tumors fulfilling these criteria are rare. If there is sufficient doubt about the presence of invasion the case should be classified as DCIS. Areas of true invasion are most easily identified at low power microscopy when the preserved organoid architecture of the involved expanded ductal and lobular system can be appreciated (Fig. 14.10). Islands of invasive tumor can be identified in the intervening non-specialized stroma and worrisome in situ extension into lobules, 'cancerization', can be disregarded. Cases of pure high or intermediate nuclear grade DCIS and those with comedo type necrosis should be sampled extensively to exclude foci of established invasion. Stains for a smooth muscle actin may assist in the diagnosis, as may stains for basement membrane components such as laminin. Alpha smooth muscle reactive myoepithelial cells will invariably be absent on invasion fronts (Fig. 14.11).

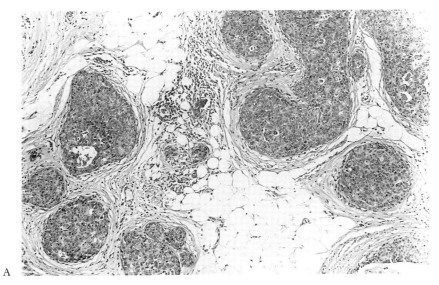

A

Fig. 14.10A See caption overleaf.

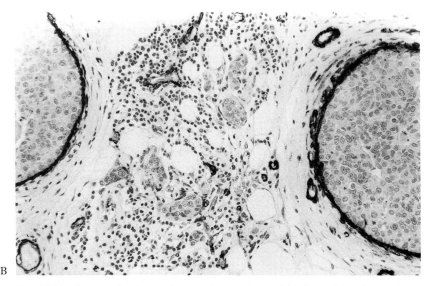

Fig. 14.10 An example of true microinvasive carcinoma. The focus of invasion can be seen between two expanded lobular units (A). The lack of smooth muscle actin reactive myoepithelial cells helps to distinguish these cells from the adjacent in situ component (B). Hematoxylin–eosin, A × 57; immunostaining for smooth muscle actin, B × 185.

In true microinvasive carcinomas of the breast the incidence of metastatic disease in axillary lymph nodes is very low and the condition is generally managed clinically as a form of DCIS. It is relevant also to note that one recent study using a PCR technique showed evidence of metastatic breast carcinoma in axillary lymph nodes in one of 14 cases of DCIS,[66] presumably representing occult invasive disease. DCIS with PCR evidence of metastatic disease, but without microscopic evidence of nodal tumor deposits, should probably be assigned to an 'indeterminate' category.

RARER SUBTYPES OF DCIS

A variety of rare but morphologically distinct subtypes of DCIS are recognized. There is currently no firm evidence to support the distinction of special DCIS types from commoner DCIS subtypes with the exception of encysted papillary carcinoma in situ and apocrine DCIS. However, the practical problem of interobserver disagreement in distinction of some special DCIS subtypes, particularly apocrine and micropapillary DCIS, caused one group in a preliminary study to suggest a working classification of DCIS with five sub-types; high, intermediate, and low grade, with additionally apocrine and micropapillary DCIS.[67] Simultaneous use of the grading system described above and subtyping is suggested. A fuller account of rare subtypes of DCIS is given by Tavassoli.[68]

Apocrine DCIS

Apocrine change is of course frequent in breast biopsy material and is recognized to show nuclear atypia which should not be interpreted as DCIS. Apocrine metaplasia and atypia are in general readily diagnosed with classic cytological features including finely granular eosinophilic cytoplasm and a moderately large, sometimes vesicular nucleus with a single nucleolus (see also Chs 2 and 5). Overtly malignant apocrine lesions are also readily diagnosed and often distend and distort the underlying breast parenchymal elements in the same way as other types of DCIS (Fig. 14.12). The tumor cells show abundant granular cytoplasm, moderate to severe cytological atypia and there is accompanying central necrosis. Apical snouting (cytoplasmic protrusions) is not always seen.

The diagnosis of apocrine DCIS should be made with caution, particularly in the absence of comedo type necrosis[69] (see below), and some

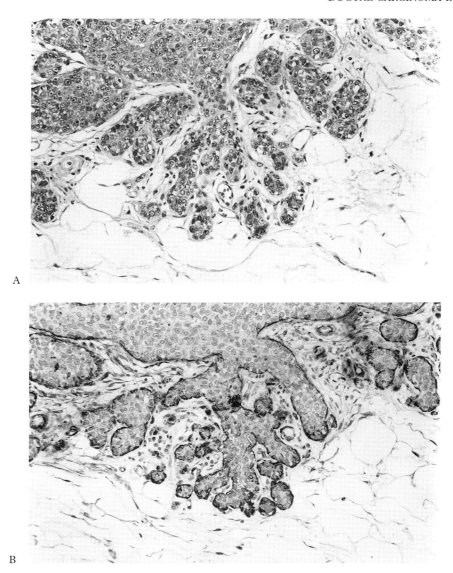

Fig. 14.11 Cancerization of lobular units by high grade DCIS can appear invasive or microinvasive (A). In this example the true in situ nature of the process was confirmed by identification of the residual myoepithelial cell population in the acinar units (B). Hematoxylin–eosin, A × 125; immunostaining for smooth muscle actin, B × 125.

authors have not attempted to separate atypical apocrine hyperplasias from apocrine DCIS.[70] However, the well recognized patterns of growth of ADH or DCIS are not always seen in atypical apocrine proliferations and a complex papillary pattern of apocrine change which is extensive or shows cytological atypia can cause significant dilemmas in classification (see also Ch. 5).

O'Malley and colleagues utilized nuclear pattern (usual, borderline and overtly atypical as seen in DCIS) and extent of lesion (<4 mm, 4 to 8 mm, and 8 mm) to categorize these difficult apocrine lesions.[71] They classified lesions which were composed of overtly malignant hyperchromatic cells with an irregular nuclear outline, coarse chromatin and multiple nucleoli as apocrine DCIS (Fig. 14.12). Apocrine DCIS was also diagnosed if the disease process was greater than 8 mm in extent but formed predominantly from atypical apocrine cells, the nuclei of which showed

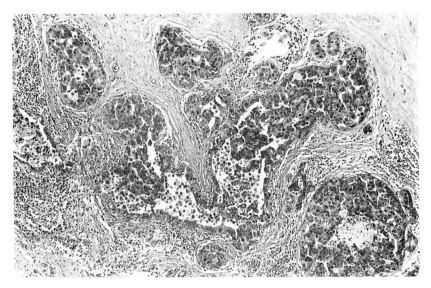

Fig. 14.12 High grade apocrine DCIS can be recognized by the highly abnormal cytonuclear morphology, but with coexisting apocrine cellular structure, and the association of necrosis, inflammation and fibrosis. Hematoxylin–eosin × 57.

moderate atypia with nuclei two to three times the normal size, irregular outlines and two to three nucleoli (Fig. 14.13). If the abnormality measured 4 to 8 mm and more than half the nuclei were moderately atypical or if the lesion measured more than 8 mm and the majority of cells were of usual apocrine appearance with a small proportion (at least 25%) of cells showing markedly enlarged nuclei, then a category of 'borderline apocrine DCIS' was suggested. These authors defined lesions smaller than 4 mm in size where less than half the nuclei were of borderline atypical appearance as 'apocrine atypia'.[71] Using these parameters of lesion size and degree of atypia, few

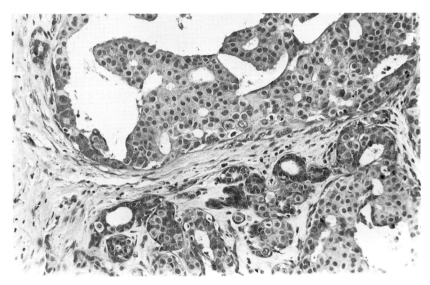

Fig. 14.13 Low grade apocrine DCIS is difficult to distinguish from apocrine hyperplasia. There is usually some cytomorphological atypia, but the size of the lesion is used by authorities to distinguish benign apocrine proliferations from low grade apocrine DCIS. Hematoxylin–eosin × 185.

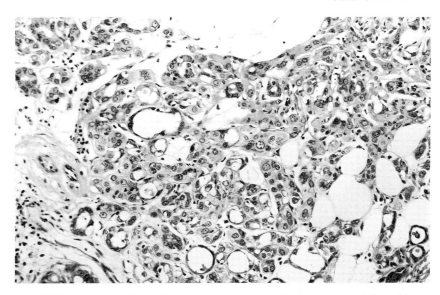

Fig. 14.14 Apocrine cells showing cytonuclear atypia can be found in association with sclerosing adenosis and should not be mistaken for apocrine DCIS or invasive carcinoma. Hematoxylin–eosin × 185.

cases in their series of difficult apocrine lesions were of 'borderline' classification.

Similar criteria to those of O'Malley et al were applied by Tavassoli and Norris[69] who defined atypical apocrine proliferations into three broad categories: atypical apocrine metaplasia, atypical apocrine hyperplasia and apocrine intraduct carcinoma. The former was diagnosed if a single layer of markedly pleomorphic apocrine cells (with a 3-fold variation in nuclear size) replaced the normal breast epithelium. In our experience this process generates the most concern when it is found in association with sclerosing adenosis (Fig. 14.14). A classification of atypical apocrine hyperplasia was used if markedly pleomorphic apocrine cells (with a 3-fold variation in nuclear size) formed a tufted, papillary or stratified growth pattern, but where no epithelial bridging was seen. In common with ADH atypical apocrine hyperplasia was also diagnosed if minimal cytological changes were present, but epithelial bridges or a complete cribriform architecture were seen involving all of the duct space in a lesion less than 2 mm in size histologically (Fig. 14.15). Although the group of apocrine DCIS was further divided by Tavassoli and Norris into non-comedo (non-necrotic), papillary (non-necrotic) and comedo (necrotic) types, these authors found that the majority of cases (32 of

37) of apocrine DCIS were of high histological grade based on cytological atypia and the presence of necrosis (Fig. 14.12). The remainder were all of intermediate grade. Two of these five non-comedo cases were admixed with non-apocrine DCIS.

Tavassoli et al summarized that 'in the absence of significant atypia and necrosis, a diagnosis of apocrine intraduct carcinoma should be made cautiously to avoid overdiagnosis of pronounced, but benign, apocrine hyperplasia'.[69] On reviewing the published data there is general agreement that high grade apocrine DCIS can be recognized by marked cytological atypia, abundant mitoses and necrosis. We regard apocrine proliferations which do not show significant cytological atypia or those which are small but severely atypical cytologically (but do not fulfil all the criteria for DCIS) as 'apocrine atypia'. These may or may not show the architectural changes seen in other forms of ADH/DCIS such as a cribriform or micropapillary growth pattern. Care should be taken that minor degrees of abnormal apocrine change, particularly those forming complex papillary tufts, but with minimal atypia, should not be classified as atypical. Agreement on the diagnostic criteria for apocrine atypia is required in order to achieve reproducibility of diagnosis and reach a better

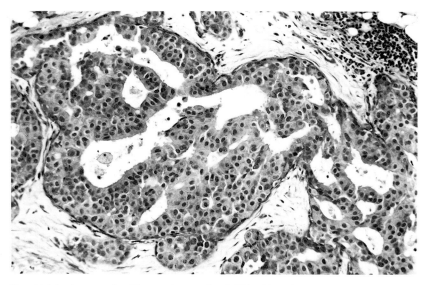

Fig. 14.15   An example of low grade apocrine DCIS with a distinct cribriform architecture helping to distinguish it for papillary apocrine hyperplasia. Hematoxylin–eosin × 185.

understanding of the significance of these lesions. At the present time the clinical importance of apocrine atypia and the risk of invasive breast carcinoma which it may confer is unclear.

Small cell solid DCIS

The duct spaces are filled by a uniform population of cells which resemble the cells found in cribriform or micropapillary DCIS but without the structured architectural arrangement of the latter (Fig. 14.16). This condition, if it extends to involve terminal duct lobules, may be indistinguishable from LCIS (see above). In this situation an overall diagnosis of LCIS/small cell solid DCIS can be made[72] and we currently report these as tumors showing combined features of DCIS and LCIS (Fig. 14.8) (see also p. 98).

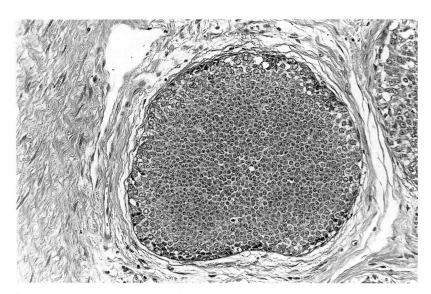

Fig. 14.16   An example of small cell solid DCIS. Hematoxylin–eosin × 125.

Encysted papillary carcinoma in situ

This rare but distinctive form of DCIS, which we describe in more detail in Chapter 8, is more common in older women and recognized to carry an excellent prognosis if confined within the capsule without surrounding DCIS.[73] It is usually circumscribed and accompanied by a fibrous wall giving an encysted appearance. It has a papillary structure with fibrovascular cores which are usually fine and may be absent in at least part of the lesion. It may be accompanied by other forms of DCIS, usually of micropapillary or cribriform type. There is also frequently hemosiderin (or hematoidin) pigment in the adjacent fibrous tissue.

Clear cell DCIS

This is a proliferation of cells with optically clear cytoplasm and distinct cell margins forming cribriform structures. Central necrosis may be present. A solid pattern may also be present.[68]

Signet ring DCIS

A very rare variant characterized by the prolifera-tion of signet ring cells in solid or papillary growth patterns (Fig. 14.17). The cytoplasm shows posi-tive staining with diastase-resistant-PAS or alcian blue.[74]

Neuroendocrine DCIS

The lesion and invasive counter part is described in more detail in Chapter 16. It has an organoid appearance with prominent argyrophilia, resem-bling a carcinoid tumor. The neoplastic cells may be in a solid configuration, or may be papillary, forming tubules, pseudorosettes, palisades or rib-bons.[75] The cytoplasmic granularity and organoid spindle morphology suggest a neuroendocrine phenotype. Because of the lack of microcalcifica-tion these tumors tend to present symptomati-cally, most commonly in elderly patients with bloodstained nipple discharge.

Cystic hypersecretory DCIS and mucocele-like lesion

This type of DCIS is a variant of micropapillary DCIS.[76–78] The cells produce mucinous secretions which distend involved duct spaces giving a cystic appearance (Fig. 14.18), and microcalcifications

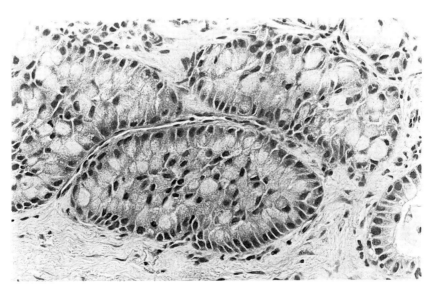

Fig. 14.17 An example of signet ring cell DCIS. Note that the cells do not contain dilated intracytoplasmic lumina. Their appearance is due to cytoplasmic distension by mucin-filled organelles. Hematoxylin–eosin × 400.

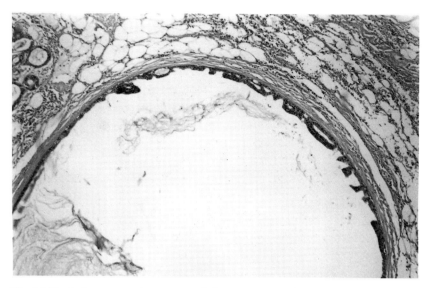

Fig. 14.18 At low power microscopy cystic hypersecretory DCIS is very distinctive with distended mucous-filled dilated duct spaces. Hematoxylin–eosin × 57.

are often a very prominent feature. The distended cystic ducts contain gelatinous eosinophilic material resembling colloid of the thyroid.[76] The cells lining these spaces may form micropapillary structures, but have more cytoplasm than those of true micropapillary DCIS (Fig. 14.19). Often the epithelium is attenuated making examination of cytological features difficult but secretory changes may be identified within the neoplastic cells. Mucus may be extruded into adjacent stroma (Fig. 14.20), producing a mucocele-like lesion[77] (see also Ch. 11).

Clinging carcinoma

This is a controversial entity recognized by some

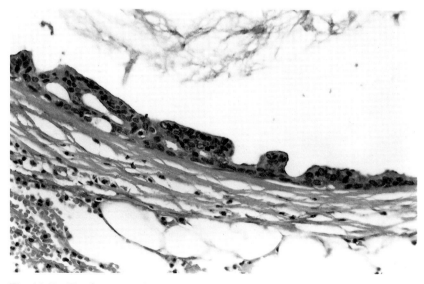

Fig. 14.19 The duct spaces in cystic hypersecretory DCIS are lined in part by a micropapillary arrangement of cells usually of low or intermediate grade. Hematoxylin–eosin × 185.

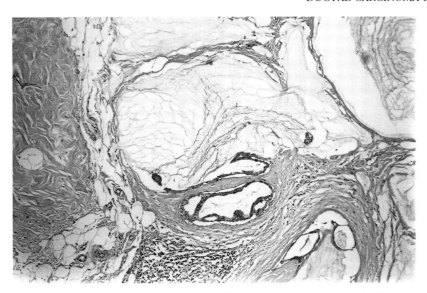

Fig. 14.20 Expulsion of mucus into surrounding tissue, a 'mucocele-like lesion', is a common feature in cystic hypersecretory DCIS and should not be misdiagnosed as invasive carcinoma of mucinous type. Hematoxylin–eosin × 57.

authorities as a variant of ADH or DCIS.[5,79] It is described as being composed of cells adherent ('clinging') to the basement membrane attached to or replacing the normal epithelium (Fig. 14.21). The cells may be bland and essentially similar to those of micropapillary ADH or DCIS or large and pleomorphic like those of high grade DCIS.[80]

Clinging 'DCIS' should probably be regarded as a risk factor equivalent to atypical ductal hyperplasia rather than a lesion conferring a risk equivalent to other forms of DCIS. This assertion is based on the published rates of local recurrence and development of invasive breast carcinoma in so-called clinging DCIS.[79] We believe that at the

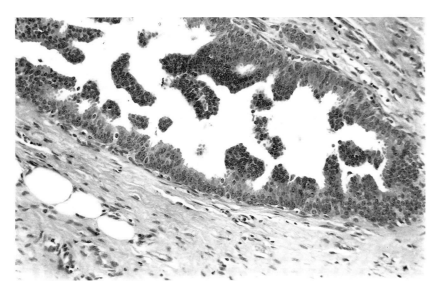

Fig. 14.21 An example of micropapillary DCIS exhibiting a clinging growth pattern. The nests of tumor cells appear to rest on top of a layer of normal duct lining cells. Hematoxylin–eosin × 185.

present time there is little evidence that this is truly a specific entity as opposed to a variant of ADH or DCIS and do not currently recommend the use of the term. The use of grading systems for DCIS also reduces the value of recognition of such entities.

Male breast DCIS

This is a rare entity with only about 90 cases reported in the world literature and accounting for slightly more than 7% of all male breast cancers in published series.[81] It typically presents with a retroareolar mass and may require mastectomy.

PATHOLOGICAL EXAMINATION OF SPECIMENS

WHAT IS A CLEAR MARGIN?

It is probable that the most crucial information pathologists can currently provide from their examination of local resection surgical specimens of DCIS is accurate evaluation of the excision margin status. The EORTC advocate 2 cm as a 'clear' margin with 1–2 cm indicating 'uncertain' margin status and less than 1 cm 'incomplete' tumor excision.[82] It has been further suggested (Holland, personal communication) that the presence of benign breast acini between the tumor and the margin may be helpful since this should imply complete excision with a boundary of normal tissue; there is no conclusive proof of this view thus far.

At the 3rd EORTC DCIS consensus meeting in 1994[82] Faverly and colleagues[27] described three-dimensional studies of DCIS distribution within the breast tissue in 60 mastectomy specimens, using a stereomicroscopic subgross method.[29] This technique requires slicing of the breast tissue at 5 mm intervals, with a radiograph being made of each macrosection. Tissue blocks are taken from radiologically and grossly suspicious areas. Blocks containing histologically identified areas of DCIS are de-paraffinized and prepared for stereomicroscopy allowing direct three-dimensional viewing of the mammary glandular tree. The stereomicroscopic analysis[27] showed a range of growth patterns including massively filled duct

system with cells arranged solidly (solid and comedo subtypes), and as delicate endoluminal blebs or coraliform-like structures (clinging/micropapillary types). A total of 90% of cases of poorly-differentiated DCIS (largely equivalent to high nuclear grade DCIS and types with comedo type necrosis) showed continuous growth along the duct system, compared with discontinuous growth in 70% of well-differentiated DCIS (largely equivalent to low nuclear grade DCIS and cases which would be classified as cribriform or micropapillary DCIS). In 92% of the cases examined gaps were <10 mm long. A tumor-free margin of 10 mm should therefore suffice to achieve adequate clearance of disease in the majority of cases. One other study of the three-dimensional distribution of DCIS using a different backprocessing method for subgross examination of paraffin wax blocks has shown much smaller 'gaps' of approximately 100 μm or more in cases of high nuclear grade comedo type DCIS.[83]

Current routine methods of examining excision margins can be inaccurate. A recent US study has shown that when a pathologist reports that a margin is uninvolved and tumor is at least 1 mm distant there will be residual tumor in the breast in 43%; in contrast 76% will have residual disease when the tumor was reported to be less than 1 mm from the nearest excision plane.[84] A further smaller study showed that in patients undergoing wide local excision and radiotherapy the risk of recurrence was 38% (three of eight patients) when the tumor extended histologically within 5 mm of the resection margins, compared to only 6% (two of 33 patients) when the width of the microscopically tumor-free margin was greater than 5 mm.[85] Adoption of a wider surgical excision policy coupled with diligent histological examination of excision margins can reduce local recurrence rates. The results from the combined Van Nuys/Lagios series show that where the margins are >10 mm clear, the likelihood of recurrence after 8 years follow-up is very low (4%).[53] Similarly, since adopting a wide excision policy (>10 mm) for DCIS with detailed assessment of margins and margin distance coupled with re-excision of cavity walls for lesions <10 mm distant our group in Nottingham have shown a low frequency of local recurrence (6%).[86]

The appearance of 'recurrence' of DCIS following local excision, with or without additional radiotherapy, is in the majority of cases really the detection of persistent residual disease. This view is supported by the observation of a high frequency of residual DCIS in patients undergoing mastectomy following 'curative' local excision[84] and also by finding that 95% of local recurrences occur at the site of previous surgery. Detection of DCIS recurrence in cases of intermediate and high nuclear grade DCIS may be facilitated by their association with early calcification of comedo necrotic debris which is clearly visible mammographically. Low grade forms of DCIS may show calcification of luminal or microacinar secretions.

This latter form of calcification is believed to occur slowly and is often present as fine particles which may be below the resolution of conventional mammography. For this reason the pathological extent of some DCIS lesions can be substantially larger than that of the radiological abnormality. As combined mammographic, specimen radiology, and microscopic examination of random specimen margins are the usual means of assessing margin status it is probably not surprising that DCIS is frequently 'left behind' after apparent complete local excision of mammographically detected DCIS.[84]

In summary there are no absolute guidelines to ensure total confidence about completeness of surgical excision. We would suggest a tumor clear surgical margin of between 10 and 20 mm coupled with meticulous histological examination of the excised specimen, in the ways suggested below.

PATHOLOGY EXAMINATION METHODS FOR DCIS (see also Ch. 2)

DCIS managed by breast conservation requires diligent assessment of margins, as well as classification of the pathological subtype and size of the lesion. Various suggestions have been proposed or applied for routine margin assessment. One is the 'onion skinning' of margins, originally suggested by Carter and advocated in modified form in our own practice (see Chs 2,5). A cylinder excision technique is adopted by the surgeon (see Ch. 22), the cylinder of tissue extending from the subcutaneous tissues to the deep pectoral fascia. The anterior (subcutaneous) and posterior (deep fascial) excision margins are irrelevant as no further breast tissue can be removed and margin assessment is directed at the radial excision margins.[86]

Alternatively, the whole specimen may be embedded and processed for histological examination and all the margins examined tangentially.[87] This method requires many more blocks, particularly if the excised lesion is large, weighing more than 20–30 grams. A variation on this theme is the use of large tissue blocks, embedding the whole of specimen as performed in Guildford, UK.[88] Estimation of the distance to the various circumferential excision margins can be achieved by taking 'radial' blocks which include both tumor and peripheral margins (see Chs 2,5).

Block selection is also targeted at establishing the character of the lesion and its size. If possible the tumor blocks with specimen and mammographic correlation at the time of specimen cut-up may be necessary to give an accurate assessment of tumor excision. It can be helpful to embed blocks in serial numbered sequence, allowing reconstruction of the lesion and better microscopic documentation of the overall pathological size of the lesion, a key fact which should be specified in the report. Processing and reporting of large block macrosections can be more helpful in assessing the extent of DCIS than conventionally sized blocks[88] but this type of preparation is time consuming and more expensive than conventional processing techniques and is not essential.

DCIS of over 4 cm extent, assessed clinically or radiographically, is widely regarded as unsuitable for conservative surgery and mastectomy is the usual form of treatment. Selection of blocks for mastectomy specimens should aim to establish the diagnosis and determine the extent of disease. It should be borne in mind that the frequency of associated foci of invasion increases with increasing size of DCIS; adequate numbers of blocks should be taken to exclude the presence of metastatic carcinoma. For the same reason it is also recommended that any axillary lymph nodes sampled should be examined to exclude the presence of invasive carcinoma.

AXILLARY NODE EXAMINATION IN DCIS

The frequency of axillary node metastases in screening detected localized DCIS is extremely low, and for this reason the value of axillary sampling for prognostication or axillary node treatment is questionable.[9] At present the existing preoperative diagnostic systems do not appear accurate enough to allow a definite preoperative diagnosis of DCIS without an invasive element thus avoiding the necessity of an axillary node sampling procedure at the time of initial surgery if a one stage treatment policy is adopted. The alternative is a multi-step process; for example multiple core biopsy (showing DCIS with no evidence of invasion) followed by complete local excision with subsequent axillary node clearance/sampling if invasion is then identified.

SUMMARY

Our knowledge of DCIS is expanding and answers to some important questions are becoming apparent. Margin status, size and nuclear grade seem to be the most important pathological indicators in DCIS predictive of likelihood of recurrence after breast conservation. All other biomarkers are probably related to lesion size (and grade), and hence ease of local excision. The value of margin status still requires prospective evaluation in clinical trials, and should be treated with caution until this is available. Prognostic indices for DCIS such as the Van Nuys DCIS Prognostic Index[55] may be helpful in guiding but not dictating patient management. The practical and cost implications of meticulous pathological margin assessment (an average of 30–40 tissue blocks or shave blocks of excision margins) requires serious consideration. Newer molecular biological markers although currently investigative tools, will, in the future, undoubtedly assist in quantifying risk in certain cases. The MIN concept, or at least the idea that proliferative changes, ADH and DCIS form a spectrum of disease is now borne out by numerous molecular studies. The adoption of MIN in routine practice requires evaluation of its reproducibility and evidence of clinical or prognostic importance.[24]

DCIS is a form of unifocal in situ neoplasia which carries a high risk for development of invasive breast cancer. Whilst considerable advances have been made in the understanding of DCIS, in terms of both the pathology and molecular biology, we do not yet have clear views of its ideal management. It may be that there will be a trend away from conservation back to mastectomy or very wide local excision, unless better imaging techniques can be devised to assess accurately and reliably the extent of DCIS in vivo. Newer DCIS classification and prognostic index systems may help to some extent in predicting patients likely to suffer recurrent disease, but their value remains to be shown conclusively in prospective randomized trials. Recurrence of DCIS is, in reality, a manifestation during follow-up of persistence of DCIS after previous treatment, with or without development of invasive carcinoma.

PAGET'S DISEASE OF THE NIPPLE

CLINICAL FEATURES

Paget's disease of the nipple is now believed by most authorities to be a manifestation of large cell comedo ductal carcinoma in situ, which when involving subareolar ducts can extend within the confines of the duct, and epidermal basement membrane into the epidermis. This view is supported by the fact that DCIS of large cell type is virtually always identified in at least one subareolar nipple duct. Between 35% and 50% of patients will have associated invasive adenocarcinoma.[90] Paget's disease occurs in around 2% of patients with breast cancer, presenting clinically as an erythematous or eczematous rash of the nipple.[90] The clinical features may be indistinguishable clinically from eczema or other chronic forms of dermatitis. Any nipple lesion with such features, particularly if it fails to heal rapidly, should be regarded as suspicious of Paget's disease and biopsied.

MACROSCOPIC FEATURES

The skin of the nipple area bears a moist erythematous or eczematous eruption which may be encrusted or scaly.

HISTOLOGICAL FEATURES

The epidermis contains an infiltrate of single or small groups of large pleomorphic cells, usually having abundant clear staining cytoplasm which may be vacuolated (Fig. 14.22A). Some larger groups of cells may form acinar structures. There is usually an accompanying infiltrate of small mature lymphoid cells which extends to involve the epidermal layers; acute inflammatory cells may also be present. The epidermis may be hyperplastic and show parakeratosis.

The tumor cell population may show positive staining for PAS diastase resistant mucins but immunohistology now appears to be a more sensitive method for diagnosis.[94] Paget's cells can be distinguished from the surrounding keratinocytes using immunocytochemical staining for low molecular weight cytokeratins (Fig. 14.22b) and EMA. The antibody CAM 5.2 has been shown to be particularly useful in this context.[94] Amplificiation of the c-erbB-2 gene is associated with large cell types of DCIS and occurs in over 90% of mammary Paget's disease.[94] The tumor cells show

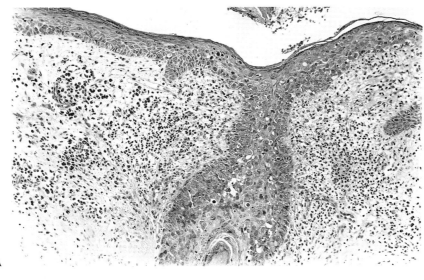

A

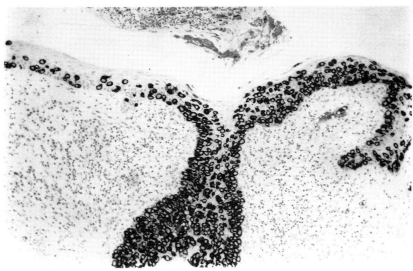

B

Fig. 14.22A & B   See caption overleaf.

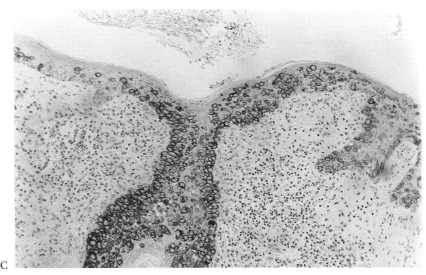

C

Fig. 14.22 An example of mammary Paget's disease showing infiltration of the epidermis by a population of adenocarcinoma cells (A). Their glandular epithelial nature is confirmed by staining with low molecular weight cytokeratin (antibody CAM 5.2) (B) and their association with high grade DCIS by membrane staining for c-erbB-2 protein (C). Hematoxylin–eosin, A × 125; immunostaining for CAM 5.2, B × 125; immunostaining for c-erbB-2, Dako, C × 125.

positive membrane immunoreactivity for c-erbB-2 oncoprotein and can also be useful for diagnosis (Fig. 14.22C).

DIFFERENTIAL DIAGNOSIS

In a severely inflamed nipple it may be difficult to identify the infiltrate of neoplastic cells. These cells may also prove difficult to distinguish from melanocytes and in cases where the cytoplasm is not particularly vacuolated or clear they may resemble atypical keratinocytes such as those seen in other forms of chronic dermatitis. The use of mucin stains is an unreliable special technique in difficult cases. Immunocytochemistry using antibodies to low molecular weight cytokeratins and c-erbB-2 is the preferred method for demonstration of Paget's disease.[94]

REFERENCES

1. Evans AJ, Pinder S, Ellis IO et al. Screening-detected and symptomatic ductal carcinoma in situ: mammographic features with pathologic correlation. Radiology 1994; 191: 237–240.
2. Fechner RE. One century of mammary carcinoma in situ. What have we learned? Am J Clin Pathol 1993; 100: 654–661.
3. Bloodgood JC. Comedo carcinoma (or comedo adenoma) of the female breast. Am J Cancer 1934; 22: 842–853.
4. Lewis D, Geschickter CF. Comedo carcinomas of the breast. Arch Surg 1938; 36: 225–244.
5. Azzopardi JG. Problems in Breast Pathology. Philadelphia: Saunders, 1979.
6. Page DL, Dupont WD, Rogers LW, Landenberger M. Intraductal carcinoma of the breast: follow-up after biopsy only. Cancer 1982; 49: 751–758.
7. Lagios MD. Duct carcinoma in situ: pathology and treatment. Surg Clin North Am 1990; 70: 853–871.
8. Lagios MD, Margolin FR, Westdahl PR, Rose MR. Mammographically detected duct carcinoma in situ. Frequency of local recurrence following tylectomy and prognostic effect of nuclear grade on local recurrence. Cancer 1989; 63: 618–624.
9. van Dongen J, Holland R, Peterse JL et al. Ductal carcinoma in-situ of the breast; second EORTC consensus meeting. Eur J Cancer 1992; 28: 626–629.
10. Rosai J. Borderline epithelial lesions of the breast. Am J Surg Pathol 1991; 15: 209–221.
11. Page DL, Jensen RA. Evaluation and management of high risk and premalignant lesions of the breast. World J Surg 1994; 18: 32–38.
12. Micale MA, Visscher DW, Gulino SE, Wolman SR. Chromosomal aneuploidy in proliferative breast disease. Hum Pathol 1994; 25: 29–35.

13. Lakhani SR, Slack DN, Hamoudi RA, Collins N, Stratton MR, Sloane JP. Detection of allelic imbalance indicates that a proportion of mammary hyperplasia of usual type are clonal, neoplastic proliferations. Lab Invest 1996; 74: 129–135.

14. Lakhani SR, Collins N, Stratton MR, Sloane JP. Atypical ductal hyperplasia of the breast: clonal proliferation with loss of heterozygosity on chromosomes 16q and 17p. J Clin Pathol 1995; 48: 611–615.

15. Pandis N, Heim S, Bardi G, Idvall I, Mandahl N, Mitelman F. Chromosome analysis of 20 breast carcinomas: cytogenetic multiclonality and karyotypic-pathologic correlations. Genes Chromosomes Cancer 1993; 6: 51–57.

16. Nielsen KV, Andersen JA, Blichert TM. Chromosome changes of in situ carcinomas in the female breast. Eur J Surg Oncol 1987; 13: 225–229.

17. Nielsen KV, Blichert TM, Andersen J. Chromosome analysis of in situ breast cancer. Acta Oncol 1989; 28: 919–922.

18. Harrison M, Magee H, O'Loughlin J, Gorey T, Dervan P. Chromosome 1 aneusomy identified by interphase cytogenetics in mammographically detected ductal carcinoma in situ of the breast. J Pathol 1995; 175: 303–309.

19. Murphy DS, McHardy P, Coutts J et al. Interphase cytogenetic analysis of erbB2 and topoIIa co-amplification in invasive breast cancer and polysomy of chromosome 17 in ductal carcinoma in-situ. Int J Cancer 1995; 64: 18–26.

20. Murphy DS, Hoare S, Going JJ et al. Characterization of extensive genetic alterations in ductal carcinoma in-situ by fluorescence in situ hybridization and molecular analysis. J Natl Cancer Inst 1995; 87: 1694–1704.

21. Munn KE, Walker RA, Varley JM. Frequent alterations of chromosome 1 in ductal carcinoma in-situ of the breast. Oncogene 1995; 10: 1653–1657.

22. Visscher DW, Wallis TL, Crissman JD. Evaluation of chromosome aneuploidy in tissue sections of preinvasive breast carcinomas using interphase cytogenetics. Cancer 1996; 77: 315–320.

23. Radford DM, Fair K, Thompson AM et al. Allelic loss on a chromosome 17 in ductal carcinoma in situ of the breast. Cancer Res 1993; 53: 2947–2949.

24. Lininger RA, Tavassoli FA. Atypical intraductal hyperplasia of the breast. In: Silverstein MJ, Lagios MD, Poller DN, Recht A, eds. Ductal carcinoma in situ of the breast. Baltimore: Williams and Wilkins, 1997: 195–222.

25. Wellings SR, Jensen MH, Marcum RG. An atlas of subgross pathology of the human breast with special reference to possible precancerous lesions. J Natl Cancer Inst 1975; 55: 231–273.

26. Holland R, Hendriks JH, Vebeek AL, Mravunac M, Schuurmans SJ. Extent, distribution, and mammographic/histological correlations of breast ductal carcinoma in situ. Lancet 1990; 335: 519–522.

27. Faverly DR, Burgers L, Bult P, Holland R. Three dimensional imaging of mammary ductal carcinoma in situ: clinical implications. Semin Diagn Pathol 1994; 11: 193–198.

28. Nielsen M, Thomsen JL, Primdahl S, Dyreborg U, Andersen JA. Breast cancer and atypia among young and middle-aged women: a study of 110 medicolegal autopsies. Br J Cancer 1987; 56: 814–819.

29. Faverly D, Holland R, Burgers L. An original stereomicroscopic analysis of the mammary glandular tree. Virchows Arch A Pathol Anat Histopathol 1992; 421: 115–119.

30. Stratton MR, Collins N, Lakhani SR et al. Loss of heterozygosity in ductal carcinoma in situ of the breast. J Pathol 1995; 175: 195–201.

31. Nowell PC. The clonal evolution of tumor cell populations. Science 1976; 194: 23–28.

32. Lennington WJ, Jensen RA, Dalton LW, Page DL. Ductal carcinoma in situ of the breast. Heterogeneity of individual lesions. Cancer 1994; 73: 118–124.

33. Sloane JP, Ellman R, Anderson TJ et al. Consistency of histopathological reporting of breast lesions detected by screening: findings of the U.K. National External Quality Assessment (EQA) Scheme. U.K. National Coordinating Group for Breast Screening Pathology. Eur J Cancer 1994; 30: 1414–1419.

34. Lampejo OT, Barnes DM, Smith P, Millis RR. Evaluation of infiltrating ductal carcinoma with a DCIS component: correlation of the histological type of the insitu component with grade of the infiltrating component. Sem Diag Pathol 1994; 11: 215–222.

35. Poller DN, Roberts EC, Bell JA, Elston CW, Blamey RW, Ellis IO. p53 protein expression in mammary ductal carcinoma in situ: relationship to immunohistochemical expression of estrogen receptor and c-erbB-2 protein. Hum Pathol 1993; 24: 463–468.

36. Bobrow LG, Happerfield LC, Gregory WM, Springall RD, Millis RR. The classification of ductal carcinoma in situ and its association with biological markers. Semin Diagn Pathol 1994; 11: 199–207.

37. Broders AC. Carcinoma in situ contrasted with benign penetrating epithelium. JAMA 1992; 99: 1670–1674.

38. National Coordinating Group for Breast Cancer Screening Pathology. Pathology Reporting in Breast Cancer Screening. Second Edition. NHS Breast Screening Program Publications, 1995.

39. Schnitt SJ, Connolly JL, Tavassoli FA et al. Interobserver reproducibility in the diagnosis of ductal proliferative breast lesions using standardized criteria. Am J Surg Pathol 1992; 16: 1133–1143.

40. Page DL, Rogers LW. Carcinoma in situ (CIS). In: Page D, Anderson, TJ, eds. Diagnostic histopathology of the breast. New York: Churchill Livingstone, 1987; pp 157–192.

41. Page DL, Salhany KE, Jensen RA, Dupont WD. Subsequent breast carcinoma risk after biopsy with atypia in a breast papilloma. Cancer 1996; 78: 258–266.

42. Tavassoli FA, Norris HJ. A comparison of the results of long-term follow-up for atypical intraductal hyperplasia and intraductal hyperplasia of the breast. Cancer 1990; 65: 518–529.

43. Tavassoli FA. Atypical hyperplasia: a morphologic risk factor for subsequent development of invasive breast carcinoma. Cancer Invest 1992; 10: 433–441.

44. Masood S, Sim SJ, Lu L. Immunohistochemical differentiation of atypical hyperplasia vs. carcinoma in situ of the breast. Cancer Detect Prev 1992; 16: 225–235.

45. Bocker W, Bier B, Freytag G et al. An immunohistochemical study of the breast using antibodies to basal and luminal keratins, alpha-smooth muscle actin, vimentin, collagen IV and laminin. Part II: Epitheliosis and ductal carcinoma in situ. Virchows Arch A Pathol Anat Histopathol 1992; 421: 323–330.

46. Poller DN, Ellis IO. Ductal carcinoma in situ (DCIS) of

the breast. In: Kirkham NL, Lemoine NR, eds. Progress in pathology. New York: Churchill Livingstone, 1995; Vol 2, pp 47–87.

47. Holland R, Peterse JL, Millis RR et al. Ductal carcinoma in situ: a proposal for a new classification. Semin Diagn Pathol 1994; 11: 167–180.

48. Bellamy CO, McDonald C, Salter DM, Chetty U, Anderson TJ. Noninvasive ductal carcinoma of the breast: the relevance of histologic categorization. Hum Pathol 1993; 24: 16–23.

49. Poller DN, Silverstein MJ, Galea M et al. Ideas in pathology. Ductal carcinoma in situ of the breast: a proposal for a new simplified histological classification association between cellular proliferation and c-erbB-2 protein expression. Mod Pathol 1994; 7: 257–262.

50. Ottesen GL, Graversen HP, Blichert TM, Zedeler K, Andersen JA. Ductal carcinoma in situ of the female breast. Short-term results of a prospective nationwide study. The Danish Breast Cancer Cooperative Group. Am J Surg Pathol 1992; 16: 1183–1196.

51. Silverstein MJ, Poller DN, Waisman J et al. Prognostic classification of breast ductal carcinoma in situ. The Lancet 1995; 345: 1154–1157.

52. Douglas-Jones AG, Gupta SK, Attanoos RL, Morgan JM, Mansel RE. A critical appraisal of six modern classifications of ductal carcinoma in situ of the breast (DCIS): Correlation with grade of associated invasive carcinoma. Histopathology 1996; 29: 397–409.

53. Poller DN, Silverstein MJ, Lagios MD, Craig PH, Waisman JR. Use of a prognostic index for breast ductal carcinoma in situ: Is excision margin status still the most crucial factor in predicting disease recurrence? J Pathol 1996; 178 (Suppl): 6A.

55. Silverstein MJ, Lagios MD, Craig PH et al. A prognostic index for ductal carcinoma in situ of the breast. Cancer 1996; 77: 2267–2274.

56. Baird RM, Worth A, Hislop G. Recurrence after lumpectomy for comedo-type intraductal carcinoma of the breast. Am J Surg 1990; 159: 479–481.

57. Kuske RR, Bean JM, Garcia DM et al. Breast conservation therapy for intraductal carcinoma of the breast. Int J Radiat Oncol Biol Phys 1993; 26: 391–396.

58. Schwartz GF, Carter DL, Conant EF, Gannon FH, Finkel GC, Feig SA. Mammographically detected breast cancer. Nonpalpable is not a synonym for inconsequential. Cancer 1994; 73: 1660–1665.

59. Solin LJ, Yeh IT, Kurtz J et al. Ductal carcinoma in situ (intraductal carcinoma) of the breast treated with breast-conserving surgery and definitive irradiation. Correlation of pathologic parameters with outcome of treatment. Cancer 1993; 71: 2532–2542.

60. Sneige N, McNeese MD, Atkinson EN et al. Ductal carcinoma in situ treated with lumpectomy and irradiation: histopathological analysis of 49 specimens with emphasis on risk factors and long term results. Human Pathol 1995; 26: 642–649.

61. De Potter CR, Schelfhout A, Verbeeck P et al. neu overexpression correlates with extent of disease in large cell ductal carcinoma in situ of the breast. Hum Pathol 1995; 26: 601–606.

62. Evans A, Pinder S, Wilson R et al. Ductal carcinoma in situ of the breast: correlation between mammographic and pathologic findings. Ajr Am J Roentgenol 1994; 162: 1307–1311.

63. Patchefsky AS, Schwartz GF, Finkelstein SD et al.

Heterogeneity of intraductal carcinoma of the breast. Cancer 1989; 63: 731–741.

64. Zafrani B, Leroyer A, Fourquet A et al. Mammographically-detected ductal in situ carcinoma of the breast analyzed with a new classification. A study of 127 cases: correlation with estrogen and progesterone receptors, p53 and c-erbB-2 proteins, and proliferative activity. Semin Diagn Pathol 1994; 11: 208–214.

65. European Community. European Guidelines for Quality Assurance in Mammographic Screening. 2nd edn. Luxembourg: Office for Official Publications of the European Communities, 1996.

66. Noguchi S, Aihara T, Motomura K, Inaji H, Imaoka S, Koyama H. Histologic characteristics of breast cancers with occult lymph node metastases detected by keratin 19 mRNA reverse transcriptase-polymerase chain reaction. Cancer 1996; 78: 1235–1240.

67. Scott MA, Lagios MD, Axelsson K, Rogers LW, Anderson TJ, Page DL. Ductal carcinoma in situ of the breast. Reproducibility of histologic subtype analysis. Cancer 1996; (in press).

68. Tavassoli FH. Pathology of the breast. Norwalk: Appleton and Lange, 1992, pp 229–261.

69. Tavassoli FA, Norris HJ. Intraductal apocrine carcinoma: a clinicopathologic study of 37 cases. Modern Pathol 1994; 7: 813–818.

70. Seidman JD, Ashton M, Lefkowitz M. Atypical apocrine adenosis of the breast: a clinicopathologic study of 37 patients with 8.7-year follow-up. Cancer 1996; 77: 2529–2537.

71. O'Malley FP, Page DL, Nelson EH, Dupont WD. Ductal carcinoma in situ of the breast with apocrine cytology: definition of a borderline category. Hum Pathol 1994; 25: 164–168.

72. Ellis IO, Elston CW. Tumors of the breast. In: Fletcher C, ed. Diagnostic Histopathology Of Tumors. New York: Churchill Livingstone, 1995; pp 635–689.

73. Carter D, Orr S, Merino M. Intracystic papillary carcinoma of the breast after mastectomy, radiotherapy and excisional biopsy alone. Cancer 1983; 52: 14–19.

74. Fisher ER, Brown R. Intraductal signet ring carcinoma. A hitherto undescribed form of intraductal carcinoma of the breast. Cancer 1985; 55: 2533–2537.

75. Cross AS, Azzopardi JG, Krausz T, Polak JM. A morphological and immunocytochemical study of a distinctive variant of ductal carcinoma in-situ of the breast. Histopathology 1985; 9: 21–37.

76. Guerry P, Erlandson RA, Rosen PP. Cystic hypersecretory hyperplasia and cystic hypersecretory duct carcinoma of the breast. Pathology, therapy, and follow-up of 39 patients. Cancer 1988; 61: 1611–1620.

77. Rosen PP, Scott M. Cystic hypersecretory duct carcinoma of the breast. Am J Surg Pathol 1984; 8: 31–41.

78. Bena HD, Cranor ML, Rosen PP. Mammary mucocele-like lesions. Am J Surg Pathol 1996; 20: 1081–1085.

79. Eusebi V, Feudale E, Foschini MP et al. Long-term follow-up of in situ carcinoma of the breast. Semin Diagn Pathol 1994; 11: 223–235.

80. De Potter CR, Foschini MP, Schelfhout AM, Schroeter CA, Eusebi V. Immunohistochemical study of neu protein overexpression in clinging in situ duct carcinoma of the breast. Virch Arch A Pathol Anat Histopathol 1993; 422: 375–380.

81. Camus MG, Joshi MG, Mackarem G et al. Ductal

carcinoma in situ of the male breast. Cancer 1994; 74: 1289–1293.

82. Recht A, Fentiman IS, Holland R, Peterse JL. Third meeting of the DCIS Working Party of the EORTC (Fondazione Cini, Isola S. Giorgio, Venezia, 28 February 1994) — Conference report. Eur J Cancer 1994; 28: 626–629.

83. Armstrong JS, Davies JD, Hronkova B. Backprocessing paraffin wax blocks for subgross examination. J Clin Pathol 1992; 45: 1116–1117.

84. Silverstein MJ, Gierson ED, Colburn WJ et al. Can intraductal breast carcinoma be excised completely by local excision? Clinical and pathologic predictors. Cancer 1994; 73: 2985–2989.

85. Arnesson LG, Smeds S, Fagerberg G et al. Follow-up of two treatment modalities for ductal cancer in situ of the breast. Br J Surg 1989; 76: 672–675.

86. Sibbering DP, Pinder SE, Obuszko Z, Ellis IO, Elston CW, Morgan DAL, Robertson JFR, Blamey RW. Local excision with a 10 mm margin as sole treatment for ductal carcinoma in situ of the breast. Eur J Cancer 1997; in press.

87. Lagios MD. Pathologic procedures for mammographically detected ductal carcinoma in situ. In: Silverstein MJ, Lagios MD, Poller DN, Recht A, eds.

Ductal carcinoma in situ. Baltimore: Williams and Wilkins, 1997; pp 189–193.

88. Jackson PA, Merchant W, McCormick CJ, Cook MG. A comparison of large block macrosectioning and conventional techniques in breast pathology. Virchows Arch 1994; 425: 243–248.

89. Farrow FH. Current concepts in the detection and treatment of the earliest of early breast cancers. Cancer 1970; 25: 468–477.

90. Haagensen CD. Diseases of the breast. Philadelphia: WB Saunders, 1986.

91. Millis RR, Thynne GSJ. In situ intraduct carcinoma of the breast: a long-term follow up study. Br J Surg 1975; 62: 957–962.

92. Rosen PP Jr, Kinne DW. The clinical significance of preinvasive breast carcinoma. Cancer 1980; 46: 919–925.

93. Page DL, Dupont WD, Rogers LW, Jensen RA, Schuyler PA. Continued local recurrence of carcinoma 15–25 years after a diagnosis of low grade ductal carcinoma in situ of the breast treated only by biopsy. Cancer 1995; 76: 1197–1200.

94. Hitchcock A, Topham S, Bell J, Gullick W, Elston CW, Ellis IO. Routine diagnosis of mammary Paget's disease. A modern approach. Am J Surg Pathol 1992; 16: 58–61.

Invasive carcinoma — usual histological types

GENERAL INTRODUCTION

Our philosophy for the morphological classification of invasive carcinomas of the breast has already been discussed in Chapter 13. In this chapter, which should be read in conjunction with Chapter 13, we provide a detailed account of the histological patterns which are encountered most frequently in routine clinical practice. The classification is based to a large extent on that published by WHO[1–2] but we have also taken into consideration the contributions to the literature of other breast pathologists,[3–5] the Royal College of Pathologists' publication 'Pathology reporting in breast cancer screening',[6] the numerous papers on special morphological types and our own observations from the Nottingham Tenovus Primary Breast Cancer Study (NTPBCS).[7]

In order to avoid undue repetition the correlation between histological type and prognosis is considered in a separate section at the end of the chapter.

CLINICAL FEATURES

These are considered in more detail in Chapter 22, but some general points are pertinent here. In the absence of mammographic screening the great majority of invasive carcinomas are diagnosed because the patient has felt a lump in the breast. These vary markedly in size from approximately 1 cm to several centimeters in diameter. The palpable mass is usually firm or even hard, and the edge may be well or poorly defined. Less commonly, especially if breast self-examination is being practised, the patient may notice a diffuse thickening or an ill-defined change in texture of the breast tissue. The mass may be present anywhere in the breast, but the outer upper quadrant is the most frequent site. Breast pain is very rarely a manifestation of malignancy and virtually all breast carcinomas are, in themselves, painless. Nipple discharge is an infrequent presenting sign, but it should also be noted that Paget's disease of the nipple, which presents as nipple eczema and indicates an underlying in situ carcinoma, is also associated with an invasive carcinoma in up to 40% of cases.

In the United Kingdom the introduction of a National Breast Screening Programme (NHSBSP) has significantly altered the pattern of presentation and in the target age group of 50–64 years many cases are now detected because of a mammographic abnormality. However, it is of interest that in the *prevalent* round of screening more than 50% of the carcinomas identified are palpable.[8]

Apart from the fact that most tubular carcinomas are relatively small, mucinous carcinomas tend to be well-defined and relatively soft and a minority of infiltrating lobular carcinomas are diffuse and ill-defined, there are no specific clinical features by which any of the subtypes can reliably be identified.

HISTOLOGICAL TYPES

INVASIVE CARCINOMA OF NO SPECIAL TYPE (DUCTAL NST)

Introduction

As the name implies the diagnosis of ductal NST carcinoma is one of exclusion, since the group includes those tumors in which the morphological features do not satisfy the criteria for inclusion in any of the other categories. It is the most common 'type' of invasive carcinoma of the breast comprising between 41 and 75% of published series (see Table 13.2). The main reasons for this wide range are the lack of application of strict criteria for inclusion in the special types and the reluctance by some groups to recognize tumors having a combination of ductal NST and special type patterns as a mixed category. Although it was

suggested by Murad[9] on the basis of histochemical and ultrastructural studies that ductal NST carcinomas were derived from myoepithelial cells their epithelial origin is now firmly established.

A wide variety of terms has been used for this type of breast carcinoma including scirrhous carcinoma, carcinoma simplex and spheroidal cell carcinoma. Infiltrating ductal carcinoma is used in the Armed Forces Institute of Pathology fascicle[5,10] and was the nomenclature adopted in the WHO classification.[1,11] This perpetuates the traditional concept that these tumors are derived exclusively from mammary *ductal* epithelium in distinction from lobular carcinomas which were deemed to have arisen from within lobules. However, as Azzopardi[12] stressed, the work of Wellings and colleagues[13] has shown that the terminal duct-lobular unit (TDLU) should be regarded as a single entity from the point of view of the site of origin of most ductal carcinomas. Fisher and colleagues[14–15] have retained the term ductal but added the phrase 'not otherwise specified (NOS)', whilst Page and colleagues[3] preferred to use 'no special type (NST)' to emphasize their distinction from special type tumors. We are in agreement with this latter view, but since 'ductal' is still widely used throughout the world our favored term is ductal NST.

Macroscopic appearances

Since ductal NST carcinoma is a diagnosis of exclusion these tumors have no specific gross features. There is a marked variation in size from 2 or 3 mm to 1.5 cm if detected 'early', and up to 10 cm or more in advanced cases. In Nottingham the average size at presentation of a palpable tumor mass is 2 cm, whilst in the prevalent round of breast screening 40% of tumors measure 1 cm or less.[8] Tumors usually have an irregular, stellate outline, but not surprisingly some have a nodular configuration. The tumor edge is only moderately or ill-defined and lacks the sharp circumscription of mucinous or medullary carcinomas (see below). Classically ductal NST carcinomas are firm or even hard on palpation, and have a curious 'gritty' feel when cut with a knife. These features are due to the presence of a varying proportion of desmoplastic fibrous stroma and gave rise to one of the original descriptive terms for this tumor type, scirrhous or schirrus carcinoma (Skirrhos, Gr = hard). The cut surface is grey-white in color and often finely granular with slightly raised, yellowish particles or streaks that are usually no more than 0.5 mm or so across; the firmness and gross appearance are traditionally, and with some justification, likened to those of the cut surface of a ripening pear.

Microscopic appearances

The morphological features vary considerably from case to case depending to a large extent on the relative proportions of tumor cells and stroma. Overall the appearances lack the regularity of structure associated with the tumors of special type. The tumor cells may be arranged in cords and trabeculae whilst some tumors are characterized by a predominantly solid or syncytial infiltrative pattern with little associated stroma (Figs 15.1–15.3). In a small proportion of cases glandular differentiation may be apparent as poorly formed tubular structures with central lumina (Fig. 15.4A and B). Occasionally areas with single file infiltration or targetoid features are seen; they should not be mistaken for infiltrating lobular carcinoma (Fig.15.5A and B) (see below). At the periphery tumor cells infiltrate into adjacent adipose or fibrous connective tissue (Fig. 15.6). The carcinoma cells also have a variable appearance, but abundant eosinophilic cytoplasm is usually present. Nuclei may be regular or highly pleomorphic with prominent, often multiple, nucleoli (Figs 15.1C, 15.2, 15.5B). In most cases, after adequate sampling foci of associated ductal carcinoma in situ (DCIS) will be present. However, even after an exhaustive search an in situ component may be lacking in up to 20% of cases.[4,12] The DCIS is often of high grade comedo type, but all other patterns may be seen. Some authorities recognize a subtype of ductal NST carcinoma, infiltrating ductal carcinoma with extensive in situ component; this is discussed in Chapter 18.

The stromal component is extremely variable. There may be a highly cellular desmoplastic fibroblastic proliferation, a scanty connective tissue element or marked hyalinization (Figs 15.1B, 15.2). Foci of elastosis may also be present, especially in a periductal distribution around residual ductal structures. Focal necrosis may be present and this is occasionally extensive; the poor prognostic significance of this feature is discussed further in Chapter 18. In a minority of cases a distinct lymphoplasmacytoid infiltrate can be identified (Fig. 15.7).

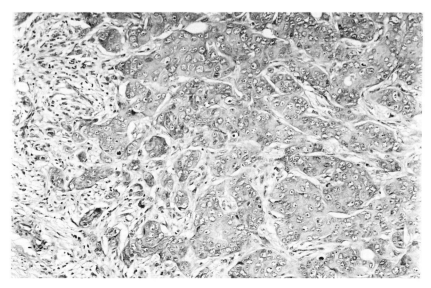

Fig. 15.1A   Invasive carcinoma, ductal NST. In this example the tumor has a broad trabecular pattern. Hematoxylin–eosin × 125.

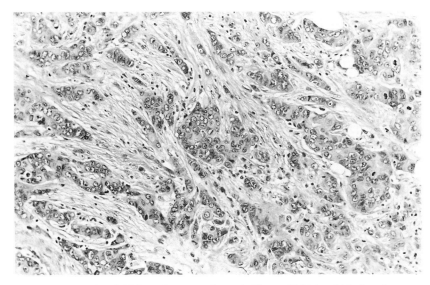

Fig. 15.1B Another field from the tumor shown in Figure 15.1A in which there is a densely cellular desmoplastic stroma. Hematoxylin–eosin × 125.

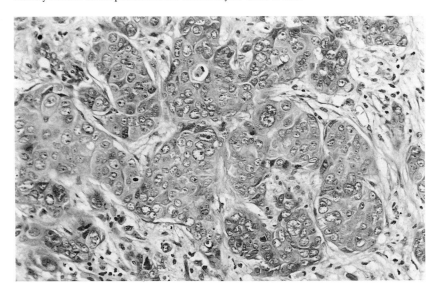

Fig. 15.1C Higher magnification of tumor shown in Figure 15.1A and B. There is marked nuclear pleomorphism. Hematoxylin–eosin × 185.

Differential diagnosis

For a tumor to be typed as ductal NST it must show that non-specialized pattern in over 90% of its mass as judged by thorough examination of representative sections. If the ductal NST pattern comprises between 10 and 90% of the tumor, the rest being of a recognized special type, then it will fall into one of the mixed groups — tubular mixed, mixed ductal and special type or mixed ductal and lobular carcinoma. These are discussed below.

Apart from these considerations there are very few lesions that should be confused with ductal NST carcinomas. The distinction from infiltrating lobular carcinoma is discussed on page 15. In rare cases the cellular features may raise the possibility of a neuroendocrine carcinoma; this

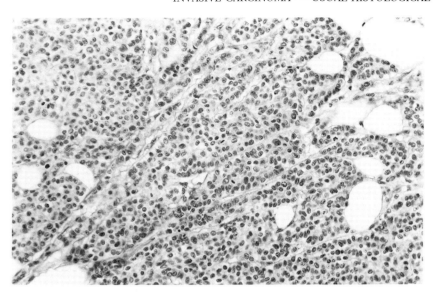

Fig. 15.2 Ductal NST carcinoma. Another example with a mixture of narrow trabeculae and cord-like structures. Nuclei are relatively uniform in size and shape. Hematoxylin–eosin × 185.

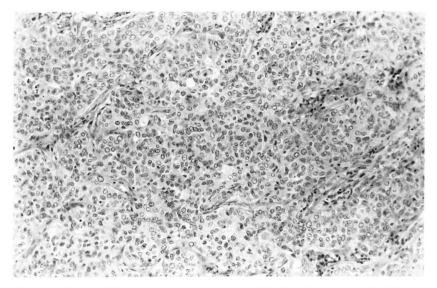

Fig. 15.3 Ductal NST carcinoma showing a more solid infiltrative pattern, with little intratumoral stroma. Hematoxylin–eosin × 125.

entity can be confirmed or excluded by appropriate immunostaining for markers such as PGP 9.5, NSE and S-100 (see Ch. 16). Similarly examples of ductal NST carcinoma in which the nuclei are large and vesicular, and tumor is arranged in solid sheets, may bear a superficial resemblance to malignant lymphoma. Immunostaining for epithelial and lymphoid markers will usually resolve the problem (see Ch. 19). A number of benign entities may cause diagnostic problems, in particular sclerosing lesions such as sclerosing adenosis and radial scar, but in these cases the differential diagnosis usually lies with the special type carcinomas rather than ductal NST.

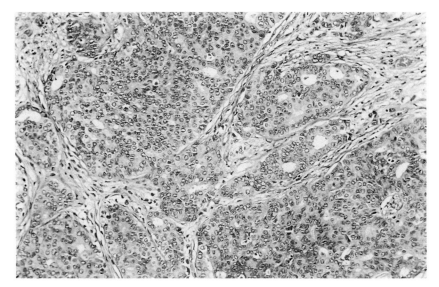

Fig. 15.4A Ductal NST carcinoma in which focal glandular structures are present. Hematoxylin–eosin × 125.

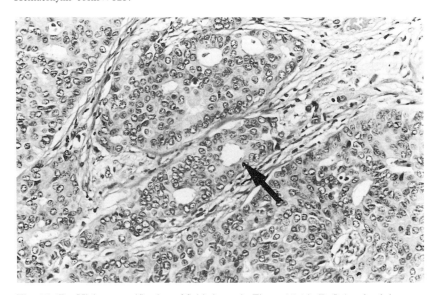

Fig. 15.4B Higher magnification of field shown in Figure 15.4A. Definite glandular structures are seen, one with apical snouts (arrowhead). Hematoxylin–eosin × 185.

INFILTRATING LOBULAR CARCINOMA (ILC)

Introduction

According to Tavassoli[4] the first accounts of invasive carcinoma of the breast composed of small cells with a linear growth pattern which we recognize today as infiltrating lobular carcinoma were traced to intralobular carcinoma in the 19th century by Cornil[16] and Waldeyer.[17] Interestingly Haagensen and colleagues[18] attributed the first description of carcinoma arising within acini to Ewing,[19] although he (Ewing) did not give the lesion a name.

It is Foote and Stewart who are usually credited with the introduction of the terms lobular

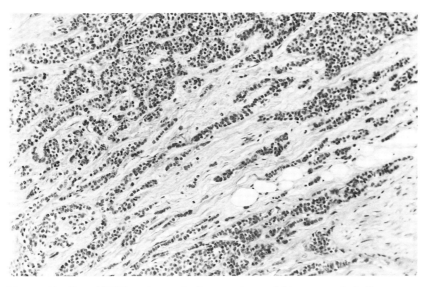

Fig. 15.5A Ductal NST carcinoma. In the central part of this tumor a single file infiltrative pattern is seen, but elsewhere there is a trabecular structure which rules out a diagnosis of infiltrating lobular carcinoma. Hematoxylin–eosin × 125.

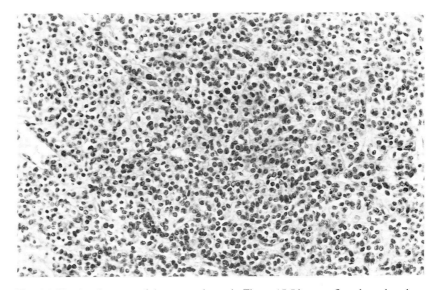

Fig. 15.5B Another area of the tumor shown in Figure 15.5A to confirm the trabecular and solid NST structure. Note the relative regularity of nuclei with little pleomorphism. Hematoxylin–eosin × 185.

carcinoma in situ (LCIS)[20] and infiltrating lobular carcinoma (ILC).[21] In their first study[20] sections from 300 cases from patients treated by mastectomy for carcinoma were examined; they found two cases in which there was LCIS alone. There were a further 12 cases in which LCIS was accompanied by an infiltrating carcinoma. Subsequently Foote and Stewart[21] showed that the classical single file small cell infiltrating carcinoma was accompanied by LCIS in over 60% of cases and therefore coined the term infiltrating lobular carcinoma for this type of invasive carcinoma. The

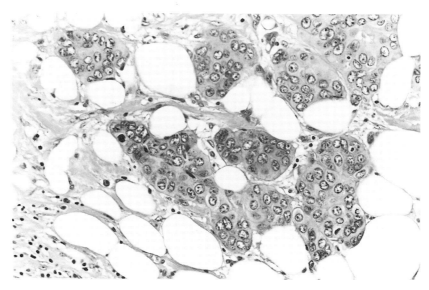

Fig. 15.6   Infiltrating edge of a ductal NST carcinoma showing trabeculae of tumor cells extending into adjacent adipose tissue. Hematoxylin–eosin × 185.

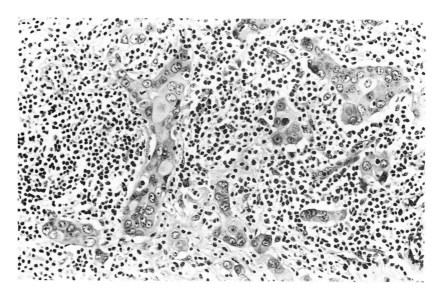

Fig. 15.7   Ductal NST carcinoma with prominent lymphoplasmacytic infiltrate in the stroma. Care must be taken to distinguish these appearances from medullary carcinoma; in this case the trabecular pattern rules out that diagnosis. Hematoxylin–eosin × 185.

definition and diagnostic criteria for classical ILC were thoroughly reviewed by Wheeler and Enterline in 1976,[22] but since then a number of variants have been described including solid lobular and mixed lobular carcinoma,[23] alveolar lobular carcinoma,[24] and tubulo-lobular carci-noma.[25] In addition Dixon et al[26] and Page et al[3] recognized a subgroup within the mixed category which has been termed pleomorphic lobular carci-noma.[27–28] The term lobular carcinoma has been justified for all these variants because of the pres-ence of associated lobular carcinoma in situ in between 40 and 90% of cases.[3,26] Whether all such carcinomas are derived directly from the epithelial cells of the lobular acini remains unproven, but there are sufficient morphological and clinical differences from ductal NST carcinomas to warrant their separate classification.

The reported frequency of infiltrating lobular carcinoma varies considerably, from as little as 0.7% up to 15%[7,24] (see also Table 13.2). This is almost certainly due to differences in interpretation of diagnostic criteria rather than true differences in frequency. The recognition of further variants may also have contributed to the apparent higher percentage of cases in more recent studies.

Macroscopic appearances

Because of the microscopic characteristics of diffuse tumor cell infiltration it is widely believed that infiltrating lobular carcinomas usually form an ill-defined mass. In the NTPBCS the majority of lobular carcinomas form a stellate 'schirrhous' mass indistinguishable from ductal NST carcinoma,[29] and the finding of an ill-defined diffuse area of induration is relatively uncommon. The latter cases may be difficult to detect by clinical palpation, other than as a vague thickening in the breast and may not produce an abnormal pattern on mammography, although we have found no significant difference in mammographic features between infiltrating lobular and ductal NST carcinomas.[30] Gross examination of such cases may reveal little or no discernible abnormality.[3] In rare cases the whole breast may become infiltrated diffusely by tumor before an abnormality becomes apparent clinically.

Microscopic appearances

Page and colleagues[3] have emphasized the two most important identifying features of infiltrating lobular carcinoma. These are the cytological characteristics of the tumor cells which are generally small and regular with darkly staining round or oval nuclei, and the pattern of invasion which is diffusely infiltrative. The inter-relationships between these features vary in the different subtypes; their histological appearances are described below:

a. Classical

The classical subtype is the most common pattern and accounts for approximately 40% of infiltrating lobular carcinomas.[7,26] The term 'classical' is used because the pattern of diffusely infiltrating small, round regular cells in single lines (Fig. 15.8A and B) is that first described by Foote and Stewart.[21] The tumor cells infiltrate the mammary stroma, often appearing to engulf normal ductal structures, surrounding them in a targetoid fashion (Fig. 15.9A and B). They exhibit round or ovoid nuclei which are often eccentrically placed in a manner reminiscent of plasmacytoid cells. They display little nuclear pleomorphism and mitoses are usually infrequent (Fig. 15.9C). Although intracytoplasmic lumina may be found in all types of invasive breast carcinoma they are most frequent in ILC and may be a prominent feature.[31] These structures may be visible on hematoxylin and eosin staining, but are more easily visualized histochemically with the Alcian Blue-Periodic acid Schiff (AB-PAS) stain or by immunostaining for epithelial mucin antigen (Fig. 15.10A, B and C). The classical type of ILC is associated with lobular neoplasia in approximately 90% of cases.[26]

b. Alveolar

In our experience this is an uncommon variant, accounting for only 4–5% of ILC.[7] The cells have the same uniform cytological appearances as those of the classical type, but the infiltrative pattern is different. The characteristic cells, instead of infiltrating diffusely, are clustered in rounded aggregates of 20 or more cells (Fig. 15.11).

c. Solid

Approximately 10% of cases are of this subtype.[7,26] The tumors are composed of typical lobular cells, but these infiltrate diffusely in large solid sheets rather than single cords, and there is little intervening stroma (Fig. 15.12A and B).

d. Mixed

Cases of ILC are only included in one of the specific subtypes above if 80% or more of the tumor

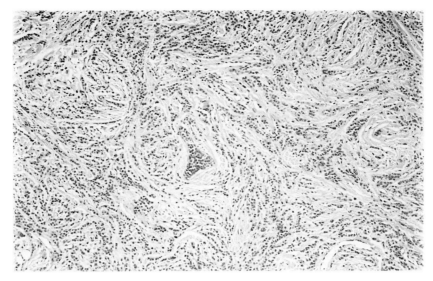

Fig. 15.8A Infiltrating lobular carcinoma, classical type. This low power view shows the diffuse infiltrative nature of the tumor, with its distinctive single file pattern. Hematoxylin–eosin × 100.

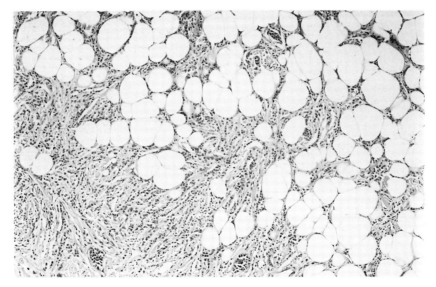

Fig. 15.8B Another field from the same case as Figure 15.8A showing diffuse extension of tumor into adipose tissue. It is this diffusely infiltrative pattern, without a significant desmoplastic reaction which accounts for the impalpability of such tumors. Hematoxylin–eosin × 100.

area has a single pattern, e.g. classical. Where there is a mixture of patterns, each amounting to less than 80%, cases are placed in the mixed group, which accounts for approximately 40% of ILC. Dixon and colleagues[26,32] recognized another category which they included in the

mixed category, the pleomorphic pattern. Tumor cells infiltrate in the same diffuse manner as in the classical type, but are less regular with more cellular atypia and nuclear pleomorphism. The cells are also larger than is usual in ILC with more cytoplasm (Fig. 15.13A, B and C). Other groups

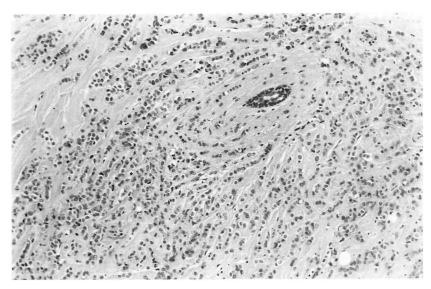

Fig. 15.9A   Infiltrating lobular carcinoma, classical type. Single cords of tumor cells surround a normal duct in a 'targetoid' fashion. Hematoxylin–eosin × 125.

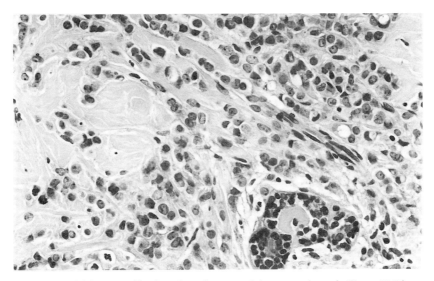

Fig. 15.9B   Higher magnification of another area of the tumor shown in Figure 15.9A. Hematoxylin–eosin × 185.

have also reported on this variant[7,27–28] and the morphology is discussed further in Chapter 16 in the section on apocrine carcinoma. The extremely uncommon signet ring variant (Fig. 15.14A and B) is also included in the mixed group by Page and colleagues.[32]

e. Tubulo-lobular

This is another uncommon variant first described by Fisher et al.[25] It accounts for up to 2% of ILC.[7,25,32] The tumor is characterized by an infiltrative pattern similar to that of the classical ILC,

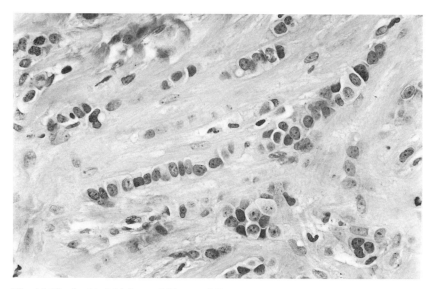

Fig. 15.9C   In this field the nuclei have a delicate chromatin pattern, with small nucleoli. There is little nuclear pleomorphism. From the same case as Figure 15.9A and B. Hematoxylin–eosin × 400.

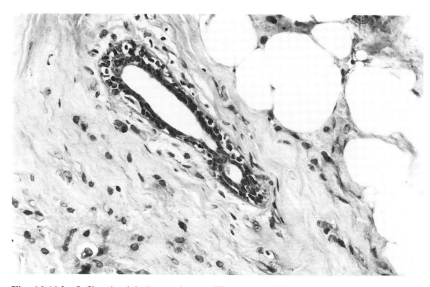

Fig. 15.10A   Infiltrating lobular carcinoma. The tumor cells are seen rather indistinctly around a normal duct. Hematoxylin–eosin × 400.

but to a variable degree the cells in some of the cords form distinct microtubules (Fig. 15.15A and B). These are much smaller than the tubules found in pure tubular carcinoma (compare Fig. 15.15A with Fig. 15.17A and B) but also consist of a single layer of epithelial cells. The lumen is small and may be indistinct and cells are regular, lacking nuclear atypia. In situ carcinoma, usually of ductal type with a micropapillary or cribriform pattern, is often present. To be typed as tubulo-lobular carcinoma a tumor must display this pattern over at least 90% of its area.

Although we have included tubulo-lobular carcinoma within the broad lobular category, it should be noted that there is still a lack of agreement concerning its assignment as a variant of

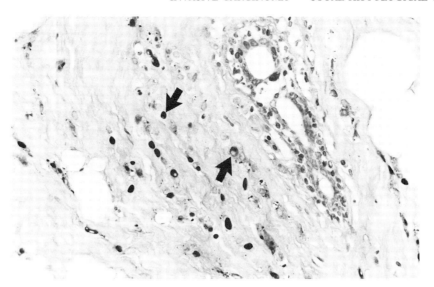

Fig. 15.10B   Infiltrating lobular carcinoma. Intracytoplasmic lumina (arrowheads) are identified in some of the tumor cells by mucin histochemistry. This is the same field as that shown in Figure 15.10A. Alcian Blue/Periodic acid Schiff × 400.

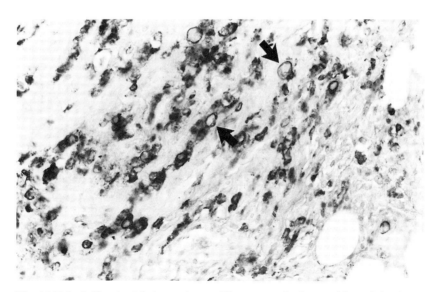

Fig. 15.10C   Infiltrating lobular carcinoma. The tumor cells show positive staining for epithelium mucin antigen (B55 antibody); intracytoplasmic lumina are clearly visible (arrowheads). This field is from the same case as those shown in Figure 15.10A and B. Immunostaining for epithelial mucin antigen × 400.

ILC. Following the first description by Fisher et al,[25] Martinez and Azzopardi[24] recognized a similar tubular variant within ILC. However, Page and Anderson[32] recorded tubulo-lobular carcinoma as a separate entity under 'uncommon types of invasive carcinoma' and expressed doubts as to how it should be classified. Tavassoli[4] is rather dismissive of the entity and refuses to accept a tumor forming tubules as a variant of ILC; she adds the somewhat confusing rider that it can be regarded as a tumor displaying both ductal and lobular patterns of invasion.

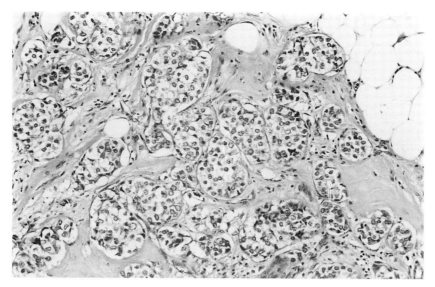

Fig. 15.11 Infiltrating lobular carcinoma, alveolar type. The tumor nuclei show the typical features of a lobular carcinoma but the diffuse infiltrative pattern is replaced by clustered groups of 20 or more cells. Hematoxylin–eosin × 125.

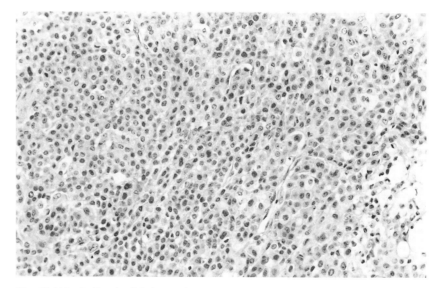

Fig. 15.12A Infiltrating lobular carcinoma, solid type. Note the sheet-like infiltrative pattern. Hematoxylin–eosin × 125.

Differential diagnosis

In tumors which are composed of both lobular and ductal NST elements more than 90% of the area must be of lobular type or mixed lobular pattern to be included in the ILC category. Those cases exhibiting a true biphasic pattern, but with less than 90% lobular pattern are classified as mixed ductal NST and lobular carcinomas (see p. 330).

As Martinez and Azzopardi[24] pointed out 'the division into invasive lobular and ductal carcinomas is not as easy as most of the literature

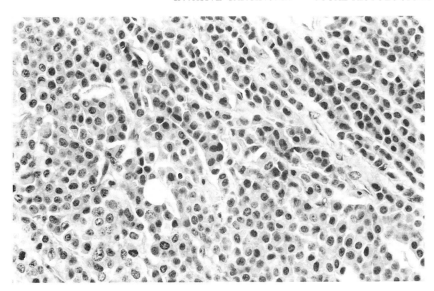

Fig. 15.12B Higher magnification of another field from the case shown in Figure 15.12A. Single cords of carcinoma cells are seen at the top right but most of the tumor is composed of solid sheets with little intervening stroma. Hematoxylin–eosin × 400.

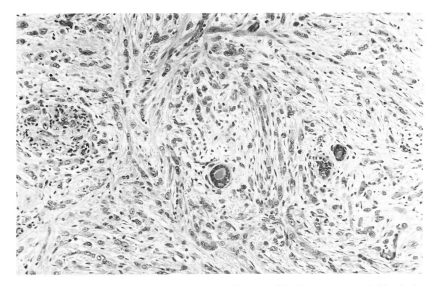

Fig. 15.13A Pleomorphic lobular carcinoma. The overall infiltrative pattern is identical with that seen in the classical subtype. Hematoxylin–eosin × 57.

implies'. Whilst little difficulty should be experienced in establishing a diagnosis of the classical lobular type in well fixed specimens, problems are sometimes posed by ductal NST carcinomas with a diffuse infiltrative pattern, especially if specimen preparation is suboptimal. The distinction between ductal NST and pleomorphic lobular carcinoma may be particularly difficult and examination of multiple blocks is advisable before the latter diagnosis is made. The presence of abundant eosinophilic cytoplasm favours a diagnosis of ductal NST carcinoma and in any case in which a trabecular pattern is displayed a potential diagnosis of ILC should be reconsidered.

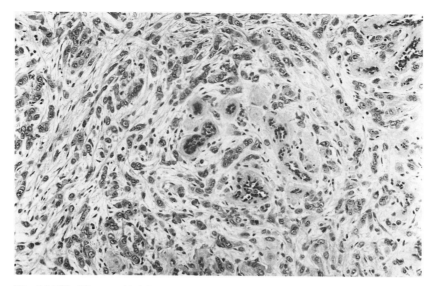

Fig. 15.13B   Pleomorphic lobular carcinoma. Another field from the case illustrated in Figure 15.13A. Note the 'targetoid' pattern of infiltration. Hematoxylin–eosin × 125.

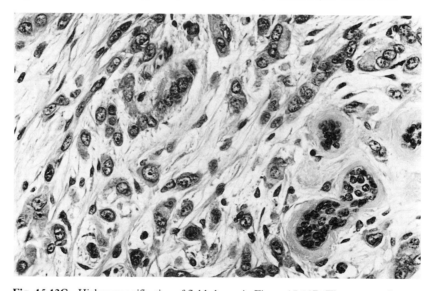

Fig. 15.13C   Higher magnification of field shown in Figure 15.13B. The tumor cells exhibit marked nuclear pleomorphism, in comparison with the normal ductule at the lower right. Hematoxylin–eosin × 400.

Infiltrating lobular carcinoma, and in particular the solid variant, may mimic the appearances of malignant lymphoma, especially in poorly prepared specimens or needle core biopsies (see also Ch. 2). The presence of intracytoplasmic lumina can be identified in ILC by the AB-PAS stain, but immunostaining has proved to be much more useful. Combination of an epithelial marker such as Cam 5.2, an antibody to epithelial mucins (EMA) and a lymphoid marker such as CD 45 should render the distinction between ILC and malignant lymphoma relatively straightforward (see also Ch. 19).

Inflammatory processes such as periductal fibrosis and its associated lesions such as plasma cell mastitis may also simulate ILC, and this is

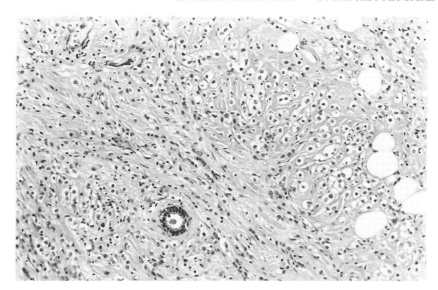

Fig. 15.14A   Infiltrating lobular carcinoma, signet ring pattern. A normal duct is surrounded by diffusely infiltrating lobular carcinoma cells. A signet ring pattern is prominent at the top right. Hematoxylin–eosin × 125.

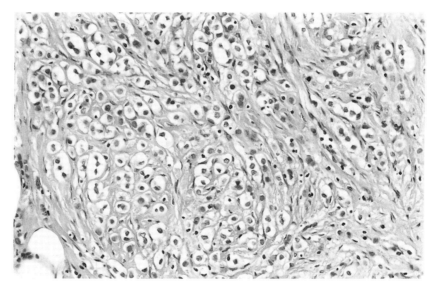

Fig. 15.14B   Higher magnification of another field from the case shown in Figure 15.14A to illustrate the signet ring pattern in more detail. Hematoxylin–eosin × 400.

especially true in frozen sections.[33] If there is any doubt about the diagnosis the prudent pathologist will defer his or her decision until paraffin sections are available.

Tubulo-lobular carcinomas must be distinguished from pure tubular and tubular mixed carcinomas. The major point of difference, as indicated above, is the size of the tubular structures, which in tubulo-lobular carcinoma are very small and rarely larger than the adjacent cords of tumor cells; the presence of a targetoid pattern is also helpful. In tubular mixed carcinoma (see p. 313) a lobular component may be present, but again, the tubules are larger than in tubulo-lobular carcinoma and are placed centrally in the tumor.

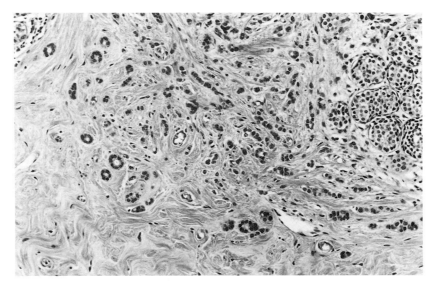

Fig. 15.15A   Tubulo-lobular carcinoma. The tumor is composed of a diffuse infiltration of small, regular cells, most in single files with an admixture of microtubular structures. A focus of lobular carcinoma in situ is seen at the top right. Hematoxylin–eosin × 125.

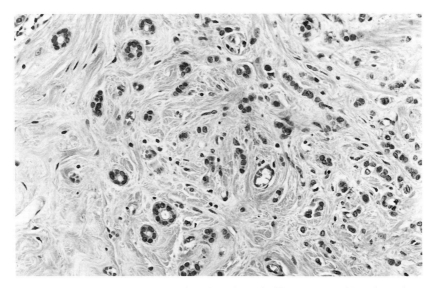

Fig. 15.15B   Higher magnification of the field shown in Figure 15.15A. Note the typical lobular infiltrative pattern with associated microtubules. Hematoxylin–eosin × 185.

MEDULLARY CARCINOMA

Introduction

This specific type of invasive breast cancer was first defined properly by Moore and Foote in 1949.[34] It was established as a separate entity because of its distinctive morphological appearances and the apparently favorable prognosis.

Since then considerable controversy has been generated in relation both to the prognosis and the diagnostic criteria. It has become established dogma that medullary carcinoma carries a good prognosis[4,32,35] based on data from a relatively small number of studies.[10,36–39] This is despite the fact that a similar number of studies have failed to establish any more than an average prognosis.[7,40–42] Furthermore, an unacceptable inter- and intra-observer variability in diagnosis, using the criteria proposed by Fisher et al[14] and Ridolfi et al,[37] has been shown in several reproducibility studies.[43–45] This lack of specificity of the diagnostic criteria has undoubtedly contributed to the wide variation in the reported frequency of medullary carcinoma (see Table 13.2), from 2% up to 10%.

Macroscopic appearances

The gross features of a typical medullary carcinoma are quite distinctive. The tumors form well, often sharply, circumscribed masses with a soft fleshy consistency which may be confused clinically with a fibroadenoma. The cut surface is usually of a uniform gray-white appearance, although small foci of necrosis may be apparent. They usually measure between 1 and 4 cm in diameter.

Microscopic appearances

The criteria for the histological diagnosis of medullary carcinoma have been reviewed repeatedly,[14,37,39,41] but it has been generally accepted that there are three key morphological features:

1. The tumor is composed of interconnecting sheets of large epithelial cells with abundant cytoplasm, forming a syncytial network (Fig. 15.16A and B), rather than a trabecular pattern. Nuclei are pleomorphic with a proportion of bizarre forms and there is a high mitotic count, i.e., the appearances are those of a poorly differentiated (grade 3) carcinoma (Fig. 15.16C).

2. Between these sheets of tumor cells the stroma contains moderate or large numbers of lymphocytes and plasma cells which do not infiltrate extensively between individual tumor cells (Fig. 15.16B and C). The stroma itself is scanty.

3. In keeping with the circumscription visible grossly the border of the tumor is pushing rather than infiltrative, giving a sharply defined tumor margin (Fig. 15.16A).

The presence of associated ductal carcinoma in situ does not preclude a diagnosis of medullary carcinoma, but it should only be present to a limited degree. In addition small foci of necrosis may be present, but vascular invasion is not usually seen.

This pattern must be consistent throughout the entire tumor in order for it to be typed as medullary.

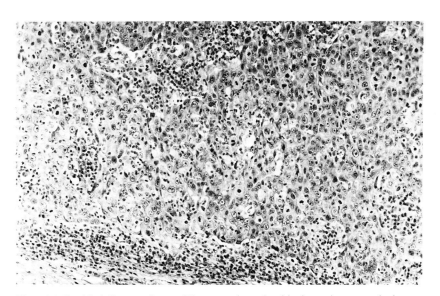

Fig. 15.16A   Medullary carcinoma. The tumor has a 'pushing' margin seen at the lower part of the field with a syncytial growth pattern. Even at this power the associated lymphoplasmacytoid infiltrate can be visualized. Hematoxylin–eosin × 125.

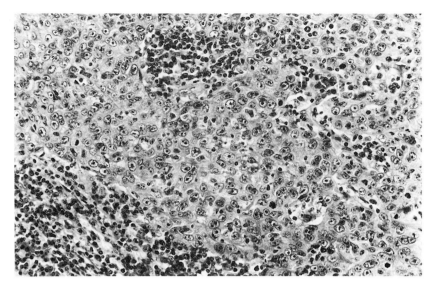

Fig. 15.16B   Another field from the case shown in Figure 15.16A to emphasize the syncytial growth pattern. Note the lymphoplasmacytic infiltrate at the lower left and top center. Hematoxylin–eosin × 185.

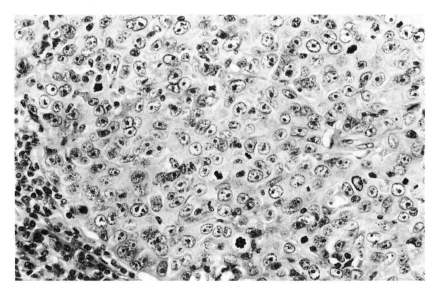

Fig. 15.16C   Higher magnification of the field shown in Figure 15.16B. The carcinoma cell nuclei are markedly pleomorphic with prominent nucleoli and several mitotic figures are present. Hematoxylin–eosin × 400.

Differential diagnosis

It is recognized that a proportion of invasive carcinomas of breast have some but not all the features of medullary carcinoma. These have been designated as *atypical medullary carcinoma* by both Fisher et al[14] and Ridolfi et al.[37] These tumors are well circumscribed but show a lesser degree of lymphoplasmacytoid infiltrate, several points of microscopic invasion beyond the main border or dense areas of fibrosis, whilst retaining the other features of medullary carcinoma such as the syncytial growth pattern. A well circumscribed tumor is also classified as atypical medullary if up to 25% of its area is composed of a ductal NST pattern provided that the rest shows classical medullary features. Based on these criteria atypical medullary carcinoma accounts for approximately 5% of invasive carcinomas.[7]

Tumors in which the classical medullary component is less than 75% should be designated as ductal NST carcinomas. It should also be noted that the presence of a lymphoid infiltrate alone does not qualify a tumor for inclusion in the medullary category. This is, in fact, a common phenomenon in invasive carcinomas, occurring in at least 50% of cases.[46–47] Wargotz and Silverberg[39] have proposed that the category of atypical medullary carcinoma be abolished altogether. Based on a study of 53 cases they found that tumors with only one of the atypical features described above had the same 'good' prognosis as pure medullary carcinoma. They have therefore suggested that these cases be included in the medullary category and all other cases with atypical features be designated as ductal NST carcinomas. It must be emphasized that their clinical follow-up was short and the apparent differences in survival were not statistically significant.

It was pointed out above that Pedersen et al[43] found poor reproducibility in the diagnosis of medullary carcinoma, using the criteria described above. They have now produced a simplified histopathological definition based on two criteria only, a syncytial growth pattern and diffuse moderate or marked mononuclear cell infiltrate.[42] They claim that these criteria are reproducible with consistency, and Gaffey et al,[45] who compared the method with those of Ridolfi et al[37] and Wargotz and Silverberg,[39] found it to be the most reproducible. However, they also found that a diagnosis of medullary carcinoma with any of the systems was unassociated with other prognostic factors such as tumor size or lymph node stage nor with overall survival. Further studies are clearly required but for the present time we use the diagnostic criteria described on page 301.

TUBULAR CARCINOMA

Introduction

As McDivitt and colleagues[48] have pointed out,

the morphological features of tubular carcinoma were recognized over 100 years ago, but until comparatively recently the tumor has received little attention because of its relative rarity in symptomatic practice. Tubular carcinoma of the breast is, in fact, a readily recognizable subtype composed as it is of distinct tubular structures with open lumina lined by a single layer of epithelial cells. There has been considerable debate concerning the precise morphological criteria, and in particular the proportion of tubular structures required to establish the diagnosis; this is discussed in more detail below. In general symptomatic practice tubular carcinoma is uncommon, with a recorded frequency of 1–7% (see Table 13.2). However, a much higher frequency is found in cases detected by mammographic screening, from 9 to 19%,[8,49–52] due to the detection of small impalpable lesions.

Macroscopic appearances

Grossly there are no specific features which can be used to distinguish a tubular carcinoma from the commoner ductal NST or mixed types, other than the overall tumor size. Tubular carcinomas usually measure between 2 mm and 2 cm in diameter; the majority are 1 cm or less[8,48,53] whilst most ductal NST carcinomas measure more than 1.5 cm in diameter. Nevertheless, despite this general rule we have encountered occasional cases of pure tubular carcinoma measuring more than 2 cm, and one which was 3 cm in diameter. Two basic morphological subtypes have been described, the 'pure' type in which the stellate nature is pronounced, with central yellow flecks due to elastosis and radiating arms, and the 'sclerosing' type characterized by a more diffuse, ill-defined structure.[54–55] In our experience it is the latter type which is more likely to be of a larger size.

Microscopic appearances

The single most important identifying feature of tubular carcinoma is, as the name implies, the dominant presence of open tubules which, by definition, are composed of a single layer of epithelial cell enclosing a clear lumen (Fig. 15.17A, B, C and D). The tubules are generally oval or

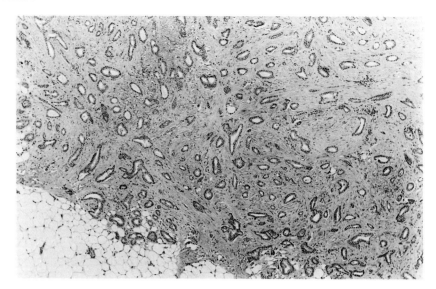

Fig. 15.17A   Tubular carcinoma, 'pure' type. The tumor is composed entirely of tubular structures which extend out to the periphery. Hematoxylin–eosin × 57.

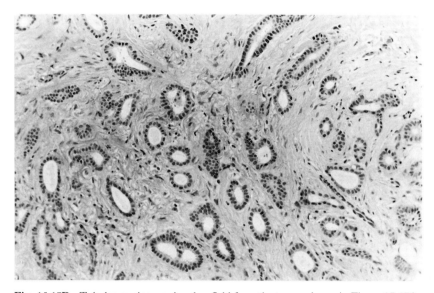

Fig. 15.17B   Tubular carcinoma. Another field from the tumor shown in Figure 15.17A to show the open tubular structure and cellular desmoplastic stroma. Hematoxylin–eosin × 125.

rounded and characteristically, a proportion appears angulated (Fig. 15.17B and C). The epithelial cells are small and regular with little nuclear pleomorphism and only scanty mitotic figures (Fig. 15.17D). Apical snouts (Fig. 15.18) are seen in up to a third of cases,[4] but are by no means pathognomonic and cannot be used to distinguish tubular carcinoma from benign lesions. Fine speckled microcalcifications are frequently found within the tubular lumina (Fig. 15.19).

A secondary but important feature of tubular carcinoma is the cellular desmoplastic stroma which accompanies the tubular structures (Fig. 15.17A, B and C). In the *pure* type there is often central rather hyalinized fibrosis, usually with associated elastosis, which contains scanty tubules. The

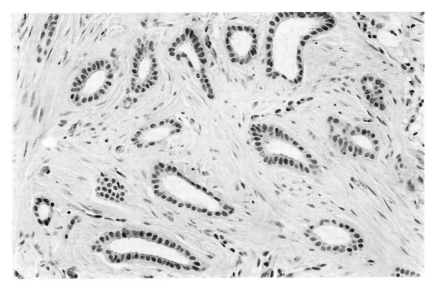

Fig. 15.17C Tubular carcinoma. There is a mixture of oval and angulated tubular structures. From the same case as that shown in Figure 15.17A and B. Hematoxylin–eosin × 185.

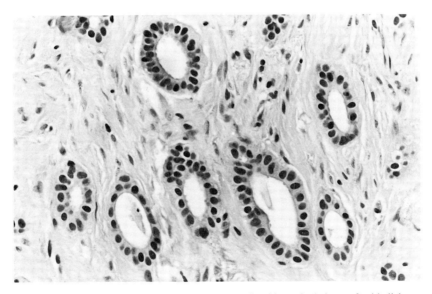

Fig. 15.17D Tubular carcinoma. The tubules are lined by a single layer of epithelial cells, which show minimal nuclear pleomorphism. Hematoxylin–eosin × 400.

latter radiate outwards and are usually more abundant peripherally. The *sclerosing* type has much less apparent central hyalinization and elastosis, with a diffuse and rather haphazard infiltration of tubules within the desmoplastic stroma (Fig. 15.20A and B). In both types tubular structures at the periphery infiltrate into adjacent adipose tissue, often without significant accompanying fibrous tissue (Fig. 15.21). Residual normal lobules and ductular elements may become surrounded by neoplastic tubules; these may be a useful point of reference in assessing nuclear pleomorphism within the tumor cells. Ductal carcinoma in situ is found in association with tubular

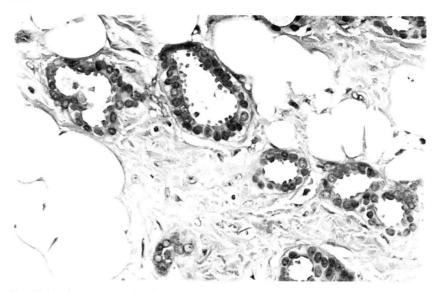

Fig. 15.18   Another example of pure tubular carcinoma, in which there are well formed apical snouts. Hematoxylin–eosin × 400.

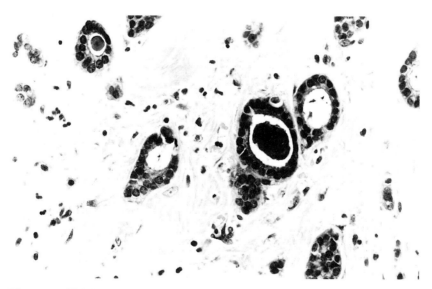

Fig. 15.19   Tubular carcinoma. Foci of microcalcification are seen within the lumina of tubular structures. Hematoxylin–eosin × 400.

carcinoma in the majority of cases; this is usually of low grade type with a cribriform or micro-papillary pattern.

Whilst the description given above implies that the morphological criteria for tubular carcinoma are relatively straightforward there has in fact been considerable disagreement in the past concerning the proportion of tubular structures required to establish the diagnosis. In the WHO classification[1–2] and a number of published studies[10,53,55] no specific cut-off point is indicated although there is an assumption that all the tumor is of a tubular configuration. Some authors have applied a strict 100% rule for pure tubular carcinoma,[54,56–57] some set the proportion of tubular structures at 75%[5,48,58–59] and yet others at 90%.[3,51] For purely

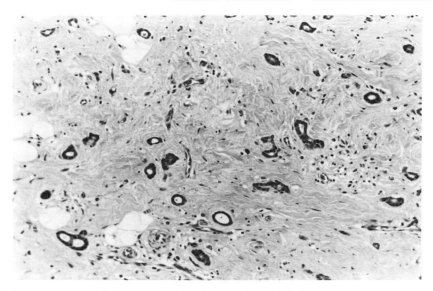

Fig. 15.20A Tubular carcinoma, sclerosing type. Islands of adipose tissue are incorporated into the tumor mass. Hematoxylin–eosin × 125.

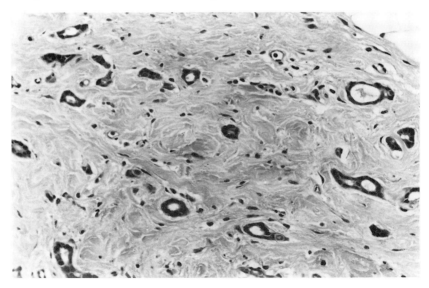

Fig. 15.20B Higher magnification of case shown in Figure 15.20A. Small tubules infiltrate diffusely within a dense stroma. Hematoxylin–eosin × 185.

pragmatic reasons we have opted to follow the latter view, on the basis that a thorough search of most pure tubular carcinomas will reveal some closed epithelial structures and to expect 100% purity is unrealistic. It is our view then that a tumor may be categorized as tubular carcinoma if more than 90% of its area is composed of open tubular structures, provided that the non-tubular

component has the same well differentiated nuclear morphology. If a tumor consists of less than 90% tubular carcinoma it enters the tubular mixed, ductal NST and special type or miscellaneous categories (these are discussed below). The only exception to the above rule is the combination of tubular and cribriform elements; in these cases a tumor is typed as tubular if more

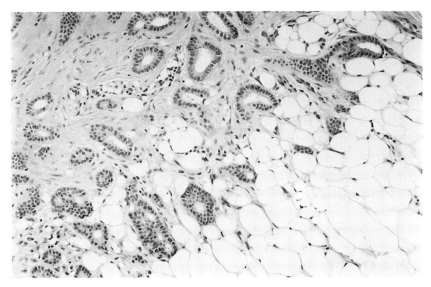

Fig. 15.21 Periphery of a tubular carcinoma. Tubular structures invade into adjacent adipose tissue. Hematoxylin–eosin × 125.

than 50% of the area is occupied by a tubular pattern.

Differential diagnosis

As indicated above care must be taken to distinguish tubular carcinoma from other types of invasive carcinoma in which tubular structures may be found. This is based on two features, the morphological characteristics of the tubular structures and their relative proportion. A significant minority of ductal NST carcinomas contain tubular areas, but these usually lack the regular well differentiated pattern of tubular carcinoma (see Fig. 15.4A and B). In any event, if they occupy less than 90% of the tumor then tubular carcinoma is excluded and a diagnosis of tubular mixed carcinoma should be considered (as discussed on p. 313). The distinction from tubulo-lobular carcinoma has been discussed previously.

It is also extremely important that benign conditions such as sclerosing adenosis, microglandular adenosis and radial scar/complex sclerosing lesion (CSL) are not mistaken for tubular carcinoma.[60] The distinguishing features are discussed in some detail in Chapter 7. It is sufficient to re-iterate two points here: the absence of immunostaining with an antibody to smooth muscle actin is extremely useful in confirming the single layer of epithelial cells of tubular carcinomas; CSLs must be examined very carefully to exclude the possibility of an associated tubular carcinoma.

INVASIVE CRIBRIFORM CARCINOMA (ICC)

Introduction

This specific type of invasive breast carcinoma has been a source of considerable terminological confusion in the past. The tumor was originally identified because of its combination of low grade DCIS of cribriform type with invasive elements and its significantly better prognosis than ductal NST carcinoma. It was incorrectly named infiltrating papillary carcinoma by McDivitt, Stewart and Berg,[10] as pointed out by Azzopardi[12] who introduced the term infiltrating cribriform carcinoma. Page et al[61] were the first to describe the characteristics of these tumors in detail, particularly emphasizing their distinction from adenoid cystic carcinoma. It appears that invasive cribriform carcinoma shares considerable homology with the papillo-tubular carcinomas described by the Japanese Mammary Cancer Society.[62]

Invasive cribriform carcinomas of the breast are

uncommon, accounting for between 0.8 and 3.5% of cases presenting with symptomatic disease.[7,61,63] However, in common with other special type carcinomas the frequency is increased in mammographic screening.[8,51]

Macroscopic appearances

In general there are no specific gross features. The tumors form a firm mass similar to that of a ductal NST carcinoma, and may have a stellate configuration. They are usually larger than tubular carcinomas, measuring between 1 and 3 cm in diameter.

Microscopic appearances

The key defining feature of this type is the presence of invasive cords and islands of small regular epithelial cells exhibiting the same morphological pattern as that seen in DCIS of cribriform type (Fig. 15.22A and B). The nuclei are generally dark staining, show little pleomorphism and infrequent mitoses (Fig. 15.22B). The invasive islands demonstrate typical geometric 'punched out' spaces and arches (Figs 15.22A and B, 15.23); apical 'snouting' of the epithelial cells is a common occurrence (Fig. 15.24A). Foci of genuinely in situ

carcinoma of cribriform type are usually present (Fig. 15.24A). In most cases there is an admixture of tubular structures, similar to those seen in tubular carcinoma, and having the same nuclear features as the cribriform areas (Fig. 15.24B). We have followed the convention used for tubular carcinoma so that for a tumor to be classified as invasive cribriform this pattern must form at least 90% of the area of the lesion, and the rest must have a low grade appearance. The only exception to this rule is made when the other component in a tumor is pure tubular in type; in this case over 50% of the tumor must be cribriform to be so designated.[61] A similar desmoplastic stroma to that associated with tubular carcinoma is frequently present (Fig. 15.23).

A rare but distinctive variant of ICC has been described in which the stroma contains osteoclast-like giant cells.[64–66] We have encountered two such cases. In each the tumor mass appeared soft and hemorrhagic on gross examination, whilst microscopically the typical low grade invasive cribriform pattern was accompanied by prominent stromal giant cells (Fig. 15.25A and B). This phenomenon is not restricted to ICC and has been described in several tumor types (see Ch. 18).

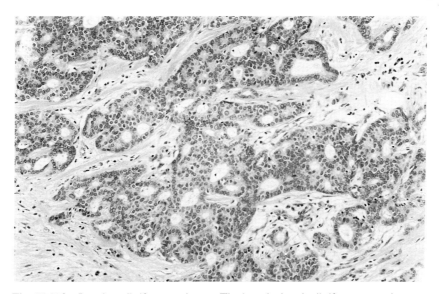

Fig. 15.22A Invasive cribriform carcinoma. The 'punched out' cribriform pattern is apparent, even in this low power view. Hematoxylin–eosin × 125.

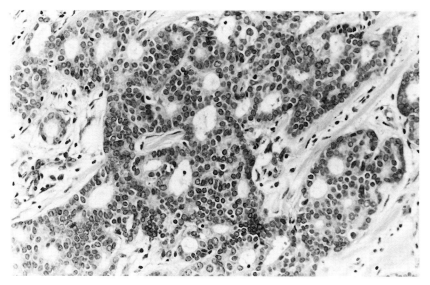

Fig. 15.22B Invasive cribriform carcinoma. Note the well defined cribriform structure, with regular small nuclei showing little pleomorphism. From the same case as that illustrated in Figure 15.22A. Hematoxylin–eosin × 185.

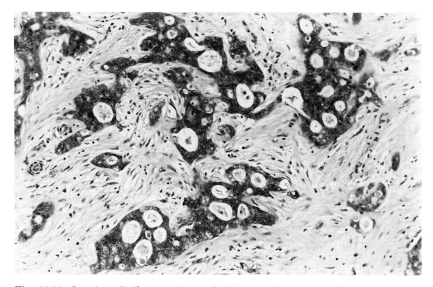

Fig. 15.23 Invasive cribriform carcinoma. In this example the tumor islands are set within a prominent desmoplastic stroma. Hematoxylin–eosin × 125.

Differential diagnosis

The distinction of ICC from tubular carcinoma has been described above. Page et al[61] recognize a 'mixed' type of ICC in which cribriform elements are associated with areas of less differentiated carcinoma of ductal NST type. Rather confusingly, Venable et al[63] include in their 'mixed' group cases in which the other element is tubular in type and which by the criteria of Page et al[61] qualify for the pure ICC group. We agree with Page et al[61] on this latter point, but prefer to designate cases with less than 90% ICC combined with ductal NST elements in our mixed ductal

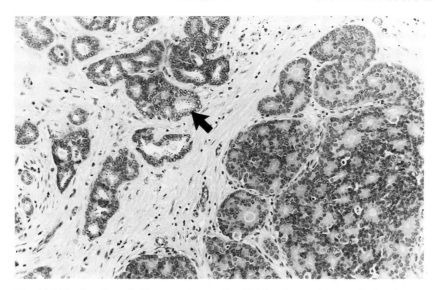

Fig. 15.24A   Invasive cribriform carcinoma. A well defined area of low grade ductal carcinoma in situ, cribriform pattern, is seen at the right of the field, with invasive cribriform carcinoma to the left. Note the apical snouts in the latter (arrowhead). Hematoxylin–eosin × 185.

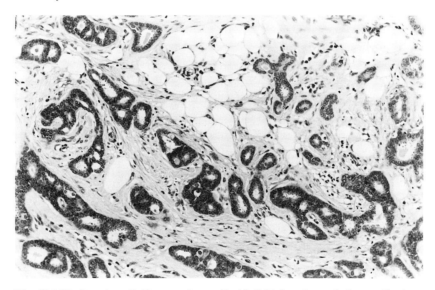

Fig. 15.24B   Invasive cribriform carcinoma. In this field there is an admixture of both cribriform and tubular structures, the former predominating. From the same case as that shown in Figure 15.24A. Hematoxylin–eosin × 125.

and special type category (see below). As Page et al[3] have pointed out many such cases go unrecognized as being of a special type and are consigned to the ductal NST group. This is unfortunate as potentially useful prognostic information is lost.

Occasionally problems are encountered in distinguishing an invasive cribriform carcinoma from a purely in situ carcinoma of low nuclear grade, cribriform type. It is difficult to lay down absolute criteria for such cases, but preservation of normal anatomical ducto-lobular structures

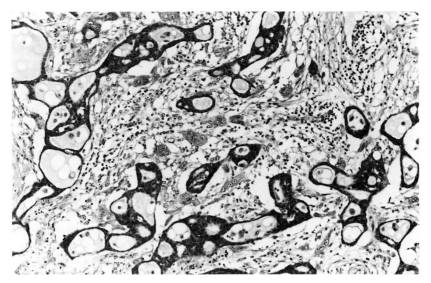

Fig. 15.25A Invasive cribriform carcinoma. The stroma contains an infiltrate of inflammatory cells including multinucleated giant cells. Hematoxylin–eosin × 125.

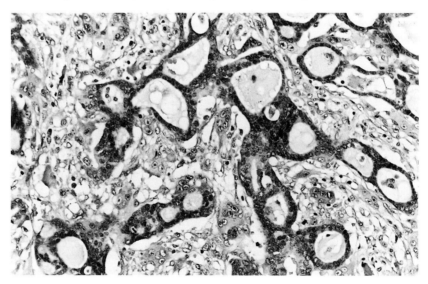

Fig. 15.25B Higher magnification of another area from the case illustrated in Figure 15.25A. The stromal giant cells are seen to be in close contact with the epithelial cells of the tumor. Hematoxylin–eosin × 185.

favors an in situ diagnosis, and the presence of irregular, often sharply angulated cribriform islands, are suggestive of invasion. Multiple blocks should be examined and a careful search made for extension of cords of tumor into adjacent connective or adipose tissue.

Adenoid cystic carcinoma poses an even more difficult differential diagnosis since there are close similarities with ICC. This is dealt with in more detail in Chapter 16; it is sufficient to point out here that the glandular spaces are more sharply defined in adenoid cystic carcinoma, there is a prominent basement membrane component and biphasic cellularity is usually evident.

TUBULAR MIXED CARCINOMA

Introduction

Whilst there is now general agreement that to establish a diagnosis of tubular carcinoma it must be composed of at least 90% tubular structures, categorization of tumors with a smaller tubular component has proved more controversial. Parl and Richardson,[54] following criteria established by Carstens et al,[55] used the term 'tubular mixed' carcinoma for such cases, but set a lower level for the proportion of tubules of 75%. Subsequently, in a long-term follow-up study, Carstens et al[56] confirmed the fact that patients with tubular mixed carcinoma defined in this way had a reduced survival compared with patients having pure tubular carcinoma. They also concluded that there was no difference in survival between tumors with 50–75% tubular structures and those with less than 50%; all were included in the ductal NST group. This definition of tubular mixed carcinoma has become accepted dogma[3–4] although some groups prefer to use the term 'tubular *variant* carcinoma'.[51,67] By contrast Deos and Norris[68] used an upper limit for the ductal NST component of 50%. In our own study we found that there was no significant difference in survival for patients whose tumors had less than 75% tubule formation compared with those with 75–90% tubule formation, but all had a better prognosis than ductal NST carcinoma.[7] In order not to lose valuable prognostic information by consigning these cases to the ductal NST category we have proposed a broader definition for our category of tubular mixed carcinoma.

Because of the differences in diagnostic criteria for tubular mixed carcinoma it is difficult to give a general estimate of its frequency. In the NTPBCS this type accounts for 14% of patients presenting symptomatically;[7] this increases up to 26% in the prevalent round of mammographic screening.[8]

Macroscopic appearances

Since they form an intermediate group between tubular and ductal NST carcinoma the gross features are similar to these types. Tumors generally measure between 1.5 and 3 cm in diameter with an average size of approximately 2 cm. They are firm or hard in consistency, with an overall stellate structure and may be moderately or ill-defined.

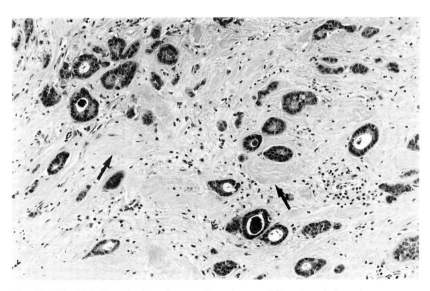

Fig. 15.26A Tubular mixed carcinoma. There is central fibrosis and elastosis (arrowheads) infiltrated by a mixture of open and closed tubular structures. Hematoxylin–eosin × 125.

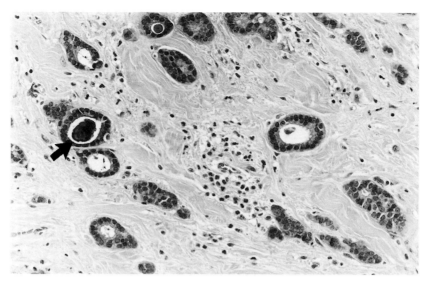

Fig. 15.26B Tubular mixed carcinoma. Higher magnification of field shown in Figure 15.26A. Note the oval open tubules and regular nuclei with little pleomorphism. Microcalcification is seen in some tubules (arrowhead). Hematoxylin–eosin × 185.

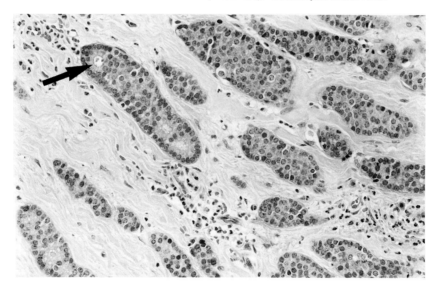

Fig. 15.26C Tubular mixed carcinoma. This field is from the periphery of the tumor shown in Figure 15.26A and B. Here there are solid trabeculae more in keeping with a ductal NST structure, although some small lumina are apparent (arrowhead). Hematoxylin–eosin × 185.

Microscopic appearances

To qualify for inclusion in the tubular mixed category a tumor must have the following features:

1. The overall structure is that of a stellate mass with central fibrosis and, usually, elastosis.

2. Well differentiated tubules are present centrally (Fig. 15.26A and B) identical in appearance to those seen in tubular carcinoma.

3. There is a peripheral border of variable thickness composed of less differentiated infiltrating adenocarcinoma (Fig. 15.26C).

The two morphological patterns merge one

into the other, there being a graded progression from the well differentiated centre to a less differentiated structure at the periphery. The peripheral tumor is usually of ductal NST type (Fig. 15.26C), but may be a mixture of ductal NST and ILC, or even classical ILC alone. There is no definite minimum cut-off point for the proportion of tumor occupied by tubules; even if the number is very small, provided that the characteristic distribution described above is seen then a tumor may be typed as tubular mixed carcinoma. In practice the lower limit is usually of the order of 5–10%.

An in situ element is usually present in these tumors and may be of low or high nuclear grade. Necrosis and lymphocytic infiltration are not features of this type.

Differential diagnosis

The main distinction is, not surprisingly, from tubular carcinoma at one end of the spectrum and ductal NST at the other. The distinguishing criteria for tubular carcinoma have already been discussed, and rest on the proportion of tubular structures present. Some ductal NST carcinomas may exhibit focal tubule formation, but if these do not have a well differentiated appearance similar to tubular carcinoma and they are distributed throughout the tumor rather than in a central position then a designation of tubular mixed carcinoma is not appropriate (see Fig. 15.4A and B).

MUCINOUS CARCINOMA

Introduction

This special type of invasive carcinoma is also referred to as gelatinous, mucoid and colloid carcinoma. These names reflect uncertainty in the past concerning the origin and nature of the characteristic mucinous component, but there can be no doubt that the mucin is produced by the tumor cells themselves. As the name implies these are tumors in which the mucinous component is apparent to the naked eye. They are relatively uncommon, accounting for between 1 and 3% in symptomatic series (see Table 13.2). Interestingly this tumor, regarded as being of special type because of its relatively favorable prognosis,[7] is not found with increased frequency in mammographic screening,[8,51] possibly because its relatively slow growth and lack of spiculation on imaging may lead to an erroneous diagnosis of benignity.[69]

Macroscopic appearances

Mucinous carcinomas form rounded, soft masses which have a characteristic glistening gelatinous cut surface. The edge is usually well, if not sharply, defined, but may be bosselated. They vary in size from about 1 cm up to 4 cm, but occasional examples of much larger tumors are sometimes encountered.[4]

Microscopic appearances

Histologically these tumors consist of small islands or clusters of epithelial cells (comprising between 10 and 100 cells) set within extensive lakes of extracellular mucin (Fig. 15.27A, B and C). The cells are of relatively small size, with regular darkly staining nuclei which usually exhibit little nuclear pleomorphism (Figs 15.27B, 15.28, 15.29). In some cases tubular or cribriform structures are seen within the epithelial islands (Fig. 15.29). Mitoses are variable in number but usually scanty. At the periphery of the tumor which is usually sharply defined, the epithelial islands may be embedded in a loose connective tissue stroma (Fig. 15.28). An associated in situ component is found in up to 30% of cases; this has the same cytological characteristics as the invasive component.[70] Necrosis is an uncommon feature, but may be present in larger tumors. Both neutral and acidic mucopolysaccharides may be identified in the extracellular mucins and also as intracytoplasmic vacuoles, using the Alcian Blue-Periodic acid Schiff stain. Argyrophilia has been identified in up to 25% of mucinous carcinomas[71] but this appears to carry no prognostic significance.

Some tumors are composed of a mixture of mucinous carcinoma and ductal NST carcinoma. In the past there has been a lack of agreement on how such tumors should be classified, and in practice many pathologists used the term mucinous carcinomas for cases showing any mucinous

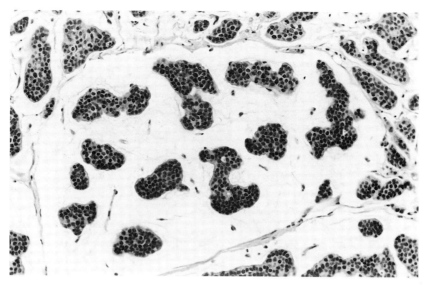

Fig. 15.27A Mucinous carcinoma. Small 'islands' of tumor cells appear to float within a 'sea' of mucin. Hematoxylin–eosin × 125.

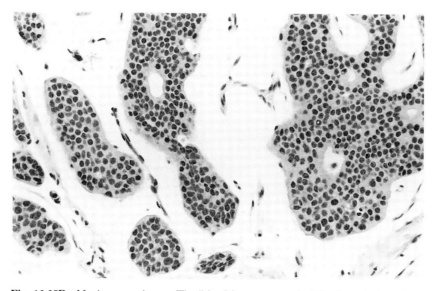

Fig. 15.27B Mucinous carcinoma. The 'islands' are composed of closely packed regular cells showing mild nuclear pleomorphism. Note the luminal spaces within some islands. Hematoxylin–eosin × 185.

features. There is now general acceptance of the rule that the term mucinous carcinoma should only be applied to tumors in which at least 90% of the structure is of pure mucinous appearance.[3–4,7,70,72–73] It follows that the presence of more than 10% of a ductal NST element excludes a tumor from this category. Some authors have placed such tumors in a 'mixed mucinous' group[4,72–74] but we prefer to include them in the larger mixed ductal NST/Special type category.

Differential diagnosis

The distinction of pure mucinous carcinoma from cases with a mixed pattern is relatively easy, as long as there is strict adherence to the 90% rule.

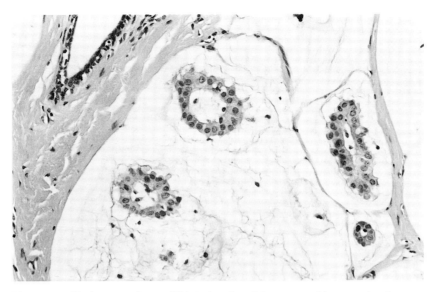

Fig. 15.28   Mucinous carcinoma. This is the edge of the tumor, with connective tissue stroma and a normal duct to the top left. The tumor cells form tubular structures and nuclei show little pleomorphism. Hematoxylin–eosin × 185.

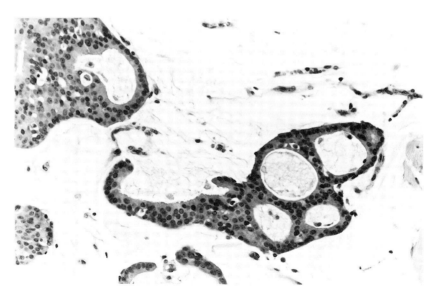

Fig. 15.29   Mucinous carcinoma. In this example a well formed cribriform structure is seen. Hematoxylin–eosin × 185.

At the other end of the spectrum some ductal NST carcinomas contain small areas with extra-cellular mucin production. Such cases may be included in the mixed ductal NST/Special type category, but if the area of mucinous differentia-tion is insignificant they are better designated simply as ductal NST.

There are few benign lesions which are likely to be confused with pure mucinous carcinoma. Tavassoli[4] provides anecdotal evidence that fibro-adenomas with marked myxoid change in the stroma have caused diagnostic problems, both grossly and microscopically. The arrangement of the epithelial elements in cleft-like spaces, however attenuated, should distinguish the structure of a fibroadenoma from the much looser rounded epithelial islands of mucinous carcinoma.

The rather rarer mucocele-like lesion described by Rosen[75] is a source of greater diagnostic difficulty. Mucin lakes are usually found in association with fibrocytic change, and are due to rupture of mucin-containing cysts with discharge of the

contents into the adjacent stroma (Fig. 15.30A and B). They are usually very small (less than 2 mm) and rarely contain any cells. However, occasionally much larger mucin lakes occur and these may contain scanty epithelial cells. The only way to distinguish these benign mucocele-like lesions from a paucicellular mucinous carcinoma is by assessment of the epithelial cells, especially if

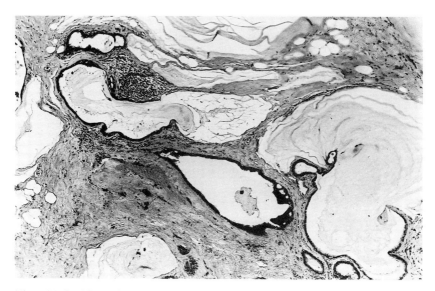

Fig. 15.30A Mucocele-like lesion. There is a background of cystic structures with associated mucin lakes. Hematoxylin–eosin × 57.

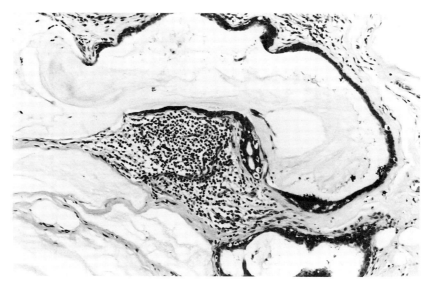

Fig. 15.30B Mucocele-like lesion. Higher magnification of the field shown in Figure 15.30A. The point of rupture of a cyst is seen at the top left with a mucin lake at the lower left. Apart from the epithelial lining of the cyst there are no epithelial structures within the mucin. Compare with Figure 15.28. Hematoxylin–eosin × 125.

both epithelial and myoepithelial cells are present. We have encountered anecdotal cases of mucocele-type lakes in association with both atypical ductal hyperplasia and low grade ductal carcinoma in situ; in this situation it is virtually impossible to exclude a tiny invasive mucinous element.

INVASIVE PAPILLARY CARCINOMA

Introduction

In the past the term papillary carcinoma has been used in a broad sense, with little attempt to distinguish in situ from invasive types. However, as Fisher et al[76] have pointed out, it is important in terms of prognosis and management to make the distinction clear and the appropriate prefix should always be applied. There are two distinct subgroups, dominantly invasive carcinomas with a papillary structure and papillary carcinoma in situ with a definite invasive component. In practice invasive papillary carcinomas are uncommon, occurring in less than 2% in most symptomatic series,[7,67,76] although they may be more frequent in the elderly.[76]

Macroscopic appearances

The gross appearances are variable. They may be soft and well circumscribed, or indistinguish-able from ductal NST carcinoma. They measure between 1 and 3 cm in diameter.

Microscopic appearances

The distinguishing feature of the dominantly invasive subtype is the presence within an invasive tumor of papillary structures composed of fibrovascular cores lined by malignant epithelial cells (Fig. 15.31A and B). In many cases these structures are so closely packed that their papillary nature may be relatively obscured (Fig. 15.31A) whilst in others a definite fronded pattern is easily made out (Fig. 15.32). Cytological appearances are varied and nuclear pleomorphism and increased number of mitoses may be seen (Fig. 15.33). Many papillary carcinomas exhibit mucin secretion, (two thirds of the cases in the series described by Fisher et al[76]) and foci in which tumor cells float in a mucinous lake, resembling pure mucinous carcinoma, may be seen. At the tumor margin an infiltrative pattern may be seen, although in some cases the degree of obvious invasion is limited (Fig. 15.34).

Invasive papillary carcinomas are rarely 'pure' and there is usually an admixture with other morphological patterns such as ductal NST, mucinous or invasive cribriform carcinoma. The defining limits for the relative proportions of these

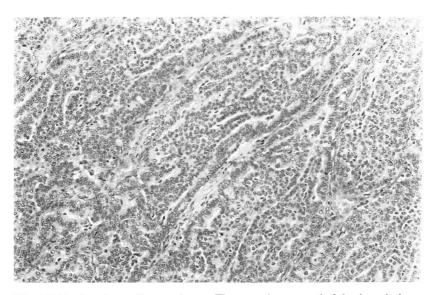

Fig. 15.31A   Invasive papillary carcinoma. The tumor is composed of closely packed epithelial structures with associated fibrovascular cores. Hematoxylin–eosin × 125.

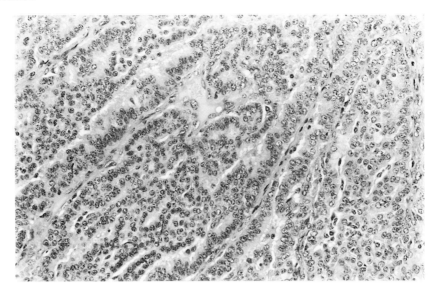

Fig. 15.31B   Invasive papillary carcinoma. Higher magnification of the tumor shown in Figure 15.31A. Hematoxylin–eosin × 185.

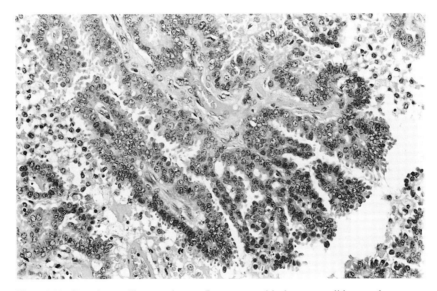

Fig. 15.32   Invasive papillary carcinoma. In contrast with the more solid example illustrated in Figure 15.31A and B, there is a well marked fronded structure in this case. Hematoxylin–eosin × 185.

types have not been set (Fisher and colleagues[76] referred to their cases as 'pure' without further clarification) but we feel that it is sensible to follow the 90% rule used for other specific tumor types. In most cases low nuclear grade micropapillary or cribriform DCIS is present in adjacent ducts.

In the second subtype the basic lesion is a papillary carcinoma in situ (encysted papillary carcinoma) (see also Ch. 8) in which associated invasive carcinoma is present. In such cases the invasive component is not necessarily of papillary pattern and is frequently of ductal NST type with high grade or poorly differentiated features.

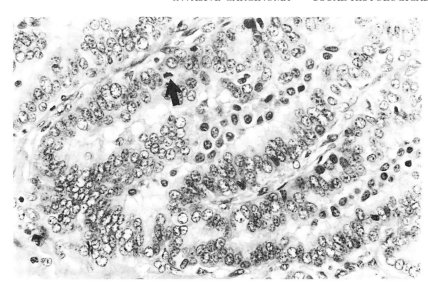

Fig. 15.33 Invasive papillary carcinoma. The nuclei are open and vesicular with visible nucleoli and a moderate to marked degree of pleomorphism. A single mitosis is seen in this field (arrowhead). Hematoxylin–eosin × 400.

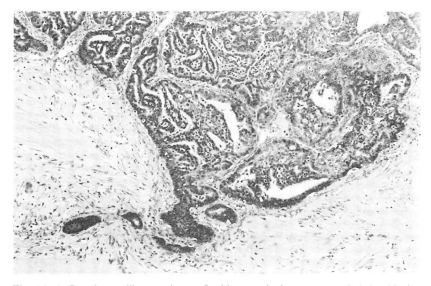

Fig. 15.34 Invasive papillary carcinoma. In this example the tumor margin is 'pushing' with relatively limited stromal invasion in the lower part of the field. Hematoxylin–eosin × 100.

Differential diagnosis

There are two main areas where the differential diagnosis of invasive papillary carcinoma requires consideration, distinction from other invasive carcinomas including metastases and from papillary carcinoma in situ.

As noted above, in invasive papillary carcinoma there may be an admixture of other morphological types and in these cases the 90% rule should be used. For example, in some ductal NST carcinomas areas with a papillary pattern may be encountered; such 'impure' cases should not be included as invasive papillary carcinomas and we use the designation 'ductal NST carcinoma with papillary features'.

Since primary invasive papillary carcinoma of the breast is relatively uncommon the possibility of a metastasis should always be considered. The presence of associated ductal carcinoma in situ confirms the primary nature of a breast tumor, but in its absence a metastasis from other sites such as the ovary should be excluded. This is covered in more detail in Chapter 19.

Distinction from papillary carcinoma in situ may pose more difficult practical problems. Again, this is dealt with in more detail elsewhere (Chs 8 and 14). Suffice it to emphasize here that before a diagnosis of invasion is made in a case of papillary carcinoma in situ multiple blocks should be examined and care taken not to mistake the pseudo-infiltrative entrapped tubules in the capsule for true invasion.

Invasive micropapillary carcinoma

By definition papillary carcinomas have a fronded structure with supportive fibrovascular cores *within* the papillary processes. The term invasive micropapillary carcinoma has now been applied to an uncommon and unusual variant of invasive breast carcinoma in which epithelial tufts forming micropapillae *without* a fibrovascular core are located within clear spaces (Fig. 15.35A and B).[77–78] On low power scanning the pattern is suggestive of fixation artefact or vascular space invasion (Fig. 15.35A), but more detailed examination including mucin histochemistry and immunostaining for epithelial membrane antigen (EMA) and endothelial markers shows that the spaces frequently contain mucin and the epithelial cells exhibit reverse polarity with microvilli in a peripheral position (Fig. 15.35C and D). Nuclear appearances are variable and mitoses may be frequent (Fig. 15.35E). Tubular structures may also be seen and in many cases there is an admixture with ductal NST, mucinous and true papillary areas.[78] Whilst the morphological pattern is certainly distinctive enough to warrant the separate identification of this tumor type we are uncertain whether micropapillary carcinoma should be regarded as a variant of papillary or mucinous carcinoma. Siriaunkgul and Tavassoli[77] identified nine cases of invasive micropapillary carcinoma in the files of the AFIP between 1985 and 1992 and, given this relatively small number, came to the tentative conclusion that the behavior was not significantly different from that of ductal NST carcinoma. We have identified rather more cases in the NTPBCS and have come to the same conclusion (unpublished data). However, Luna More and colleagues,[78] who found 27 cases which

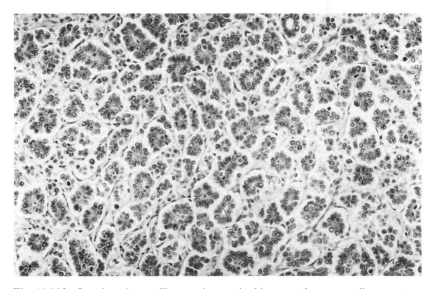

Fig. 15.35A   Invasive micropapillary carcinoma. At this power the tumor cells appear to be grouped within spaces caused by shrinkage artefact. Hematoxylin–eosin × 125.

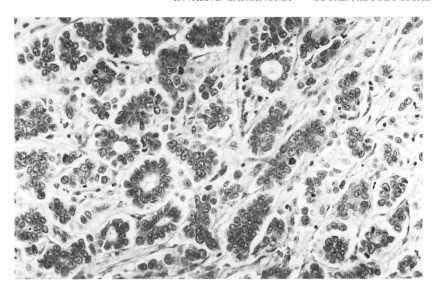

Fig. 15.35B Invasive micropapillary carcinoma. Higher magnification of the case shown in Figure 15.35A. A micropapillary structure is clearly apparent, but some tubular structures are also present. Hematoxylin–eosin × 185.

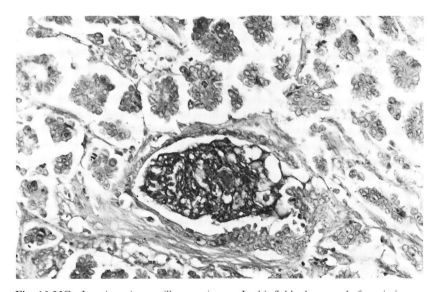

Fig. 15.35C Invasive micropapillary carcinoma. In this field a large pool of mucin is seen within a tubular structure. From the same case as that shown in Figure 15.35A. PAS/Alcian Blue × 185.

showed micropapillary differentiation out of 986 cases of invasive carcinoma, consider this tumor type to be particularly aggressive. Vascular invasion was present in two thirds of the cases, all had lymph node metastases and six of the 12 patients in which follow-up was available had died within a mean of 22 months. It is clear that confirmatory studies are required to establish the clinical importance of this entity.

METAPLASTIC CARCINOMA

Introduction

The term 'metaplastic carcinoma' covers a hetero-

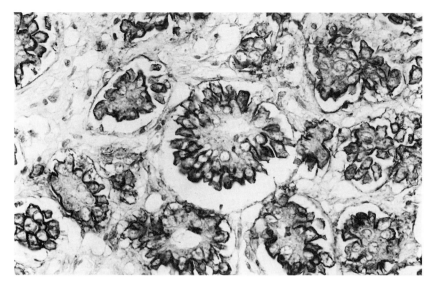

Fig. 15.35D Invasive micropapillary carcinoma. Tumor cells show positive peripheral membrane immunopositivity with an antibody to epithelial mucin antigen. From the same case as that shown in Figure 15.35A. Immunostaining with B55 × 400.

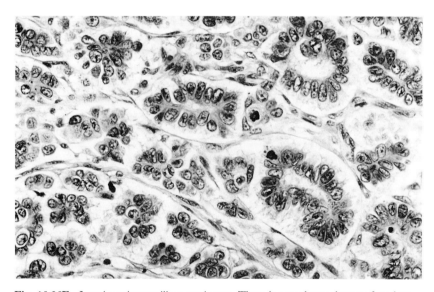

Fig. 15.35E Invasive micropapillary carcinoma. There is a moderate degree of nuclear pleomorphism; two mitotic figures are seen in this field. From the same case as that shown in Figure 15.35A. Hematoxylin–eosin × 400.

geneous range of uncommon entities and has been used loosely by many authors to refer to a variety of breast malignancies of mixed epithelial and mesenchymal appearance. The use of a large number of synonyms has not helped to provide clarity in the definition of these lesions. For example, some authors have included primary squamous and adenosquamous carcinomas of the breast in the category of metaplastic carcinoma, based on a putative origin from metaplastic epithelium in breast ducts. These two tumors are described in Chapter 16 and will not be discussed here.

We include in the category of metaplastic carcinoma two main groups of lesions with a spectrum of appearances: (a) monophasic 'sarcomatoid' or spindle cell carcinomas and (b) biphasic 'sarcomatoid' carcinomas (which have also been classified as 'carcinosarcomas' or 'malignant mixed tumors') with discrete foci of malignant epithelial and mesenchymal elements. Some authors have categorized these biphasic lesions according to the immunohistochemical reactivity of the mesenchymal elements; if positive immunostaining with cytokeratin markers is seen they would class the tumor as a metaplastic carcinoma and if none is present the tumor would be grouped as a 'carcinosarcoma'. Metaplastic carcinomas are currently believed to arise from either myoepithelial or epithelial cells; the ultrastructural and immunohistochemical appearances support an epithelial origin and tight junctions, although rare, may be seen in the sarcomatous portion of 'carcinosarcomas'.[79] The components of these latter lesions are intimately intermingled within the main tumor mass and show similar immunohistochemical profiles suggesting an epithelial origin; we include them in the category of metaplastic carcinoma.

Macroscopic appearances

These lesions show no specific macroscopic features, but over 60% of cases of metaplastic carcinoma have been reported to be circumscribed.[80] The size may vary from 1 to 20 cm in maximum extent.[79,81] The appearance of the cut surface reflects the microscopic components of the tumor and may be fleshy or firm with areas of necrosis present in large tumors.

Microscopic appearances

Multiple histological sections should be examined to determine whether the tumor is truly monophasic of pure spindle cell pattern or of biphasic epithelial and mesenchymal morphology. The spindle cell variant of metaplastic carcinoma is composed of malignant elongated plump cells of relatively monotonous morphology in a fibrocollagenous stroma[80,82] (Fig. 15.36A, B and C). The latter varies in degree from abundant and fibroblastic to scanty, less cellular and more collagenous. Mitoses are also variable in number, but are usually plentiful in the tumor cells.

The epithelial component of the biphasic sarcomatoid type of metaplastic carcinoma may have squamous features, but is more commonly of ductal NST pattern and usually of grade 2 or 3 morphology.[81] Apocrine, mucinous and medullary patterns of carcinoma have also been

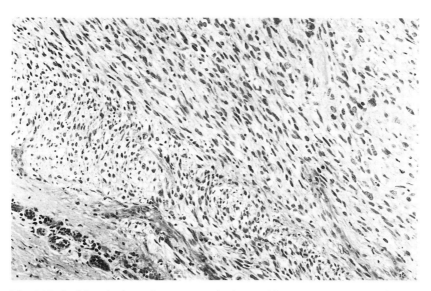

Fig. 15.36A Metaplastic carcinoma, monophasic type. The tumor is composed of spindle cells arranged in a 'herringbone' pattern resembling a spindle cell sarcoma. Normal breast tissue is present at the lower left of the field. Hematoxylin–eosin × 125.

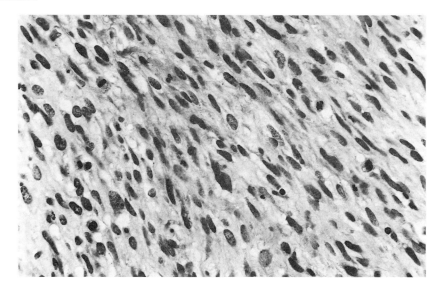

Fig. 15.36B Metaplastic carcinoma, monophasic type. Higher magnification from the field shown in Figure 15.36A. There is marked nuclear pleomorphism and several mitotic figures are present. Hematoxylin–eosin × 400.

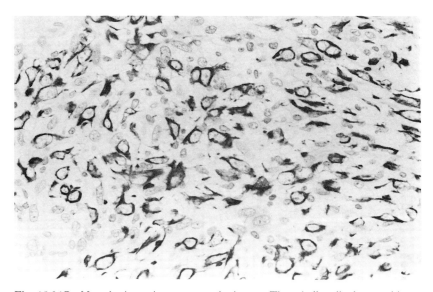

Fig. 15.36C Metaplastic carcinoma, monophasic type. The spindle cells show positive cytoplasmic expression with anti-cytokeratin antibodies. Immunostaining for Cam 5.2 × 400.

described[83–84] but invasive lobular carcinoma has not been reported. Associated DCIS is present in up to 50% of cases (Fig. 15.37A and B) but intraduct sarcomatous foci are not seen.[81,85]

The mesenchymal elements in biphasic metaplastic carcinoma of the breast are usually fibrosarcomatous, or 'malignant-fibrohistiocytoma-like'

in appearance; more rarely angiosarcomatous, leiomyosarcomatous, osteosarcomatous, chondrosarcomatous (Fig. 15.38A and B), or rhabdomyosarcomatous patterns are present. Some authors have distinguished metaplastic carcinomas with a direct transition from the epithelial to a chondroid or osteoid stromal component without inter-

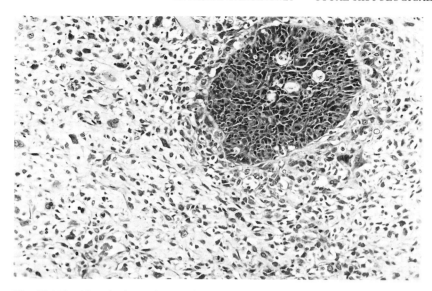

Fig. 15.37A   Metaplastic carcinoma, biphasic type. The tumor is composed of islands of high grade ductal carcinoma in situ with an invasive element of pleomorphic spindle cells. Hematoxylin–eosin × 125.

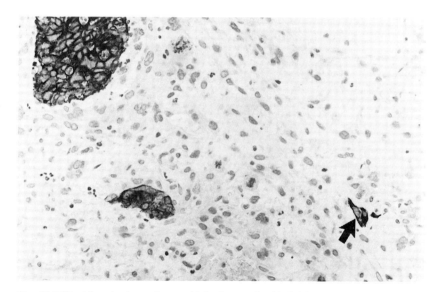

Fig. 15.37B   Metaplastic carcinoma, biphasic type. In this field there is positive expression of low molecular weight cytokeratin in both the in situ element (top left) and, focally, in the malignant stromal cells (arrowhead). Immunostaining for Cam 5.2 × 185.

spersed spindled or giant cell areas, as a separate entity of 'matrix-producing' carcinoma.[85]

Differential diagnosis

The differential diagnosis of metaplastic carcinoma includes other breast malignancies such as the extremely rare true primary sarcomas of the breast including angiosarcoma (Fig. 15.39A–D) and metastatic sarcoma, lymphoma and malignant phyllodes tumors. These tumors and benign spindle cell lesions such as fibromatoses are readily excluded by the presence of immunoreactivity with anti-cytokeratin antibodies and epi-

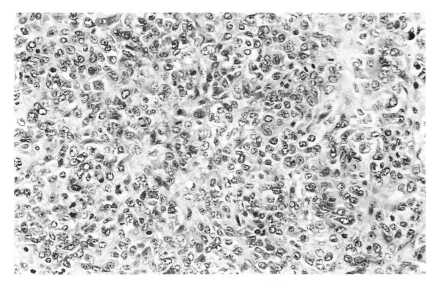

Fig. 15.38A Metaplastic carcinoma, biphasic type. In this field there is a pleomorphic spindle cell pattern, with numerous mitotic figures. Hematoxylin–eosin × 185.

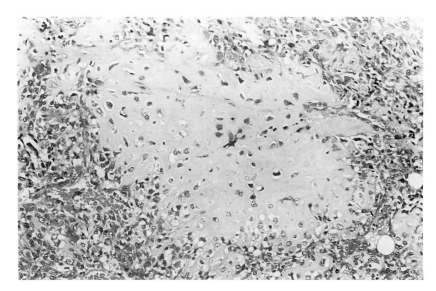

Fig. 15.38B Metaplastic carcinoma, biphasic type. This field, from the same case as that shown in Figure 15.38A, shows an island of chondrosarcoma within a background spindle cell element. Hematoxylin–eosin × 125.

thelial mucin antigen (EMA) in metaplastic carcinomas (Figs 15.36C, 15.39D). Immunopositivity may also be seen with CEA. In those cases in which cytokeratin reactivity is not confirmed initially investigation with a broader range of keratin antibodies is indicated. Currently we use a panel of antibodies including Cam 5.2, MNF 116, CK 7, CK 19 and CK 20. In addition focal positivity is often seen with cytokeratin markers in the mesenchymal areas of biphasic metaplastic carcinomas (Fig. 15.37B). Vimentin positivity is always seen in the sarcomatous portions of these tumors and may also be present in epithelial foci, as in any breast carcinoma of ductal NST type. Focal S-100, smooth muscle actin and desmin immunostaining may also be seen in all areas of these tumors.

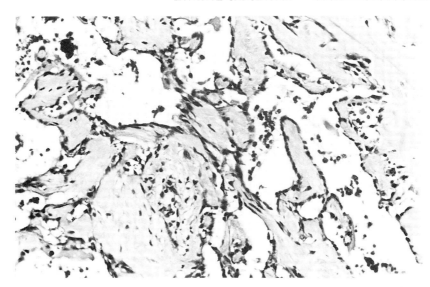

Fig. 15.39A Metaplastic carcinoma, pseudoangiosarcomatous pattern. In this part of the tumor there are apparent irregular spaces lined by flattened hyperchromatic cells. The tumor, from a 69-year-old female, measured 3.5 cm in diameter, and had a markedly hemorrhagic cut surface. Reproduced with kind permission from Dr H Emmamy. Hematoxylin–eosin × 185.

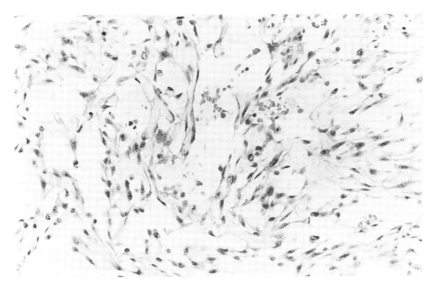

Fig. 15.39B Metaplastic carcinoma, pseudoangiosarcomatous pattern. Another field from the tumor shown in Figure 15.39A. The cells lining the apparent vascular spaces show moderate nuclear pleomorphism. Although the appearances in Figure 15.39A and 15.39B are strongly suggestive of an angiosarcoma, immunostains for endothelial markers (factor VIII, CD 31, CD 34) were all negative. Hematoxylin–eosin × 185.

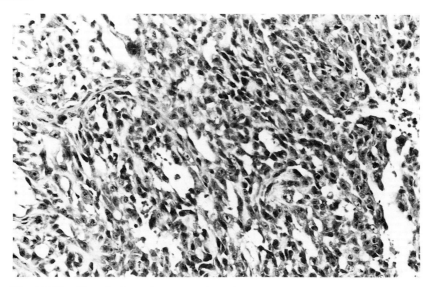

Fig. 15.39C Metaplastic carcinoma, pseudoangiosarcomatous pattern. The structure of the tumor is more solid in this area, with a pronounced spindle cell appearance. From the same case as that shown in Figure 15.39A and B. Hematoxylin–eosin × 185.

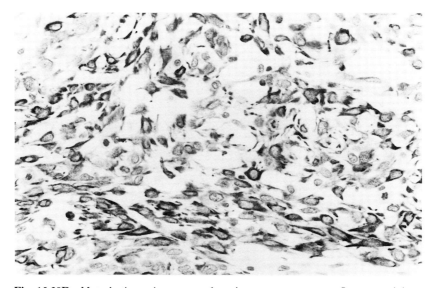

Fig. 15.39D Metaplastic carcinoma, pseudoangiosarcomatous pattern. Immunostaining for a range of epithelial markers including several cytokeratin antibodies (e.g. Cam 5.2, MNF 116, CK 7) showed positive expression in both the 'vascular' and the spindle cell areas (illustrated in this field). From the same case as that shown in Figure 15.39A, B and C. Immunostaining for Cam 5.2 × 400.

MIXED TYPES

Excluding tubular mixed carcinoma, which we regard as a specific tumor type closely allied to pure tubular carcinoma, we recognize two mixed types of invasive carcinoma with a biphasic pattern.[7]

Tumours which are composed of distinct and separate elements of ductal NST and infiltrating lobular carcinoma are entered into the *mixed*

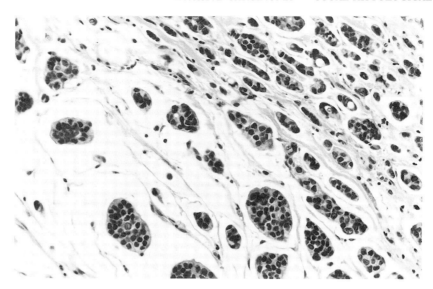

Fig. 15.40 Invasive carcinoma, mixed ductal NST and special type. In this example there is a mucinous element at the lower left which merges with a trabecular ductal NST pattern at the upper right. Overall the latter formed approximately 25% of the tumor area. Hematoxylin–eosin × 185.

ductal and *lobular* category, if the former accounts for between 10 and 90% of the area. These tumors must be distinguished from infiltrating lobular carcinomas of mixed type and also from those ductal NST carcinomas which have an infiltrative pattern resembling ILC. In the NTPBCS this type amounted to just under 5% of cases.

Tumors which are composed of a mixture of tubular, invasive cribriform or mucinous carcinoma with ductal NST, where the latter forms more than 10% of the area are termed *mixed ductal NST* and *special type* (Fig. 15.40). This group therefore includes cases which others might label as mixed invasive cribriform carcinoma[61,63] and mixed mucinous carcinoma.[4,72–74] The main reason for including them all together in one group is to obtain sufficient numbers of cases in an unselected series to assess their prognostic significance. In the NTPBCS this category accounts for 2.5% of cases.

REPRODUCIBILITY AND CONSISTENCY OF DIAGNOSIS

In marked contrast with the comparatively large number of publications concerned with the reproducibility and consistency of histological grading (see Ch. 17) very few formal studies have been carried out in relation to histological type. Histological typing is equally as subjective as grading and it is surprising that so little attention has been paid to this aspect of the subject. The need for such studies is abundantly clear from the marked variation in the reported frequency of the different morphological types referred to in Chapter 13 and illustrated in Table 13.2. Whilst differences in the use of 'mixed' categories may account for some of the variation the wide range for the reported frequency of such special types as infiltrating lobular, medullary and tubular carcinoma can only be explained by differences in interpretation of histological criteria. As noted earlier this view has been reinforced for one type, medullary carcinoma, by a number of studies[43–45] which have found poor reproducibility using the criteria laid down by Fisher et al[14] and Ridolfi et al.[37]

Further evidence is supplied by the results of the UK National External Quality Assessment (EQA) scheme in breast screening pathology[86] (see also Ch. 24). This involved the circulation of sets of 12 histological sections to between 186 and 251 histopathologists associated with the NHS BSP. Over a 3-year period a total of 72 slides were circulated. As one part of this scheme participants were asked to record histological type on a standardized proforma and reproducibility was measured using Cohen's kappa statistic.[87] The overall kappa value for histological type was 0.21, indicating very poor agreement. This result must be interpreted with some caution as the study had not been designed to focus specifically on this aspect of breast screening pathology, but it is, nonetheless, rather worrying.

Further studies are undoubtedly required. These should focus on the reproducibility of the criteria for individual histological types and on typing in general. In the meantime pathologists should follow the relatively strict criteria outlined in this chapter and in other standard works.[3–6]

PROGNOSIS

There is little merit in subdividing invasive carcinoma of the breast into the morphological categories described above unless the exercise has some clinical relevance. There have been surprisingly few comprehensive long-term follow-up studies relating histological type to survival. Dawson and colleagues[88] found a relative excess of tubular, mucinous, medullary and infiltrating lobular carcinomas in patients who had survived at least 25 years after mastectomy compared with those having a survival of less than 10 years. These findings were substantially confirmed in a similar study from Edinburgh[67] with the addition of papillary and invasive cribriform carcinoma among the long-term survivors. A relative excess of special type carcinomas, and in particular the tubular, invasive cribriform and tubular variant or tubular mixed categories, has also been shown amongst tumors detected in the prevalent round of mammographic breast screening.[8,51] Whilst this is interesting information it is more important to establish the actual prognostic implications of each histological type or group of types in terms of long term survival for an individual patient.

There is no doubt that patients with pure tubular carcinoma have an excellent prognosis.[7,53–54,56–57,59] In most studies, including our own, the 10-year survival is at least 90% whilst Cooper et al[57] recorded a 15-year survival of 100%. This is, of course, considerably better than the survival data for ductal NST carcinoma, which at 10 years ranges from 33 to 48%.[7,10,56–57] A similar prognosis has been observed with invasive cribriform carcinoma. Although the data must be interpreted with a little caution because of the relatively small number of cases reported the long-term survival appears to be at least 90%[7] and both Page et al[61] and Venable and colleagues[63] found 100% survival at 10 and 5 years respectively. This is an important, if uncommon, type of breast cancer since it can readily be separated morphologically from ductal NST carcinoma and which offers the same excellent prognosis as tubular carcinoma despite the fact that these tumors are usually larger at presentation.[61] The third tumor type to carry a very good prognosis is the pure mucinous carcinoma, although reported 10-year survival data is more variable, ranging from 68% up to 90%.[7,70,73–74] Even in the study with the poorest survival (68%) Clayton[70] found that the average length of survival was over 11 years, which is in accordance with data presented by Rosen and Wang[89] who concluded that the crude long-term survival of mucinous carcinoma (16-year follow-up) was approximately 70%, but with a median survival of nearly 12 years for those with fatal tumors.

In the section detailing the morphological features of tubular mixed carcinoma we referred briefly to the previous lack of agreement concerning the diagnostic criteria. Much of the debate has related to the prognostic significance of the percentage of tubules present in a tumor, and a number of authorities have accepted a cut-off point of 75% as the lower defining limit for tubular mixed or tubular variant carcinoma.[3–4,54,56] However, in the NTPBCS we investigated the influence on prognosis of percentage tubule formation in several groups, 90–75% (group 1), 75–50% (group 2) and 50–5% (group 3). No significant difference was found between the survival curves of these groups, and a significant survival advantage was identified for groups 2 and 3 combined (< 75% tubule formation) compared with ductal NST carcinoma. We therefore feel justified in using our rather broader definition for tubular mixed carcinomas, especially since the 10-year survival of 69% implies a good prognosis, intermediate between that of pure tubular carcinoma and ductal NST carcinoma.

The position of tubulo-lobular carcinoma is more difficult to establish, partly because there is still a lack of agreement concerning its assignment as a variant of tubular or infiltrating lobular carcinoma[3-4] and partly because of inadequate long-term follow-up data. For example, in Fisher's study[25] clinical details are rather scanty and the only prognostic statement made is that 'treatment failure' was intermediate between that for tubular carcinoma and that for ductal NST carcinoma. Page et al[3] came to a similar conclusion. In our series from the NTPBCS only one death occurred in 15 patients after 10 years follow-up. Although this is a small number of cases the long term survival of 91% points to an excellent prognosis, but it is clear that further confirmatory studies are required.

Despite earlier reports to the contrary[10,90] it has been found that patients with infiltrating lobular carcinoma have a better prognosis than patients with ductal NST carcinoma,[7,26,91] although the 10-year survival of 54% in our own study implies only an average category. Further prognostic information can be obtained by analyzing survival data according to morphological subtype. Thus the classical lobular variant carries a relatively good prognosis[26] with a survival in the NTPBCS of 60%.[7] The mixed lobular group has an average prognosis[26] with a 10-year survival of 55%.[7] Data on pleomorphic lobular carcinoma are limited. They are included within the mixed lobular group by Dixon et al[26] and Ellis et al.[7] Weidner and Semple[28] found a trend towards a poorer prognosis compared with classical ILC, but this was not statistically significant due to the small number of cases studied. Eusebi et al[27] considered pleomorphic lobular carcinoma to be an aggressive tumor; six of the 10 cases in their study died within 42 months of diagnosis and three others developed recurrence or distant metastases. Further data on this uncommon subtype are required, and it may prove to be inappropriate to include it within the mixed group because of its relatively poorer prognosis. Although Fechner[23] suggested that ILC with a solid pattern might have a more favorable prognosis than classical lobular carcinoma this was only based on the absence of lymph node involvement in the six cases described. Both the Edinburgh[26] and the Nottingham[7,92] groups have found that solid lobular carcinoma carries a poor prognosis with a 10-year survival of under 50%. Too few cases of alveolar lobular carcinoma have been reported to provide accurate survival data, but prognosis is probably at the better end of the range, 10-year survival of between 70 and 80% having been recorded.[7,26]

As pointed out earlier it has become widely accepted that medullary carcinoma of the breast carries a good prognosis since the early reports of Moore and Foote[34] and Bloom, Richardson and Field.[36] In this respect the most widely quoted and influential study has been that of Ridolfi et al.[37] They found an overall 84% 10-year survival for medullary carcinoma, compared with 63% for ductal NST carcinoma; the prognosis for atypical medullary carcinoma was intermediate, at 74%. Whilst these figures undoubtedly indicate a significant difference in survival it should be noted that the data for ductal NST indicate a very much better prognosis than that usually recorded for this type (less than 50% survival at 10 years), which raises the possibility of selection bias in the construction of the study. However, Rapin et al,[38] using the diagnostic criteria laid down by Ridolfi et al,[37] have recorded an even higher 10-year survival of 92%, closely similar to that for special type carcinomas; furthermore the comparable survival for 'non-medullary carcinoma' was only 51%, in keeping with most data for ductal NST carcinoma. Similar results have also been recorded by Wargotz and Silverberg[39] although their survival figure of 95% for medullary carcinoma was for 5-year survival only. It should be noted that the number of cases in these latter two studies, 26 and 24, is relatively small.

In contrast with these results a number of other studies have failed to demonstrate a significant survival advantage for medullary carcinoma[7,40–42,45] especially in comparison with the special type carcinomas. The study from Fisher et al[41] is particularly worthy of comment because of the relatively large number of patients included; 332 with typical and 273 with atypical medullary carcinoma. They found that typical medullary carcinoma conveyed a 17% survival advantage at 10 years for patients with node negative disease given no adjuvant systemic therapy, and a closely similar survival advantage for patients with node positive disease treated with adjuvant chemotherapy. On the basis of this data they concluded that the prognosis of medullary carcinoma is not as 'good' as previously perceived. Our own data from the NTPBCS support this contention.[7] Using strict diagnostic criteria we did not find a significant difference in survival between medullary and atypical medullary carcinomas nor between these two groups and ductal NST carcinoma (10-year survival respectively 51, 55 and 47%). The only improvement in survival for medullary carcinoma was in its comparison with grade 3 ductal NST carcinoma which carried only a 40% 10-year survival.

One possible explanation for these conflicting results may be a lack of agreement on the appropriateness of the diagnostic criteria.[43–45] Pedersen et al[42] have taken their work a step further and proposed a simplified histopathological definition based on only two criteria, a syncytial growth pattern and diffuse moderate or marked mononuclear infiltrate. They suggest that these criteria are reproducible with consistency and claim that medullary carcinoma defined in this way has a significantly better prognosis than ductal NST carcinomas of grade 2 or 3. Although Gaffey et al[45] have confirmed that the Pedersen method is reasonably reproducible they found no correlation with survival and it is clear that further studies are required to test these proposals. In the meantime we believe that medullary carcinoma should be regarded as having a moderate rather than a good or excellent prognosis.

It is difficult to obtain accurate estimates of the prognosis of invasive papillary carcinoma partly because many studies have failed to make a distinction between the invasive groups and papillary carcinoma in situ and partly due to their comparative rarity. In the only substantial series of pure invasive papillary carcinoma published to date, Fisher et al[76] concluded that the tumor carries a favorable prognosis. Axillary node metastasis was found in only 32% of the 22 cases in which node sampling was carried out and only four of the 35 patients died, three of unrelated causes. In the NTPBCS we have encountered insufficient cases to provide reliable data, but our anecdotal experience is entirely in keeping with that of Fisher et al.[76]

The prognosis of metaplastic carcinomas is unclear since much of the data is derived from small series of cases. However, they are generally believed to carry a poorer prognosis than more common types of breast carcinoma.[93] Patients with the biphasic sarcomatoid type of metaplastic carcinoma appear to have a very poor prognosis; Wargotz et al reported that the 5-year survival for patients with 'carcinosarcoma' was about 50% overall and fell as low as 35% for women with TNM stage 3 disease.[81] The same authors have, however, reported a 5-year survival of 64% for the 'matrix-producing' subtype of metaplastic carcinoma.[85]

As we pointed out above, in order to assess the prognostic information which can be obtained from histological type in as much depth as possible we have recognized a number of mixed patterns in the NTPBCS.[7] The tubular mixed carcinomas have already been discussed; they carry a good prognosis, intermediate between that of the special types and ductal NST carcinoma. A closely similar prognosis was found for tumors which were designated as mixed ductal NST/Special type, 64% 10-year survival. This is in agreement with data obtained for the mixed variant of invasive cribriform carcinoma[61,63] and the mixed type of mucinous carcinoma,[73] both of which are included in our overall mixed ductal NST/Special type category. Although this group is relatively small (2.5% of the total in the NTPBCS) it is worth separating from ductal NST carcinomas as it can be considered to carry a relatively good prognosis.

We have found the mixed ductal and lobular group to have less prognostic value. The majority of these cases showed over 50% lobular features (including a mixture of lobular subtypes) admixed with ductal NST carcinoma. However, no significant improvement in survival over ductal NST carcinoma was found, and it is therefore doubtful whether such cases are worth classifying as a separate entity.

In summary, it is clear that assessment of histological type can provide valuable prognostic information. Further discussion of its relative value, especially in comparison with histological grade, is provided in Chapter 18.

REFERENCES

1. World Health Organization. International histological classification of tumours. Histologic types of breast tumours. Geneva: World Health Organization, 1981.

2. Azzopardi JG, Chepick OF, Hartmann WH et al. The World Health Organization histological typing of breast tumors. 2nd ed. Am J Clin Pathol 1982; 78: 806–816.

3. Page DL, Anderson TJ, Sakamoto G. Infiltrating carcinoma: major histological types. In: Page DL, Anderson TJ, eds. Diagnostic histopathology of the breast. London: WB Saunders, 1987; 193–235.

4. Tavassoli FA. Infiltrating carcinomas, common and familiar special types. In: Tavassoli FA, ed. Pathology of the breast. Norwalk: Appleton and Lange, 1992; 293–294.

5. Rosen PP, Oberman HA. Tumors of the mammary gland. Atlas of tumor pathology. Washington: Armed Forces Institute of Pathology 1993. 7th series, fascicle 3.

6. National Co-ordinating Group for Breast Screening Pathology. Pathology Reporting in Breast Cancer Screening. 2nd ed. NHSBSP Publication No 3, 1995.

7. Ellis IO, Galea M, Broughton N et al. Pathological prognostic factors in breast cancer. II. Histological type. Relationship with survival in a large study with long-term follow-up. Histopathol 1992; 20: 479–489.

8. Ellis IO, Galea MH, Locker A et al. Early experience in breast cancer screening: Emphasis on development of protocols for triple assessment. The Breast 1993; 2: 148–153.

9. Murad TM. A proposed histochemical and electron microscopic classification of human breast cancer according to the cell of origin. Cancer 1971; 27: 288–299.

10. McDivitt RW, Stewart FW, Berg JW. Tumors of the breast. Atlas of tumor pathology. Washington: Armed Forces Institute of Pathology 1968. 2nd series, fascicle 2.

11. Scarff RW, Torloni H. Histological typing of breast tumours (International histological classification of tumours, no 2). Geneva: World Health Organization, 1968.

12. Azzopardi JG. Classification of primary breast carcinoma. In: Azzopardi JG, ed. Problems in breast pathology. Philadelphia: Saunders, 1979; 240–257.

13. Wellings SR, Jensen HM, Marcum RG. An atlas of subgross pathology of the human breast with special reference to possible precancerous lesions. J Natl Cancer Inst 1975; 55: 231–273.

14. Fisher ER, Gregorio RM, Fisher B. The pathology of invasive breast cancer. A syllabus derived from findings of the National Surgical Adjuvant Breast Cancer Project (protocol no 4). Cancer 1975; 36: 144–156.

15. Fisher ER, Sass R, Fisher B et al. Pathologic findings from the National Surgical Adjuvant Project for breast cancer (protocol no 4). Discrimination for tenth year treatment failure. Cancer 1984; 53: 712–723.

16. Cornil A-V. Contributions à l'histoire du développement histologique des tumeurs epitheliales (squirrhe, encephaloide, etc). J Anat Physiol 1865; 2: 266–273.

17. Waldeyer W. Die Entwickelung der Carcinome. Arch Pathol Anat Phys Klin Med 1867; 4: 470–523.

18. Haagensen CD, Lane N, Lattes R, Bodian C. Lobular neoplasia (so-called lobular carcinoma in situ) of the breast. Cancer 1978; 42: 737–767.

19. Ewing J. Neoplastic diseases. 1st ed. Philadelphia: Saunders, 1919.

20. Foote FW Jr, Stewart FW. Lobular carcinoma in situ. A rare form of mammary cancer. Am J Pathol 1941; 7: 491–496.

21. Foote FW Jr, Stewart FW. A histologic classification of carcinoma in the breast. Surgery 1946; 19: 74–99.

22. Wheeler JE, Enterline HT. Lobular carcinoma of the breast in situ and infiltrating. Pathol Annu 1976; 11: 161–188.

23. Fechner RE. Histological variants of infiltrating lobular carcinoma of the breast. Hum Pathol 1975; 6: 373–378.

24. Martinez V, Azzopardi JG. Invasive carcinoma of the breast: incidence and variants. Histopathol 1979; 3: 467–488.

25. Fisher ER, Gregorio RM, Redmond C et al. Tubulolobular invasive breast cancer: A variant of lobular invasive cancer. Hum Pathol 1977; 8: 679–683.

26. Dixon JM, Anderson TJ, Page DL et al. Infiltrating lobular carcinoma of the breast. Histopathol 1982; 6: 149–161.

27. Eusebi V, Magalhaes F, Azzopardi JG. Pleomorphic lobular carcinoma of the breast: an aggressive tumour showing apocrine differentiation. Hum Pathol 1992; 23: 655–662.

28. Weidner N, Semple JP. Pleomorphic variant of invasive lobular carcinoma of the breast. Hum Pathol 1992; 23: 1167–1171.

29. O'Rourke S. Personal communication, 1995.

30. Cornford EJ, Wilson ARM, Athanassiou E. Mammographic features of invasive lobular and invasive ductal carcinoma of the breast: a comparative analysis. Br J Radiol 1995; 68: 450–453.

31. Quincey C, Raitt N, Bell J et al. Intracytoplasmic lumina — a useful diagnostic feature of adenocarcinomas. Histopathol 1991; 19: 83–87.

32. Page DL, Anderson TJ. Uncommon types of invasive carcinoma. In: Page DL, Anderson TJ, eds. Diagnostic histopathology of the breast. Edinburgh: Churchill Livingstone, 1987; 236–252.

33. Underwood JCE, Parsons MA, Harris SC et al. Frozen section appearances simulating invasive lobular carcinoma in breast tissue adjacent to inflammatory lesions and biopsy sites. Histopathol 1988; 13: 232–234.

34. Moore OS Jr, Foote FW Jr. The relatively favourable prognosis of medullary carcinoma of the breast. Cancer 1949; 2: 635–642.

35. Pedersen L, Holck S, Schiødt T. Medullary carcinoma of the breast. Cancer Treat Rev 1988; 15: 53–63.

36. Bloom HJC, Richardson WW, Field JR. Host resistance and survival in carcinoma of the breast: a study of 104 cases of medullary carcinoma in a series of 1411 cases of breast cancer followed for 20 years. Br Med J 1970; 3: 181–188.

37. Ridolfi RL, Rosen PP, Port A et al. Medullary carcinoma of the breast — a clinicopathologic study with a ten year follow-up. Cancer 1977; 40: 1365–1385.

38. Rapin V, Contesso G, Mouriesse H et al. Medullary breast carcinoma. A re-evaluation of 95 cases of breast carcinoma with inflammatory stroma. Cancer 1988; 61: 2503–2510.

39. Wargotz ES, Silverberg SG. Medullary carcinoma of the

breast. A clinicopathologic study with appraisal of current diagnostic criteria. Hum Pathol 1988; 19: 1340–1346.

40. Cutler SJ, Black MM, Fried GH et al. Prognostic factors in cancer of the female breast II. Reproducibility of histopathologic classification. Cancer 1966; 19: 75–82.

41. Fisher ER, Kenny JP, Sass R et al. Medullary carcinoma of the breast revisited. Br Cancer Res Treat 1990; 16: 215–229.

42. Pedersen L, Zedeler K, Holck S et al. Medullary carcinoma of the breast, proposal for a new simplified histopathological definition. Br J Cancer 1991; 63: 591–595.

43. Pedersen L, Holck S, Schiødt T et al. Inter- and intraobserver variability in the histopathological diagnosis of medullary carcinoma of the breast, and its prognostic implications. Br Cancer Res Treat 1989; 14: 91–99.

44. Rigaud C, Theobald S, Noël P. Medullary carcinoma of the breast. A multicenter study of its diagnostic consistency. Arch Path Lab Med 1993; 117: 1005–1008.

45. Gaffey MJ, Mills SE, Frierson HF et al. Medullary carcinoma of the breast: interobserver variability in histopathologic diagnosis. Mod Pathol 1995; 8: 31–38.

46. Elston CW, Gresham GA, Rao GS et al. The Cancer Research Campaign (Kings/Cambridge) trial for early breast cancer — pathological aspects. Br J Cancer 1982; 45: 655–669.

47. Hamlin IME. Possible host resistance in carcinoma of the breast: a histological study. Br J Cancer 1968; 22: 383–401.

48. McDivitt RW, Boyce W, Gersell D. Tubular carcinoma of the breast. Am J Surg Pathol 1982; 6: 401–411.

49. Patchefsky A, Shaber GS, Schwartz GF et al. The pathology of breast cancer detected by mass population screening. Cancer 1977; 40: 1659–1670.

50. Anderson TJ, Lamb J, Alexander FE et al. Comparative pathology of prevalent and incident cancers detected by breast screening. Lancet 1986; i: 519–522.

51. Anderson TJ, Lamb J, Donnan P et al. Comparative pathology of breast cancer in a randomized trial of screening. Br J Cancer 1991; 64: 108–113.

52. Rajakariar R, Walker RA. Pathological and biological features of mammographically detected invasive breast carcinomas. Br J Cancer 1995; 71: 150–154.

53. Oberman HA, Fidler WJ. Tubular carcinoma of the breast. Am J Surg Pathol 1979; 13: 387–395.

54. Parl FF, Richardson LD. The histologic and biologic spectrum of tubular carcinoma of the breast. Hum Pathol 1983; 14: 694–698.

55. Carstens PHB, Huvos AG, Foote FW Jr. Tubular carcinoma of the breast: a clinicopathologic study of 35 cases. Am J Clin Pathol 1972; 58: 231–238.

56. Carstens PHB, Greenberg RA, Francis D, Lyon H. Tubular carcinoma of the breast. A long-term follow-up. Histopathol 1985; 9: 271–280.

57. Cooper HS, Patchefsky AS, Krall RA. Tubular carcinoma of the breast. Cancer 1978; 42: 2334–2342.

58. Linell F, Ljungberg O, Andersson I. Breast carcinoma. Aspects of early stages, progression and related problems. Acta Pathol Microbiol Scand 1980; 272: 1–233.

59. Peters GN, Wolff M, Haagensen CD. Tubular carcinoma of the breast — clinical pathologic correlations on 100 cases. Am J Clin Pathol 1981; 58: 138–149.

60. Eusebi V, Foschini MP, Betts CM et al. Microglandular adenosis, apocrine adenosis and tubular carcinoma of the breast. Am J Surg Pathol 1993; 17: 99–109.

61. Page DL, Dixon JM, Anderson TJ et al. Invasive cribriform carcinoma of the breast. Histopathol 1983; 7: 525–536.

62. Sakamoto G, Sugano H, Hartmann WH. Comparative pathological study of breast carcinoma among American and Japanese women. In: McGuire WL, ed. Breast cancer. Advances in research and treatment, vol 4. New York: Plenum, 1981; 211–231.

63. Venable JG, Schwartz AM, Silverberg SG. Infiltrating cribriform carcinoma of the breast: a distinctive clinicopathologic entity. Hum Pathol 1990; 21: 333–338.

64. Tavassoli FA, Norris HJ. Breast carcinoma with osteoclast-like giant cells. Arch Pathol Lab Med 1986; 110: 636–639.

65. Saout L, Leduc M, Suy-Beng PT, Meignie P. Présentation d'un nouveau cas de carcinoma mammaire cribriforme associé à une réaction histocytaire giganto-cellulaire. Arch Anat Cytol Pathol 1985; 33: 58–61.

66. Holland R, Van Haelst UJGM. Mammary carcinoma with osteoclast-like giant cells. Cancer 1984; 53: 1963–1973.

67. Dixon JM, Page DL, Anderson TJ et al. Long term survivors after breast cancer. Br J Surg 1985; 72: 445–448.

68. Deos PH, Norris HJ. Well-differentiated (tubular) carcinoma of the breast. A clinicopathologic study of 145 pure and mixed cases. Am J Clin Pathol 1982; 78: 1–7.

69. Chopra S, Evans AJ, Pinder SE et al. Pure mucinous breast cancer — mammographic and ultrasound findings. Clin Radiol 1996; 51: 421–424.

70. Clayton F. Pure mucinous carcinomas of the breast: morphologic features and prognostic correlates. Hum Pathol 1986; 17: 34–38.

71. Rasmussen BB, Rose C, Thorpe SM et al. Argyrophilic cells in 202 human mucinous carcinomas. Relation to histopathologic and clinical factors. Am J Clin Pathol 1985; 84: 737–740.

72. Rasmussen BB, Rose C, Christensen JB. Prognostic factors in primary mucinous breast carcinoma. Am J Clin Pathol 1987; 87: 155–160.

73. Komaki K, Sakamoto G, Sugano H et al. Mucinous carcinoma of the breast in Japan. A prognostic analysis based on morphologic features. Cancer 1988; 61: 989–996.

74. André S, Cunha F, Bernardo M et al. Mucinous carcinoma of the breast: a pathologic study of 82 cases. J Surg Oncol 1995; 58: 162–167.

75. Rosen PP. Mucocele-like tumors of the breast. Am J Surg Pathol 1986; 10: 464–469.

76. Fisher ER, Palekar AS, Redmond C et al. Pathologic findings from the National Surgical Adjuvant Breast Project (Protocol No 4). VI. Invasive papillary cancer. Am J Clin Pathol 1980; 73: 313–322.

77. Siriaunkgul S, Tavassoli FA. Invasive micropapillary carcinoma of the breast. Mod Pathol 1993; 6: 660–662.

78. Luna More S, Gonzalez B, Acedo C et al. Invasive micropapillary carcinoma of the breast. A new special type of invasive mammary carcinoma. Pathol Res Pract 1994; 190: 668–674.

79. Tavassoli FA. Classification of metaplastic carcinomas of the breast. Pathol Annu 1992; 27: 89–119.

80. Foschini MP, Dina RE, Eusebi V. Sarcomatoid neoplasms of the breast: proposed definitions for biphasic and monophasic sarcomatoid mammary carcinomas. Semin Diagn Pathol 1993; 10: 128–136.

81. Wargotz ES, Norris HJ. Metaplastic carcinomas. III. Carcinosarcoma. Cancer 1989; 64: 1490–1499.

82. Wargotz ES, Deos PH, Norris HJ. Metaplastic carcinomas. II. Spindle cell carcinoma. Hum Pathol 1989; 20: 732–740.

83. Eusebi V, Cattani MG, Caccarelli C et al. Sarcomatoid carcinomas of the breast: An immunocytochemical study of 14 cases. Progr Surg Pathol 1989; 10: 83–99.

84. Banerjee SS, Eyden BP, Wells S et al. Pseudoangiosarcomatous carcinoma: a clinicopathological study of seven cases. Histopathol 1992; 21: 13–23.

85. Wargotz ES, Norris HJ. Metaplastic carcinomas of the breast. I. Matrix-producing carcinoma. Hum Pathol 1989; 20: 628–635.

86. Sloane JP, National Coordinating Group for Breast Screening Pathology. Consistency of histopathological reporting of breast lesions detected by screening: findings of the UK National External Quality Assessment (EQA) Scheme. Eur J Cancer 1994; 30A: 1414–1419.

87. Cohen JA. A coefficient of agreement for nomimal scales. Educ Psychol Measurements 1960; 20: 37–46.

88. Dawson PJ, Ferguson DJ, Karrison T. The pathologic findings of breast cancer in patients surviving 25 years after radical mastectomy. Cancer 1982; 50: 2131–2138.

89. Rosen PP, Wang T-Y. Colloid carcinoma of the breast. Analysis of 64 patients with long-term follow-up. Am J Clin Pathol 1980; 73: 304.

90. Ashikari R, Huvos AG, Urban JA, Robbins GF. Infiltrating lobular carcinoma of the breast. Cancer 1973; 31: 110–116.

91. Haagensen CD. Small cell carcinoma. In: Haagensen CD, ed. Diseases of the breast. 3rd ed. Philadelphia: Saunders, 1986; 815–832.

92. Du Toit RS, Locker AP, Robertson JFR et al. An evaluation of differences in prognosis and recurrence patterns between invasive lobular and ductal carcinoma. Eur J Surg Oncol 1991; 17: 251–257.

93. Oberman HA. Metaplastic carcinoma of the breast. A clinicopathologic study of 29 patients. Am J Surg Pathol 1987; 11: 918–929.

Rare carcinomas of the breast

GENERAL INTRODUCTION

The difficulty in describing rare tumors of the breast resides not only in the relative lack of acquaintance with these lesions, but also on the definition itself of the term rare. A study of dictionaries is not very helpful since in most cases the word rare is defined as 'not very frequent'! Consequently, to establish the line below which a specific type of carcinoma of the breast is not frequent would be the object of endless discussions. We have decided, therefore, only to include entities of which most pathologists have not had direct experience and which have been the subject of relatively few papers in the literature. We are conscious that we have not included all the rarities reported in breast in the world literature, but have chosen only those of which we have had personal experience, or have seen by the courtesy of various colleagues who were kind enough to let us study part of their material.

SQUAMOUS CELL CARCINOMA (SCC)

INTRODUCTION

The incidence of SCC of the breast is very variable in different series depending on the selection criteria used. In some series SCC of the skin overlying the breast have been grouped with identical tumors arising in the breast parenchyma.[1] In others SCC have been lumped together with 'sarcomatoid' carcinomas and with mixed adenosquamous carcinomas,[2] or grouped with cases of phyllodes tumor showing features of squamous carcinoma in the glandular component.[3] In addition, squamous differentiation in invasive carcinoma of no special type (ductal NST) is not uncommon, being recognized in 3.6% of the 1000 cases reviewed by Fisher,[4] whilst squamous cell areas were seen in up to 16% of the cases of medullary carcinoma reported by Ridolfi.[5] All five cases of pure squamous cell carcinoma diagnosed on light microscopy by Woodard[6] displayed areas of glandular differentiation when observed at ultrastructural level. It appears then that the definition of SCC resides on the criteria used. If these are strict and only primary SCC which has not arisen in phyllodes tumors and does not show glandular differentiation is accepted, the real incidence is less than 0.1%.[7] If these strict criteria are followed, it appears that only 10 published cases are well enough documented to be accepted as pure squamous cell carcinomas of the breast.[3,7-11,19]

MACROSCOPIC APPEARANCES

Pure squamous cell carcinomas of the breast are usually large tumors. With the exception of two of the cases reported by Fisher[3] all measure more than 4 cm in their greatest axis and have infiltrative margins. Cysts of variable size may be visible on the cut surface.

MICROSCOPIC APPEARANCES

These tumors show large sheets or strands of moderately to well differentiated squamous cell carcinoma (Fig. 16.1) which surround cystic spaces. In the lumina of the cysts there is nuclear debris, together with globoid atypical keratotic cells, reminiscent of those seen in acantholytic SCC (Figs 16.2 and 16.3).[6] No intracytoplasmic mucosubstances are seen. In contrast abundant stromal mucopolysaccharides may be present, as cases of SCC with abundant myxoid stroma (Fig. 16.4) have been described.[13] The neoplastic cells express only high molecular weight keratins (HWK) as opposed to ductal NST carcinomas with squamous differentiation which in addition express low molecular weight keratins (LWK).[11]

It has been suggested that SCC of the breast originate from epidermal or dermoid cysts, in view of the finding that they frequently show central

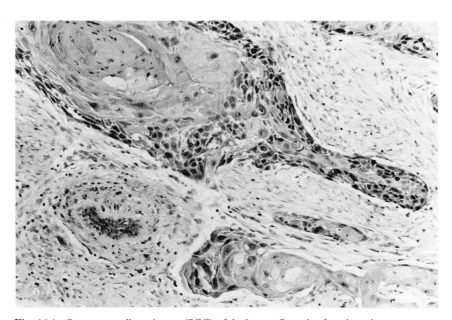

Fig. 16.1   Squamous cell carcinoma (SCC) of the breast. Strands of moderately differentiated squamous cell carcinoma are adjacent to an atrophic mammary duct. Hematoxylin–eosin × 125.

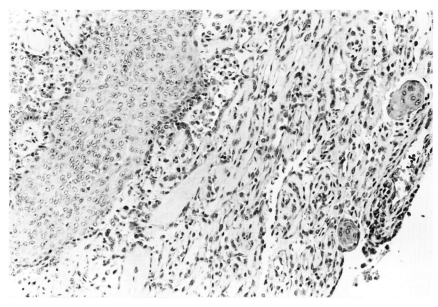

Fig. 16.2 Acantholytic SCC. Squamous neoplastic cells dissect the connective tissue, creating pseudovascular channels. Hematoxylin–eosin × 40.

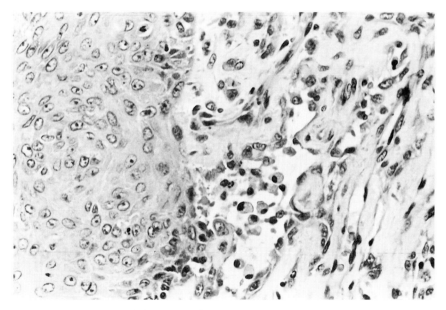

Fig. 16.3 Acantholytic SCC. Microcystic spaces contain cellular debris and atypical keratinocytes. Hematoxylin–eosin × 250.

cavitations. However, it would be difficult to explain the presence of necrotic and acantholytic atypical elements within the lumen of an epidermoid cyst. On the contrary it is more likely that the cyst formation inside a SCC is the result of necrotic cavitation of the tumor.[7]

PROGNOSIS AND MANAGEMENT

Whether pure SCC are very aggressive tumors[7] or have the same degree of malignancy as invasive ductal NST carcinomas[3–4] is still uncertain due to the very limited number of cases reported.

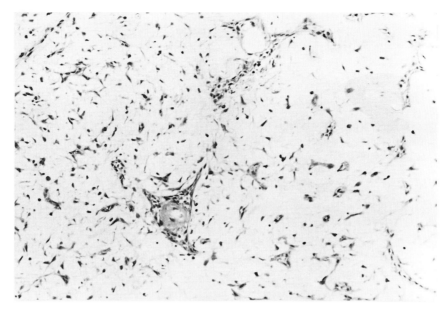

Fig. 16.4   SCC. On rare instances SCC may contain abundant stromal mucopolysaccharides, in which the neoplastic cells are floating. Hematoxylin–eosin × 40.

Management of individual patients should be based on the criteria set out in Chapters 18 and 22.

MUCOEPIDERMOID CARCINOMA (MEC)

MEC were described in salivary glands for the first time in 1945 by Stewart et al.[14] They defined these tumors as frequently cystic and formed by at least three types of cells: mucus producing, intermediate elements and cells with abundant, opaque cytoplasm, possessing squamoid characteristics. If these criteria are applied, MECs of the breast are one of the rarest tumors of this organ, and we believe that only five cases reported in the literature can be accepted as such.

Two low-grade MECs were described by Patchefsky;[15] these had a cystic structure on macroscopic examination. One was the only example of this type in a series of 636 consecutive carcinomas. The two cases reported by Hanna and Kahn[17] also appear consistent with the diagnosis of MEC. In their ultrastructural study, the intermediate cells had at the same time features of myoepithelial and squamous elements which led these authors to suggest a myoepithelial origin for the epidermoid cells. Of the five cases reported by Fisher[3] only one was consonant with the description of Stewart et al,[14] while the remaining cases appear to be invasive carcinomas with divergent squamous and mucinous differentiation. A similar type of divergent differentiation is probably represented by those cases reported by Kovi[16] as high-grade MEC of the breast. This statement is further reinforced by the admission of the authors themselves that the morphological appearance of their cases of high-grade MECs of the breast was somewhat similar histologically to infiltrating ductal NST carcinoma. The age range of the five patients reported to date is 31 to 70 years.[15,17] Mastectomy was carried out in all cases with the exception of Case 2 of Patchefsky[15] which was treated by wide local excision. No axillary lymph node deposits were present and, although overall follow-up was short, all the patients were disease free at the time of publication.

LOW GRADE ADENOSQUAMOUS CARCINOMA (LASC)

This tumour was reported for the first time by Rosen and Ernsberger in 1987 who presented data on 11 cases.[18] It is the breast counterpart of identical skin tumors variously termed microcystic adnexal carcinoma, sclerosing duct carcinoma or sweat gland carcinoma.[19]

The average age of the patients was 59 years (range 42–76). The tumors measured 1.5 to 3.4 cm (average 2.3) and *macroscopically* were firm in consistency, tan yellow in color with an infiltrative edge.

Microscopically the tumors are composed of solid cords and glandular structures with angulated profiles and the infiltrative nature of the margin is confirmed (Figs 16.5 and 16.6). The stroma is frequently 'desmoplastic', characterized by proliferating fibroblasts with plump, elongated, tortuous nuclei. Small lymphocytes either clumped or diffusely dispersed through the lesion are an additional feature. The cytoplasm of the epithelial cells is strongly eosinophilic, reminiscent of 'squamoid' elements. Clear squamous pearls, together with squamous cysts, are seen only infrequently. On close analysis the epithelial tubules have a flattened layer of myoepithelial cells which surround the 'squamoid' elements. By courtesy of Dr H L Peterse we have had the opportunity to study two examples of this tumor, in which the presence of myoepithelial cells was confirmed by the immuno-

localization of actin. The two cases were associated respectively with a ductal adenoma and an adenomyoepithelioma.

Tubular carcinoma can easily be distinguished from LASC as the former lacks myoepithelial cells. In contrast the *differential diagnosis* between LASC and syringomatous adenoma of the nipple is very difficult,[20] if not impossible, especially when LASC, as in one of the cases of Rosen and Ernsberger's series,[18] is located in the subareolar region.

The *prognosis* appears to be relatively good if adequate surgical excision is achieved.[18] No cases recurred after radical mastectomy and no lymph node metastases were seen. In contrast, in four of eight patients treated by local excision alone, the lesion recurred.

ADENOID CYSTIC CARCINOMA (ACC)

INTRODUCTION

Adenoid cystic carcinoma of the breast is a very rare tumor with an extremely good prognosis in contrast with tumors of similar morphology in the salivary glands.[21] Consequently, it is important that stringent criteria are adopted, otherwise

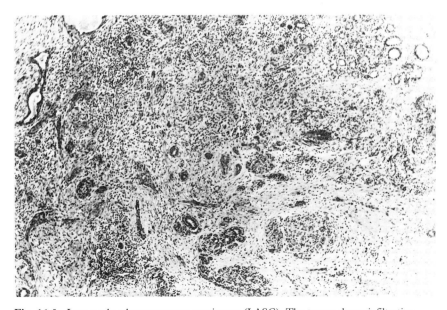

Fig. 16.5 Low grade adenosquamous carcinoma (LASC). The tumor shows infiltrative margins. Hematoxylin–eosin × 40.

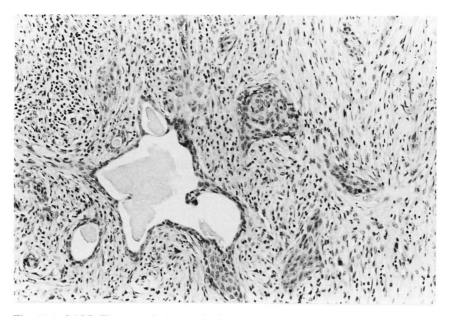

Fig. 16.6   LASC. The tumor is characterized by angulated glands, bordered by cells with eosinophilic cytoplasm, immersed in a desmoplastic stroma containing lymphocytes. Hematoxylin–eosin × 125.

the diagnosis of adenoid cystic carcinoma of the breast loses much of its significance.[22,31]

The literature published before 1979 on the subject was reviewed by Azzopardi,[22] who accepted an incidence of 0.1% for these tumors. An identical incidence was reported by Lamovec et al[23] who found six examples of ACC in a total of 5994 consecutive cases of breast cancer. The histological pattern was predominantly cribriform in two (Fig. 16.7), trabecular-tubular in one (Fig. 16.8) and solid in the remaining cases, showing similar histological features to the analogous tumors of salivary glands. Most of these breast tumors reported in the literature are microinvasive. The size of the cribriform spaces varies and the largest are referred as microcysts.

CLINICAL FEATURES

At least 50% of ACC arise in the sub- or peri-areolar region.[22] They may be painful or tender and unexpectedly cystic. They vary in size from 0.7 to 10 cm, with an average in most reported cases of the order of 3 cm.

MICROSCOPIC APPEARANCES

The neoplastic cellular component is of two types. One is composed of basaloid elements. These have scanty cytoplasm and are grouped in nests or line the cribriform spaces. The other cellular component forms the minority of the total neoplastic proliferation and must be searched for carefully. It has abundant eosinophilic cytoplasm, and lines very small ductule-like structures (Fig. 16.9).

The content of the cribriform spaces comprises two types of mucin. Most of the mucosubstances are alcianophilic, but there are also areas of PAS positive material.[22]

Within the microcysts there are eosinophilic cylinders which are also PAS positive. A thick PAS and collagen IV positive basal lamina outlines the cribriform spaces and the microcystic areas.[24] Epithelial mucin antigen (EMA) and high molecular weight cytokeratin antisera stain the cytoplasm of the cells with abundant eosinophilic cytoplasm, especially when they form glandular structures.[23] In contrast the basaloid cells appear unstained by EMA antiserum.[24] A third type of cell is revealed by immunostaining with anti-smooth

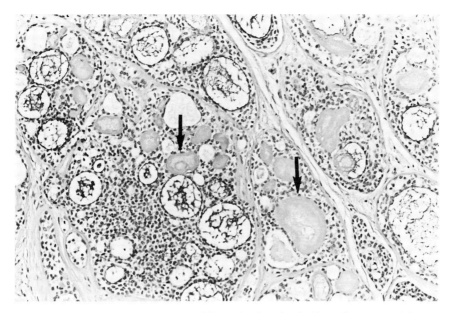

Fig. 16.7 Adenoid cystic carcinoma (ACC) predominantly cribriform. Spaces containing mucins are adjacent to round areas filled with basal lamina-like material (arrow). Hematoxylin–eosin × 125.

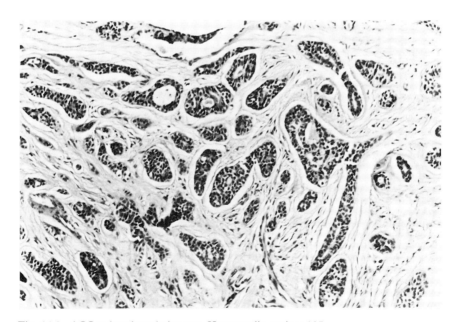

Fig. 16.8 ACC trabecular-tubular type. Hematoxylin–eosin × 125.

muscle actin which demonstrates elements mostly located at the periphery of the basaloid nests.[23] These actin rich elements have been interpreted as myoepithelial cells[23] and this has been con-

firmed at ultrastructural level by Ro et al.[25] Squamous metaplasia was identified in two instances by Lamovec et al[23] who also found several foci of DCIS in one case. Perineural inva-

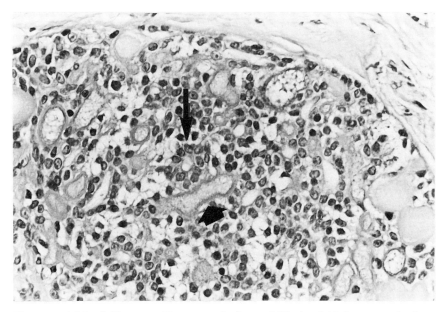

Fig. 16.9 ACC cribriform type. Two types of cells are visible: basaloid elements and cells with eosinophilic cytoplasm (arrow) lining small ductule-like structures. Some spaces are lined by thick basal lamina (arrowhead). Hematoxylin–eosin × 250.

sion and areas of necrosis are very rare. Mitoses are infrequent. No estrogen receptor positivity has ever been found.[24–25]

PROGNOSIS AND MANAGEMENT

Ro et al[25] reported that it is important to grade ACC using the system adopted in salivary glands. All five patients in their series with grade I tumors were either alive without evidence of disease or had died of unrelated causes. Among the six patients with grade II tumors, one developed a local recurrence and pulmonary metastases 5 years after diagnosis, and one died of metastatic ACC 13 years after diagnosis. Finally the only patient with a grade III tumor showed metastatic deposits in four axillary lymph nodes at mastectomy and died of disease with multiple metastases 2 years after surgery.

The same grading system was adopted by Lamovec et al[23] but it appeared of very limited value as no recurrences nor metastases were observed in their cases. No patients in Peters and Wolff's[26] series died of disease, but two developed local recurrence 5 and 8 years after surgery. A third patient was alive after 10 years with radiological evidence of lung and liver metastases. One patient, reported by Lusted,[27] developed a recurrence 22 years after surgery. Therefore, since recurrences may develop 10 to 20 years after initial excision, there is a need for longer follow-up studies than are mostly available.[22]

Since local excision alone may lead to local recurrence and as lymph node metastases are very rare[25,28] it appears that simple mastectomy is the best treatment for ACC.

ADENOMYOEPITHELIOMA (ADMY)

INTRODUCTION

Adenomyoepithelioma is a rare tumor which can occur in the skin, salivary glands and very rarely in the breast.[22,29–30] In salivary glands this tumor is generally termed epimyoepithelial carcinoma.[32]

The entity in the breast was illustrated for the first time by Hamperl[29] and was fully documented by Kiaer et al.[33] The latter authors reported a case in which the disease spanned 18 years and was preceded by a lesion they called adenomyoepithelial adenosis. Eusebi et al[34] reported two cases which

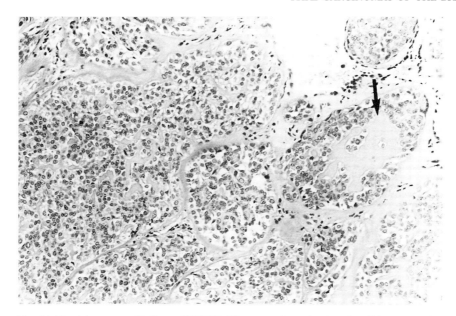

Fig. 16.10 Adenomyoepithelioma (ADMY). The tumor is predominantly solid, composed of nests of both eosinophilic and clear cells. Hyaline basal-like material is abundant (arrow). Hematoxylin–eosin × 125.

also showed the same features described by Kiaer et al[33] including adenomyoepithelial adenosis which was named, for reasons illustrated later, as apocrine adenosis.

Three further cases were reported by Young and Clement,[35] two by Weidner and Levine[36] and one case each by Toth,[37] Zarbo and Oberman,[38] and Jabi et al.[39] Larger series have been reported by Rosen[40] (18 patients) and by Tavassoli[41] (27 cases). However, these latter authors have probably included cases of ductal adenoma in their series.[42]

CLINICAL FEATURES

The age at presentation of ADMY ranges between 27 and 82 years,[40–41] the majority of patients being over 50. The lesion usually presents as a palpable mass.[34,40–41] In one remarkable case reported by Tavassoli,[41] the lesion had been present for 18 years. The nodules are circumscribed and range in size from 1 to 7 cm in diameter.

MICROSCOPIC APPEARANCES

The architecture of these tumors is predominantly solid (Fig. 16.10); in a minority of cases glandular structures are the main element. Whatever the growth pattern, two cell types are constantly seen (Fig. 16.11). One type of cell is basaloid or spindle-shaped with cytoplasm which varies from clear to eosinophilic. These cells constitute the majority of the total neoplastic proliferation, especially when the tumor displays a solid pattern (Fig. 16.12). They form the outer cell layer where glandular structures are present. The cells are glycogen rich, contain actin demonstrable both by immunostaining and electron microscopy,[33] are S-100 protein positive, but are devoid of EMA. The nuclei are round with inconspicuous nucleoli (Fig. 16.13). The glandular structures are lined by columnar to cuboidal cells showing a finely granular eosinophilic to faintly foamy cytoplasm. Their nuclei are globoid with, in general, a prominent nucleolus. These cells stain strongly with EMA and display immunochemical and ultrastructural evidence of apocrine differentiation.[33] In cases showing a solid pattern, confluent areas of necrosis are seen in about 40% (Fig. 16.14).[41]

Mitoses are infrequent and usually do not exceed three mitotic figures/10 HPF.

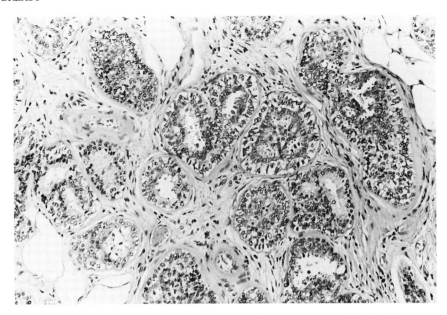

Fig. 16.11   ADMY. In a minority of cases the tumor is predominantly of the glandular type. Two cell types are readily visible. Hematoxylin–eosin × 125.

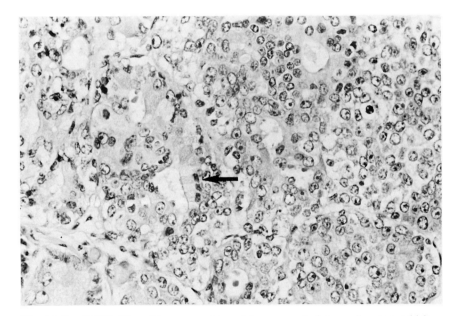

Fig. 16.12   ADMY. The solid component is mainly composed of clear cells among which eosinophilic columnar elements are seen (arrow). Hematoxylin–eosin × 250.

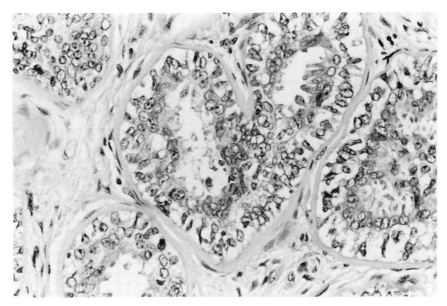

Fig. 16.13   ADMY glandular type. The eosinophilic columnar cells line the lumina of the neoplastic glands, while the clear elements constitute the outer layer. Hematoxylin–eosin × 250.

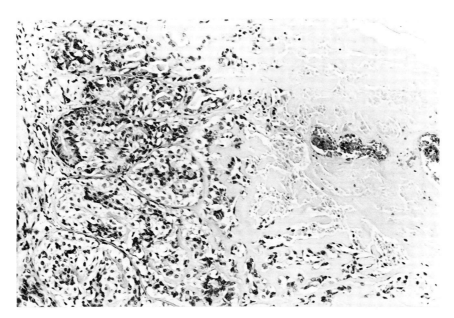

Fig. 16.14   ADMY solid type. This type often shows areas of necrosis. Hematoxylin–eosin × 125.

DIFFERENTIAL DIAGNOSIS

ADMYs differ from clear cell glycogen-rich carcinoma described by Hull and Warfel.[43] Such cases lack a biphasic pattern. Adenoid cystic carcinoma, while showing a biphasic cellular pattern, has a characteristic cribriform structure, the basal lamina lines the microcysts, no apocrine differentiation is seen and, finally, exhibits two types of mucins which are not present in ADMYs.[34]

APOCRINE ADENOSIS

Eusebi et al[34] described a glandular proliferation which was observed in both their cases of ADMY. It was very similar to adenomyoepithelial adenosis which preceded the case reported by Kiaer et al.[33] Apocrine adenosis is formed by glands with large open lumina containing a faintly eosinophilic granular material (Fig. 16.15). The glands are usually lined by two layers of cells. The outer layer is composed of cuboidal cells usually showing clear cytoplasm (Fig. 16.16). These same cells contain smooth cell actin and lie on a prominent and usually thickened basal lamina. The cells lining the

lumina are columnar, have glandular eosinophilic cytoplasm and show ultrastructural and immunological evidence of apocrine differentiation;[34] hence the descriptive name of apocrine adenosis.

Whether this lesion is hyperplastic or neoplastic is very much a matter for debate. In one case it preceded ADMY.[33] In the six instances in which it has been observed by the authors it was adjacent to typical areas of ADMY, with zones of transition between the two. On this evidence it is very likely that this glandular proliferation is part of the spectrum of ADMY. Apocrine adenosis (AA) can mimic microglandular adenosis as well as tubular carcinoma.[44-46] In microglandular adenosis there are smaller and more regular glandular structures with small lumina, while AA displays glands of variable size with large, irregular lumina. In addition, in most cases of microglandular adenosis there is a lack of myoepithelial cells, the gland consisting only of a single layer of epithelial elements which lie on a well formed basal lamina (but see also Ch. 7). Apocrine differentiation is only seen in AA (Table 16.1).[47] In tubular carcinoma (TC) the glands are also lined by a single cell type, and lack both myoepithelial cells and basal lamina. No apocrine differentiation is seen in tubular carci-

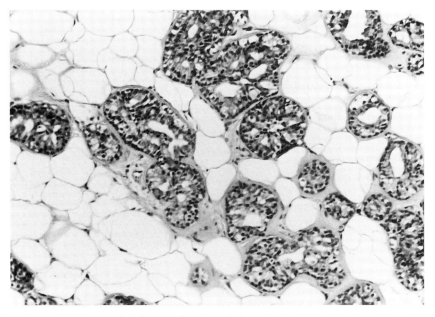

Fig. 16.15   Apocrine adenosis (AA). Large glandular structures are present within adipose tissue. Hematoxylin–eosin × 125.

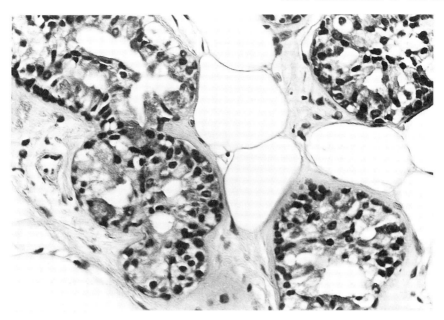

Fig. 16.16   AA. At higher magnification there are two cell layers and the cytoplasm of the luminal epithelial cells is granular. Same case as Figure 16.15. Hematoxylin–eosin × 250.

Table 16.1   Comparison of main diagnostic features of apocrine adenosis, microglandular adenosis and tubular carcinoma

	Apocrine adenosis	Microglandular adenosis	Tubular carcinoma
Size and shape of glands	Large variable	Small round	Variable angular
Myoepithelial cells	+	–	–
Basal lamina	+	+	–
Apocrine differentiation	+	–	–

Modified from Eusebi et al.[47]

noma. The stromal reaction in tubular carcinoma is also useful in distinguishing it from AA, as in TC the stroma is desmoplastic and perivascular elastosis is the rule.[48]

PROGNOSIS AND MANAGEMENT

The behaviour of ADMY of the breast is difficult to predict in view of the very limited number of cases reported. Kiaer et al[33] regarded their case as a carcinoma of low grade malignancy, both on the basis of cytological features and of the multiple recurrences, despite apparently adequate excision. However, there have been few recurrences in most of the cases reported in the literature. Two of 17 women treated by local excision had recurrent

ADMY in the same breast.[40] Apparently these two patients differed from the others as a more florid ductal hyperplasia was present around the lesions. Three out of 27 patients reported by Tavassoli,[41] who had all been treated by local excision, developed recurrences. One of these patients presented the ADMY in the axillary tail. The tumor had areas of anaplasia and the patient had axillary node metastases at the time of presentation. A fourth patient in this same series developed invasive ductal carcinoma in the same breast two and a half years after the excision of the ADMY. Three patients reported by Loose et al,[48] developed recurrences. Their Case 6 had six local recurrences over 52 months treated with re-excisions, mastectomy and radiation therapy. The same patient developed a lung metastasis at 54 months and brain metastases were identified at 60 months. Death occurred at 64 months.

In summary it appears that ADMY in the breast is a tumor of a low malignant potential. Metastases are uncommon and to date only one fatal case has been reported.[48] No recurrences are seen if the patient is treated with mastectomy, with the exception of one case in the series of Loose and colleagues.[48]

MALIGNANT MYOEPITHELIOMA (MM)

If the two cases showing anaplastic areas within ADMY[41] are excluded, there are only three well documented cases of MM of the breast reported so far, two of which developed subsequent metastasis.[49–50] In these cases no epithelial component was present. The neoplastic proliferation was composed of spindle cells which, by definition, showed immunoreactivity for actin and keratin. It appears extremely difficult, if not impossible, to separate these tumors from the monophasic variant of metaplastic (sarcomatoid) carcinoma,[51] especially in view of the fact that no fewer than 10 out of 14 cases with sarcomatoid carcinoma studied by us,[52] displayed actin positive cells in the 'sarcoma-like' component.

It is pertinent that the authors have had the opportunity to examine two cases of ADMY which also had adjacent spindle cell malignant tumor; it seems possible that transitions exists between classical ADMYs and spindle cell pure myoepithelioma which makes the dividing line with sarcomatoid carcinomas extremely subtle.

APOCRINE CARCINOMA

INTRODUCTION

Notable discrepancies exist in the literature concerning the incidence of apocrine carcinomas of the breast. This is partly due to the use of differing morphological criteria with variable levels of stringency. In addition, in recent years additional objective means of diagnosis, such as immunohistochemistry, have been added to conventional diagnostic criteria. This has led to a widening of the spectrum of apocrine carcinoma.

Diagnosis based on light microscopy, sometimes aided by ultrastructural studies, has led to conflicting statements. Frable and Kay[53] found that apocrine carcinomas constitute 1% of mammary carcinomas. A lower incidence of only 0.3% was suggested by Azzopardi.[22] The latter accepted as apocrine carcinoma only those tumors composed largely of easily recognizable apocrine type epithelium, in which the distinctive PAS-positive granules can be found. Mossler et al,[54] in an ultrastructural study, found that apocrine carcinomas constituted 0.4% of their prospective series.

Eusebi et al,[55] in an immunocytochemical and electron microscopical study, reported a 12% incidence of apocrine differentiation in their series of breast carcinomas. These latter authors used an immunoperoxidase technique to localize the antigen GCDFP-15, a unique 15 000 Kd molecular weight glycoprotein, which has become an established marker of apocrine differentiation. 4% of their tumors were dominantly apocrine, at both structural and immunological levels, while in the remaining cases the apocrine differentiation was focal only.

MICROSCOPIC APPEARANCES

Definition by conventional morphology: as Eusebi et al[55] have pointed out, patches of apocrine cell differentiation can be seen in practically any type of carcinoma of the breast, including papillary carcinoma,[58] medullary carcinoma[55] and adenomyoepitheliomas.[34] Ductal carcinoma in situ (DCIS) of comedo, cribriform and micropapillary patterns showing apocrine changes have been reported by Abati et al[57] and apocrine lobular carcinoma in situ has been described by Eusebi et al.[59] Invasive apocrine carcinomas of ductal type were the first type of apocrine carcinoma documented.[54,57] Finally, invasive lobular carcinomas showing apocrine differentiation have also been described.[56]

Apocrine carcinomas, whatever their origin, are usually composed of two intermingled cell types. One type (type A) has been long recognized as apocrine by various authors. It has abundant granular eosinophilic cytoplasm (Fig. 16.17). The granules are PAS positive after diastase digestion.

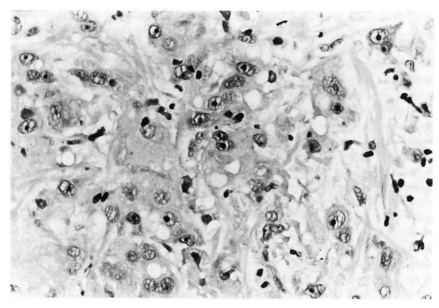

Fig. 16.17 Apocrine carcinoma mainly composed of large cells with eosinophilic granular cytoplasm. Nuclei are globoid with prominent nucleoli. Hematoxylin–eosin × 250.

Mucosubstances are absent in these cells, especially in cases of invasive duct apocrine carcinomas. Their nuclei are globoid with prominent nucleoli. Not infrequently nuclei are hyperchromatic.

The second type of cell (type B) displays abundant cytoplasm in which fine empty vacuoles are seen. This cell appears conspicuously foamy and superficially may resemble histiocytes (Fig. 16.18). The nuclei are similar to those seen in type A cells. In pleomorphic lobular apocrine carcinoma (PLAC) the two types of cell are present in varying degrees. They are very irregular in shape, frequently arranged in single files and show very variable nuclear size, often with multinucleation, hence the definition of pleomorphic (Figs 16.19–16.22). In rare instances only one type of cell forms the major component of the tumor. When the tumoral elements are formed by foamy type B cells, the name of histiocytoid carcinoma has been used.[59]

Definition by ultrastructure: apocrine carcinomas have been defined ultrastructurally as possessing an extensive rough endoplasmic reticulum and numerous (400–600 μ) osmiophilic granules. Ultrastructural study of a case of invasive lobular carcinoma with immunohistochemical evidence of apocrine differentiation[59] showed that only 5% of neoplastic elements exhibited osmiophilic membrane-bound granules, whereas most of the cells contained numerous empty vesicles, a prominent Golgi apparatus and large mitochondria with incomplete cristae. In these, characteristic osmiophilic granules, which measured 303–727 mm, were seen in about 10% of the overall neoplastic cell population. In contrast the majority of the neoplastic cells contained numerous empty vesicles of about the same dimensions as the osmiophilic granules. Mazoujan et al[61] demonstrated by an immunogold technique that the GCDFP-15 is localized to the ultrastructural vesicles as well as to the osmiophilic granules.

Definition by immunohistochemistry: Mazoujan et al[62] using an immunoperoxidase technique, were able to localize an apocrine gland related antigen to specific tissue sites. This antigenic marker called Gross Cystic Disease Fluid Protein (GCDFP-15) is a unique glycoprotein initially isolated from the fluid of breast cysts. It is present in apocrine glands at all sites, including the apocrine glands of the axilla and 'metaplastic' apocrine epithelium in the breast. Salivary glands are also positive for this marker. Using a polyclonal anti-

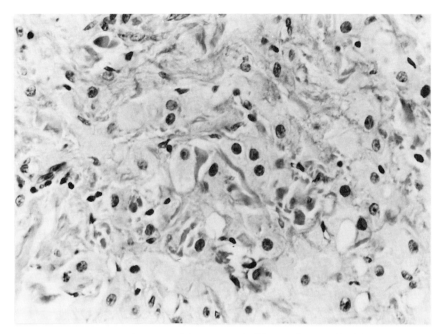

Fig. 16.18 Apocrine carcinoma, mainly composed of foam cells, superficially resembling histiocytes. Hematoxylin–eosin × 250.

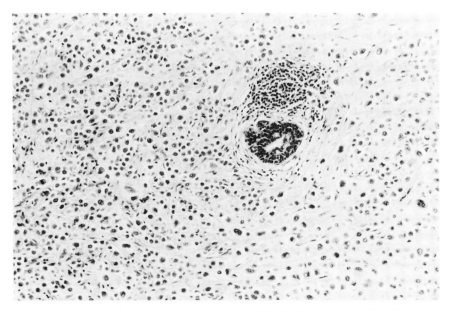

Fig. 16.19 Pleomorphic lobular apocrine carcinoma (PLAC). Pleomorphic cells infiltrate the breast tissue, in a single file, non-cohesive pattern. Hematoxylin–eosin × 40.

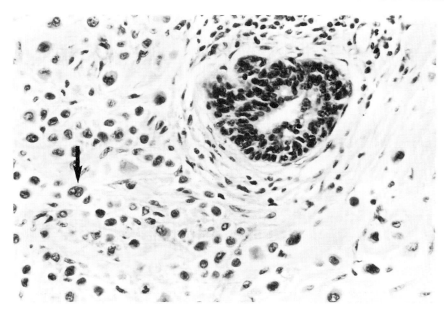

Fig. 16.20   PLAC. Cells show irregular size and shape, nuclei are irregular in size. Binucleated cells are present (arrow). Hematoxylin–eosin × 250.

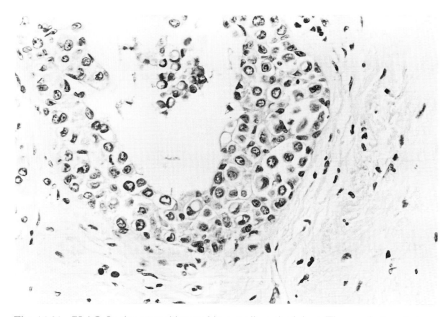

Fig. 16.21   PLAC. In situ pagetoid spread in a medium sized duct. The neoplastic cells have the same cytological characteristics as the invasive component. Hematoxylin–eosin × 250.

serum Mazoujan et al,[62] demonstrated that 14 of 30 (46%) breast carcinomas they studied were of apocrine type, including 12 of 16 cases diagnosed as apocrine carcinomas on morphologic grounds.

Later Eusebi et al,[55] using the same antiserum as employed by Mazoujan et al,[62] found only 12% of positive cases of which the positivity was patchy in eight cases. The higher percentage found by

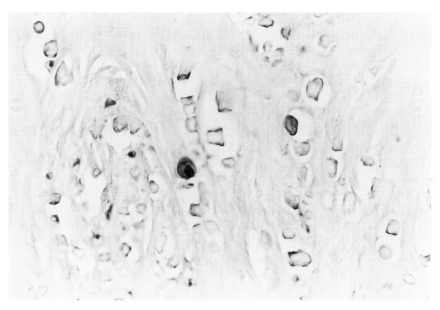

Fig. 16.22 PLAC. Neoplastic cells contain alcianophilic mucins. These are distributed within intracytoplasmic lumina or at one pole of the cell in a crescent-like fashion. (Alcian Blue pH 2.5/PAS after diastase digestion × 400.

Mazoujan et al[62] was probably in part due to an element of case selection. In their series 16 cases were selected because they showed apocrine features in H&E sections. In addition, eight cases were pure in situ carcinomas. The series of Eusebi et al[55] consisted of unselected consecutive tumors and the number of cases was greater.

More recently Wick et al,[63] using a monoclonal antibody directed to the same antigen, studied 105 breast cancers and 585 non-mammary malignancies. It was found that overall, the rates of specificity and sensitivity and the predictive value of a positive result for GCDFP-15 were 95% and 74% respectively. In addition 72% of the 105 breast neoplasms manifested GCDFP-15 immunoreactivity, which in most of the cases was extended to the majority of the neoplastic cellular proliferation.

It appears therefore that a great discrepancy exists in terms of positivity found in the cases of these latter authors and those of Eusebi et al.[55] The higher percentage of positivity in the series of Wick et al[63] is probably due to the fact that the monoclonal antibody they employed recognizes an antigen specific for breast tissue, but different from the one recognized by the polyclonal antibody. Before accepting 74% as a real percentage

of apocrine carcinomas of the breast on the basis of this latter monoclonal antiserum, further studies are required, at least at immunoelectron-microscopical level.

PROGNOSIS AND MANAGEMENT

No age, size, site, prognosis (with the exception of PLAC[56]), nor estrogen or progesterone receptors analysis has been found specific for this form of carcinoma.[55] Survival analysis of 17 patients with invasive ductal carcinomas and apocrine features compared with non-apocrine ductal NST carcinoma cases matched for stage, revealed no statistical difference in estimated recurrence-free survival nor estimated survival probability.[57] Recently Eusebi et al[56] reported 10 cases of PLAC showing apocrine differentiation. Six of the 10 patients died within 42 months of diagnosis. Three other patients developed recurrences or distant metastases at short intervals. These authors concluded that since grading of lobular carcinoma may be difficult, recognition of the pleomorphic apocrine subtype was useful in identifying a lethal variant.

PRIMARY OAT CELL (NEUROENDOCRINE) CARCINOMA (OCC)

Primary oat cell carcinomas of the breast are one of the rarest forms of breast carcinoma. To accept an OCC as primary in the breast, the possibility of a metastasis from a bronchial OCC must be excluded since it is well known that lung is the most common site of origin of secondary deposits to the breast.[68] To date only six cases have been reported in the literature.[64–66] With the exception of Case 1 from the series described by Papotti et al[66] in which the patient was free of disease 44 months after operation, in all the other cases these tumors appeared fatal. The age of the patients varied from 41 to 69 years old, and the average size was 3 cm, with the exception of the case reported by Wade et al[64] which measured 10 cm in diameter. Vascular invasion was visible in all cases and in situ lesions, cytologically similar to the invasive area, were present in all four cases described by Papotti and colleagues.[66] Histologically all tumors showed features compatible with those currently accepted for oat cell carcinoma (Fig. 16.23).[69] In addition at least one case displayed cells with round 'clear' nuclei, suggestive of Merkel cell carcinoma. The endocrine differentiation of these tumors was proven at electron microscopic, immunocytochemical and genetic levels;[66] two of the cases showed endocrine-like granules ultrastructurally as seen by Hattori[67] in oat cell carcinomas of the lung. In addition three cases were immunocytochemically positive for neuron specific enolase, gastrin-releasing peptide/bombesin (GRP), serotonin, synaptophysin and leu 7. Chromogranin A and B were demonstrated in two of such cases respectively at both protein and gene levels by immunohistochemistry and in situ hybridization.

The acceptance of endocrine neoplasms in breast, in contrast with other sites, has generated more than a decade of debate. The scientific evidence, including genetic proof, all points towards the existence of neoplastic endocrine tumors. Their denial can lead only to sterile discussion. It seems more appropriate to investigate the way in which endocrine tumors of breast differ from those of other organs.

CLEAR CELL CARCINOMA (GLYCOGEN RICH) (CCC)

Clear cell glycogen rich carcinoma (CCC) was depicted by Azzopardi in 1979,[22] who defined it

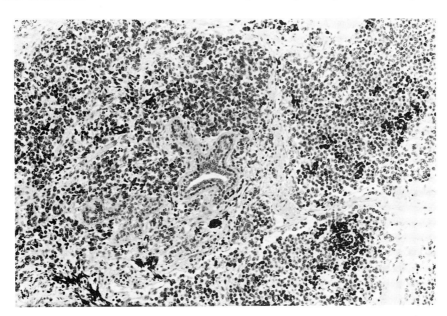

Fig. 16.23 Oat cell carcinoma (OCC). A proliferation of small neoplastic cells surrounds a mammary duct. Focally filamentous degeneration of the nuclei is seen. Hematoxylin–eosin × 40.

as a bulky, usually well circumscribed tumor showing extensive necrosis. The clear cells may be so numerous that the possibility of metastatic carcinoma, especially from the kidney, must be considered. The in situ component is usually inconspicuous. The neoplastic cells show abundant cytoplasmic glycogen and lack mucins. Lipofuscin-rich PAS positive cytoplasmic globules are also a feature of this tumor. Among the neoplastic cells a modest amount of stroma is present and no elastosis is seen. Benisch et al[70] reported on a case histologically identical to those described by Azzopardi.[22] Ultrastructurally the neoplastic elements showed open spaces where glycogen had been found. Hull and Warfel[43] reported on 10 cases structurally and cytologically identical to those previously described, with the exception of one case which appeared partly papillary. They also referred to another similar case of their own which had been reported previously,[71] and which also displayed a papillary type of growth.

The incidence of CCC is 0.9% according to Hull et al[71] which is probably an overestimate. Fisher et al[72] reported on 45 cases of CCC which constituted an incidence of 3% of their 1510 cases. This exceedingly high incidence is probably due to the inclusion of invasive histiocytoid apocrine carcinomas, which superficially may appear similar as a consequence of their foamy clear cytoplasm. CCC should be distinguished from clear cell adenomyoepitheliomas. These latter tumors show a biphasic type of growth and glandular apocrine differentiation. The possibility of a metastatic deposit from kidney or thyroid must also be considered. The clinical history together with immunohistochemistry are often helpful. Renal clear cell carcinoma is a vimentin rich tumor. Vimentin was lacking in two of our cases of CCC. Immunostaining for thyroglobulin is extremely helpful in establishing the correct diagnosis in metastatic clear cell carcinomas of thyroid.[73] Finally, histiocytoid carcinomas differ from CCC both on structural and immunohistochemical grounds. Glycogen is a normal constituent of invasive carcinoma of the breast.[72] For an invasive tumor of the breast to qualify as CCC the criteria of a mainly solid tumor composed of a majority of clear cells must be met. Unfortunately it does not seem that these features are of prognostic relevance and the clinical behavior of this lesion is no different from that of invasive carcinomas of ductal NST type.[43,72]

SECRETORY (JUVENILE) CARCINOMA

INTRODUCTION

It is a curious feature in pathology that whenever a lesion is defined by the term 'juvenile', cases occurring in older patients are seen. This applies in breast to juvenile papillomatosis as described by Rosen et al,[74] juvenile fibroadenoma[75] and lastly to juvenile carcinoma.

This entity, first reported in children by McDivitt and Stewart,[76] was later described in adults,[77-78,80] including an 87-year-old patient.[80] To date, fewer than 100 cases have been published, of which approximately two thirds are in adults. In a survey of 5000 cases of breast carcinoma Norris and Taylor[77] found 135 tumors in women less than 30 years old, and six of this latter group were of juvenile secretory type, an incidence of only 4%, even in this highly selected group. Most of the cases have been described in females, but cases seen in male children[81-82] and in two adult men[83-84] have also been reported.

MACROSCOPIC APPEARANCES

Secretory carcinomas usually present as circumscribed, mobile masses, which are frequently in a subareolar location. Their size varies from 0.5 to 12 cm. Larger tumors are seen in adult patients only.[85] In most cases there is central fibrosis. Multifocality is very uncommon. Nevertheless in a case reported by Krausz et al[83] about 20 nodules measuring between 1 and 4 mm in diameter were found in the excised breast.

MICROSCOPIC APPEARANCES

Microscopically the tumors are mostly circumscribed in outline. Focal areas of invasion of adipose tissue are seen. Three patterns are present in varying combination: honeycombed, compact and tubular.[83] The tubular pattern is mostly present in

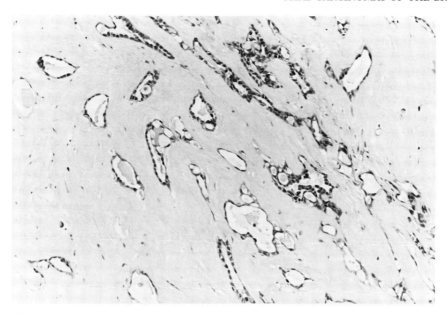

Fig. 16.24 Secretory (juvenile) carcinoma, tubular pattern. The lesion is composed of elongated and angulated glands, immersed in a fibrous stroma. Hematoxylin–eosin × 40.

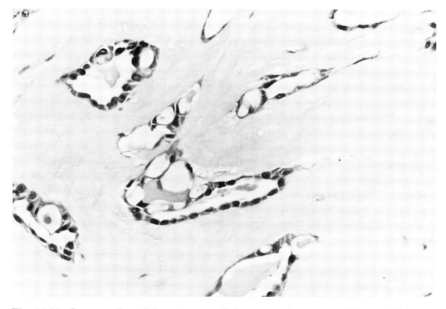

Fig. 16.25 Secretory (juvenile) carcinoma, tubular pattern (same case as Figure 16.24). The tubules are lined by cuboidal to flat cells. Hematoxylin–eosin × 125.

the central fibrotic areas (Figs 16.24 and 16.25). Tubules are angulated and lined by cuboidal to flat cells. The honeycomb pattern is composed of follicular and microcystic structures which give a spongy appearance at low power, superficially resembling an acinic cell carcinoma of the salivary glands (Fig. 16.26). This structure merges with the solid pattern in which occasional microcysts

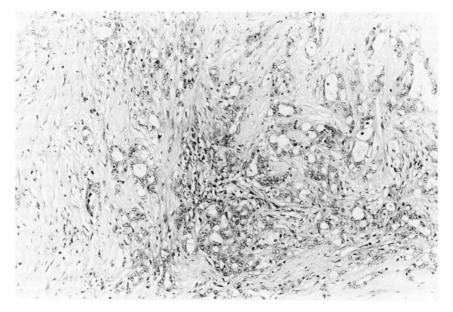

Fig. 16.26 Secretory (juvenile) carcinoma, honeycomb pattern: follicles and microcystic structures give a spongy appearance to the tumor. Hematoxylin–eosin × 40.

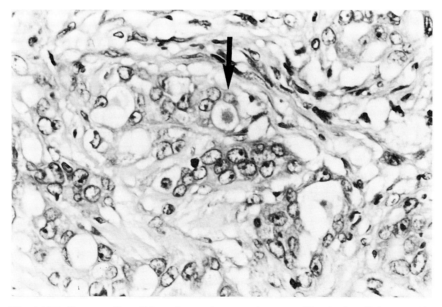

Fig. 16.27 Secretory (juvenile) carcinoma, honeycomb pattern. Neoplastic cells have ovoid nuclei with small nucleoli. Intracytoplasmic lumina are present (arrows). Hematoxylin–eosin × 250.

are seen. The neoplastic cells have a large amount of pale staining cytoplasm. The nuclei are ovoid and have a small nucleolus (Fig. 16.27). Intracytoplasmic lumina (ICL), of variable size, are

frequent; fusion of the larger ICL probably generates the microcystic structures. Mitoses are very scanty and necrotic areas are practically absent. The secretion in the honeycombed spaces, as well as in the ICL, is PAS positive after diastase digestion and stains with Alcian Blue at pH 2.5. An abundance of sialomucins has been demonstrated[83] and human alpha lactalbumin has been localized by Botta et al.[85]

Ductal carcinoma in situ has been reported in association with the main tumor.[83,86] When present the DCIS has the same histological features as the invasive counterpart.

ULTRASTRUCTURE

The neoplastic cells are characterized by large cytoplasmic electron-dense secretory granules as well as intracytoplasmic lumina.[78] Numerous microvilli abut into the ICL lumina. Microcysts are also lined by microvilli. The lumina are filled with a densely granular secretory material with electron dense central spheres.

PROGNOSIS AND MANAGEMENT

Secretory breast carcinomas appear to have an extremely favorable prognosis in children and adolescents. Isolated recurrences in children are the exception[87] although, interestingly, the risk of nodal involvement is similar in young and old patients (Fig. 16.28).[80] Systemic metastases or deaths attributable to this tumor are unknown in childhood.[83] Secretory carcinomas in adult women are more aggressive. The first case of recurrent secretory carcinoma was reported by Sullivan et al.[87] Other cases with recurrent disease were described by Krausz et al[83] and Rosen and Cranor.[80] Simple mastectomy, as opposed to excision of the tumor, has led to cure, with the exception of the case reported by Meis[88] in which tumor recurred several years after removal of the breast. Axillary lymph node metastases are also seen in adults[78,80,83,89] although they rarely involve more than three lymph nodes.[78,80,83,90]

As recurrence of the tumor may appear after 20 years,[83,86] prolonged follow-up is advocated to assess accurately the biological behavior of the tumor. Two cases only, up to the present, have proved fatal. One died of disseminated tumor within 10 months of radical mastectomy for a 6 cm tumor with involvement of lymph nodes.[78] The second case occurred in an adult male who had a 4 cm tumor.[83] He was treated with simple mastectomy and radiotherapy and survived for 20 years before developing distant metastases.

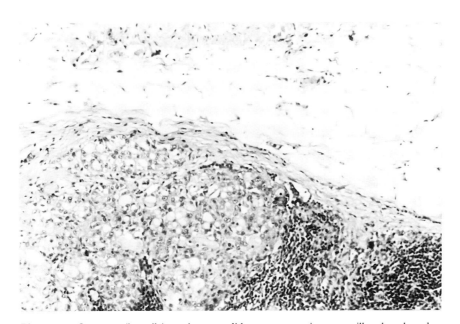

Fig. 16.28 Secretory (juvenile) carcinoma, solid type, metastatic to an axillary lymph node. Hematoxylin–eosin × 250.

Mastectomy appears necessary for large primary tumors to control recurrent disease. There is no evidence at the present that radiotherapy is effective.[80]

REFERENCES

1. Cornog JL, Mobini J, Steiger E, Enterline HT. Squamous carcinoma of the breast. Am J Clin Pathol 1971; 55: 410–417.
2. Dalla Palma P, Parenti A. Squamous breast cancer: report of two cases and review of the literature. Appl Pathol 1983; 1: 14–24.
3. Fisher ER, Gregorio RM, Palekar AS, Paulson JD. Mucoepidermoid and squamous cell carcinomas of breast, with reference to squamous metaplasia and giant cell tumors. Am J Surg Pathol 1983; 7: 15–27.
4. Fisher ER, Gregorio RM, Fisher B. The pathology of invasive breast cancer. A syllabus derived from findings of the National Surgical Adjuvant Breast Project (Protocol 4). Cancer 1975; 36: 1–85.
5. Ridolfi RL, Rosen PP, Port A et al. Medullary carcinoma of the breast. A clinicopathologic study with 10 year follow-up. Cancer 1977; 40: 1365–1385.
6. Woodard BH, Brinkhous AD, McCarty KS Sr, McCarty KS Jr. Adenosquamous differentiation in mammary carcinoma. An ultrastructural and receptor study. Arch Pathol Lab Med 1980; 104: 130–133.
7. Toikkanen S. Primary squamous cell carcinoma of the breast. Cancer 1981; 48: 1629–1632.
8. Arffmann E, Hojgaard K. Squamous carcinoma of the breast: report of a case. J Pathol 1965; 90: 319–320.
9. Essex WB, Rigg BM. Squamous carcinoma of the breast: report of a case. Austral N Zealand J Surg 1965; 34: 207–210.
10. Hasleton PS, Misch KA, Vasudev KS, George D. Squamous carcinoma of the breast. J Clin Pathol 1978; 31: 116–124.
11. Cattani MG, Ceccarelli C. Carcinoma squamoso della mammella. Studio immunocitochimico. Pathologica 1987; 79: 457–468.
12. Eusebi V, Lamovec J, Cattani MG et al. Acantholytic variant of squamous cell carcinoma of the breast. Am J Surg Pathol 1986; 10: 855–861.
13. Foschini MP, Fulcheri F, Baracchini P et al. Squamous cell carcinoma with prominent myxoid stroma. Hum Pathol 1990; 21: 855–859.
14. Stewart FW, Foote FW Jr, Becker WF. Mucoepidermoid tumors of salivary glands. Ann Surg 1945; 122: 820–844.
15. Patchefsky AS, Frauenhoffer CM, Krall RA, Cooper HS. Low-grade mucoepidermoid carcinoma of the breast. Arch Pathol Lab Med 1979; 103: 196–198.
16. Kovi J, Duong HD, Leffall LD Jr. High grade mucoepidermoid carcinoma of the breast. Arch Pathol Lab Med 1981; 105: 612–614.
17. Hanna W, Kahn HJ. Ultrastructural and immunohistochemical characteristics of mucoepidermoid carcinoma of the breast. Hum Pathol 1985; 16: 941–946.
18. Rosen PP, Ernsberger D. Low-grade adenosquamous carcinoma. A variant of metaplastic mammary carcinoma. Am J Surg Pathol 1987; 11: 351–358.
19. Santa Cruz DJ. Sweat gland carcinomas: a comprehensive review. Sem Diagn Pathol 1987; 4: 38–74.
20. Rosen PP. Syringomatous adenoma of the nipple. Am J Surg Pathol 1983; 7: 739–745.
21. Anthony PP, James PD. Adenoid cystic carcinoma of the breast: prevalence, diagnostic criteria and histogenesis. J Clin Pathol 1975; 28: 647–655.
22. Azzopardi JG. Problems in breast pathology. WB Saunders: London, 1979.
23. Lamovec J, Us-Krasovec M, Zidar A, Kljun A. Adenoid cystic carcinoma of the breast: a histologic, cytologic and immunohistochemical study. Sem Diagn Pathol 1989; 6: 153–164.
24. Due W, Herbst H, Loy V, Stein H. Characterization of adenoid cystic carcinoma of the breast by immunohistology. J Clin Pathol 1989; 42: 470–476.
25. Ro JY, Silva EG, Gallager HS. Adenoid cystic carcinoma of the breast. Hum Pathol 1987; 18: 1276–1281.
26. Peters GN, Wolff M. Adenoid cystic carcinoma of the breast. Report of 11 new cases: review of the literature and discussion of biological behaviour. Cancer 1982; 52: 680–686.
27. Lusted D. Structural and growth patterns of adenoid cystic carcinoma of the breast. Am J Clin Pathol 1970; 54: 419–425.
28. Wells CA, Nicoll S, Ferguson DJP. Adenoid cystic carcinoma of the breast: a case with axillary lymph node metastasis. Histopathol 1986; 10: 415–424.
29. Hamperl H. The myothelia (myoepithelial cells) normal state; regressive changes; hyperplasia tumors. Curr Top Pathol 1970; 53: 161–213.
30. Collina G, Gale N, Visona A et al. Epithelial-myoepithelial carcinoma of parotid gland: a clinicopathologic and immunohistochemical study of 7 cases. Tumori 1991; 77: 257–263.
31. Tavassoli FA. Infiltrating carcinoma, special types. In: Tavassoli FA, ed. Pathology of the breast. Norwalk: Appleton and Lange, 1992; 349–423.
32. Seifert G, Brocherious C, Cardesa A, Eveson JW. WHO International Classification of Tumours. Tentative histological classification of salivary gland tumours. Path Res Pract 1990; 186: 555–581.
33. Kiaer H, Nielsen B, Paulsen S et al. Adenomyoepithelial adenosis and low-grade malignant adeno-myoepithelioma of the breast. Virchows Archiv (A) Pathol Anat 1984; 405: 55–67.
34. Eusebi V, Casadei GP, Bussolati G, Azzopardi JG. Adenomyoepithelioma of the breast with a distinctive type of apocrine adenosis. Histopathol 1987; 11: 305–315.
35. Young RH, Clement PB. Adenomyoepithelioma of the breast. A report of three cases and review of the literature. Am J Clin Pathol 1988; 89: 308–314.
36. Weidner N, Levine JD. Spindle-cell adenomyoepithelioma of the breast. A microscopic, ultrastructural and immunocytochemical study. Cancer 1988; 62: 1561–1567.

37. Toth J. Benign human mammary myoepithelioma. Virchows Archiv (A) Pathol Anat 1977; 374: 263–269.

38. Zarbo RJ, Oberman HA. Cellular adenomyoepithelioma of the breast. Am J Surg Pathol 1983; 7: 863–870.

39. Jabi M, Dardick I, Cardigos N. Adenomyoepithelioma of the breast. Arch Pathol Lab Med 1988; 112: 73–76.

40. Rosen PP. Adenomyoepithelioma of the breast. Hum Pathol 1987; 18: 1232–1237.

41. Tavassoli FA. Myoepithelial lesions of the breast. Myoepitheliosis, adenomyoepithelioma and myoepithelial carcinoma. Am J Surg Pathol 1991; 15: 554–568.

42. Lammie GA, Millis RR. Ductal adenoma of the breast. A review of fifteen cases. Hum Pathol 1989; 20: 903–908.

43. Hull MT, Warfel KA. Glycogen-rich clear cell carcinoma of the breast. A clinicopathologic and ultrastructural study. Am J Surg Pathol 1986; 10: 553–559.

44. Clement PB, Azzopardi JG. Microglandular adenosis of the breast — a lesion simulating tubular carcinoma. Histopathol 1983; 7: 169–180.

45. Rosen PP. Microglandular adenosis. A benign lesion simulating invasive mammary carcinoma. Am J Surg Pathol 1983; 7: 137–144.

46. Tavassoli FA, Norris HG. Microglandular adenosis of the breast. A clinicopathologic study of 11 cases with ultrastructural observations. Am J Surg Pathol 1983; 7: 713–737.

47. Eusebi V, Foschini MP, Betts MC et al. Microglandular adenosis of the breast: an immunohistochemical comparison with apocrine adenosis and tubular carcinoma. Am J Surg Pathol 1993; 17: 99–109.

48. Loose JH, Patchefsky AS, Hollander IJ et al. Adenomyoepithelioma of the breast. A spectrum of biologic behaviour. Am J Surg Pathol 1992; 16: 868–876.

49. Schurch W, Potvin C, Seemayer TA. Malignant myoepithelioma (myoepithelial carcinoma) of the breast: an ultrastructural and immunohistochemical study. Ultrastructural Pathol 1985; 8: 1–11.

50. Thorner PS, Kahn HJ, Baumal R et al. Malignant myoepithelioma of the breast. An immunohistochemical study by light and electron microscopy. Cancer 1986; 57: 745–750.

51. Foschini MP, Dina R, Eusebi V. Sarcomatoid neoplasms of the breast: proposed definitions for biphasic and monophasic sarcomatoid mammary carcinomas. Sem Diagn Pathol 1993; 10: 128–136.

52. Eusebi V, Catanni MG, Ceccarelli C, Lamovec J. Sarcomatoid carcinomas of the breast: an immunocytochemical study of 14 cases. Progr Surg Pathol 1989; 10: 83–99.

53. Frable WJ, Kay S. Carcinoma of the breast. Histologic and clinical features of apocrine tumors. Cancer 1968; 21: 756–763.

54. Mossler JA, Barton TK, Brinkhous AD et al. Apocrine differentiation in human mammary carcinoma. Cancer 1980; 46: 2463–2471.

55. Eusebi V, Millis RR, Cattani MG et al. Apocrine carcinoma of the breast. A morphologic and immunocytochemical study. Am J Pathol 1986; 123: 532–541.

56. Eusebi V, Magalhaes F, Azzopardi JG. Pleomorphic lobular carcinoma of the breast: an aggressive tumor showing apocrine differentiation. Hum Pathol 1992; 23: 655–662.

57. Abati A, Kimmel M, Rosen PP. Apocrine mammary carcinoma. A clinicopathologic study of 72 cases. Am J Clin Pathol 1990; 94: 371–377.

58. Papotti M, Eusebi V, Gugliotta P, Bussolati G. Immunohistochemical analysis of benign and malignant papillary lesions of the breast. Am J Surg Pathol 1983; 7: 451–461.

59. Eusebi V, Betts CM, Haagensen DE Jr et al. Apocrine differentiation in lobular carcinoma of the breast. A morphologic, immunologic and ultrastructural study. Hum Pathol 1984; 15: 134–140.

60. Hood CI, Font RL, Zimmerman LE. Metastatic mammary carcinoma in the eyelid with histiocytoid appearance. Cancer 1973; 31: 793–800.

61. Mazoujian G, Warhol MJ, Haagensen DE Jr. The ultrastructural localization of gross cystic disease fluid protein (GCDFP-15) in breast epithelium. Am J Pathol 1984; 116: 305–310.

62. Mazoujian G, Pinkus GS, Davis S, Haagensen DE Jr. Immuno-histochemistry of a breast gross cyst disease fluid protein (GCDFP-15): a marker of apocrine epithelium and breast carcinomas with apocrine features. Am J Pathol 1983; 110: 105–112.

63. Wick MR, Lillemoe TJ, Copland GT et al. Gross Cystic Disease Fluid Protein-15 as a marker for breast cancer: Immunohistochemical analysis of 690 human neoplasms and comparison with alpha-lactalbumin. Hum Pathol 1989; 20: 281–287.

64. Wade PM Jr, Mills SE, Read M et al. Small cell neuroendocrine (oat cell) carcinoma of the breast. Cancer 1983; 52: 121–125.

65. Jundt G, Schulz A, Heitz PhU, Osborn M. Small cell neuroendocrine (oat cell) carcinoma of the male breast. Immunocytochemical and ultrastructural investigations. Virchows Archiv (A) Pathol Anat 1984; 404: 213–222.

66. Papotti M, Gherardi G, Eusebi V et al. Primary oat cell (neuroendocrine) carcinoma of the breast. Report of four cases. Virchows Archiv (A) Pathol Anat 1992; 420: 103–108.

67. Hattori S, Matsuda M, Tateishi R et al. Oat-cell carcinoma of the lung. Clinical and morphological studies in relation to its histogenesis. Cancer 1972; 30: 1011–1024.

68. Kelly C, Henderson D, Corris P. Breast lumps: rare presentation of oat cell carcinoma of the lung. J Clin Pathol 1988; 41: 171–172.

69. Azzopardi JG. Oat cell carcinoma of the bronchus. J Pathol Bacteriol 1959; 78: 513–519.

70. Benisch B, Peison B, Newman R et al. Solid glycogen-rich clear cell carcinoma of the breast (A light and ultrastructural study). Am J Clin Pathol 1983; 79: 243–245.

71. Hull MT, Priest JB, Broadie TA et al. Glycogen-rich clear cell carcinoma of the breast. A light and electron microscopic study. Cancer 1981; 48: 2003–2009.

72. Fisher ER, Tavares J, Bulatao IS et al. Glycogen-rich clear cell breast cancer: with comments concerning other clear cell variants. Hum Pathol 1985; 16: 1085–1090.

73. Carcangiu ML, Sibley RK, Rosai J. Clear cell change in primary thyroid tumours. A study of 38 cases. Am J Surg Pathol 1985; 9: 705–722.

74. Rosen PP, Holmes G, Lesser ML et al. Juvenile papillomatosis and breast carcinoma. Cancer 1985; 55: 1345–1352.

75. Fekete P, Petrek J, Majmudar B et al. Fibroadenomas with stromal cellularity. Arch Pathol Lab Med 1987; 111: 427–432.

76. McDivitt RW, Stewart FW. Breast carcinoma in children. JAMA 1966; 195: 388–390.

77. Norris HJ, Taylor HB. Carcinoma of the breast in women less than thirty years old. Cancer 1970; 26: 953–959.

78. Tavassoli FA, Norris HJ. Secretory carcinoma of the breast. Cancer 1980; 45: 2404–2413.

79. Oberman HA. Secretory carcinoma of the breast in adults. Am J Surg Pathol 1980; 4: 465–470.

80. Rosen PP, Cranor ML. Secretory carcinoma of the breast. Arch Pathol Lab Med 1991; 115: 141–144.

81. Hartman AW, Magrish P. Carcinoma of the breast in children: case report: six year old boy with adenocarcinoma. Ann Surg 1955; 141: 792–797.

82. Karl SR, Ballantine TVN, Zaino R. Juvenile secretory carcinoma of the breast. J Pediatr Surg 1985; 20: 368–371.

83. Krausz T, Jenkins D, Grontoft O et al. Secretory carcinoma of the breast in adults: emphasis on late recurrence and metastasis. Histopathol 1989; 14: 25–36.

84. Roth JA, Discafani C, O'Malley M. Secretory breast carcinoma in a man. Am J Surg Pathol 1988; 12: 150–154.

85. Botta G, Fessia L, Ghiringhello B. Juvenile milk protein secreting carcinoma. Virchows Archiv (A) Pathol Anat 1982; 395: 145–152.

86. Oberman HA, Stephens PJ. Carcinoma of the breast in childhood. Cancer 1972; 30: 470–474.

87. Sullivan JJ, Magee HR, Donald KJ. Secretory (juvenile) carcinoma of the breast. Pathol 1977; 9: 341–346.

88. Meis C. Recurrent secretory carcinoma in residual mammary tissue after mastectomy. Am J Surg Pathol 1993; 17: 715–721.

89. Akhtar M, Robinson C, Ali MA, Godwin JT. Secretory carcinoma of the breast in adults. Light and electron microscopic study of three cases with review of the literature. Cancer 1983; 51: 2245–2254.

90. Byrne MP, Fahey MM, Gooselaw JG. Breast cancer with axillary metastasis in an eight and one-half year old girl. Cancer 1973; 31: 726–728.

Assessment of histological grade

INTRODUCTION

One of the most fundamental tenets of oncological pathology has been the observation that differing degrees of malignancy of tumors are reflected in their morphological structure. This was certainly recognized by Virchow,[1] and the idea was further developed by von Hansemann[2] who introduced the term 'anaplasia' to indicate the process by which carcinoma cells come to differ from the normal cells of the organ or tissue concerned. The term implies a loss of differentiation and an increase in cell proliferation so that the malignant cells fulfil only in an abortive way the structure and function of that tissue. It is a short step in theoretical terms to make the connection between the morphological structure of tumors and their clinical behavior, but it was not until 1920 that the first formal studies were carried out, by Broders.[3–4] He found a good correlation between the loss of differentiation in squamous carcinomas of the lip and skin and clinical outcome.

The credit for introducing this same concept to breast cancer must go to Greenhough[5] working at the Massachusetts General Hospital in Boston, USA. Stimulated by Broder's studies[3–4] he was the first to evaluate histological grading, and all modern methods stem from his original work. In this chapter the development of the current methods for assessing differentiation in breast cancer is traced from Greenhough's initial studies,[5] and particular emphasis is placed on the contribution which histological grade makes to the management of patients with breast cancer.

HISTORY AND BACKGROUND

The power of histological grading in breast cancer is evident from the outset since Greenhough[5] was able to obtain conclusive results from the comparatively small sample of 73 patients whose initial treatment was radical mastectomy. Greenhough and a colleague[5] reviewed histological sections from all the tumors and assessed eight morphological factors, namely the amount of gland formation, the presence of secretory vacuoles, cell size, nuclear size, variation in the size of both cells and nuclei, the degree of nuclear hyperchromatism and the number of mitoses. Tumors were then allocated to one of three grades; 1 — low malignancy, 2 — medium malignancy, 3 — high malignancy, although no details were given for the criteria used for each category. A clear association between grade and clinical outcome was obtained, although follow-up was short (between 5 and 7 years) and the end-point, 'cure', was not defined (grade 1, 19 cases — 68% cure; grade 2, 33 cases — 33% cure; grade 3, 21 cases — 0% cure).

The next landmark is provided by the studies carried out by Scarff and his colleagues at the Middlesex Hospital, London.[6–7] He followed Greenhough's method,[5] but placed most emphasis on the amount of tubule formation, inequality in the size of nuclei and hyperchromatism; mitoses were noted but considered to be of less importance. In each tumor it was decided whether the factors were absent or present in slight, moderate or marked degree and tumor placed in three grades of malignancy, low, moderate and marked. A broad correlation with clinical behavior was found but the number of cases studied, 50, was too small for formal analysis. However, 10 years later, using the same criteria, Scarff and Handley[8] studied 172 patients and showed a clear correlation between histological grade and survival; 31% of patients with grade 1 tumors were alive at 10 years compared with only 13% of patients with grade 3 tumors.

Scarff[8] therefore demonstrated that by using a relatively simple morphological method, based on a small number of factors to assess the degree of malignancy of a tumor, valuable clinical information was obtained.

Unfortunately little clinical interest was generated by these studies, due in part to the fact that at that time prognostic information was not used to determine the type of treatment received by a patient, and also to an innate scepticism in the medical community. For example, Willis,[9] a very influential figure in pathology, stated that attempts at precise numerical histological grading of tumors were arbitrary, unscientific and wasted effort! Paradoxically, to the shame of the pathology profession, it was left to a radiotherapist, Bloom, to revive interest in histological grading.[10–11] He started with the premise that a reliable system for classifying breast cancer was essential for appropriate management and then made a detailed review of the literature, especially that relating to histological aspects. Bloom chose to follow the Patey and Scarff method[6] (this decision may have been related in part to the fact that he too was based at the Middlesex Hospital) and applied it to 470 patients. He seems to have paid more attention to mitotic figures than Patey and Scarff,[6] but otherwise used the same rather subjective criteria to divide tumors into three grades of malignancy, low, moderate and high. He found a clear correlation with prognosis, and was one of the first clinicians to recognize that in breast cancer the long-term outlook is equally as important as short-term survival. He, therefore, expressed his results in terms of both 5- and 10-year survival; 45% of patients with grade 1 tumors were alive at 10 years compared with 28% of patients with grade 2 tumors and 13% of patients with grade 3 tumors.

Together with Richardson, a surgical research fellow, Bloom is also responsible for the next advance in histological grading, the addition of a numerical scoring system.[12] Each of the three factors assessed was scored on a scale of 1 to 3 to indicate whether it was present in slight, moderate or marked degree, giving a possible total of 3–9 points. Grade was allocated by an arbitrary division of the total points as follows:

			Points				
3	4	5	6	7		8	9
Low (Grade I)			Intermediate (Grade II)			High (Grade III)	

The point scoring system was not meant to ascribe mathematical accuracy to the method but to serve as an aid to grading. Its introduction was certainly a step on the way to providing greater objectivity in an essentially subjective method. Bloom and Richardson[12] confirmed the earlier correlation between grade and survival and in a later study Bloom showed that the effect persisted in the same group of patients with up to 20-year follow-up.[13]

The Patey and Scarff method,[6] modified by Bloom and Richardson,[12] has subsequently been used in a substantial number of studies and all have shown a powerful correlation between grade and prognosis.[14–20] The method was also adopted as the preferred grading system by the WHO.[21] Despite this other groups have not found the Scarff–Bloom–Richardson (SBR) method to be entirely satisfactory and alternative methods of grading breast carcinomas have been developed,[22–26] most of which have concentrated on nuclear characteristics.

Black's method[22] has been used almost exclusively in the United States where it is referred to as 'nuclear grading'. It is, in fact, derived from the work of Bloom.[10] Black and colleagues[22] re-evaluated the multifactorial method which Bloom[10] advocated, but assessed tubular structures and nuclear features separately. They concluded that tubular differentiation made no contribution to the prediction of prognosis, but that nuclear morphology was important. They devised four grades of malignancy, based on the regularity of the nuclear outline, delicacy of chromatin strands, presence or absence of nucleoli and mitotic figures. It is unfortunate that Black and colleagues[22] reversed the numerical order of their grades in comparison with the Scarff–Bloom–Richardson studies, so that nuclear grades 0–1 apply to poorly differentiated carcinomas and grades 3–4 to well-differentiated tumors. Black and his colleagues[22] used the nuclear grading method in a number of studies and found a significant correlation with survival.[27–29] This has been confirmed by Russo et al[30] although Kister et al[31] did not find nuclear grading to be of value.

The method devised by Hartveit[23] was based partly on examination of primary tumors and partly on necropsy material. The criteria used were essentially cytological, and included the definition of cell borders, nuclear crowding, nuclear lobula-tion and nuclear diameter; mitoses were not considered. Three grades of differentiation were used, but unfortunately, as in the Black nuclear grading system,[29] the order was the reverse of conventional histological grade. Very few other groups seem to have used the Hartveit system,[23] but neither Turner and Berry[32] nor Stenkvist et al[33] found it to be as accurate in assessing prognosis as the Bloom and Richardson[12] and WHO[21] methods respectively.

Fisher and associates have proposed a method which combines elements of both histological grade as originally devised by Patey and Scarff[6] and nuclear grade.[34] They showed a satisfactory correlation with survival[35] and later introduced a further modification by considering the degree and type of tubule formation.[24] However, it should be noted that approximately two-thirds of cases, even in the modified system, are placed in the poorly differentiated grade, so that stratification with this method is poor, and its utility in clinical practice must be doubtful.

Le Doussal and colleagues[25] have taken a slightly different approach. They began by using multivariate analysis to test the prognostic value of histological grading and did, in fact, confirm that the SBR method together with nodal status were the most important factors in predicting metastasis-free survival. They then went on to try and improve the SBR system by analyzing each component separately. Like Black et al[22] before them they found that nuclear pleomorphism and mitotic count were the most predictive elements. Using only these two factors they rearranged the scores to produce five modified SBR categories (MSBR) and claimed that this new grading method produced better separation of prognostic groups. Furthermore, MSBR eliminated the SBR in multivariate analysis. Since the allocation of points in both methods is purely arbitrary, the comparison of five grades versus three grades is hardly valid. In order to obtain a fair comparison both methods should have been analyzed with three grade divisions and five grade divisions separately, and the conclusions of Le Doussal and colleagues[25] that MSBR is a more discriminating method must remain in doubt. A closely similar system has been devised by Schumacher and colleagues,[36] based on studies in patients with node negative breast cancer. They too found that a combination of nuclear pleomorphism and mitotic count gave the most significant results.

Parham et al[26] have proposed yet another variation from a retrospective analysis of only 105 cases, a rather small sample. In addition to the three conventional components of histological grade they also assessed stromal fibrosis and tumor necrosis. They concluded that mitotic count and tumor necrosis correlated best with survival and proposed that these two factors be combined to form a new 'simplified grading method for breast cancer'. Unfortunately, as pointed out by Elston and Ellis,[37] the details of the methodology supplied in the paper are so imprecise that the proposed method must be virtually impossible to reproduce.

It will be clear from this review that two main types of grading method have emerged from Greenhough's[5] original concept, one based on use of multiple morphological factors and the other on nuclear features. Both types of method have been shown to provide significant prognostic information but relatively few comparisons have been made. Eichner, Lemon and Friedell[38] specifically examined the Bloom and Richardson[12] and Black[22] methods. They found little difference between the two in prediction of survival and concluded that both provide a useful means of estimating the neoplastic potential of breast cancer. Similar results have since been obtained by Stenkvist et al[33] and Russo et al.[30] However, Le Doussal et al[25] and Parl and Dupont[18] came to completely opposite conclusions. Le Doussal et al[25] produced their MSBR method based on nuclear factors because they found that tubule formation was the least contributory factor analyzed, whilst Parl and Dupont,[18] from a multivariate analysis of all the factors in the Bloom[10–11] and Black[22] methods, concluded that tubule formation was, in fact, the most powerful.

It can only be concluded that selection of a particular grading method is to a large extent a matter of personal choice. In practice the choice of method up to the present has emerged mainly along geographical lines, the nuclear grading technique of Black[22] being more popular in the United States and the SBR method in Europe and Australasia. It was partly for this reason that when

it was decided that pathological data should be incorporated into the analysis of the multicenter Cancer Research Campaign Trial of the treatment of early breast cancer, the Working Party chose to use the Bloom and Richardson method[12] for histological grading.[17] Four pathologists were involved in this study, and it quickly became apparent that consistency of grading would be difficult without modifications to the rather imprecise descriptions in the Bloom and Richardson method.[12] The assessment of mitotic counts was improved, and in this large study a clear and significant association between grade and survival was confirmed.

The importance of pathological prognostic information was recognized from the outset in the Nottingham Tenovus Primary Breast Cancer Study (NTPBCS). Because one of us (CWE) had previous experience with the modification of the Bloom and Richardson[12] method it was decided to evaluate histological grading further as part of the pathology data set. During the time that we were evolving the Nottingham method a number of reports appeared in the literature claiming that existing grading methods had poor reproducibility (see below). This further stimulated us to take a critical approach to the method in order to introduce greater objectivity to the assessment of the component factors. The method is described in some detail below.

NOTTINGHAM METHOD[39]

TISSUE PREPARATION

The first prerequisite for accurate histological grading is careful specimen preparation. We use 10% phosphate buffered formalin which gives good preservation of cytological detail but other fixatives such as B55 also give good results.[40] It is now well established that formalin penetrates tissues rather poorly, and certainly not more than 3.8 mm from a surface in 24 h.[41–42] More specifically Start and colleagues[43] have investigated the effect of delay in fixation on histological grade in breast cancer. They found that with a 6-hour delay the number of mitoses was reduced by up to 76%, which may therefore cause a reduction in assigned histological grade. These data confirm the importance of incising tumor masses in the *fresh state* immediately after resection (see also Ch. 2). This requires discussion and liaison with surgical colleagues, and special arrangements may have to be made, the simplest of which is to ensure that specimens are sent to the laboratory fresh. In any event the traditional practice of immersion of the whole specimen into fixative unsliced, whether it is a mastectomy or an excision biopsy, should be actively discouraged. Adequate tumor sampling is equally important. In Nottingham a skilled laboratory scientific officer has been specially trained to carry out this procedure. The tumor is sliced in a cruciate manner, and at this point the first measurement of tumor diameter is made in three planes (Fig. 17.1). This measurement is recorded and checked later after fixation (see Ch. 18). Segments may then be removed for snap freezing (for receptor assay, immunochemistry, molecular techniques and archival storage), leaving the majority of the tumor for routine histology. After adequate time for fixation tumor blocks are then cut from the faces of the segments (Fig. 17.1). Blocks obtained in this way provide a good representation of the whole tumor from the center to the periphery. The total number of blocks which can be obtained depends on overall tumor size, but, bearing in mind the potential value of archival material, no upper limit should be set; we prefer to examine a minimum of 3–4 blocks, but often obtain 6–10 blocks overall. Careful tissue processing of paraffin blocks is required, and this may necessitate the use of special processing cycles. Sections are cut at 4–6 μm; nuclear detail is obscured if sections are too thick. Conventional staining with hematoxylin and eosin is sufficient and special stains are not required.

TECHNIQUE

Histological grading may be carried out in all cases of invasive mammary adenocarcinoma; tumours which are entirely of in situ type, or those in which the invasive component is minimal, are not suitable for grading. It is our policy to grade all histological types of invasive adenocarcinoma; the reasons for this will be discussed later, but assessment is not limited to tumors of no special type (ductal/NST).

As indicated previously our method is derived from that originally described by Patey and Scarff[6] and modified by Bloom and Richardson,[12] the so-called SBR system. Grade is therefore based on assessment of three morphological features, tubule formation, nuclear pleomorphism and mitotic counts. A score of 1–3 is given for each, as summarized in Table 17.1.

TUBULE FORMATION

In the SBR methods the allocation of points for tubule formation was based on a subjective assessment of whether tubules were 'well marked', 'moderately well formed' or present in only a 'slight degree'. In our method more objective

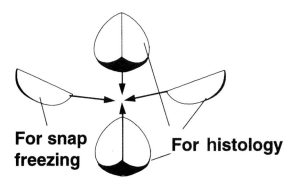

For snap freezing   **For histology**

Fig. 17.1 Method for incision and sampling of tumor specimens. After fixation blocks for histology are taken from the segment faces.

Table 17.1 Summary of semi-quantitative method for assessing histological grade in breast carcinoma

Feature	Score
Tubule formation	
Majority of tumor (>75%)	1
Moderate degree (10–75%)	2
Little or none (<10%)	3
Nuclear pleomorphism	
Small, regular uniform cells	1
Moderate increase in size and variability	2
Marked variation	3
Mitotic counts	
Dependent on microscope field area (see Table 17.2 and Fig. 17.12)	1–3

criteria are used. Qualitatively tubular structures must exhibit clear central lumina; care must be taken not to mistake clefts induced by shrinkage artefact for tubules (this is one area in which good fixation is important) (Figs 17.2, 17.3). Quantitatively all parts of each tumor block are scored and the proportion occupied by such tubular structures is assessed semiquantitatively. A score of one

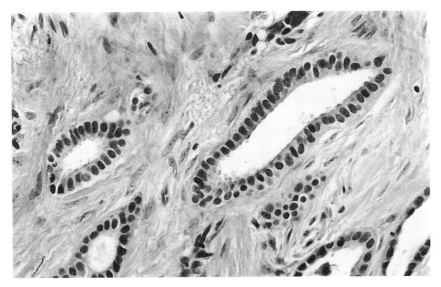

Fig. 17.2 Tubule formation. In the assessment of tubule formation only structures in which there is a clearly defined lumen, as shown here, should be counted. A tumor in which more than 75% of its area exhibits such structures will score 1 point for tubule formation. Hematoxylin–eosin × 185.

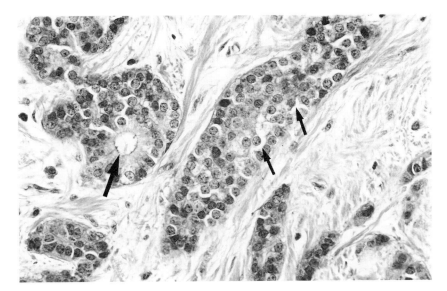

Fig. 17.3 Tubule formation. The structure on the left shows a clearly defined central lumen (large arrowhead). The other structures are solid cords of tumor cells; the irregular spaces (small arrowheads) are artefactual and should not be counted as luminal spaces. This section is from a tumor which scored 2 points for tubule formation. Hematoxylin–eosin × 185.

point is allocated when more than 75% of the area is composed of definite tubules. Two points are appropriate for tumors in which between 10 and 75% of the area shows tubule formation. Where tubules occupy 10% or less of the tumor three points are assigned.

These cut-off points are to some extent arbitrary. The upper limit of 75% was originally chosen to conform with the definition used by McDivitt et al[44] in their definition of tubular carcinoma. Subsequently we carried out a pilot study on the prognostic significance of the proportion of tubular structures in invasive breast cancer which supports the use of the above criteria.[45]

NUCLEAR PLEOMORPHISM

Evaluation of nuclear pleomorphism is the least satisfactory element of any grading system. In the SBR methods vague terms such as 'fairly uniform in size, shape and staining' were used. The only way in which differences in nuclear features can be assessed with complete accuracy is by use of morphometry or image analysis, which are expensive and time-consuming processes, impractical for routine diagnostic practice.

In order to introduce a degree of objectivity we have suggested that the size and shape of normal epithelial cells present in breast tissue adjacent to the tumor should be used as a reference point. If normal epithelial structures are not present in the tumor sections, then it is usually possible to find inflammatory cells such as lymphocytes for comparative purposes. Allowance should be made for the fact that lymphoid cells have a relatively smaller overall size than epithelial cells. When the tumor nuclei are small, with little increase or variation in size compared with normal nuclei and have regular outlines and uniformity of nuclear chromatin, one point is appropriate (Fig. 17.4). A score of 2 points is given when the nuclei are larger than normal, have more open vesicular nuclei with visible, usually single, nucleoli, and there is a moderate variation in size and shape (Figs 17.5, 17.6). A marked variation in size and shape, especially when very large and bizarre nuclei are present, scores 3 points; nuclei are vesicular with prominent enlarged and often multiple nucleoli (Figs 17.7, 17.8). It is interesting that Helpap[46] has correlated increasing numbers and size of nucleoli with worsening SBR grade, confirming our use of this aspect of pleomorphism.

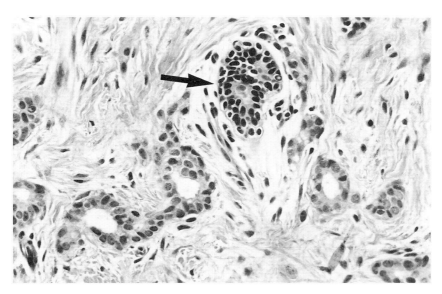

Fig. 17.4 Nuclear pleomorphism. The structure in the upper central part of the field is a normal ductule (arrowhead). This serves as a reference point for the nuclei in the adjacent infiltrating carcinoma. These are only slightly larger than the normal nuclei, and vary little in size and shape. The score is therefore 1 point. Hematoxylin–eosin × 185.

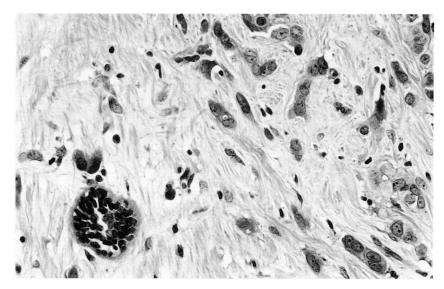

Fig. 17.5 Nuclear pleomorphism. A normal ductule is seen at the bottom left of the field. The nuclei of the adjacent infiltrating carcinoma are larger and exhibit a moderate variation in size and shape. The score is 2 points. Hematoxylin–eosin × 185.

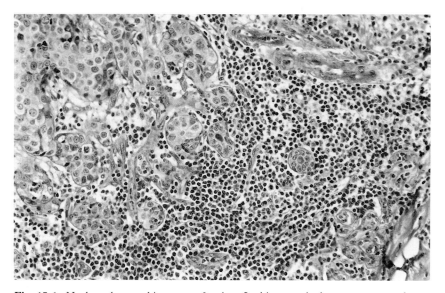

Fig. 17.6 Nuclear pleomorphism, score 2 points. In this example there are no normal structures for comparison. In such cases the presence of normal lymphoid cells, as seen here, may be used as a surrogate reference point to assess nuclear size and shape in the adjacent tumor cells. Hematoxylin–eosin × 125.

MITOTIC COUNTS

It is in the assessment of mitotic counts that we have made the most significant modifications to the SBR methods.[6,12] They assessed both hyper- chromatic nuclei and mitotic figures but it has been established that hyperchromicity is more likely to indicate individual cell necrosis (apop- tosis) than proliferation, and such nuclei should therefore be excluded from the counts. Further-

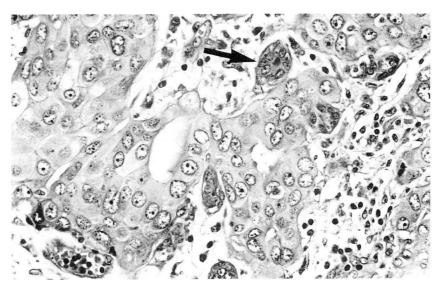

Fig. 17.7 Nuclear pleomorphism. A normal ductule (arrowhead) is surrounded by invasive carcinoma. Comparison between the nuclei of the normal cells and those of the carcinoma cells shows a marked variation in size and shape in the latter. The score is therefore 3 points. Hematoxylin–eosin × 185.

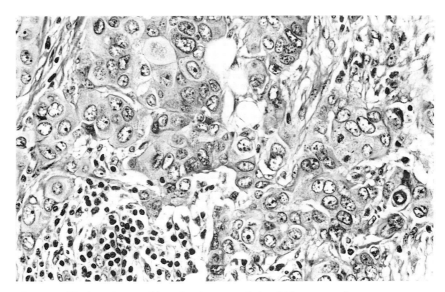

Fig. 17.8 Nuclear pleomorphism. Another example in which no normal structures are available for reference. However, there are numerous normal lymphoid cells in the adjacent stroma and in comparison with these there is marked variation in the size and shape of tumor nuclei. The appropriate score is 3. Hematoxylin–eosin × 185.

more, qualitatively it is our practice only to include figures which clearly fulfill the morphological criteria for the various stages of mitosis, prophase, metaphase, anaphase and telophase (Figs 17.9–17.11); in particular confusion with

apoptic nuclei and intratumoral lymphocytes can be avoided by very strict application of criteria for prophase nuclei.

The SBR method was also rather imprecise in the numerical allocation for point scoring; phrases

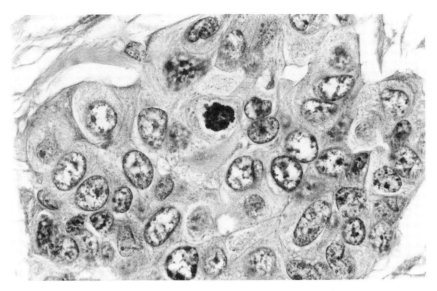

Fig. 17.9 Apoptosis. The nucleus in the upper central part of the field shows coarse clumping of nuclear material with a surrounding halo; these are the features of apoptosis and such appearances should not be confused with a prophase mitosis. Hematoxylin–eosin × 800.

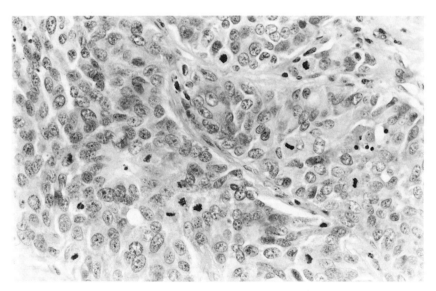

Fig. 17.10 Mitoses. In this field several putative mitoses are seen, including those in prophase and metaphase. Higher magnification is required to distinguish the prophase figures from apoptotic cells. Hematoxylin–eosin × 400.

such as 'an occasional mitosis per high-power field' and 'about two or three figures per high-power field' were used, the high-power field was not further defined and no advice given as to how many fields should be counted. It is now appreciated that the size of a so-called high-power field (HPF) varies up to six-fold from microscope to microscope[47] and it has been calculated that the count for the same tumor assessed by different instruments may vary from 3–20 mitoses per 10 HPF.[48] We have, therefore, standardized our counts to a defined field area; using this conven-

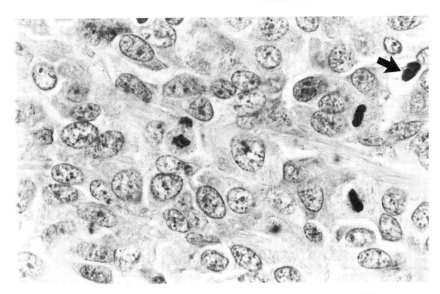

Fig. 17.11 Mitoses. Two cells in metaphase and one in anaphase are seen. The hyperchromatic nucleus at the top right (arrowhead) is probably apoptotic and should not be counted. Hematoxylin–eosin × 800.

tion any microscope can be calibrated to produce comparable data (Table 17.2 and Fig. 17.12). To our knowledge, in only one other grading method, that of Contesso et al,[49] is reference made to expression of mitotic count per defined field area. The count in the Contesso method[49] is based on the maximum number of mitoses in a *single* field rather than an overall count which means comparison with other methods of assessing proliferation is impossible. Furthermore, no attempt was made in this method to increase precision in the assessment of tubules and nuclear pleomorphism, and it therefore remains as subjective as the SBR system on which it is based.

Table 17.2 Assignment of points for mitotic counts according to the field area, using several microscopes

	Microscope		
	Leitz Ortholux	Nikon Labophot	Leitz Diaplan
Objective	×25	×40	×40
Field diameter (mm)	0.59	0.44	0.63
Field area (mm²)	0.274	0.152	0.312
Mitotic count★			
1 point	0–9	0–5	0–11
2 points	10–19	6–10	12–22
3 points	>20	>11	>23

★Assessed as number of mitoses per 10 fields at the tumor periphery.

Quinn and Wright[48] quite correctly point out that the most accurate way of counting mitoses in hematoxylin and eosin sections of tumors is the Mitotic Index (MI), in which the number of mitoses is expressed as a percentage of the total number of tumor cells and this has been confirmed by van Diest et al.[50] Assessing MI eliminates problems related to the variability in cellularity of tumors and differences in tumor cell/stromal proportions. Unfortunately, it is also an extremely tedious and time-consuming exercise and although a somewhat simpler modification of MI, in which tumor cellularity is taken into account, has been proposed by Simpson, Dutt and Page[51] we have felt that use of mitotic index in the routine setting was an impractical procedure which would render the grading method unacceptable to most diagnostic histopathologists. Initially we carried out a pilot study to establish appropriate cut-off points for the counting of mitoses per defined HPF, based on a detailed comparison with mitotic index.[52] A minimum of 10 fields is counted at the periphery of the tumor where it has been demonstrated that proliferative activity is greatest.[53–54] If there is a perceived variation in the number of mitoses in different areas of the tumor further groups of 10 fields should be counted to establish the correct (highest) count.

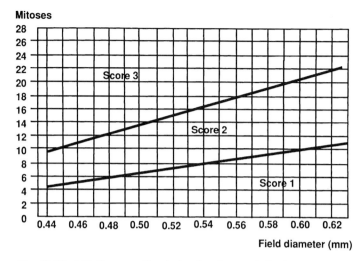

Fig. 17.12   Mitotic count. Graph showing the correlation between microscope field diameter and number of mitoses. The correct point score is obtained by plotting the actual mitotic count against the field diameter, e.g. a count of 10 mitoses per 10 fields at a field diameter of 0.62 mm gives a score of 2 for mitoses.

In our pilot study the assignment of points was originally carried out using a Leitz Ortholux microscope with wide angle eye pieces and a ×25 objective. This gives an HPF area of 0.274 mm². Up to nine mitoses per 10 HPF scores 1 point, 10–19 scores 2 points and more than 20 scores 3 points. As pointed out above this point scoring system can be adapted for use with any other microscope, once the field area has been measured, by a simple proportional calculation. Some examples of appropriate scores are shown in Table 17.2. Alternatively the graph shown in Fig. 17.12 may be found easier to use.[55] After measurement of the field diameter at the appropriate magnification the correct point score is obtained by plotting the actual mitotic count per 10 fields against diameter.

Support for the validity of counting mitoses per specific field area in this way is provided by several studies which have shown a good correlation with prognosis.[56–58]

POINT SCORING SYSTEM

It was Bloom and Richardson[12] who introduced the point scoring system. Their motive was not to ascribe mathematical accuracy to the grading method, but to induce a degree of discipline in the pathologist. In normal practice pathologists usually make an initial instinctive and subjective judgment of the overall degree of differentiation; using the numerical system each factor must be analyzed separately and its relative value assessed independently. One potential problem with the point scoring system for the assessment of tubules and nuclear pleomorphism is that it is still possible to 'play safe' and faced with a choice of 1–3 opt for the middle, i.e. 2. This can easily be obviated by making an initial decision to reduce the available options to two. Thus in a tumor with a large tubular component the tubule score can only be 1 or 2; the score of 3 is eliminated and the decision is immediately made more straightforward. Similarly when assessing nuclear pleomorphism the presence of large, irregular nuclei, more than twice the size of a normal epithelial cell, rules out a score of one; the number of these nuclei then influences the choice between a score of 2 or 3. When used in this way it is a relatively simple exercise to concentrate on each factor one at a time in an objective rather than a subjective fashion.

ALLOCATION OF GRADE

To obtain the overall tumour grade the scores for each factor are added together, giving a possible total of 3–9 points. Tumor grade is then allocated on the following basis:

3–5 points: grade 1–well differentiated.
6–7 points: grade 2–moderately differentiated.
8–9 points: grade 3–poorly differentiated.

It is recognized that the separation into three grades along these lines is arbitrary, since it is highly likely that there is, in fact, a continuous scale of malignancy. Indeed there has recently been some speculation on the appropriateness of this point allocation.[59] From a reproducibility study it has been suggested that 'clustering' of grades occurs, with very well differentiated tumors (3, 4 points), very high grade tumors (9 points) and three intermediate groups, 5–6, 6–7 and 7–8 point tumors.

These are interesting data which clearly need confirmation. In the meantime, as will be shown, a highly significant correlation with survival is achieved using the original three grades.[39]

VALIDATION

Despite the objective improvements which we have made to the grading method, any assessment of morphological characteristics must retain a subjective element. For this reason it is advisable, where possible, to validate results. In our own department tumors are graded independently by two histopathologists. In cases where assessment of grade differs (and this is rarely by more than one point) disagreements are resolved by consensus after joint review using a conference microscope. With increasing experience this may become less necessary, and for single-handed pathologists it may be sufficient to re-check a sample of cases without knowledge of the prior result.

TUMOR HETEROGENEITY

In some breast carcinomas there may be a variation in appearance from one part of the tumor to another; this is particularly true of tumors of mixed type (see Ch. 15) and is one of the main reasons for examining multiple blocks before arriving at a final grade. Assessment of tubule formation is made on the overall appearances of

the tumor and so account is taken of any regional variation. Nuclear pleomorphism is also assessed throughout the tumor and the points allocated are based on the highest degree of variation encountered. So far we have not quantified in a prospective fashion the minimum area of a tumor to show marked pleomorphism before a score of 3 is given; this is a matter for personal judgment, but as a general guide this should probably be at least one quarter. Certainly the finding of only occasional bizarre nuclei should not be used to allocate a score of 3. Mitoses are counted at the periphery of the tumor to obviate differences between the growing edge and the less active center.[54] In the small group of cases where equivocal counts may be obtained further areas should be assessed until a consistent count is obtained. For genuinely biphasic tumors, for example, of Mixed Ductal NST/Mucinous type, the least differentiated area should be assessed. In practice we have found that tumor heterogeneity rarely poses a serious problem in assigning an accurate grade.

CORRELATION WITH PROGNOSIS

Since Greenhough[5] first proposed the multifactorial histological grading method there has been a large volume of publications confirming the powerful predictive value of histological grade in terms of both disease free interval and long-term survival. The list is too extensive to cite each study, but the key references are shown in Table 17.3. These studies include both multifactorial methods (combined histological grade) and nuclear grading methods; some are from single centers and others are based on multicenter collaboration.

Table 17.3 List of key studies which have shown a significant correlation between histological grade and survival

- Patey and Scarff, 1928[6]
- Bloom, 1950 a and b[10,11]
- Bloom and Richardson, 1957[12]
- Black et al, 1975[22]
- Elston et al, 1982[17]
- Fisher et al, 1984[24]
- Davis et al, 1986[19]
- Contesso et al, 1987[49]
- Le Doussal et al, 1989[25]
- Hopton et al, 1989a[20]
- Elston and Ellis, 1991[39]
- Schumacher et al, 1993[36]

In our view the fact that such a diverse group of methods and study types all show correlation with survival adds strength to the power of histological grade. As Henson has pointed out (see below) perceived problems with reproducibility should not be used to detract from the validity of histological grade as a prognostic factor.[60]

The method described above has been fully evaluated in the NTPBCS. Nineteen percent of tumors are grade 1 (342 cases), 34% grade 2 (631 cases) and 47% grade 3 (857 cases). Initial results, based on life table analysis of over 1800 patients, confirmed conclusively the highly significant relationship between histological grade and prognosis.[39] We have recently re-examined the data with longer follow-up from six to 20 years and the correlation is confirmed. Both recurrence free interval and overall survival are significantly worse in patients with poorly differentiated (grade 3) tumors compared with those with moderately (grade 2) and well differentiated (grade 1) tumors (Fig. 17.13).

In summary, there can now be no doubt that histological grading of primary breast carcinoma provides important independent prognostic information. However, over 40 years ago Bloom[10–11] suggested that its predictive value is improved by combination with histological lymph node stage. We have made a comprehensive study of the interrelationships of multiple prognostic factors in breast cancer; this is covered briefly below and more fully in Chapter 18.

CONSISTENCY AND REPRODUCIBILITY

Despite the data presented in the previous section there has been a great reluctance by clinicians to use histological grading in patient management, and one of the reasons most frequently cited is the perceived lack of reproducibility of the method. This is highlighted by the wide variation in the proportion of each grade in published series (Table 17.4). Part of this variation may be due to real differences in the populations of patients studied, but other factors must also be considered. Although some of the earlier studies were carried out by clinicians rather than pathologists[12,15,61]

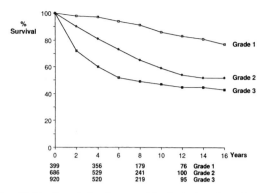

Fig. 17.13 Correlation between histological grade and overall survival in 2005 patients with primary operable carcinoma of the breast: $\chi^2 = 238.8$, 2 d.f.: $P<0.0001$.

their data is not significantly different from those in studies performed by histopathologists.[19–20,24–25,49,62] Little information is given in most of these studies concerning the validation of results by double or cross-checking, essential in a subjective method. As noted previously observers inexperienced in histological grading, faced with a choice of three grades, have a tendency to 'play for safety', and allocate too high a proportion in the middle; this is certainly true of some of the series shown in Table 17.4.

These data raise the possibility that the methods used for histological grading are insufficiently precise to achieve satisfactory consistency and reproducibility. In this respect Greenhough's original publication makes fascinating reading.[5] Although a formal reproducibility study was not carried out he observed that when the 73 cases in his series were examined independently by a colleague (Dr J Homer-Wright) there was disagreement in only seven cases, that is, 10%. Further-

Table 17.4 Comparison of the relative percentage of cases in each grade in a number of different studies

Study	Grade		
	1	2	3
*Bloom and Richardson, 1957[12]	26	45	29
*Tough et al, 1969[61]	11	51	38
*Champion, Wallace and Prescott, 1972[15]	23	52	25
Fisher et al, 1984[24]	11	23	66
Elston, 1984[62]	17	37	46
Davis et al, 1986[19]	22	49	29
Contesso et al, 1987[49]	21	50	29
Hopton et al, 1989a[20]	29	45	26
Le Doussal et al, 1989[25]	11	55	46

*Studies carried out by clinicians.

more, after discussion they 'were able to eliminate these differences' and come to substantial agreement. In our view these figures indicate more than adequate reproducibility, and it is a pity that this aspect of Greenhough's work has been completely overlooked.[5] Subsequent literature on consistency and reproducibility has been contradictory, but it is interesting that those studies which have claimed that agreement is poor have been the most widely quoted and influential, especially in studies promoting the newer molecular prognostic factors. Cutler et al,[63] using nuclear grading, found that only 60% agreement was reached between an experienced observer and a pathologist who had not classified tumors previously. In the same study Black,[29] who had devised the method, obtained only 70% agreement between his first and second evaluations. The most frequently quoted studies are those of Stenkvist and colleagues,[33] Delides et al[64] and Gilchrist et al.[65] In Stenkvist's study[33] a comparison was made of the WHO,[12,21] nuclear grade[27] and Hartveit methods[23] by two observers. The WHO and nuclear grading methods were found to stratify tumors into three categories whilst the Hartveit method[23] did not, but all three methods were considered to have poor inter- and intra-observer reproducibility when the study was repeated after an interval of 6 months. Delides et al[64] assessed the WHO method using five trainee pathologists and one tutor; of 158 tumors complete agreement was reached in only 23 cases (14.5%) and the kappa value (0.3) for overall agreement was low. Least agreement was found in grade 2 tumors and the authors concluded that prognostication should be restricted to grade 1 and 3 tumors. In the study published by Gilchrist and colleagues[65] the participants were 12 pathologists from the multicenter Eastern Co-operative Oncology Group (ECOG) Breast Pathology Committee in the United States. Inter-observer reproducibility of nuclear grade was assessed as part of a broader study of histopathological factors. The method of analysis was rather complex, but the authors concluded that agreement on three categories of nuclear grade was only marginally better than would have been expected by chance.

In contrast other studies, less widely quoted, have obtained acceptable levels of consistency and reproducibility. Fisher et al[34] found approximately 90% agreement on histological grade within one center and only a 6% discrepancy by the same reviewer on different occasions.[35] Hopton et al[66] evaluated the WHO method on a regional basis in the United Kingdom as part of a Yorkshire Breast Group study. Sections from 10 centers were graded independently by the contributing pathologist and a coordinating pathologist. The inter-observer variation of 22% for 874 tumors was considered to be satisfactory. The same group have also confirmed the significant association between histological grade and overall survival.[20] Taken together these two studies provide very important evidence concerning the value of histological grading, since they demonstrate that clinically useful data can be obtained by pathologists and clinicians in general hospitals; none of the participating pathologists were specialists in breast disease. Closely similar results were obtained by Theissig et al[67] using the Bloom and Richardson[12] method. Three pathologists, one an 'expert', obtained a satisfactory level of agreement (72%) in grading 166 invasive carcinomas of no special type. Finally, Chouinard and colleagues[68] have found good reproducibility and consistency amongst three teaching hospital pathologists in a study based on the Bloom and Richardson[12] and Contesso[49] methods.

An important feature of all the studies referred to above is the extremely subjective nature of the methods which were evaluated, a point already discussed previously. Furthermore, few details were supplied concerning the protocols used nor was any indication given concerning specimen quality (e.g., fixation, processing, section thickness). It was for precisely these reasons that we introduced the modifications on which the Nottingham method is based[39,69] in order to introduce greater objectivity with a relatively strict protocol. A number of studies which have tested reproducibility using our method have now been reported, and the results are extremely encouraging. Interestingly Dalton et al[59] used our intermediate system[69] in which the grading criteria were not as precisely defined as in our final version.[39] Nevertheless, when a single slide from 10 invasive carcinomas was submitted to 25 pathologists from six different (private) practices, none of whom were expert breast pathologists, there was greater than 87% agreement on final grade. The median weighted kappa statistic of 0.7 indicated very good inter-observer agreement. Before the study the pathologists were expected to learn the method and a written description accompanied the slides, but no formal training exercise was carried out. Frierson et al[70] have tested reproducibility using the updated version of the Nottingham method. Sections from 75 infiltrating ductal carcinomas were circulated amongst six pathologists from four separate laboratories. Each participant was furnished with a copy of the publication describing the method[39] and was referred to the photomicrographs in the chapter by Elston in *Diagnostic Histopathology of the Breast*.[69] In addition a clear written protocol was provided. Pairwise kappa values for agreement ranged from moderate to substantial (0.43–0.74) and consensus agreement (four out of six pathologists) was 88.5%. A rather different approach was taken in the study published by Robbins et al[40] which involved collaboration between the Sir Charles Gairdner Hospital (SCGH), Perth, Western Australia and the City Hospital Nottingham (CHN) including the authors of the Nottingham method. Fifty consecutive cases of invasive carcinoma of the breast were selected and sections from both buffered formal saline and B5 (mercuric chloride–formalin mixture) fixed blocks were examined. Grading was carried out by a consensus of three pathologists at SCGN and two at NCH using the Nottingham method. Complete agreement between the centers was reached in 83% of B5 fixed cases and 74% of formalin fixed cases with relative disagreement rates of 0.15 and 0.58 and kappa values of 0.73 and 0.58 respectively. The NCH pathologists assessed section quality independently and considered that in this study B5 gave better preservation of nuclear morphology and mitoses. Review of discrepant cases at SCGH allowed some to be reclassified in line with the NCH opinion, leading to a potential complete agreement of over 90%. These results represent a considerable improvement over a preliminary study carried out previously in Perth[71] and this was considered to be due mainly to the use of the strict protocol recommended by Elston and Ellis.[39] The method has now been shown to maintain validity, despite some technical limitations, when retrospective review and grading were undertaken on cases derived from eight different sources, including private laboratories.[72]

The studies described above have all demonstrated that histological grading can be carried out with satisfactory reproducibility, provided that a strict protocol, such as that recommended by Elston and Ellis,[39] is followed.[73] In this respect it is disappointing that the results of the UK National External Quality Assessment Scheme of the NHSBSP[74] showed only average overall consistency for coordinators (kappa value 0.46) and poor consistency for other pathologists (kappa value 0.26) involved in breast screening. These data almost certainly indicate that many of the participants were failing to adhere to the published criteria. As Scarff and Torloni[21] pointed out over 25 years ago experience and dedication are essential requirements for accurate histological grading, and the method should only be undertaken by trained histopathologists. Ideally results should be double checked, preferably by another pathologist so that a consensus view is obtained, but if this is not possible, by the same pathologist on a separate occasion. This becomes less important once a pathologist has gained sufficient experience with the method. It is, perhaps, self-evident but still worth stressing that accurate results will only be obtained from a professional approach with proper attention to detail.

GRADE AND TUMOR TYPE

At the present time, in order to conform with the requirements of the Nottingham Prognostic Index (see p. 381), histological grading is performed in all cases of invasive carcinoma of breast, regardless of morphological type. As described in Chapter 15 it is recognized that the special types, such as pure tubular, invasive cribriform and mucinous carcinoma, carry an excellent prognosis, whilst infiltrating lobular and medullary carcinomas have an intermediate prognosis compared with the common infiltrating ductal NST carcinomas. In view of this many pathologists only assess histological grade in the latter group of tumors, but a number of practical points should be taken into account.

When grade is analyzed in tumors of particular histological types it is usually found to be appropriate.[75] For example, the special tumor types such as pure tubular and invasive cribriform carcinoma invariably have an excellent prognosis comparable with their grade 1 status. Most infiltrating lobular carcinomas, especially those of classical subtype, are designated as grade 2, and interestingly the overall survival curve of lobular carcinoma overlies that of all other grade 2 carcinomas (Fig. 17.14). However, a minority fall into the grade 1 or grade 3 category, and as shown in Fig. 17.15, the survival curves show an appropriate and significant separation. Interestingly, Ladekarl and Sorensen[76] have recently proposed a morphometric grading system for infiltrating lobular carcinoma, based on nuclear volume and

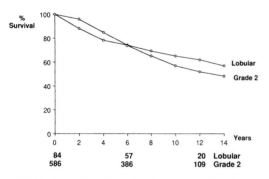

Fig. 17.14   Overall survival of patients with infiltrating lobular carcinoma compared with that of patients with grade 2 carcinomas of other histological types. $\chi^2 = 0.298$, 1 d.f.: n.s.

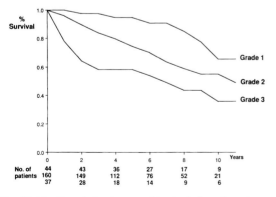

Fig. 17.15   Correlation between histological grade and overall survival in 341 patients with infiltrating lobular carcinoma. $\chi^2 = 21.5$, 2 d.f.: $P<0.001$.

mitotic index which gives good prognostic separation between poor and favorable types. Their study was based on a small number of cases, and further investigations are clearly required.

Medullary carcinoma is perhaps the only subtype for which this approach might not be appropriate. By definition these tumors are histological grade 3, but have been considered by some to have a more favorable prognosis than this degree of differentiation would imply.[77] In the NTPBCS, however, despite the use of very strict criteria, we have been unable to demonstrate a significant survival advantage for patients with medullary carcinoma when compared with other grade 3 tumors.[78]

It should also be noted that morphological typing is equally as subjective as histological grading, as demonstrated by the wide variation in the recorded frequency of special types[79] and the results of the NHSBSP Quality Assurance Scheme.[74] Furthermore, up to a quarter of tumors in a series may be of mixed or combined type[34,78] and the prognostic significance of these cases is unclear. For example, although patients with tubular mixed carcinomas have a survival intermediate between those with pure tubular and ductal NST carcinoma[78] prognosis within the tubular mixed group also varies according to histological grade. If grading is restricted to the ductal NST group alone then in a symptomatic series at best 75%[80] and at worst only 53%[34] of cases will be assessed and valuable prognostic information lost. We believe, therefore, that both grading and typing should be carried out in all invasive breast carcinomas.[73,75]

COMBINATION WITH OTHER FACTORS

Although it has now been established clearly that histological grade is a powerful independent prognostic factor it has also been recognized that its predictive value is improved by combination with other factors. This was first shown for the combinations of grade and axillary lymph node involvement in Greenhough's original study[5] and later confirmed by Bloom.[10-11] In the latter study the 5-year survival for patients with grade 1 tumors fell from 94% for those with uninvolved nodes to 65% for those with involved nodes; for grade 3 tumors the figures were 55 and 16% respectively.

In the NTPBCS a comprehensive study has been made of potential prognostic factors in both univariate and multivariate analysis. This is discussed in detail in Chapter 18, but it is pertinent here to give a brief summary of the Nottingham Prognostic Index (NPI). Analysis of a range of prognostic factors, using the multiple regression technique of Cox,[81] showed that only tumor size (pathological measurement), histological lymph node stage and histological grade gave a significant correlation with overall survival.[82] Based on the coefficients of significance produced in the Cox[81] analysis a simple composite prognostic index has been devised as follows:

$$NPI = 0.2 \times \text{tumor size} + \text{lymph node stage } (1–3) + \text{histological grade } (1–3)$$

Prognosis worsens as the numerical value of NPI increases, and by using cut-off points of 3.4 and 5.4 patients may be stratified into good, moderate and poor prognostic groups having an annual mortality of 3, 7 and 30% respectively.[83] The strength of the NPI has been confirmed after long-term (15-year) follow-up,[84] and validated independently by the Yorkshire Breast Group.[85]

REFERENCES

1. Virchow R. Form and nature of pathological new formations. In: Cellular pathology. 2nd ed. Philadelphia: Lippincott (republished by Dover Publications, New York, 1971), 1863; 507–534.
2. von Hansemann D. Ueber assymetrische Zelltheilung in Epithelkrebsen und deren biologische Bedeutung. Virchows Arch (A) Pathol Anat 1890; 119: 299–326.
3. Broders AC. Squamous-cell epithelioma of the lip. JAMA 1920; 74: 656–664.
4. Broders AC. Squamous-cell epithelioma of the skin. Ann Surg 1921; 73: 141–160.
5. Greenhough RB. Varying degress of malignancy in cancer of the breast. J Cancer Res 1925; 9: 452–463.
6. Patey DH, Scarff RW. The position of histology in the prognosis of carcinoma of the breast. Lancet 1928; 1: 801–804.
7. Patey DH, Scarff RW. Further observations on the histology of carcinoma of the breast. Lancet 1929; ii: 492–494.
8. Scarff RW, Handley RS. Prognosis in carcinoma of the breast. Lancet 1938; ii: 582–583.
9. Willis RA. Pathology of tumours. London: Butterworths, 1948; 129.
10. Bloom HJG. Prognosis in carcinoma of the breast. Br J Cancer 1950a; 4: 259–288.
11. Bloom HJG. Further studies on prognosis of breast carcinoma. Br J Cancer 1950b; 4: 347–367.
12. Bloom HJG, Richardson WW. Histological grading and prognosis in breast cancer. A study of 1409 cases of which 359 have been followed for 15 years. Br J Cancer 1957; 11: 359–377.
13. Bloom HJG, Field JR. Impact of tumor grade and host resistance on survival of women with breast cancer. Cancer 1971; 28: 1580–1589.
14. Hamlin IME. Possible host resistance in carcinoma of the breast: a histological study. Br J Cancer 1968; 22: 382–401.
15. Champion HR, Wallace IWJ, Prescott RJ. Histology in breast cancer prognosis. Br J Cancer 1972; 26: 129–138.
16. Andersen JA, Fischermann K, Hou-Jensen K et al. Selection of high risk groups amongst prognostically favorable patients with breast cancer. Ann Surg 1981; 195: 1–3.
17. Elston CW, Gresham GA, Rao GS et al. The Cancer Research Campaign (Kings/Cambridge) trial for early breast cancer — pathological aspects. Br J Cancer 1982; 45: 655–669.
18. Parl FF, Dupont WD. A retrospective cohort study of histologic risk factors in breast cancer patients. Cancer 1982; 50: 2410–2416.
19. Davis BW, Gelber RD, Goldhirsch A et al. Prognostic significance of tumor grade in clinical trials of adjuvant therapy for breast cancer with axillary lymph node metastasis. Cancer 1986; 58: 2662–2670.
20. Hopton DS, Thorogood J, Clayden AD, Mackinnon D. Histological grading of breast cancer: significance of grade on recurrence and mortality. Eur J Surg Oncol 1989; 15: 25–31.
21. Scarff RW, Torloni H. Histological typing of breast tumours (International histological classification of tumours, no 2). Geneva: World Health Organization, 1968.
22. Black MM, Opler SR, Speer FD. Survival in breast cancer cases in relation to structure of the primary tumor and regional lymph nodes. Surg Gynecol Obstet 1955; 100: 543–551.
23. Hartveit F. Prognostic typing in breast cancer. Br Med J 1971; 4: 253–257.
24. Fisher ER, Sass R, Fisher B et al. Pathologic findings from the National Surgical Adjuvant Project for breast cancer (protocol no 4). Discrimination for tenth year treatment failure. Cancer 1984; 53: 712–723.
25. Le Doussal V, Tubiana-Hulin M, Friedman S et al. Prognostic value of histologic grade nuclear components of Scarff Bloom Richardson (SBR). An improved score modification based on a multivariate analysis of 1262 invasive ductal breast carcinomas. Cancer 1989; 64: 1914–1921.
26. Parham DM, Hagen N, Brown RA. Simplified method of grading primary carcinomas of the breast. J Clin Pathol 1992; 45: 517–520.
27. Black MM, Speer FD. Nuclear structure in cancer tissues. Surg Gynecol Obstet 1959; 105: 97–102.
28. Cutler SJ, Black MM, Mork T et al. Further observations on prognostic factors in breast cancer of the female breast. Cancer 1969; 24: 653–657.

29. Black MM, Barclay THC, Hankey BR. Prognosis in breast cancer utilizing histologic characteristics of the primary tumor. Cancer 1975; 36: 2048–2055.

30. Russo J, Frederick J, Ownby HE et al. Predictors of recurrence and survival of patients with breast cancer. Am J Clin Pathol 1987; 88: 123–131.

31. Kister SJ, Sommers SC, Haagensen CD et al. Nuclear grade and sinus histiocytosis in cancer of the breast. Cancer 1969; 21: 570–575.

32. Turner D, Berry CL. A comparison of two methods of prognostic typing in breast cancer. J Clin Pathol 1972; 25: 1053–1055.

33. Stenkvist B, Westman-Naeser S, Vegelius J et al. Analysis of reproducibility of subjective grading systems for breast carcinoma. J Clin Pathol 1979; 32: 929–985.

34. Fisher ER, Gregorio RM, Fisher B. The pathology of invasive breast cancer. A syllabus derived from findings of the National Surgical Adjuvant Breast Cancer Project (protocol no 4). Cancer 1975; 36: 144–156.

35. Fisher ER, Redmond C, Fisher B. Histologic grading of breast cancer. Pathol Annu 1980; 15: 239–251.

36. Schumacher M, Schmoor C, Sauerbrei W. The prognostic effect of histological tumor grade in node-negative breast cancer patients. Br Cancer Res Treat 1993; 25: 235–245.

37. Elston CW, Ellis IO. Method for grading breast cancer (letter). J Clin Pathol 1993; 46: 189–190.

38. Eichner WJ, Lemon HM, Friedell GH. Tumor grade in the prognosis of breast cancer. Nebr Med J 1970; 55: 405–409.

39. Elston CW, Ellis IO. Pathological prognostic factors in breast cancer. I. The value of histological grade in breast cancer: experience from a large study with long-term follow-up. Histopathol 1991; 19: 403–410.

40. Robbins P, Pinder S, de Klerk N et al. Histological grading of breast carcinomas. A study of interobserver agreement. Hum Pathol 1995; 26: 873–879.

41. Medawar PB. The rate of penetration of fixatives. J Roy Microsc Soc 1942; 61: 46–57.

42. Baker JR. Principles of biological microtechnique. London: Methuen, 1960; 31–42.

43. Start RD, Flynn MS, Cross SS et al. Is the grading of breast carcinomas affected by a delay in fixation? Virchows Arch (A) Pathol Anat 1991; 419: 475–477.

44. McDivitt RW, Boyce W, Gersell D. Tubular carcinoma of the breast. Am J Surg Pathol 1982; 6: 401–411.

45. Ellis IO, Broughton N, Elston CW, Blamey RW. The relationship of histological type to survival and oestrogen receptor status in primary operable breast carcinoma. J Pathol 1987; 152: 219A.

46. Helpap B. Nucleolar grading of breast cancer — comparative studies on frequency and localisation of nucleoli and histology, stage, hormonal receptor status and lectin histochemistry. Virchows Arch (A) Pathol Anat 1989; 415: 501–508.

47. Ellis PSJ, Whitehead R. Mitosis counting — a need for reappraisal. Hum Pathol 1981; 12: 3–4.

48. Quinn CM, Wright NA. The clinical assessment of proliferation and growth in human tumours: evaluation of methods and application as prognostic variables. J Pathol 1990; 160: 93–102.

49. Contesso G, Mouriesse H, Friedman S et al. The importance of histologic grade in long-term prognosis of breast cancer: a study of 1010 patients, uniformly treated at the Institut Gustave-Roussy. J Clin Oncol 1987; 5: 1378–1386.

50. Van Diest PJ, Baak JPA, Matze-Cok P et al. Reproducibility of mitosis counting in 2469 breast cancer specimens: results from the Multicenter Morphometric Mammary Carcinoma Project. Hum Pathol 1992; 23: 603–607.

51. Simpson JF, Dutt PL, Page DL. Expression of mitoses per thousand cells and cell density in breast carcinomas: a proposal. Hum Pathol 1992; 23: 608–611.

52. Mann R, Elston CW, Hunter S et al. Evaluation of mitotic activity as a component of histological grade and its contribution to prognosis in primary breast carcinoma. J Pathol 1985; 146: 271A.

53. Verhoeven D, Bourgeois N, Derde MP et al. Comparison of cell growth in different parts of breast cancers. Histopathol 1990; 17: 505–509.

54. Connor AJM, Pinder SE, Elston CW et al. Intratumoural heterogeneity of proliferation in invasive breast carcinoma evaluated with MIB1 antibody. The Breast 1997; 6 (in press).

55. National Group for Breast Screening Pathology. Pathology Reporting in Breast Cancer Screening. 2nd ed. NHSBSP Publications, no 3, 1995.

56. Baak JPA, VanDop H, Kurver PHJ et al. The value of morphometry to classic prognosticators in breast cancer. Cancer 1985; 56: 372–382.

57. Biesterfeld S, Noll I, Noll E et al. Mitotic frequency as a prognostic factor in breast cancer. Hum Pathol 1995; 26: 47–52.

58. Clayton F. Pathologic correlates of survival in 378 lymph node-negative infiltrating ductal carcinomas. Mitotic count is the best single predictor. Cancer 1991; 68: 1309–1317.

59. Dalton LW, Page DL, Dupont WD. Histologic grading of breast carcinoma: a reproducibility study. Cancer 1994; 73: 2765–2770.

60. Henson E. End points and significance of reproducibility in pathology. Arch Pathol Lab Med 1989; 113: 830–831.

61. Tough ICK, Carter DC, Fraser J, Bruce J. Histological grading in breast cancer. Br J Cancer 1969; 23: 294–301.

62. Elston CW. The assessment of histological differentiation in breast cancer. Aust New Zeal J Surg 1984; 54: 11–15.

63. Cutler SJ, Black MM, Fried GH et al. Prognostic factors in cancer of the female breast II. Reproducibility of histopathologic classification. Cancer 1966; 19: 75–82.

64. Delides GS, Garas G, Georgouli G et al. Intralaboratory variations in the grading of breast carcinoma. Arch Pathol Lab Med 1982; 106: 126–128.

65. Gilchrist KW, Kalish L, Gould VE et al. Interobserver reproducibility of histopathological features in stage II breast cancer. An ECPG study. Br Cancer Res Treat 1979; 5: 3–10.

66. Hopton DS, Thorogood J, Clayden AD et al. Observer variation in histological grading of breast cancer. Eur J Surg Oncol 1989b; 15: 21–23.

67. Theissig F, Kunze KD, Haroske G, Meyer W. Histological grading of breast cancer — interobserver reproducibility and prognostic significance. Pathol Res Pract 1990; 186: 732–736.

68. Chouinard EE, Chen V, D'Souza TJ, Riddell RH. Reproducibility of pathological grading in breast cancer. The Breast 1994; 3: 124–129.

69. Elston CW. Grading of invasive carcinoma of the breast. In: Page DL, Anderson TJ, eds. Diagnostic

histopathology of the breast. Edinburgh: Churchill Livingstone, 1987; 300–311.

70. Frierson HF, Wolber RA, Berean KW et al. Interobserver reproducibility of the Nottingham modification of the Bloom and Richardson histological grading scheme for infiltrating ductal carcinoma. Am J Clin Pathol 1995; 105: 195–198.

71. Harvey JM, de Klerk NH, Sterrett GF. Histological grading in breast cancer: interobserver agreement, and relation to other prognostic factors including ploidy. Pathol 1992; 24: 63–68.

72. Cummings MC, Wright RG, Furnival CM et al. The feasibility of retrospective grading of breast cancer histology slides derived from multiple pathology services. The Breast 1995; 4: 179–182.

73. Page DL, Ellis IO, Elston CW. Histologic grading of breast cancer. Let's do it. Am J Clin Pathol 1995; 103: 123–124.

74. Sloane JP, National Coordinating Group for Breast Screening Pathology. Consistency of histopathological reporting of breast lesions detected by screening: findings of the UK National External Quality Assessment (EQA) Scheme. Eur J Cancer 1994; 30A: 1414–1419.

75. Pereira H, Pinder SE, Sibbering DM et al. Pathological prognostic factors in breast cancer. IV: Should you be a typer or a grader? A comparative study of two histological prognostic features in operable breast carcinoma. Histopathol 1995; 27: 219–226.

76. Ladekarl M, Sorensen FB. Prognostic, quantitative histopathologic variables in lobular carcinoma of the breast. Cancer 1993; 72: 2602–2611.

77. Ridolfi RL, Rosen PP, Port A et al. Medullary carcinoma of the breast — a clinicopathological study with a ten year follow-up. Cancer 1977; 40: 1365–1385.

78. Ellis IO, Galea M, Broughton N et al. Pathological prognostic factors in breast cancer. II. Histological type. Relationship with survival in a large study with long-term follow-up. Histopathol 1992; 20: 479–489.

79. Page DL, Anderson TJ, Sakamoto G. Infiltrating carcinoma: major histological types. In: Page DL, Anderson TJ, eds. Diagnostic histopathology of the breast. London: WB Saunders, 1987; 193–235.

80. Rosen PP. The pathological classification of human mammary carcinoma: past, present and future. Ann Clin Lab Sci 1979; 9: 144–156.

81. Cox DR. Regression models and life-tables. JR Stat Soc (B) 1972; 34: 187–220.

82. Haybittle JL, Blamey RW, Elston CW et al. A prognostic index in primary breast cancer. Br J Cancer 1982; 45: 361–366.

83. Todd JH, Dowle C, Williams MR et al. Confirmation of a prognostic index in primary breast cancer. Br J Cancer 1987; 56: 489–492.

84. Galea MH, Blamey RW, Elston CW et al. The Nottingham Prognostic Index in primary breast cancer. Br Cancer Res Treat 1992; 22: 187–191.

85. Brown JM, Benson EA, Jones M. Confirmation of a long-term prognostic index in breast cancer. The Breast 1993; 2: 144–147.

C. W. Elston, I. O. Ellis, H. Goulding and S. E. Pinder

Role of pathology in the prognosis and management of breast cancer

GENERAL INTRODUCTION

In a number of malignant tumors, the role of histopathology in the provision of prognostic information has been well established for many years (e.g. measurement of tumor thickness and level of invasion in malignant melanoma). Until comparatively recently the main role of the histopathologist in breast disease lay only in the establishment of a basic diagnosis of cancer. Apart from the examination of regional lymph nodes for the presence or absence of metastases it was unusual for any other prognostic information to be supplied or, indeed, requested. Invasive breast carcinoma was regarded as a single disease process, treatment was standardized and predominantly surgical and little attempt was made to stratify patients for appropriate therapy on an individual basis.

However, there are now encouraging signs that improvements in mortality may be a realistic target. Increasing breast awareness amongst women due to better health education should lead to earlier clinical detection. It is clear that population screening with mammography can achieve a significant improvement in survival,[1] and even in the short term will detect cancers which are substantially different in their biological behavior from those which present symptomatically.[2] In addition, there have been significant changes in the range and type of therapeutic options available for patients with breast cancer. These include conservation surgery, regional radiotherapy, an ever-widening range of cytotoxic agents and different forms of hormone therapy. Not surprisingly the attitude of patients is also changing and more women are exercising their right to participate in these management and therapeutic decisions.

All these developments highlight the increasing importance of prognostic factors in the management of patients with breast cancer.[3-4] A major change in approach is required by both pathologist and clinician alike. In a most perceptive review Clark[5] has recently addressed this question, in the light of the increasing tendency for oncologists, particularly in the USA, to adopt a strategy of advising the administration of adjuvant systemic therapy to all patients with breast cancer, regardless of prognostic factors. He proposed that there are three major reasons for the use of prognostic factors. The first is to identify patients whose prognosis is so good that adjuvant therapy after local surgery would not be 'cost-beneficial'. The second is to identify patients whose prognosis is so poor that a more aggressive adjuvant approach would be warranted. Thirdly, it is important to identify patients likely to be responsive or resistant to particular types of therapy.

Prognosis can be measured in a variety of different ways, and a large number of potential factors have been examined. Some of these are well established, with proven value, some are still at the development stage whilst others must be regarded as research tools. They can be divided broadly into three groups, traditional morphological factors, hormone receptors and the newer biological or molecular markers. In this chapter we will give an overview of all the available prognostic factors with particular emphasis on those which are of relevance in the routine laboratory setting, especially with respect to their clinical applications.

TRADITIONAL MORPHOLOGICAL FACTORS

INTRODUCTION

The diagnostic histopathologist is in an ideal position to supply clinical colleagues with a substantial amount of useful prognostic information from the routine examination of breast cancer specimens.[4] General guidelines for the preparation of such specimens have already been given in Chapter 2, but it is worth stressing again the importance of good fixation and processing. Most of the factors described below have a subjective element of morphological assessment and although relatively objective diagnostic criteria have now been provided these can be seriously compromised by poor specimen preparation. Many laboratories make a point of receiving specific specimens in the fresh state, such as lymph nodes, lungs, stomach and intestine and yet seem content to allow breast specimens to remain unsliced in formalin for 24 hours or more. Ideally then, breast specimens should also be incised in the fresh state so that immediate penetration of fixative into tumor slices can be achieved. A sufficient number of blocks should be taken to ensure adequate sampling, and routine, but careful, paraffin embedding is carried out. Standard 'thin' (4–6 µm) paraffin sections are then cut and in the great majority of cases routine staining with hematoxylin and eosin (H&E) is all that is necessary.

The following factors, all relatively simple to assess, have been shown to provide clinically relevant prognostic information, provided that careful attention is paid to diagnostic guidelines and protocols.

TUMOR SIZE

For correlation with prognosis the size of tumors should only be assessed on pathological specimens, as clinical measurement is notoriously inaccurate. If an estimate of clinical tumor size is required for therapeutic planning purposes, it should be checked by an ultrasonic measurement.

Pathological tumor size can be assessed in a number of ways. We recommend that the tumor diameter is initially measured to the nearest millimeter in three planes when the tumor is incised in the fresh state, as described in Chapter 2, Figure 2.27. After fixation, when the edges of the tumor may have become more clearly defined, the measurements are rechecked and the greatest diameter is taken as the tumor size. If there is any doubt about the definition of the tumor margin the measurement should be assessed further on the histological sections, using the Vernier scale on the microscope stage micrometer. It is recognized that this may give a small underestimation of size due to shrinkage of tissues during fixation and processing, but this slight consistent difference is preferable to the larger and less predictable errors that may arise from only measuring poorly delineated tumors macroscopically.[6] Measurement of size on histological sections is particularly appropriate for those tumors in which there is a large in situ component, and for small invasive carcinomas, especially those measuring 1 cm or less in diameter detected during mammographic screening. Examples of the measurement of tumor size on histological sections in a variety of circumstances are given in Figure 18.1.

Tumor size is a time dependent prognostic factor. As such it has been shown in many studies to influence prognosis;[4,7–11] patients with smaller tumors have a better long term survival than those with larger tumors. The significant correlations found by Elston et al,[9] Fisher et al[10] and Neville et al[11] are of particular interest since the data in these large multicenter trials, including measurement of tumor size, is based on the initial pathological assessments carried out by local participating pathologists, rather than the central review pathologists. This emphasizes the inherent strength of tumor size as a prognostic factor.

The estimation of tumor size has assumed particular importance in population screening for breast cancer. The term 'minimal breast cancer' (MBC) was originally introduced to delineate certain forms of breast cancer which carry an exceedingly good prognosis.[12] MBC included all cases of in situ carcinoma (ductal and lobular) and invasive carcinomas measuring 5 mm or less in diameter. The inclusion of in situ carcinoma is not relevant to this discussion, save to reiterate that

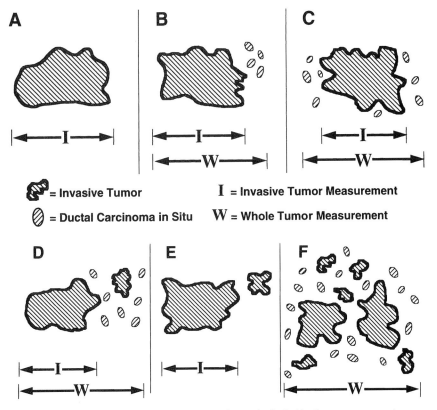

In E the satellite focus of invasive tumor is not included in the measurement

In F the best estimate of the total size of the invasive components is given

Fig. 18.1 Convention for the measurement of the maximum diameter of invasive carcinomas in a variety of circumstances.

lobular carcinoma in situ is considered nowadays to be a risk factor rather than an established malignancy (see Ch. 6). Subsequently, for no clearly defined reason (one might speculate that restriction to 5 mm simply identified too few cancers for analysis) the invasive component has been redefined by a number of different groups. The Breast Cancer Detection Demonstration Projects in the USA[13] and the American Cancer Society[14] have used 9 mm as the maximum diameter for so-called minimal invasive carcinoma (MIC) whilst the American College of Surgeons favor a measurement of up to *and including* 10 mm,[15] a figure also used in the UK National Breast Screening Programme (NHSBSP).[16] This lack of uniformity in definition causes problems in the interpretation of data from different studies, but there is little doubt that MIC are at an earlier stage than tumors which measure more than 10 mm in diameter. In most studies the frequency of axillary lymph node metastasis in MIC is 15–20%,[8,15,17] compared with over 40% in tumors measuring 15 mm or more.[17] Even more favorable results are obtained in women with breast cancer detected during the prevalent round of breast screening, axillary node metastasis ranging from 0–15%.[13,18–21]

Surprisingly it is difficult to obtain accurate data on the relationship between MIC and prognosis, but as expected survival appears to be better than that for patients with larger tumors. For example, in the long-term study from the Memorial Sloan-Kettering Cancer Centre[17] the projected relapse-free survival rates for 20 years after initial treatment were as follows:

<10 mm   — 88%
11–13 mm — 73%
14–16 mm — 65%
17–22 mm — 59%

However, our own studies from the Nottingham Tenovus Primary Breast Cancer Study (NTPBCS) suggest that the cut-off of 10 mm is not necessarily the best discriminator for MIC. Life table analysis of survival data shows that 15 mm may be a more significant watershed. The majority of the patients in this study are from symptomatic practice (i.e., those who attended a diagnostic clinic with symptoms such as breast lump) and it will be important to ascertain whether screening-detected tumors have the same pattern of prognosis.

It is clear that pathological tumor size is a valuable prognostic factor, and it has also become an important quality assurance measure for breast

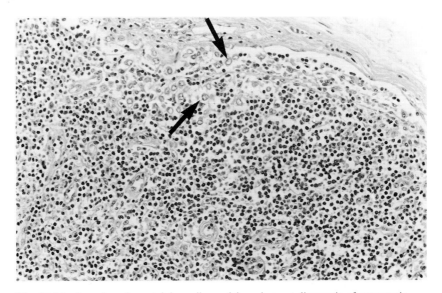

Fig. 18.2A Lymph node containing cells suspicious, but not diagnostic of, metastatic carcinoma. Grossly the node appeared normal and on this routine section the only abnormality is the presence of single large cells in the peripheral sinus (arrowheads). Hematoxylin–eosin × 185.

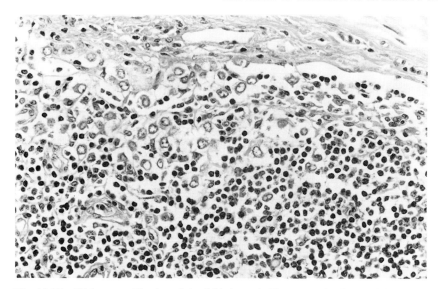

Fig. 18.2B   Higher magnification of the field shown in Figure 18.2A. The suspicious cells can be distinguished easily from normal lymphoid cells but not from macrophages. Hematoxylin–eosin × 400.

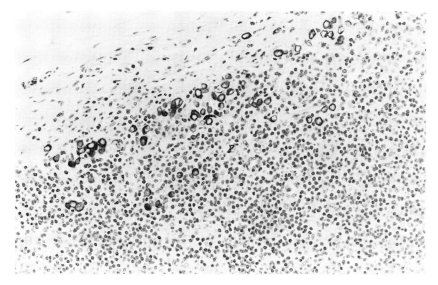

Fig. 18.2C   The epithelial nature of the suspicious cells is confirmed clearly by immunostaining with a cytokeratin marker. The primary tumor in this case was of infiltrating lobular type. Immunostaining for Cam 5.2 × 185.

screening programs[14,16,19] used in part to judge the ability of radiologists to detect impalpable invasive carcinomas in mammograms. For example, in the early years of the NHSBSP radiologists were expected to achieve a target of 15 MIC per 10 000 women screened in the prevalent round.[16] It is therefore incumbent upon pathologists to measure tumor size as accurately as possible. Paradoxically the risk of errors is greatest for smaller tumors and marked inconsistencies have been reported.[13] This has been confirmed in the UK NHSBSP during an External Quality Assessment scheme, when wide variations occurred in the measurement of tumor size in histological sections from a standard set of invasive carcinomas.[22] These data indicate that even for a relatively simple procedure such as assessment of maximum tumor diameter pathologists should use a strict protocol, as indicated in the NHSBSP document 'Pathology Reporting in Breast Cancer Screening'.[6]

DIFFERENTIATION

We have already indicated in Chapters 15–17 that until comparatively recently the histological classification of carcinoma of the breast was restricted to the main subdivision into in situ and invasive carcinoma. The majority of invasive carcinomas were designated simply as scirrhous carcinoma or mammary adenocarcinoma. It is now recognized that invasive carcinomas may be further subdivided according to their degree of differentiation. This is achieved in two ways, by more precise allocation of histological *type* according to the morphological pattern of the tumor, and by assigning a *grade* of differentiation based on evaluation of structural characteristics.

A wide range of morphological patterns may be recognized in invasive carcinoma of the breast.[23–27] These histological types have been discussed in some detail in Chapters 15 and 16, together with their prognostic implications and the data need not be repeated here. In summary, for the common histological types, patients may be stratified into four broad prognostic groups, as shown in Table 18.1. It is not possible to use the same groupings for the rare carcinomas at the present time, because for many of these tumors insufficient data is available. The reader is referred to Chapter 16 for prognostic details.

A full account of the methods for assessing histological grade in invasive carcinoma of the breast is given in Chapter 17. Essentially two main types of method have evolved, those in which multiple morphological factors are used[28–30] and those based on nuclear characteristics only.[31] Both have been shown in a large number of studies to give good correlation with overall survival (see Ch. 17), but the multifactorial method, especially with the modifications devised in Nottingham[30] has perhaps proved to be the more robust. It has been shown in three separate studies that

Table 18.1   Prognostic groups according to histological type

Excellent prognostic group: > 80% 10-year survival
    Tubular
    Invasive cribriform
    Mucinous
    Tubulolobular

Good prognostic group: 60–80% 10-year survival
    Tubular mixed
    Alveolar lobular
    Mixed ductal NST/Special type
    Atypical medullary

Moderate prognostic group: 50–60% 10-year survival
    Medullary
    Invasive papillary
    Classical lobular

Poor prognostic group: <50% 10-year survival
    Mixed lobular
    Ductal NST
    Solid lobular
    Mixed ductal NST/lobular

acceptable consistency can be achieved between different pathologists and centers[32–34] with the Nottingham method, which has been adopted for use in the UK NHSBSP,[6] by the European Breast Screening Pathology Group,[35] the Association of Directors of Anatomic and Surgical Pathology in the United States,[36] the Australian National Breast Screening Programme and in several other national studies.

In Chapter 17 we advocated the application of histological grade to all types of invasive carcinoma. We have assessed the effect of applying both tumor type and histological grade to a group of patients in the NTPBCS to determine their comparative value as prognostic factors.[37] We found that for a number of tumors the prognostic group assigned by type alone (Table 18.1) was less accurate than using type and grade combined (Table 18.2). For example, although grade 1 mucinous carcinomas behaved as predicted by type grouping with a greater than 80% 10-year survival, grade 2 mucinous carcinomas were placed more appropriately in the moderate prognostic group with a 10-year survival of 60–80%. Tubular mixed carcinomas, placed in the good prognostic group, could be re-assigned according to their grade, grade 1 tumors being more appropriate in the excellent group, grade 2 in the good group and grade 3 in the poor group. A similar pattern was found for several other types, including ductal

Table 18.2 Prognostic groups after grading and typing

Prognosis	Histological Type	Histological Grade
Excellent (>80% 10-year survival)	Tubular	Grade 1
	Invasive cribriform	Grade 1
	Tubular mixed	Grade 1
	Mixed ductal NST/special type	Grade 1
	Mixed ductal NST/lobular	Grade 1
	Tubulolobular	Grade 1
	Mucinous	Grade 1
Good (60–80% 10-year survival)	Ductal NST	Grade 1
	Mixed lobular	Grade 1
	Classical lobular	Grade 1
	Alveolar lobular	Grade 2
	Solid lobular	Grade 2
	Mucinous	Grade 2
	Tubular mixed	Grade 2
	Atypical medullary	Grade 3
Moderate (50–60% 10-year survival)	Mixed ductal NST/special type	Grades 2 and 3
	Ductal NST	Grade 2
	Mixed ductal NST/lobular	Grade 2
	Classical lobular	Grade 2
	Mixed lobular	Grade 2
	Medullary	Grade 3
Poor (<50% 10-year survival)	Mixed lobular	Grade 3
	Ductal NST	Grade 3
	Classical lobular	Grade 3
	Mixed ductal NST/lobular	Grade 3
	Solid lobular	Grade 3
	Tubular mixed	Grade 3

From Pereira et al, 1995[37]

NST and infiltrating lobular carcinoma. In multivariate analysis tumor type was found to be an independent factor, but with less weight than histological grade. In view of these data we reiterate our belief that both factors should be evaluated for each patient with invasive breast carcinoma in order to obtain the maximum prognostic information.

LYMPH NODE STAGE

It has long been recognized that involvement of loco-regional lymph nodes is one of the most important prognostic factors in breast cancer.[38–39] Clinical assessment of nodal status is notoriously inaccurate (enlarged nodes may be reactive whilst impalpable nodes may be involved by metastatic tumor) and it is now generally accepted that evaluation of lymph node stage should be based only on histological examination of excised nodes.[40] Numerous studies have shown that patients who have histologically confirmed loco-regional lymph node involvement have a significantly poorer prognosis than those without nodal involvement.[4,7–9,23,41–42] On average 10-year survival is reduced from 75% for patients with no lymph node involvement to 25–30% for those with lymph node metastases. Prognosis is also related to the overall number of loco-regional lymph nodes involved; the greater the number of nodes containing metastases the poorer the patient survival.[10,42–43] In practical terms the National Surgical Adjuvant Breast Project (NSABP) in the USA has found that it is useful to divide patients into two groups for therapeutic purposes, those with one to three positive nodes and those with four or more positive. The level of nodal involvement also provides useful prognostic information; metastasis to the 'higher' level in the axilla, and specifically the apex, carries a worse prognosis[38,42,44] as does spread to the internal mammary nodes.[44] In the NTPBCS we have demonstrated that highly significant prognostic information can be obtained by a lymph node sampling method with examination of a node from the low axilla, apex of axilla and second intercostal space.[45–47] In recent years there has been considerable debate regarding the *extent* of axillary lymph node dissection with arguments in favor of both axillary sampling[48–49] and axillary clearance.[50–51] In Edinburgh Steele et al[49] found no difference in the percentage of nodes involved in a comparison of clearance and sampling, and argued that adequate prognostic information could be obtained from the latter, provided that at least four nodes were examined. A greater number of nodes can be obtained at clearance and O'Dwyer asserted that it should be possible to examine at least 20.[50] However, the price for the additional prognostic information which may be gained by clearance is the increased risk of greater postoperative morbidity including reduced shoulder mobility and chronic lymphedema. Although Veronesi et al[42] now argue in favor of obtaining nodes from the highest level in the axilla, in practical terms we believe that a sensible compromise between the two methods should be employed. Internal mammary sampling only provides useful information in medially sited tumors and need not be performed if the tumor is in the lateral part of the breast.[52] Low axillary clearance, carried out below the level of the intercostobrachial nerve, produces enough lymph nodes (usually between four and 15) for accurate prognostication, with minimal morbidity. Apical node biopsy is additive, but to reduce the need for an additional incision should only be performed when the primary operation is mastectomy.

Since it is almost impossible to orientate axillary dissection specimens after fixation the surgeon has an obligation to identify clearly each node group (or level in a clearance sample) with sutures or clips.

The significance of the presence of metastatic carcinoma in the adipose tissue surrounding axillary lymph nodes, the so-called extranodal spread, is uncertain with conflicting data. It was suggested by Mambo and Gallager,[53] in a retrospective analysis, that this feature conveyed a poor prognosis in patients with up to three nodes involved, but not in those with four or more nodes involved. Similar results were obtained by Cascinelli et al[54] in a study of mastectomy without adjuvant radiotherapy or chemotherapy except that the effect of extranodal spread on recurrence rate was seen in patients with two or more nodes affected, irre-

spective of the total number of nodes involved. Fisher et al[55] have demonstrated in a prospective study that extranodal spread occurs significantly more frequently in patients who have four or more nodes involved by metastatic tumor, and although such patients were more likely to suffer short-term relapse they could not demonstrate that this effect was independent of nodal status. This view supports that of Hartveit[56] who found that extranodal spread had no intrinsic prognostic significance and concluded that the presence of tumor cells in efferent vessels was the only marker of poorer prognosis in patients with involved nodes.

There has also been debate on the significance of the actual size of lymph node metastases and in particular the question of so-called 'occult' metastases. A number of studies have claimed that the presence of micrometastases measuring 2 mm or less does not affect survival adversely, compared with that of lymph node negative patients.[57–59]

The data concerning the detection of tiny deposits, often consisting of scattered single cells revealed only after microscopic serial sections or immunostaining of lymph nodes with epithelial markers, are conflicting and should be interpreted with caution. Most groups have found a significantly worse prognosis for such patients[60–64] whilst others could detect no difference in survival.[58,66–67] Nasser et al[67] made a distinction between occult deposits measuring 0.2 mm or less and those greater than 0.2 mm and found that the latter conveyed a worse prognosis which did not, however, reach statistical significance. de Mascarel et al[68] in an extension of a study originally reported by Trojani et al,[69] compared serial macroscopical slicing (SMS) with immunohistochemical staining (IH). In univariate analysis patients in whom a single micrometastasis was detected by SMS had a significantly worse survival than those who were node negative, but this effect did not hold true in multivariate analysis. Using IH there was a significant difference in survival for patients with invasive ductal NST carcinomas, but not those with infiltrating lobular carcinoma. A similar study has been carried out by McGuckin and colleagues.[70] They found that step-sectioning (at 100 μm intervals) and immunohistochemistry (using the cytokeratin 'cocktail' MNF 116 and the MUC 1 antibody BC 2) identified occult metastases (OM) in 53 (25%) of 208 cases of apparently node-negative breast cancer. Most OMs were present in the subcapsular space, and in three quarters of the cases the deposits measured <1 mm in diameter and were only present in one node. Although the presence of OMs was associated with a significant reduction in survival in univariate analysis this was not the case in multivariate analysis when tumor size, histological grade and histological type were included.

Hartveit and Lilleng[71] have recently conducted a prospective study of axillary micrometastases using morphometric techniques. They used a strict definition for micrometastases (tumor deposits measuring 0.2 cm^2 or less in area) and found a rate of 15% (167 cases) in a series of 1069 patients receiving axillary dissection as part of their surgical treatment. Two different types of micrometastasis were identified: those in the capsular lymphatics or subcapsular sinus, but lacking growth in the nodal lymphoid tissue carried the same prognosis as so-called 'node positive' cases; those showing tumor growth within the lymphoid tissue, whether or not any other growth pattern was present, had a similar prognosis to node negative cases. The authors were unable to explain this apparent paradox, and, whilst interesting, their study has not settled the controversy concerning the prognostic significance of micrometastatic lymph node deposits.

Many of the studies discussed above have been based on retrospective assessment of relatively small numbers of cases and further work, preferably prospective, is clearly required to resolve the issue. For the present time it seems inappropriate to examine serial sections and carry out immunostaining in every case because of the considerable workload implications, and a sensible compromise is necessary. We agree with Hartveit et al[72] and Rosen[73] that careful manual dissection of the fixed axillary adipose tissue is the most cost-effective method for isolating lymph nodes for microscopic examination. A number of more elaborate procedures have been described including obtaining radiographs of the specimen[74] and clearing the adipose tissue with solvents.[75] Whilst these procedures will in general increase the yield of nodes found by locating very small nodes that may escape palpation the additional prognostic information obtained appears to be minimal.[72,76] We believe that the prognostic gain does not justify the considerable additional time and expense required for clearing.

Each lymph node identified should be submitted for histological examination, preferably using one cassette per node. If nodes are obviously involved on gross examination a single confirmatory section is sufficient. Nodes measuring up to 5 mm in length may be bisected and both halves embedded. For nodes measuring approximately 1 cm in length we take two separate blocks at right angles to the long axis, three blocks are made from nodes measuring 1.5 cm and a maximum of four from those up to 2 cm. Immunostaining is reserved for the small number of cases in which the morphological appearances are suspicious, but not diagnostic, of metastatic carcinoma (Fig. 18.2A–C). This protocol is very similar to that outlined in the NHSBSP guidelines for breast screening pathology.[6]

VASCULAR INVASION

The prognostic value of the estimation of the presence or absence of vascular invasion (VI) in breast cancer is disputed.[77] Some studies have found no correlation with clinical outcome[78–79] whilst others have shown that the presence of vascular invasion predicts for both recurrence[48,80–81] and long-term survival.[82–86] The most likely explanation for such discrepancies is the wide range in the reported frequency of vascular invasion, which varies from 20 to 54% and the related problem of the distinction of true vessels, especially lymphatics, from artefactual soft tissue spaces due to fixation shrinkage artefact.

In our experience tumor emboli are found only rarely in muscular blood vessels and these should not pose a diagnostic problem. In practice the great majority of vascular invasion is seen in association with thin walled channels. It is virtually impossible to determine whether such spaces are lymphatics, capillaries or post capillary venules nor, indeed, is there a compelling reason to make the distinction.[86] We believe that vascular permeation should be left unspecified and the broad term 'vascular invasion' used. VI should only be

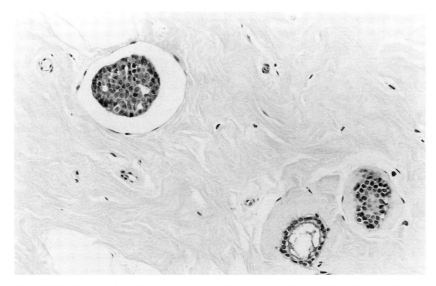

Fig. 18.3A   Vascular invasion. A tumor embolism is seen within a thin walled vascular space. Part of a normal lobule is present at the lower right. Hematoxylin–eosin × 185.

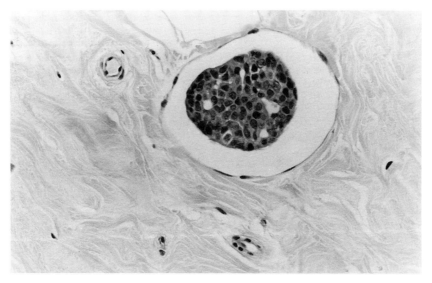

Fig. 18.3B   Higher magnification of the field shown in Figure 18.3A. The flattened endothelial lining of the vessel is clearly visible, and small arterioles are present in the adjacent connective tissue. Hematoxylin–eosin × 400.

assessed in the breast tissue adjacent to the main primary tumor and not within it; adherence to a simple but strict protocol is essential. Tumor emboli must be present within clear spaces which have a complete lining of endothelial cells (Fig. 18.3A and B). The spaces are often in close proximity to small muscular blood vessels and may also be separated from the main tumor by normal lobular units and interlobular stroma (Figs 18.4, 18.5A and B). These topographical patterns have been emphasized by Örbo and colleagues (Fig. 18.6)[87] as being helpful in distinguishing vascular invasion from artefactual spaces around cords of invasive carcinoma and foci of ductal carcinoma in situ, due to fixation shrinkage artefact (Fig. 18.7). Such problems are, of course, substantially reduced

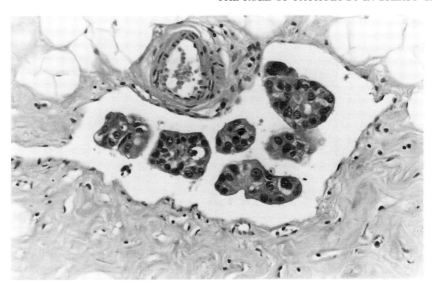

Fig. 18.4 Vascular invasion, paravascular pattern. The thin walled vessel is in close proximity to a small artery and is probably, therefore, a lymphatic channel. Hematoxylin–eosin × 185.

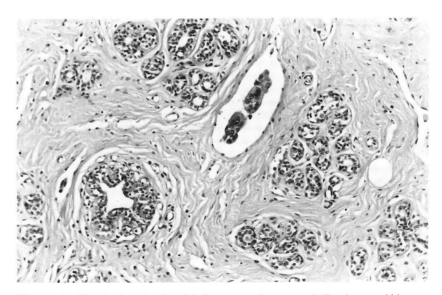

Fig. 18.5A Vascular invasion, interlobular pattern. A tumor embolism is seen within a vascular space, situated between several normal lobular units. Hematoxylin–eosin × 125.

by obtaining good fixation, as described in Chapter 2.

Special techniques have little place in the evaluation of vascular invasion. Elastic stains have been used by some groups to distinguish blood vessels from lymphatic channels; although large vessels may have elastic tissue in their walls so do breast ducts[88] and small vessels such as capillaries, venules and lymphatics have no elastic lamina. Several groups have evaluated the use of immuno-staining for endothelial markers such as laminin, type IV collagen, Factor VIII related antigen and *Ulex europaeus* agglutinin I; they are not reliable in distinguishing vessels from ductal structures, but

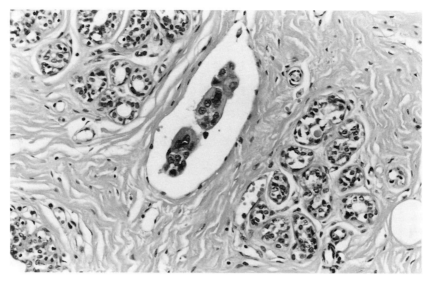

Fig. 18.5B Higher magnification of the field shown in Figure 18.5A to confirm the endothelial lining of the vascular space illustrated. Hematoxylin–eosin × 185.

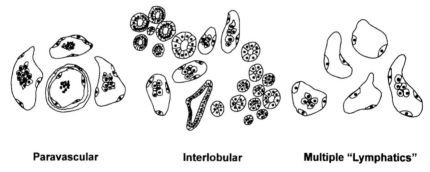

| Paravascular | Interlobular | Multiple "Lymphatics" |

Fig. 18.6 Diagram to show the different geographical patterns of vascular invasion. Reproduced, with permission, from Örbo et al.[87]

may have a place in excluding shrinkage artefact.[88–92] In summary, at the present time, it is clear that examination of hematoxylin and eosin stained sections is the most reliable method for identifying VI in breast cancer.[86,89,92] Immunostaining for endothelial markers should be reserved for equivocal cases and in this respect the newer antibodies CD 31 and CD 34 may prove to be the most useful method.

In common with other histopathological prognostic factors the assessment of VI involves a degree of subjective interpretation and its reproducibility has been questioned.[93] As indicated above, strict criteria must be followed in order to reduce inter- and intra-observer variability to a minimum. In our own study of over 1700 patients a subset of 400 cases was examined by two pathologists; overall agreement on the presence or absence of VI was 85%.[86] Other studies have also shown a similar high concurrence between pathologists.[80,84,87,94] It is interesting that although Gilchrist et al[93] concluded that the identification of intralymphatic tumor emboli was not reproducible they reported an 86% concordance for the assessment of blood vessel invasion. Many of the disagreements which were observed between the three pathologists in this study were, in fact, of a minor nature, and in our view these

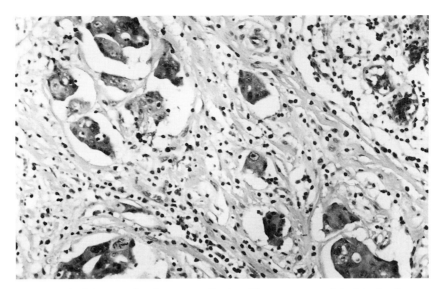

Fig. 18.7   Shrinkage artefact due to poor fixation. The spaces around the islands of tumor cells lack an endothelial lining and care must be taken not to mistake these appearances for vascular invasion. Hematoxylin–eosin × 185.

do not detract from the overall robustness of the method.

Several studies have confirmed that the presence of VI correlates very closely with loco-regional lymph node involvement[84,86,94] and it has been argued that it can provide prognostic information as powerful as lymph node stage.[81] Whilst this contention is not widely accepted it is certainly worth stressing that assessment of VI is a valuable surrogate for lymph node stage in cases where lymph nodes are not available for examination. However, the presence of VI also provides prognostic information in patients whose axillary lymph nodes are tumor free. In these patients there is a correlation between VI and early recurrence,[80–81,95] and this effect has also been shown to be independent of occult axillary node involvement. In the NTPBCS we have confirmed the significant contribution of VI to the prediction of long-term survival, but like Roses et al[80] we have also demonstrated that this effect is independent of lymph node stage, by using multivariate analysis.[86]

Despite this association with overall survival it appears that in practical management terms the most important role for the assessment of vascular invasion lies in the area of local recurrence.

Vascular invasion has been shown in a number of studies to be a powerful predictor of local recurrence following conservation therapy[48,80,86,95–96] and its presence also indicates a higher risk for flap recurrence in patients receiving mastectomy.[97] The use of VI in clinical management is discussed further in Chapter 22.

MISCELLANEOUS FACTORS

A number of other morphological features of breast carcinoma have been proposed as prognostic factors, but published data concerning their clinical significance is conflicting and they are therefore regarded as being of relatively less importance than those discussed above.

Tumor necrosis

In common with tumors in other sites carcinoma of the breast exhibits a variable degree of tumor cell necrosis. In extreme examples this may be visible on gross examination as a sharply demarcated area of dullness, usually in a central position. More frequently tumor necrosis is only apparent on microscopical examination where it is characterized, as in any tissue, by the nuclear changes of karyorrhexis, pyknosis and karyolysis and granular eosinophilic cytoplasmic degeneration resulting in loss of cellular outlines. Necrotic areas are eventually replaced by reparative fibrosis.

There is little accurate data on the proportion of invasive carcinomas which exhibit tumor necrosis, although the phenomenon appears to be confined chiefly to ductal NST carcinomas, particularly those of high grade.[65,98] Using the presence of necrosis in any group of tumor cells as the defining feature Carter et al[99] found tumor necrosis in 40% of cases in a retrospective analysis of radical mastectomy specimens. Roses et al[80] obtained a similar figure but Fisher et al[65] found tumor necrosis in 60% of cases. The latter is clearly an overestimate as the study included cases in which comedo necrosis within an associated in situ component was also counted.

The prognostic significance of tumor necrosis has been evaluated formally in relatively few studies. The conclusions are somewhat conflicting, but most have indicated that the presence of tumor necrosis is a poor prognostic feature.

Roses et al[80] assessed pathological factors in stage 1 breast cancer (T1N0M0) and found that the presence of tumor necrosis did not predict for recurrence in either univariate or multivariate analysis. In contrast tumor necrosis has been equated in other studies with 'early treatment failure'[58,65] and reduced overall survival.[99–101] It is extremely difficult to judge the relative merit of these studies, particularly as different criteria have been used to define tumor necrosis and different methods employed in assessing its extent. For example, Gilchrist et al[100] defined tumor necrosis as any 'coagulative' necrosis visible at 40× magnification, whilst Parham et al[101] used a morphometric point counting method, but then simply stated that extensive tumor necrosis was a particularly poor prognostic feature without defining 'extensive'. Parham and colleagues have proposed a new simplified method for grading breast cancer by combining tumor necrosis and mitotic counts.[102] They claim a good correlation with survival but, as Elston and Ellis[103] pointed out, little numerical data was provided, especially concerning the diagnostic criteria used, and for this reason the method seems to lack practical utility.

In summary there is some published evidence which suggests that the presence of tumor necrosis may be a poor prognostic feature. However, before tumor necrosis is accepted as a useful prognostic factor reproducible criteria for the definition of necrosis and evaluation of its extent must be devised. Tumor necrosis must also be tested in multivariate analysis against other prognostic factors, especially histological grade with which it appears to be closely associated.

Extensive in situ component (EIC)

The amount of ductal carcinoma in situ (DCIS) associated with invasive carcinomas is extremely variable and the assessment of its extent is highly subjective. Many tumors appear to have little or no associated DCIS; this was estimated as approximately three quarters of cases in one large study.[23] In a minority of tumors (approximately 10% in Fisher's study[23]) there is abundant DCIS, often associated with tiny multicentric foci of invasive carcinoma within the main tumor mass. In the World Health Organization classification of breast carcinomas[104] it was suggested that carcinomas in which the component of ductal carcinoma in situ amounted to more than four times the invasive element in area would carry a more favorable prognosis than other ductal NST carcinomas. These tumors were classified as invasive duct carcinoma with a prominent intraduct component (IDC with PIC). Few comprehensive studies have been carried out on the clinicopathological significance of the proportions of in situ and invasive components in such tumors. Linell and colleagues[105–106] divided invasive ductal carcinoma into two groups, tubuloductal and invasive comedo carcinoma. Although the invasive comedo group seems to correspond in general with the WHO IDC with PIC category, Linell and Rank[106] found that such tumors carried a worse prognosis than their tubuloductal groups. This appears to be related to the higher tumor grade of the invasive comedo type. In contrast Silverberg and Chitale[107] had shown previously that there was a significant association between a prominent in situ component and lower histological grade and increased 5-year survival. More recently Matsukuma and colleagues[108] have obtained similar results. They divided infiltrating ductal carcinomas into two main groups, those with less than 20% invasive component and those in which invasive elements exceeded 20%, and found that the former group had fewer nodal metastases and a significantly better 10-year survival. These data must, however, be interpreted with caution. It is clear from the study of Matsukuma and colleagues[108] that both the invasive and in situ components in the group with less than 20% invasive component were of lower grade, and from their illustrations some of these cases would fall into our own Tubular Mixed category.[109] It may well be that the proportion of in situ component in an invasive carcinoma is not an *independent* prognostic factor when histological grade and type are taken into account. This question would best be resolved in a multivariate analysis.

It appears that the DCIS component in invasive carcinomas is of greater importance in the management of patients considered for conservation therapy. At a meeting of the European Organization for Research into the Treatment of Cancer (EORTC) it was concluded that the principal risk factor for breast relapse after breast conserving treatment is large residual burden and the main source of this burden is EIC.[110] This statement was based on evidence from a number of studies including those of Schnitt et al[111] and Fourquet et al[112] and supported by those of Holland et al[113] and Jacquemier et al.[114] The Boston Group,[111] who have the most experience in this area, have defined EIC as the presence of DCIS within an invasive carcinoma which occupies 25% or more of the overall tumor mass and which extends beyond the confines of that main mass. They found initially that invasive carcinomas with EIC had a considerably higher local recurrence rate than those without EIC, and a significant proportion of such cases relapsed as invasive carcinoma. As yet there is no consensus agreement for the definition of EIC and some groups have not found that the presence of DCIS in invasive carcinomas is as powerful a predictor of local recurrence in multivariate analysis as other factors such as vascular invasion.[48] Furthermore, the Boston group have now shown that although the presence of EIC predicts for the likelihood of margins being involved it does not predict for recurrence in the presence of complete local excision.[115] Further studies are required to establish the precise role of EIC as a prognostic factor.

Stromal factors

A number of stromal alterations have been described in association with invasive carcinoma and are believed to result from the release of cytokines either from the tumor cells themselves or from adjacent stromal cells. Attempts have been made to correlate these with prognosis and their significance is discussed in this section.

Stromal giant cells

Benign, osteoclast-like stromal giant cells occurring in association with breast carcinoma are rare but well documented, first being reported by Leroux in 1931[116] but with several more recent descriptions[117–119] including a reported case in a male.[120] Such giant cells are found adjacent to or within the tumor cell islands and are believed to be histiocytic in origin.[117,119,121] They are also described in lymph node metastases and within intralymphatic tumor thrombi.[119] Holland and colleagues described an association with a particular type of carcinoma which often has a cribriform or 'adenocystic' architecture[119] and others have reported a similar association[122–123] (see also Ch. 15). However giant cells are also described in other tumor types.[118,124] More constantly, there is also marked stromal angiogenesis and this observation, together with the intimate association between the giant cells and the tumor cell islands, has led to the proposal that the tumor cells might elaborate some substances capable of eliciting both the giant cell formation and the marked stromal angiogenesis.[118–119] Cribriform carcinoma, with or without associated giant cells, has a good prognosis, but the prognostic implications of the finding of benign stromal giant cells in association with other types are currently unknown as so few cases with long-term follow-up have been reported. On the basis of their own series of eight and a review of previously reported cases Agnantis and Rosen[118] stated 'it seems likely that the prognosis . . . is not especially favorable when compared with that for patients who have more ordinary infiltrating lesions' and until more information becomes available, we do not feel that this somewhat vague statement can be improved upon.

Stromal elastosis

Stromal elastosis is a feature of many benign and malignant breast lesions. There has been considerable debate about the prognostic significance of tumor-associated elastosis. Shivas and Douglas, for example, found the presence of marked elastosis to be associated with prolonged survival[125] and others have noted a correlation with a lower incidence of lymph node metastases.[126] However, these observations have been disputed by groups who have shown an association with a poorer prognosis[23,127–128] and by yet others who have been unable to demonstrate any relationship between prominent elastosis and prognosis.[129–130] There does, however, appear to be a significant correlation between the presence of marked elastosis and both estrogen receptor expression by tumor cells and response of patients to endocrine therapy.[129,131–132] This is probably due to the fact that elastosis is particularly associated with tumor types having a relatively good prognosis (e.g. tubular, tubular mixed, invasive cribriform).[109] These associations suggest that elastosis is not an independent prognostic factor and assessment of its degree, difficult in itself, offers no further prognostic information over the traditional factors of tumor type and histological grade.

Stromal fibrosis

Stromal fibrosis is frequently found in varying amounts in invasive breast carcinoma.[102,133] However, as for the above mentioned stromal features, its role in influencing prognosis is not determined. Some authors have identified a favorable effect of fibrosis, or specifically, stromal hyalinization on survival.[134–135] Others have documented a lower mortality in tumors with a fibrovascular rather than dense collagenous stroma.[136–137] Still others have found no effect.[23,79,102] This may, in part, be due to the confounding effect of tumor type, in that extensive fibrosis may be found in both low and high grade tumors. Furthermore, Giani and co-workers have identified an association between fibrosis and progesterone receptor expression[138–139]

suggesting that fibrosis itself is unlikely to prove an independent prognostic factor.

HORMONE RECEPTORS

INTRODUCTION

Some tumors, notably carcinoma of the breast and prostate, are often responsive to hormones, a property which has become exploited through endocrine surgery and more recently medically using drugs which influence hormone levels or inhibit the effects of hormones on tumor cells.

Steroid hormones bind with high specificity and affinity to intracellular receptors. These steroid receptors belong to a 'superfamily' of proteins whose function is to control the transcription of a repertoire of other cellular genes.[140] Steroid receptors such as estrogen and progesterone receptor are located in the cell nucleus. Hormone is believed to diffuse or be transported to the nucleus where a steroid-receptor complex is formed with receptor dimerization. This dimer binds to specific DNA response element sequences usually located in the promoter regions of regulated genes. Some of the genes regulated by steroid receptors are involved in controlling cell growth and it is currently believed that these effects are the most relevant to estrogen receptor influences on the behavior and treatment of breast cancer.

HISTORY

The experiments of Beatson in the late 19th century first explored the influence of ovarian hormones on breast cancer growth.[141] He observed regression of metastatic lesions in premenopausal women with breast cancer following oophorectomy. This data was largely ignored, despite being confirmed by other similar studies, until further series in the 1950s demonstrated firstly that ablation of the adrenal glands could influence the behavior of postmenopausal breast cancer and prostatic cancer[142] and subsequently through the observation that similar effects could be obtained by hypophysectomy.[143] Similar effects had been observed using ovarian radiation to induce an artificial menopause.[144] For a comprehensive historical review see Seth and Allegra.[145]

In the 1940s the observation that synthetic estrogenic hormones could influence breast tumor growth[146] introduced the potential for non surgical 'hormone' treatment of breast cancer. Hormonal therapeutic agents fall into three broad categories. The first, including drugs such as Zoladex, which is a potent gonadotrophin releasing hormone agonist, act centrally to inhibit the release of gonadotrophins from the pituitary by a process of desensitization, thereby effecting a chemical castration. The second category includes inhibitors of steroid synthesis, such as the aromatase inhibitor aminoglutethamide, which reduces estrogen synthesis. Tamoxifen is currently the most widely used agent and belongs to the third category of steroid antagonists which are thought to act predominantly by inhibiting the action of hormones in their target tissues.

Approximately 30% of unselected patients with breast cancer will respond to hormone therapy such as oophorectomy (or chemical castration) or tamoxifen treatment. The demonstration that radio-labeled estradiol bound to some breast cancer specimens and that this effect was related to response to hormone ablation[147] led to the development of hormone receptor assays directed at identification of patients suitable for hormone therapy. By assay of estrogen receptor status alone, using the standard radioligand binding assay on tissue cytosol samples, a response is seen in between 50 and 60% of patients with estrogen receptor positive tumors, in contrast with a <10% response observed in patients with estrogen receptor negative tumors.[148] The threshold for designation for estrogen receptor positivity is usually 10 fmol/mg cytosol protein. Levels of response are recognized to increase to over 80% in patients with tumors having high receptor levels of several hundred or more fmol/mg protein. Prediction of response can be refined further by combining estrogen receptor assay with progesterone receptor assay;[148] ER positive PR positive tumors have a 78% response, ER negative PR positive a 45% response and ER negative PR negative 10% response.[148] It should be noted that these results relate to ligand binding assay systems and results from combined ER and PR immunocytochemical assay may differ.

The cytosol ligand binding assay has until recently been the standard assay method but has a number of disadvantages (Table 18.3). In particular it requires a relatively large amount of tissue homogenate and is affected by bound estrogen receptor from high endogenous levels of estradiol in premenopausal women. The development of monoclonal antibodies specific for the receptor protein[149] led the way to both enzyme immunoassay[150] and immunocytochemical assay development.[151-152] More recently, the immunocytochemical methods, despite being less readily quantifiable, have superseded both the ligand binding and enzyme immunobiochemical assays, as they require less tissue, allow formal histological assessment thereby reducing sampling error,[151,153-162] and may be used on very small samples such as fine needle aspirates.[163-164] All these forms of assay correlate well,[154,156,160,162-164] but there is some evidence that there is a closer association with

Table 18.3 Comparison between biochemical and immunocytochemical hormone receptor assays

	Biochemical	Immunocytochemical
Results	Objective numerical result	Subjective semiquantitative assessment
Tissue required	Fresh, relatively large volume, tissue cannot be used for anything else	Fixed, any representative cells, routine histology samples can be used
Cost	EIA expensive, tissue must be stored frozen	Cheap (with latest antibodies)
QA systems	Well established schemes	Limited QA available. No standardization available
Clinical validation	Yes	Yes
False results	Affected by tumor cellularity, cannot assess tissue quality, occupation of receptor by hormone can affect DCC result, normal tissue levels can influence result	Poor tissue fixation can affect reactivity, receptors may not be functional

response to hormone therapy using immunocyto-chemical assay results[153–154,163] probably because of avoidance of sampling error and lack of influence of tumor cellularity and type.

The early immunocytochemical methods developed required frozen material, but more recently the antibodies have been applied successfully to routinely processed formalin fixed tissue.

Initially many of the methods employed required enzyme predigestion and overnight incubation of the tissue sections.[157–158,160–161,165–166] Microwave antigen retrieval has been found by several authors[167–170] to enhance immunohistochemical staining and is becoming increasingly popular. The mechanism of antigen retrieval is uncertain but may involve disruption of protein cross-linkages in a similar way to that occurring in enzymatic predigestion.[169]

These techniques allow successful use of antibodies such as 1D5 on tissues routinely processed in any histopathology laboratory giving the potential for estimation of estrogen receptor status as part of the process of histological assessment of breast carcinoma. In our center this method[162] has now been adopted for all cases of primary breast carcinoma allowing inclusion of estrogen receptor status in the standard histological report.

IMMUNOCYTOCHEMICAL METHODS

Choice of antibody

The Abbott H222 antibody is well characterized[171] and immunohistochemical methods using this antibody have been found repeatedly to correlate well with traditional biochemical methods of assessing ER status[153–154,157,163] and to identify different prognostic groups. The antibody has been successfully applied to both frozen and formalin fixed, routinely processed tissue,[161] but the latter requires overnight incubation and careful assessment to avoid false negative results. Use of H222 has declined following development of antibodies such as 1D5 which are more successful on fixed tissues. Assessment of ER status using the 1D5 antibody with microwave pre-treatment of tissues gives comparable results with other means of assessment, but has many advantages particularly its applicability to routine

histology samples,[162] as well as methodological ease and speed. The microwave technique is technically easy and rapid to perform, not requiring an overnight incubation procedure which may be seen as a disadvantage of the methods described for the H222 antibody. 1D5 is our favored antibody for these reasons. It gives an evaluation of ER status which correlates well with the assessment made using Abbott H222 on both frozen and formalin fixed tissue.[162] However, despite the overall good correlation, in some cases a marked discrepancy has been observed between the H-scores obtained.[162] This is unlikely to have been due to interobserver error and may be the result of tumor heterogeneity, differences in individual specimen handling or to recognition of different epitopes by the two antibodies. Similar discrepancies have been observed by others using 1DS and in studies comparing the Abbott H222 antibody on frozen and formalin fixed tissue.[161]

Tissue fixation

Estrogen receptor is a thermolabile unstable nuclear protein which is water soluble and has a short half-life after surgical removal of tumor. Most tissue fixatives can be used to preserve receptor reactivity if microwave predigestion is used. It is essential, however, to ensure that rapid fixation occurs and tumor specimens should be incised immediately after resection to ensure rapid penetration of fixative (see also Ch. 2).

Staining methods and controls

The methods currently used with antibodies such as 1D5 are well described[172] and assistance is available from the commercial suppliers of these antibodies. As noted above all rely on microwave antigen retrieval.

Use of control tissue is essential in hormone receptor assays particularly because of the risk of false negative classification. Positive control tissues should include not only a block of a known strongly positive tissue but also a block of tissue showing weak expression to ensure sensitivity is maintained (Fig. 18.8). It is also useful to select a test block which includes normal breast lobules and ducts (Fig. 18.8) which provides an internal

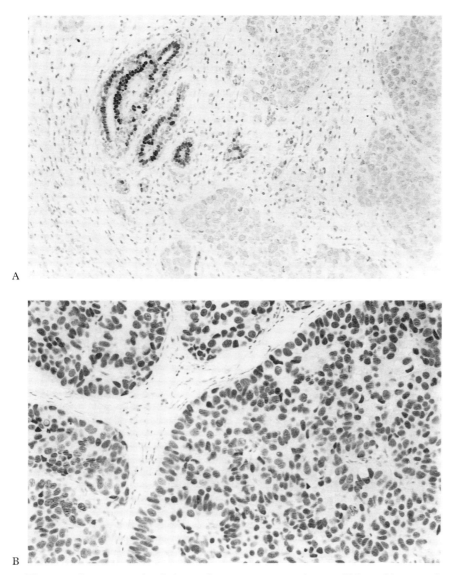

Fig. 18.8 Immunocytochemical assay for estrogen receptor is now widely used because of its benefits (see Table 18.3). Breast adenocarcinomas show a range of reactivity from negative (Fig. 18.8B), to all tumor cells being positive (Fig. 18.8B). It is important to use appropriate controls with the assay including whenever possible internal control cell in the form of normal ducts and acini (Fig. 18.8A). Antibody DAKO ID5 immunocytochemical stain, A and B × 125.

control population of cells since a proportion of the latter should show positive reactivity. Use of internal control cells in this fashion protects against the effects of poor fixation.

Evaluation of staining and scoring methods

Estrogen and progesterone receptor are located in the nucleus of breast epithelial and carcinoma cells (Fig. 18.8). There is currently no internationally accepted scoring system for hormone receptor immunocytochemical assay. The proportion of tumor cells showing positive reactivity (Abbott Laboratories data sheet), their intensity of reactivity, combinations of both of these[152] and a simple categorical system[172] have all been promoted.

Four of these methods have been reviewed recently with emphasis on their predictive abilities.[172] All showed strong association with response to hormone treatment, with the simplest categorical system having the highest statistical association, indicating that there is no clear advantage obtained by use of the more complex scoring methods for basic stratification into receptor positive and negative groups.

In our laboratory we currently provide a result in the form of an H-score and the percentage of tumor cells showing reactivity. The H-score is based on a summation of the proportion of tumor cells showing different degrees of reactivity; no reactivity = 0, weak = 1, moderate = 2, strong = 3. This gives a maximum total score of 300 if 100% of tumor cells show strong reactivity.

H-score system:
0 × % tumor cells negative
+
1 × % tumor cells weakly positive
+
2 × % tumor cells moderately positive
+
3 × % tumor cells strongly positive
= H-score (range 0–300)

For example, a tumor with all tumor cells showing positive reactivity with 20% strongly, 50% moderately and 30% weakly reactive would achieve an H-score of 190 (20 × 3 + 50 × 2 + 30 × 1). Use of semiquantitative methods, such as the H-score, which produce a numerical score influenced by the intensity of reactivity, have an association with the amount of receptor present as assessed by biochemical methods.[162] Informed clinicians are now beginning to use not only a standard result based on a common cut-off point or threshold, but some form of added quantitation of known sensitivity and specificity (Table 18.4). It is possible to assess the sensitivity and specificity of an assay at different cut-off points giving an ability to choose differing thresholds for different clinical situations.[162] For example, when selecting for adjuvant hormone therapy, sensitivity is required and a low threshold may be appropriate; in contrast, elderly patients or patients with advanced tumors being selected for primary/first line hormone treatment require specificity and a higher threshold is indicated (see also Ch. 22).

Table 18.4 Simplification of estrogen receptor immunocytochemical evaluation in the form of a positive versus negative result is common practice but is being superseded by a need to have more quantitative data for clinical situations requiring differing levels of specificity and sensitivity with regard to response to hormone therapy

H-score cut-off	Sensitivity		Specificity	
	1D5	H222	1D5	H222
30	95%	71%	49%	55%
50	90%	67%	51%	62%
100	71%	57%	59%	74%

Reproduced with permission from Goulding et al, 1995.[162]

None of the hormone receptor assays are absolute in their ability to predict response (Table 18.5). A proportion (0–10% in different studies) of ER negative tumors is found to respond to hormone therapy.[154–155,163,173] It has been postulated that estrogen receptor expression is stimulated by low levels of available estrogen[174] and it is possible that down-regulation of the ER gene to immunohistochemically undetectable levels may occur in some tumors due to high circulating levels of endogenous estrogen. This does not necessarily mean that they will not respond to hormone therapy, which has itself been shown to up-regulate ER expression in normal breast tissue.[175]

The poor specificity (Table 18.4) of the ER status in identifying tumors which will respond to hormone therapy has also been documented in many studies[154–155,162–163,173] and suggests that other factors are important. It may be that the ER receptor is present, but defective[176] or that ER production by some tumor cells is an epiphe-

Table 18.5 A typical distribution of patients showing differing levels of response to hormone therapy. Separation into ER positive and negative groups according to immunocytochemical assay scored using the H-score system allows a degree of prediction of response to treatment

	ER negative (H-score 0–49)	ER positive (H-score 50–300)	Response totals
Response (UICC 1+2)	2	18	20
Static disease (UICC 3)	1	17	18
Progression (UICC 4)	37	15	52
ER status totals	40	50	90

$\chi^2 = 35.7$, 3 df, $P < 0.0001$.
Reproduced with permission from Goulding et al, 1995.[162]

nomenon, not related to the growth requirements of the cell.

The observation that a proportion of tumors exhibit heterogeneous reactivity is well documented.[157,161–162,171] The reasons for its occurrence are not clear. It may be due to heterogeneous expression of ER by tumors as described by Poulson.[167] Similar heterogeneity is observed in normal tissue[175] and may be related to different physiological states within the cell population.[171]

MOLECULAR MARKERS

INTRODUCTION

During the last 15 years there has been considerable innovation and development of techniques which can be used to study cell biology and behavior. These include immunocytochemistry, monoclonal antibody technology, molecular biology and biomedical engineering resulting in advanced flow and image cytometric systems. The volume of research results emerging from basic scientists, pathologists and clinicians relative to these techniques is ever increasing. This generation of data demonstrates the immense interest in the potential of these methods to provide useful information of biological and clinical importance. Breast cancer is one area that has received such attention because of its frequency in Western countries and its exhibition of a wide spectrum of clinical behavior. As noted above the acceptance that conservation techniques of surgery and radiotherapy are safe alternatives to mastectomy and developments of chemotherapeutic schedules have now provided the patient, surgeon and oncologist with realistic choices of treatment. The question now being asked is whether this choice can be influenced appropriately by a knowledge of molecular processes which are present or have occurred and which may influence tumor cell behavior.

This section provides a brief overview of those techniques and molecules which have generated the most interest in the study of breast disease.

MOLECULES OF INTEREST IN BREAST DISEASE

A host of polyclonal and monoclonal antibodies have been produced to breast epithelial cells, their cell products, tumors or to common cell determinants which have associations with breast disease. The expression of antigens identified by these antibodies can be studied either by immunocytochemistry on tissue sections or cytology preparations, by enzyme linked immuno-assay (ELIZA) of body fluids or soluble cell fractions and by flow cytometry of single cell or cell fraction preparations. Antigens which vary in expression or appear at specific times during normal cell growth, function, differentiation, proliferation or neoplasia are of particular interest.

Antibodies to the following molecules have stimulated the most interest in breast cancer research.

Epithelial mucins

The primary functional role of breast epithelial cells is to produce milk during lactation. The lipid rich droplets are surrounded by a membrane derived from the epithelial cell apical membrane. This membrane is rich in carbohydrates on the external and, uniquely, on the internal cytoplasmic side. A highly immunogenic mucin component of the membrane has stimulated considerable investigation. Initially polyclonal antibodies to delipidated human milk fat globule membrane (HMFGM)[177] were produced. Following production of polyclonal antiserum many groups have produced monoclonal antisera to such high molecular weight glycoprotein mucins (see reviews[178–179]) normally expressed on the apical membrane of human breast and other epithelial cells (Fig. 18.9). The varying reactivity of some of these antibodies gave the initial impression that there may be a family of such mucins present in glandular epithelial cells and led to a variety of names such as epithelial membrane antigen (EMA),[180] the 'MAM' series 'polymorphic epithelial mucin' (PEM)[181] and episialin[182] being used to describe the mucin recognized by particular antibodies. Interlaboratory collaborative studies[183] have shown that one highly immunogenic high molecular weight glycoprotein (over 400 kD) carries most of the epitopes recognized by these antibodies. This mucin is now known as MUC 1[184] and it is a member of the heterogeneous group of at least eight highly glyco-

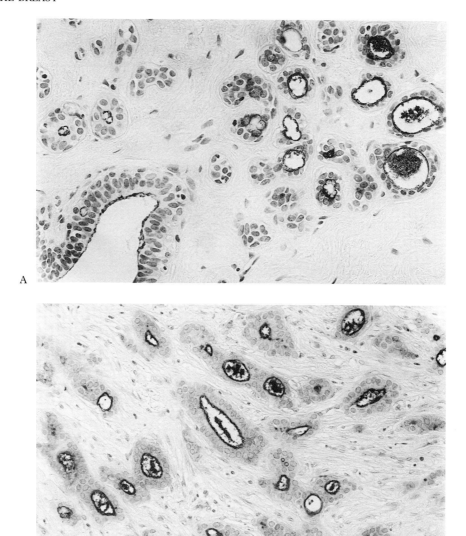

Fig. 18.9 A,B   See caption on facing page.

sylated mucin proteins (MUC 1–8), which form the major component of mucus. They have a central threadlike non-globular protein core with highly glycosylated and unglycosylated regions. MUC 1 is a transmembrane glycoprotein with a large cytoplasmic tail which interacts with the actin containing microfilaments. The core protein is made up of tandem repeats of 20 amino acids and reacts with many of the antibodies raised to HMFGM and breast cancer cells.[185] Carcinomas show a difference in glycosylation of the core protein from normal cells which could result in exposure of some epitopes in malignancy. The function of MUC 1 and other mucins is not clear but they are thought to have roles in cell protection or lubrication, maintenance of viscosity in secretions, regulation of cell growth and cellular recognition.[184,186] They are thought to facilitate tumor protection from immune attack, and influence tumor growth and metastasis.

Expression of other mucins such as MUC 2, 3 and 8 is seen in a proportion of breast carci-

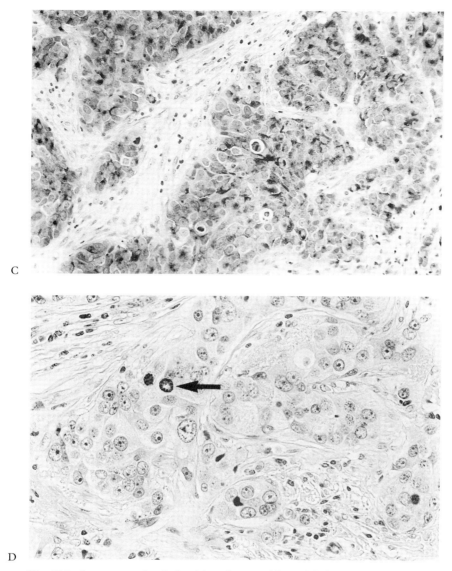

C

D

Fig. 18.9 Immunocytochemical staining of a normal breast lobular unit (Fig. 18.9A) and three breast cancers (Fig. 18.9B, C and D) with the monoclonal antibody NCRC11 which recognizes the epithelial mucin MUC 1 (epithelial membrane antigen). The mucin is present on the apical membrane surface of normal breast ducts (Fig. 18.9A) and acini. It is expressed in a similar fashion by breast carcinomas showing glandular/tubular differentiation (Fig. 18.9B) and is also expressed in the cytoplasm by a proportion of tumors (Fig. 18.9C). A proportion of poorly differentiated adenocarcinomas of the breast will show little or no reactivity (Fig. 18.9D) but as with most adenocarcinomas focal intracytoplasmic lumen staining may still be evident (arrow). Hematoxylin–eosin, A × 125, B and C × 185, D × 400.

nomas.[187] Other antisera to lower molecular weight blood group[188] and oncofetal antigens[188] have also been produced through immunization with HMFGM.

Growth factors and their receptors

Peptide growth factors

Normal and malignant breast epithelial cells co-express a number of epidermal growth factor (EGF) related peptides including EGF, transforming growth factor alpha (TGF-α), amphiregulin (AR), and cripto-1 (CR-1).[189–190] The frequency and level of expression of TGF-α, AR, and CR-1 are higher in breast cancer lines. Some of these peptides can function as autocrine and/or juxtacrine growth factors in mammary epithelial cells and they are regulated by hormones such as estrogens. The lack of expression in some normal and malignant mammary epithelial cells suggests that some of these peptides may be involved in regulating other aspects of cell behavior such as differentiation as well as proliferation.[189–190]

Type 1 growth factor receptor family

Nine different classes of tyrosine kinase growth factor receptors have been identified. They differ with respect to the structure of their extracellular ligand binding and intracellular kinase domains and the nature of their activating ligands.[191] The type 1 family includes epidermal growth factor receptor (EGFR, c-erbB-1), c-erbB-2 (HER-2, neu), c-erbB-3 (HER-3) and c-erbB-4 (HER-4) receptors, all four of which may be expressed in breast cancer.[192]

Epidermal growth factor and epidermal growth factor receptor

Epidermal growth factor (EGF) is a powerful polypeptide growth factor which is essential in the development of mammary glands in mice.[193] It has been shown to influence, and in some situations be necessary for, the growth of normal mammary epithelium,[194] breast cancer cell lines[195] and other cell lines.[196] The mitogenic effect of EGF is mediated through binding with a specific membrane receptor — epidermal growth factor receptor (EGFR).[196] It is a 170 kD transmembrane glycoprotein with a heavily glycosylated external domain responsible for ligand binding, a single transmembrane spanning sequence and an internal domain with tyrosine kinase activity.[192,197–199] Activation of the receptor induces cell division usually synergistically with other growth regulatory signals. The protein sequence for EGFR has been determined and its gene cloned. The gene and receptor show close similarity to two oncogenes and their oncoproteins, namely v-erbB-2 and c-erbB-2.[200–201] EGFRs have been found in a variety of animal and human tissues, are particularly elevated in squamous tumors of the skin[202] and have been identified in a proportion of breast cancers.[203–204] Regulation of EGFR is not clearly understood, but the level of expression in breast cells can be altered by EGF, TGF-α, phorbol esters and steroid hormones.[199] There is a striking inverse relationship between EGFR and estrogen receptor (ER) expression.[199,205]

EGFR may be measured in breast tumors by radioligand binding assay of membrane fractions and by immunohistological staining of tumor sections (Fig. 18.10). The reported frequency of expression varies from 15–60% of tumors. There is a relationship to tumor size[203,206] which could influence the frequency in individual studies. Clinical interest in EGFR has been further stimulated by the demonstration of an association between EGFR expression and poor prognosis.[204,206–208] EGFR also appears to have an influence on the processes of tumor invasion and dissemination which has led to speculation that it may be a suitable target for antimetastatic therapy.[209]

Transforming growth factors alpha and beta

The epidermal growth factor family of growth regulating peptides also includes transforming growth factor alpha (TGF-α) a related single chain polypeptide[210] which can stimulated growth by binding to and activating the EGF receptor.[190,211–212] In normal cells levels of TGF-α, EGF and EGFR are regulated and in normal breast epithelial cell lines and some breast cancer cell lines the production of TGF-α is controlled in part by estrogen which stimulates TGF-α synthesis and secretion.[213] It is secreted by all

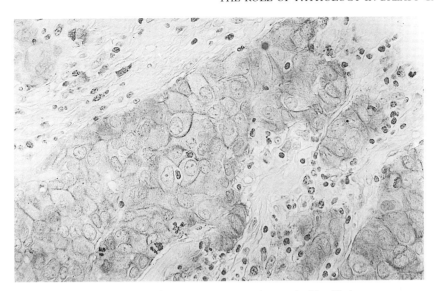

Fig. 18.10 Epidermal growth factor receptor expression can be identified immunocytochemically and shows both membrane and cytoplasmic reactivity. It is believed to relate to upregulation of the gene. Hematoxylin–eosin × 400.

tumor cell lines including breast and clinical and experimental studies have demonstrated that TGF-α is an important modulator of malignant progression of mammary epithelial cells in breast cancer.[190]

Transforming growth factor beta (TGF-β) is an unrelated two chain polypeptide which is a member of a complex structurally related family of growth and differentiation factors.[214] The various forms of TGF-β bind to a set of three structurally and functionally distinct cell surface receptors.[215] TGF-β has a growth inhibitory effect on epithelial cells, including mammary epithelium.[216–217] Some squamous cell carcinoma cell lines are not inhibited by TGF-β and it has been suggested that TGF-β may be involved in regulation of normal epithelial cell growth through negative feedback, carcinomas having altered growth due to their lack of response.[218] The evidence that both TGF-α and TGF-β are produced in situ has led to speculation that there is an autocrine growth loop, involving TGF-α and modulated by TGF-β, influencing cell proliferation in normal and malignant epithelial tissues.[214]

c-erbB-2

The proto-oncogene c-erbB-2 (also known as neu or HER-2) encodes a 190 kD transmembrane glycoprotein similar in structure to the epidermal growth factor receptor.[201] C-erbB-2 is a distinct gene but is related to the c-erbB-1 gene (epidermal growth factor receptor) and v-erb-B oncogene (avian erythroblastosis virus, AEV).[219] Other oncogenes of AEV include the homolog c-erb-A gene, a steroid receptor gene encoding a nuclear receptor for thyroid hormone.[220] In humans both c-erb-A and c-erbB-2 are located on chromosome 17q 21–22.[219–220] The extracellular domains of c-erbB-2 protein and EGFR are 40% identical in sequence and both possess two regions rich in cysteine residues which may be responsible for stabilization of their three-dimensional structure and ability to bind ligands. Monoclonal antibodies which bind to and down-regulate mutant c-erbB-2 receptor cancers inhibit tumor cell growth in vitro and in vivo[221] and overexpression of the normal c-erbB-2 protein in NIH 3T3 cells leads to transformation. Antibodies to natural human c-erbB-2 have been shown to inhibit the growth of breast cancer derived cell line SKBR-3 which expresses high levels of the protein.[222] These observations imply an important role for c-erbB-2 in at least a subset of human breast cancers.

The c-erbB-2 gene has been found to be amplified in 15–20% of invasive human breast carcinomas and gene amplification of over 3-fold appears characteristically to be associated with c-erbB-2 gene protein localization on tumor cell membranes. This localization can be detected by immunocytochemical techniques[223] (Fig. 18.11). High frequency of gene amplification of around 50% have been found in ductal carcinoma in situ (DCIS)[224] and of over 90% in Paget's disease of the nipple.[225] In DCIS there is an association with the high grade comedo subtype.[224] There has been increasing interest in the role of c-erbB-2 oncogene in breast cancer, particularly its relationship to prognosis.[226] Overexpression of c-erbB-2 oncogene is now generally accepted to correlate with poor prognosis in both primary operable and advanced breast cancer patients[227–228] and is associated with poor differentiation.[227–230]

Our knowledge of the function of c-erbB-2 oncoprotein is rudimentary. The similarities to EGFR and its persistent overexpression in a significant proportion of breast carcinomas with poorer prognosis imply an important growth regulatory role. This is further supported by the observation that monoclonal antibodies raised against the extracellular domain[231] have exerted an anti-tumor effect on mutant neu transformed NIH 3T3 cells and on a human breast tumor derived cell line. In addition it is known that EGFR expression is associated with poorer prognosis[206–208] and one might postulate that EGFR and c-erbB-2 oncoprotein are both components of a mechanism responsible for breast tumor development or progression. One group[232] has shown that c-erbB-2 oncoprotein can act as a substrate for EGFR tyrosine kinase and it has recently been demonstrated that a combination of expression of EGFR and c-erbB-2 transforms cells more efficiently than either protein alone.[233] A possible hypothesis of their role in neoplasia or tumor progression is that binding of ligand to an increasing number of receptors leads to an elevation in phosphokinase activity which would promote cell replication.

Overexpression of the c-erbB-2 protein, in the form of membrane staining by immunohistochemistry, is detected in almost 100% of cases of Paget's disease.[234–235] Apart from a growth stimulatory effect, the molecule may play an important role in cell motility of tumor cells by the activity of a motility factor, which acts as a specific ligand for the neu-protein.[234–235] This motility factor is believed to induce chemotaxis of neu-overexpressing breast cancer and may lead to an increased metastatic potential of overexpressing breast

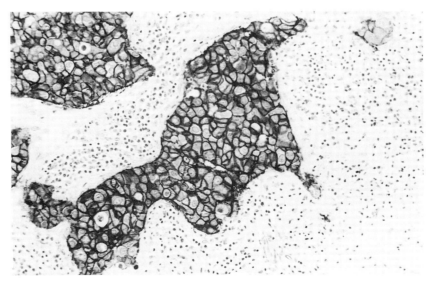

Fig. 18.11   C-erbB-2 (neu) protein is expressed on the cell membrane of a proportion of breast adenocarcinomas. Membrane localization of the protein has been shown to be associated with amplification of the gene. There is no known significance to cytoplasmic reactivity. Hematoxylin-eosin × 125.

tumors. It is also possible that in Paget's disease of the breast a motility factor secreted by epidermal keratinocytes may attract the overexpressing Paget's cells by chemotaxis and lead to invasion of the epidermis by the tumor cells.[234–235]

C-erbB-3 and heregulin

The c-erbB-3 gene produces a 180 kD trans-membrane glycoprotein product which shows considerable sequence homology to the EGFR and the c-erbB-2 protein, especially in the tyrosine kinase domain.

It has been demonstrated by Carraway and colleagues that the growth factor ligand heregulin binds to the c-erbB-3 receptor.[236] The same group have also demonstrated little or no tyrosine kinase activity following stimulation and binding of heregulin with the c-erbB-3 receptor. However in cells expressing both c-erbB-2 and c-erbB-3 a high affinity binding site is generated and on stimulation produces unique tyrosine residues.[237] This is in contrast to the interaction and complex formation between c-erbB-2 and c-erbB-4, where both receptors have active tyrosine kinase components which are capable of autophosphorylation.[238] The potential for type I tyrosine kinase receptors to produce different combinations of heregulin-stimulated heterodimeric complexes could explain some of the varied biological activities that have been demonstrated with this group of receptors.[239] We have found no association between overexpression of c-erbB-2 and c-erbB-3 assessed immunohistochemically.[240]

In breast cancer there is virtually ubiquitous cytoplasmic expression of c-erbB-3 protein at weak to strong levels.[241–242] The c-erbB-3 gene sequence codes for transmembrane types of protein, but membrane localization of c-erbB-3 protein appears to be a rare phenomenon and is much lower in frequency than EGFR and c-erbB-2 proteins in invasive breast cancer.[241–242] It is known that EGFR and c-erbB-2 are internalized by endocytosis after ligand binding. The predominant cytoplasmic localization of c-erbB-3 protein could indicate internalized non-functional or non-membrane associated protein. The c-erbB-3 protein may be an orphan receptor,[243] but if the parent of the orphan in terms of signaling were

c-erbB-2 or c-erbB-4 as has been recently suggested then the c-erbB-3 protein may be an important co-factor in the biological effects of type 1 growth factor receptors.

Breast cancer associated genes

The development and progression of a malignant phenotype of human tumors is related to abnormalities of structure or activity of proto-oncogenes[244–245] and/or mutation of tumor suppressor genes such as p53.[246] Many cellular oncogenes have been found to be activated in breast cancer and of these, c-erbB-2 (see above), c-myc and ras have excited the most interest. A variety of other oncogenes including BRCA1, BRCA2, PRAD1 and retinoblastoma gene have also been implicated in the genesis or progression of breast cancer. Their products are being actively investigated at present, but their relationships to clinical variables is not yet clear. A greater understanding of the consequences of such genetic changes and their functions may influence treatment and assessment of prognosis in the future.

p53

p53 is a tumor suppressor gene located on chromosome 17p. Mutations of p53 are the most common molecular abnormality found in human solid tumors and are present in a high proportion of breast cancers.[247–248] Normal function of p53 is regulated post-translationally and could be influenced by phosphorylation state, sub-cellular localization and interaction with many cellular proteins.[247–248] The range of functions of p53 are cell type specific and appear to be directly related to the ability of p53 to act as a specific transcriptional activator. The role that transcriptional repression plays in the function of wild type p53 is less clear. It is possible that p53 has a more direct activity in DNA regulation and repair.[247–248] Numerous roles are described, but in particular p53 appears to play a central part in cell cycle control after exposure to DNA damage.[249] Wild type p53 is a negative regulator of cell growth, thought to act by forming homodimers around DNA, allowing DNA repair to occur before cell division, or if repair does not occur then inducing cell death through apoptosis. p53 has been described as the 'guardian of the genome'.

Mutation of p53 is believed to result in more stable forms of the protein (Fig. 18.12) which form ineffective dimers around wild type p53 and lead to a failure of growth regulation.[247] Other effects of mutation include nuclear exclusion of protein and interaction with mdm2 protein. Most documented mutations result from a single amino-acid substitution with 50% of mutations occurring between exons 5–8, which are highly conserved during evolution.[250] Mutations are mainly mis-sense type and their frequency and distribution vary amongst different types of cancer.[250] p53 mutation is associated with more aggressive biological phenotypes of tumors and poorer prognosis in breast cancer patients.[248–249] Because of its role in regulation of apoptosis and response to DNA damage, p53 status could act as a predictive marker for a response to hormonal and chemotherapy.

ras

The ras family of genes c-rasH, c-rasK and N-ras are closely related.[251] They encode GTP binding proteins which act as intracellular messengers involved in transmitting signals from activated growth factor receptors to the nucleus. The most widely studied ras protein is the c-rasH p21 onco-protein which has sequence homology with the G-protein alpha subunit involved in adenylate cyclase activation. Single or small numbers of amino acid point mutations of ras genes can induce cell transformation and have been found in approximately 15% of human carcinomas[252] and ras mRNA is overexpressed in a variety of tumors including breast.[244] The mutations result in gene products deficient in GTPase reactivity and hence may influence proliferation control.

c-rasH p21 protein expression has been studied in human breast tumors by immunohistological staining. There are conflicting results, some groups finding increased p21 expression in carcinomas[253–255] and pre-malignant lesions[254–256] and others finding similar expression in benign and malignant lesions.[257–258] At present it appears that ras genes may play a role in development of a proportion of human breast cancers.

c-myc

c-myc is one of a number of cellular and viral oncogenes (myc, myb, fos, p53) which code for

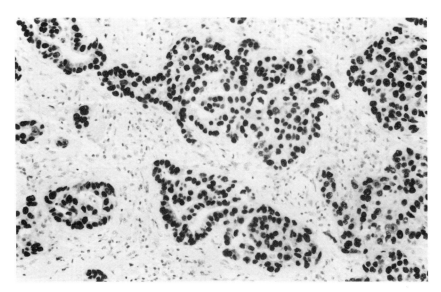

Fig. 18.12 A high proportion of p53 proteins produced by mutated p53 genes are more stable than wild type p53 protein. Antibodies to p53 do not discriminate between mutant and wild type protein but immunocytochemical detection of protein, which is located in the cell nucleus, is used to imply p53 gene mutation. Hematoxylin-eosin × 125.

nuclear proteins which appear to have a role in embryogenesis and proliferation.[259] c-myc amplification has been found in up to 30% of breast cancers.[260–261] It is a 62 kD protein product found in the nucleus during the G0 to G1 phase of the cell cycle.[251] In breast cancer an association has been found between c-myc protein expression and the histological grade of the tumor suggesting a relationship with tumor differentiation.[262] No association has been found with prognosis.[262]

Cell cycle associated molecules

Many groups have now shown that an estimate of the proliferative activity of a tumor through whatever means can give prognostic[263–264] and therapeutic[265–266] information. It must be borne in mind that true assessment of the growth rate of a tumor can only be determined by combining measurements of the proliferative fraction and the length of the cell cycle.[267] A single measurement in time of the growth fraction of a tumor should be regarded as an index of proliferation only.[267–268]

The growth fraction can be assessed by counting the number of cells in mitoses (mitotic index)[269] but this requires high quality tissue sections. Recently techniques of labeling cells which are active in the cell cycle have provided an alternative. Cells in the synthesis phase of the cycle (S phase) will take up thymidine or analogs of thymidine such as 5-Bromodeoxyuridine (BRDU). Incorporated molecules can be identified by prior radiolabeling, or in the case of BRDU by immunocytochemistry or flow cytometry using anti-BRDU antibody. Counts of the proportion of labeled cells will give an estimate of the S-phase fraction (SPF).

Two other growth fraction markers have emerged. The monoclonal antibody Ki67 was raised against a Hodgkin's disease cell line by Gerdes and colleagues and identifies cells active in the cell cycle.[270] The antigen is of unknown structure and is highly labile. It can be used to estimate a 'proliferative index' in breast cancers which can provide prognostic information.[271–273] The antibody MIB1 was raised by the same group to synthetic portions of the Ki67 molecule. It has the benefit that it recognizes a stable part of the Ki67 molecule which can be detected in formalin fixed paraffin embedded tissues (Fig. 18.13). Retrospective studies have also confirmed the prognostic significance of growth fraction assessment in this fashion.[274]

Antibodies are also available to other cell to cell cycle related proteins including a 36 kD nuclear protein named proliferating cell nuclear antigen (PCNA) or cyclin which appears in the cell nucleus in late S phase.[275] This molecule is an auxiliary protein of the DNA polymerase delta enzyme[276] and can be identified in standard histological sections.[277] It can provide information potentially analogous to, but not directly comparable with, flow cytometric estimation of SPF.

Other molecules of interest

Numerous additional molecules have been investigated in breast cancer. These include metalloproteases, intermediate filament proteins, basement membrane components, CEA, alpha lactalbumin, caseins, blood group antigens and others.[278–279] Many of these reagents have not found wide acceptance as routine tests of clinical importance, but some such as Cathepsin D have resulted in controversy and others such as p-glycoprotein potentially have therapeutic importance.

Cathepsin D

The Cathepsins D, B and L are acidic lysosomal proteinases which are involved in intracellular protein turnover. Increased levels of Cathepsin D identified by cytosol radio-immunoassay have been demonstrated in breast cancer and shown to have an association with indicators of tumor aggression such as large size, high histological grade and lymph node positivity.[280–281] More recently immunohistological studies have demonstrated that Cathepsin D can be identified not only in breast cancer cells, but also frequently in accompanying stromal tissue and particularly in infiltrating macrophages[282–286] (Fig. 18.14). Some of these studies have failed to demonstrate an independent prognostic effect,[282–283,286] whilst others have shown a prognostic effect only for stromal macrophage reactivity.[285–286] This evidence suggests that the prognostic effect of Cathepsin D is an epiphenomenon related partic-

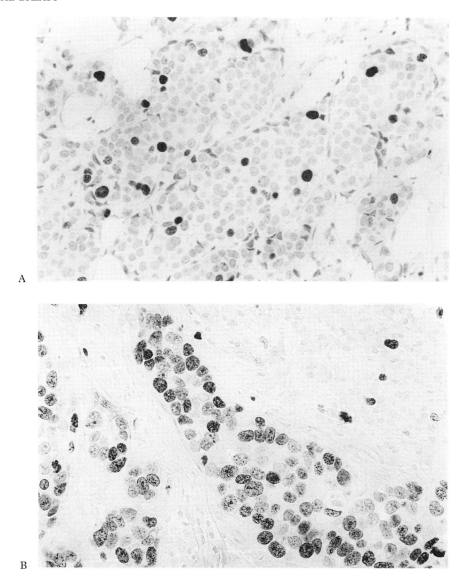

Fig. 18.13 Two breast cancers both stained immunocytochemically with antibody MIB1 raised to the cell cycle associated Ki67 protein showing a low (Fig. 18.13A) and a high (Fig. 18.13B) frequency of tumor cell nuclear labeling. The proportion of tumor cells active in the cell cycle, the 'growth fraction', can be used as an indirect marker of tumor proliferation. Such markers do not provide information about the duration of the cycle and cannot be used directly to calculate tumor growth. Hematoxylin-eosin × 400.

ularly to associated inflammation and stromal macrophage infiltration.

P-glycoprotein

A proportion of tumors of many types will develop resistance to a variety of chemotherapeutic agents.

This multidrug resistant phenotype (MDR) is associated with expression of a 170 kD membrane glycoprotein (P-glycoprotein) which acts as an energy dependent pump removing certain families of chemotherapeutic drugs.[287] Antibodies to P-glycoprotein have been produced[287] which can be used to identify expression in tumor samples. Few

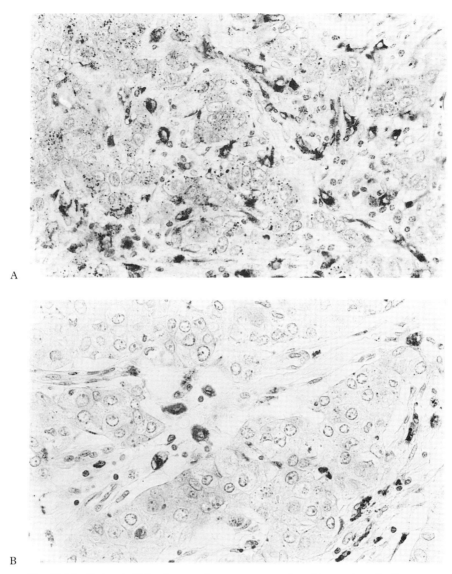

Fig. 18.14 Cathepsin D is a lysosomal protease enzyme found in a variety of cell types. High expression is seen in macrophages. These two illustrations show immunocytochemical staining for Cathepsin D of two breast cancers. In one (Fig. 18.14A) there is both tumor cell and stromal (macrophage) reactivity. In the second (Fig. 18.14B) there is only stromal cell reactivity. Biochemical assays performed on tissue homogenate samples cannot distinguish between tumor cell and stromal cell reactivity. Hematoxylin-eosin × 400.

studies have been performed in human breast cancer, but development of the MDR phenotype appears to be a late phenomenon[278] and may therefore be of limited clinical value.[288–289]

MORPHOMETRY AND CYTOMETRY

Objective measurements of the shape, arrangement and tinctorial characteristics of breast tumor cell populations can be made using a variety of simple morphometric principles or more complex computer assisted morphometric,[290–291] image cytometric[292–293] and flow cytometric equipment.[294–296] The type of morphometric information that can be obtained includes cell and nuclear size and shape, cellularity, mitotic frequency, nuclear chromatin and nucleolar texture as well as stromal characteristics, for example microvessel density as a measure of angiogenesis.

DNA

Use of fluorescent or visible stoichiometric DNA stain allows measurement of nuclear DNA content by flow cytometry and densitometry with image cytometry. DNA content can be used to assess abnormalities of ploidy[297] and to estimate the SPF.[298] Many of the variables measured by these techniques have been shown to provide prognostic information, albeit of varying importance, in breast cancer patients.[269,297–298]

At present the only technique which has shown potential as a routine system to aid diagnosis is image cytometry. By combined assessment of nuclear morphology, DNA content and possibly chromatin texture relatively acceptable levels of sensitivity and specificity for diagnosis of malignancy can be obtained.[299] Further development of preparative techniques, system hardware and feature selection criteria are imminent. This technology potentially may assist traditional cytology in diagnosis of breast disease.

ANGIOGENESIS

There is considerable experimental evidence showing that tumor growth and metastasis are dependent on neovascularization; the switch from the avascular to the vascular phase being accompanied by a rapid increase in tumor growth rate.[300–303] Tumor 'angiogenesis' refers to the growth of new vessels towards and within a tumor and some authorities have shown that unless tumor neovascularization occurs cell proliferation reaches a steady state and the tumor grows no larger than about 2 mm in maximum diameter.[301,303] Angiogenesis is also believed to be one of the important events occurring during the complex process of metastasis, with capillary ingrowth increasing the likelihood of tumor cells entering the circulation and tumor cell clumps rarely doing so in the absence of neovascularization.[304–305] It has been suggested that this may be related to increased surface area for adherence by tumor cells

and to the increased 'leakiness' of new vessels.[306] Furthermore, the ability of the tumor to evoke an angiogenic response in the surrounding stroma would increase the likelihood of survival of embolic seedlings. Thus angiogenesis appears to be important at both the beginning and end of the metastatic sequence.[307]

It would not, therefore, be surprising to find that tumors showing a high level of new vessel formation have a poorer prognosis, particularly with regard to the presence or development of metastatic disease. In the last few years, a number of authors, using semi-quantitative histological studies (Fig. 18.15), appear to have identified a significant association between high tumor vascular density and poor prognosis in several tumors,[308–309] including breast carcinoma.[300,310–315] Despite this being a plausible concept, other groups have failed to demonstrate such a prognostic effect.[316–320] Our own experience is similar to this second group of investigators; we assessed vascular density in breast tumors using both random field selection (93 cases) and preselection of the perceived area of highest vascularity (165 cases) in tumor sections immunostained for expression of the endothelial markers CD 31 and CD 34. Using a minimum follow-up time of 12 years, we were unable to identify any significant association with the presence of metastases at presentation, disease-free interval or survival.[320]

Weidner argues that to assess angiogenesis using vascular density in this way, vascular 'hot spots' must be identified[311] and it may be, therefore, that in immunostaining only one block of tissue for each tumor, we and others have failed to identify these areas. Nevertheless, Costello and colleagues[321] were unable to demonstrate any relationship between vessel density and clinical outcome using Weidner's technique. It is possible, therefore, that while angiogenesis is certainly important in tumor biology, and inhibition of angiogenesis may be an important target for chemotherapy (see below),[300] it is only one of a number of factors affecting prognosis and is not necessarily a rate-limiting step in tumor biology. Indeed, neovascularization has been described around ductal carcinoma in situ[310,319] which is clearly not capable of metastasizing, suggesting that it may be an early event in the lifetime of a

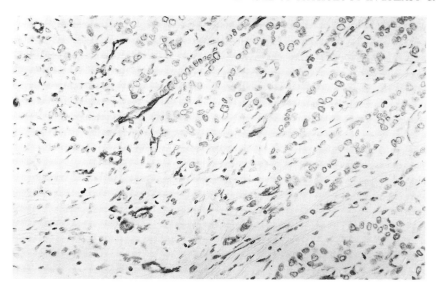

Fig. 18.15 New vessel formation is an essential phenomenon for tumor growth. The vessels have been identified immunocytochemically using the vascular endothelial marker CD 31. Hematoxylin-eosin × 125.

tumor and although necessary, is not sufficient in itself for tumor progression. We agree with Page and Jensen[322] that further work is necessary to determine the role of assessment of tumor vascularity in predicting prognosis, but we feel currently that performing vascular counts on routinely selected blocks of tumor tissue offers no advantage over traditionally accepted prognostic indicators.

Despite questions about the applicability as a prognostic factor in breast cancer, there is mounting evidence demonstrating a predictive value of angiogenesis for response to anti-cancer therapies and the essential requirement of neovascularization for tumor growth is leading to development of anti-angiogenic drugs as novel therapeutic strategies.[300,322] The presence of a well defined stromal vascular component in human breast carcinoma and the demonstration that these tumors produce angiogenic factors is leading some authorities to suggest that breast cancer may be one of the most responsive tumors to angiogenesis inhibitors given alone or in combination with conventional anti-cancer chemotherapy.[300]

MOLECULAR GENETIC ANALYSIS

At present, blotting, PCR and in situ hybridiza-tion techniques are providing important understanding of tumor cell biology, in particular gene regulation and gene abnormalities during neoplasia. The methods used can be time consuming and probes may not be widely available and expensive to purchase. Expertise in these methods is generally confined to major research institutions and for these reasons the results are not being applied directly to clinical situations. A greater understanding of the relevance of molecular changes will be required before there is wider use of these techniques for prognostic purposes in clinical laboratories but the rapidity and diversity of results currently emerging leads us to believe that there will be a future for molecular technology in clinical management of breast disease.

PRACTICAL APPLICATION OF PROGNOSTIC FACTORS

The factors described above have been shown to convey prognostic information to a greater or lesser degree, and several provide a powerful indication of the likely outcome for particular groups of patients. However, as yet no consensus has been reached on which factors should be used routinely in clinical practice, and Hawkins,[323] in a review of a large number of publications, found a staggering range of findings and conclusions. He reiterated a proposal made by McGuire and Clark[324] that the following guidelines should be utilized in deciding what constitutes a useful prognostic factor:

- an associated 'biologic' hypothesis
- methodological validation
- optimal cut-off points (derived from 'training' data)
- a pilot study
- a definitive study (plus appropriate population sample)
- avoidance of sampling bias
- multivariate analysis.

Missing from this list, perhaps because it was felt to be too obvious to need re-stating, is the most important point of all, namely *clinical relevance*.

The majority of the factors described in the previous sections can be assessed in a routine diagnostic histopathology laboratory and are therefore readily available for use in clinical management. Histopathologists are already familiar with the need to supply such information in their routine reports (e.g. Duke's staging of colo-rectal carcinoma, measurement of Breslow thickness and Clark's levels in malignant melanoma) but to avoid wasted effort they need to agree with their clinical colleagues which prognostic factors should be recorded. There is little point in pathologists writing extensive and elegant reports full of data on the latest prognostic factor if the clinicians have no intention of using the information to plan therapy for an individual patient.

COMBINATION OF FACTORS

As noted at the beginning of this chapter, until comparatively recently there has been a depressing lack of interest in the use of prognostic factors in the management of patients with breast cancer. Indeed, the only factor used consistently in most centers as a guide for therapy has been loco-regional lymph node status, and this has also been the case in patient stratification for clinical trials. Lymph node status is a time-dependent prognostic factor and the longer a tumor has been growing the more likely it is that spread to lymph nodes will have occurred. Taken alone, lymph node stage, although a powerful factor, is incapable of defining either a 'cured' group of patients or a group with a close to 100% mortality from breast cancer.[4]

Prognosis in breast cancer depends not only upon the presence of distant metastases but also on the aggressiveness or virulence of the tumor. The virulence of a tumor depends on a number of intrinsic biological characteristics, some of which can already be evaluated such as morphological features of differentiation, growth rate and hormone responsiveness and some of which are not as yet assessable, such as invasiveness or power of tissue destruction. If accurate prognostication is required on an individual patient basis then a Prognostic Index is required which uses both time-dependent factors and biological factors. This is not a new idea; when Greenhough[325] first introduced histological grading 70 years ago he noted that, even in his small series, the combination of high grade malignancy and lymph node involvement gave an exceedingly poor prognosis. Much later, when Bloom[326–327] revived interest in grading he too stressed that prediction of survival was improved by combining grade with stage. The 5-year survival of 94% for patients with grade 1 tumors and uninvolved nodes fell to 65% for those with involved nodes, and for patients with grade 3 tumors from 55% to 16%. Similar findings were subsequently reported from the multicenter Cancer Research Campaign trial.[9]

Observations such as these were largely derived from studies of sub-groups using univariate analysis. The Nottingham Tenovus Primary Breast Cancer Study (NTPBCS) was established in 1973 specifically to investigate the value of a comprehensive range of potential prognostic factors. All patients with primary operable breast cancer presenting to a single surgical team (Professor R. W. Blamey and Mr J. F. R. Robertson) are entered into the study. Initial surgical treatment includes simple or subcutaneous mastectomy, or wide local excision and post-operative radiotherapy, together with lymph node sampling and low axillary clearance. Over 3000 patients have been entered into the study which has been used both to derive and to test a prognostic index based on multiple factors, the Nottingham Prognostic Index.

NOTTINGHAM PROGNOSTIC INDEX (NPI)

From the beginning of the study data has been accumulated both prospectively and retrospectively. Basic prospective data has included age at diagnosis, menopausal status (based on menstrual history and checked by FSH levels), tumor size (measured pathologically as described previously), histological grade (assessed by the method described by Elston and Ellis[30]), estrogen receptor status (ER) (initially using the dextran coated charcoal method (DCC) and latterly based on ELIZA and ERICA monoclonal antibody methods — see pages 400 to 405) and lymph node stage. The latter is divided into three groups, based on histological examination of resected nodes, as follows:

1. No nodal involvement.
2. Involvement of up to three low axillary nodes OR an internal mammary node (for medial tumors).
3. Involvement of four or more low axillary nodes and/or the apical node, or any low axillary node and internal mammary node simultaneously.

In a preliminary study based on this data an initial group of patients with a particularly poor prognosis was identified.[45] The index (tumors >2 cm, grade 2 or 3, lymph node stage 3), although very specific, lacked sensitivity as it only identified 50% of the patients who actually had a very poor prognosis. Accordingly, in 1982, a retrospective multivariate analysis was carried out, of nine separate factors studied in 387 patients.[46] A number of factors were related to survival in univariate analysis but only three remained significant in multivariate analysis, namely tumor size, histological grade and lymph node stage. Using the coefficients of significance for these three factors an index predicting survival was calculated: NPI = Size (cm) $\times$ 0.2 + Grade (1–3; well, moderate or poor differentiation) + Stage (1–3 as shown above).

The higher the value for NPI the worse the prognosis. Curves of survival by life table analysis showed excellent separation of patient groups, depending on the index value, but since the index had been derived from these patients this was a self-fulfilling prophecy. The NPI was therefore tested prospectively in a further 320 patients and it was shown that the index based on data derived from one group of patients could be applied successfully to another entirely separate group.[47] Figure 18.16 shows the analysis based on all of the first 1662 patients entered into the NTPBCS with up to 15-year follow-up. Three groups of patients have been identified by employing (arbitrary) cut-off points of < 3.4 for the Good prognosis group (GPG), 3.41–5.4 for the Moderate group (MPG) and > 5.41 for the Poor group (PPG); the percentage of patients falling into each group in symptomatic practice, and their predicted 15-year survival, is shown in Table 18.6.

Whilst it is clear that the NPI provides extremely powerful prognostic information within the NTPBCS it is important to demonstrate its utility and reproducibility in studies from other centers, especially in view of the relatively subjective nature of one of its components, histological grade. In this respect Henson et al[328] have carried out a retrospective analysis of prognostic data in over 22 000 women as part of the SEER (Surveillance, Epidemiology and End Results) Programme of the National Cancer Institute in the United States. Despite the fact that the data was collected from a large variety of institutes and there was no standardization of methods, especially grading, they confirmed that a combination of stage and grade improved prediction of outcome. Furthermore, they argued powerfully that observer variation in grade assignment had not been proven to interfere with the estimation of prognosis in breast cancer. In a similar way to the NTPBCS

Table 18.6 NPI groups for 1662 patients showing the numbers and percentages in each group, the expected 15-year survival and for comparison the expected survival for age-matched females without breast cancer

NPI	n	%	15-year survival (%)
Age-matched females			83
GPG (<3.4)	490	29	80
MPG (3.41–5.4)	887	54	42
PPG (>5.41)	285	17	13

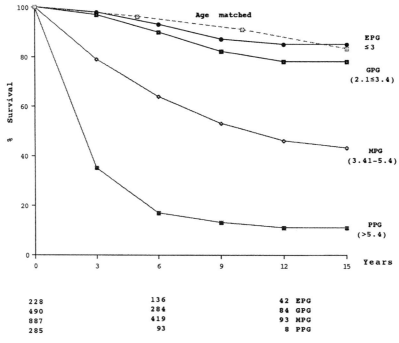

Fig. 18.16 Survival curves for 1662 patients in the Nottingham Tenovus Primary Breast Cancer Study. N.B. The EPG is a sub-group of the GPG.

Chevallier and colleagues[329] have identified young age, tumor size and histological grade as factors which added to lymph node stage in the prediction of recurrence. These factors were combined to divide lymph node negative patients into three prognostic groups.

One of the strengths of the NPI is that it has been verified prospectively in the NTPBCS.[4] Further confirmation of its value has been provided by its validation in two large multicenter studies.[330–330a] In the Yorkshire Breast Cancer Group (YBCG) study[330] the NPI was applied to 1186 patients with primary operable breast cancer and compared with their own closely similar index; both provided excellent separation into three prognostic groups. The Danish Breast Cancer Cooperative Group (DBCG) study[330a] was even larger, consisting of over 9000 patients, but unlike the original Nottingham study group some patients received adjuvant systemic therapy. Nevertheless, very similar stratification into three clearly different prognostic groups was obtained. It is also pertinent to record that in the DBCG study the histological grading was carried out as a routine in 32 different pathology departments without central review, confirming its robustness as a prognostic factor.

All these studies confirm the inherent power of the pathological prognostic factors described above. The NPI has become the most widely used index, certainly in the United Kingdom;[331] one of its main strengths lies in the fact that it is based on relatively simple data which can be provided in any routine histopathology laboratory.

IMPROVEMENTS TO THE INDEX

Although, as emphasized above, the NPI has the considerable advantage of simplicity the search continues for more objective factors which may reflect the biology of individual breast cancers more accurately than tumor morphology. These have been described in some detail in a previous section (pp. 400 to 417). Several commercial organizations are marketing prognostic indices based on such factors as hormone receptor status (ER and PR), DNA ploidy, S-phase fraction

(SPF), Epidermal Growth Factor (EGFR) and c-erbB-2 expression. The group from Guy's Hospital, London have devised one such index for node-positive patients using c-erbB-2 expression and S-phase fraction.[332] It is interesting to observe that the study from which this index was derived did not include an evaluation of histological grade.

As part of our long-term study of prognosis in breast cancer many of the biological factors described above have been evaluated in the NTPBCS. These include ER status,[173] binding of epithelial mucin antibodies,[333] proliferation markers such as Ki67 and KiS1,[273–274,334] DNA index and SPF,[335] Epidermal growth factor,[336] c-erbB-2 expression,[227] c-myc expression,[262] *Helix pomatia* lectin binding[337] and p53 expression.[336] Each relates to prognosis in univariate analysis but also to histological grade and in multivariate analysis grade emerges as the more powerful (and after its inclusion) the only significant prognostic factor.

Most of these factors have been the subject of encouraging reports in the world literature. It is worth pointing out that although some show excellent prognostic separation at, say 2 years, any significant differences may be eliminated at 5 to 10 years. Ploidy, ER status and probably EGFR are examples of this. Thus, at 18 months' follow-up patients with ER positive tumors show a 15% mortality compared with 30% for patients with ER negative tumors. There is a 100% difference in mortality, but in fact only a 5% difference in case survival, and by 10 years follow-up, the mortality is the same. In general oncological terms most breast cancer is relatively 'chronic' and analysis too early has led to many misleading publications on the value of individual prognostic factors. A further point is of relevance here; some factors carry prognostic importance not strictly related to survival. ER, for example, predicts hormone responsiveness after primary treatment failure[173] and also in the adjuvant situation.[338]

It would be fortunate indeed if a single molecular event could offer analogous prognostic power. This would provide a relatively simple objective method of assessing prognosis. It is possible to discuss some possible reasons for this lack of power. The observation that c-erbB-2 amplification is related to large cell morphology, particularly in ductal carcinoma in situ,[224,339] has prompted speculation that amplification and over-expression of certain genes may be reflected in tumor cell morphology.[340–341] Histological grading is assessed by combining the appearance of various morphological features and mitotic figure frequency[30] and as a result provides an overview of the effects of a number of inherent molecular changes which affect morphological appearance. It is unlikely therefore that a single molecular event could compete with histological grade. The future of molecular markers of prognosis will be in combination, providing information analogous to histological grade, or as predictors of response to specific forms of therapy.

The most important component of histological grade is the assessment of mitotic frequency. Objective measurements of tumor cell proliferation such as percentage of cells in mitosis, thymidine or BRDU labeling index, SPF measurement and Ki67 or MIB1 labeling index[264,274] have produced the greatest challenge to histological grade and have the advantage of objectivity of measurement. However all have some drawbacks; mitotic frequency is time consuming to perform, thymidine or BRDU labeling index requires in vivo or in vitro incorporation and subsequent measurement of labeling by flow cytometric analysis or assessment of immunocytochemical preparation, S-phase fraction requires flow cytometry equipment and Ki67 labeling index immunocytochemical staining of fresh tissue. It is difficult to justify some of these methods in a cost conscious health environment when histological grade and tumor type can be assessed rapidly on a routine histological tissue section.

In summary, whilst most of the factors referred to in this chapter have been shown to provide some prognostic information the only ones which fulfil the criteria proposed by Hawkins[323] and McGuire and Clark[324] seem to be morphological, and in particular those forming the Nottingham Prognostic Index. At the beginning of this chapter we quoted the review article written by Clark[5] in which he gave three major reasons for the use of prognostic factors in breast cancer. In the next section we will expand on this theme and demonstrate their practical application in clinical management.

PRACTICAL APPLICATION OF PROGNOSTIC FACTORS

COMPARISON OF PATIENT GROUPS

a. There are some situations in which controlled clinical trials may be considered inappropriate. For example, it is difficult to randomize between reconstructive surgery and mastectomy since this is an emotive issue, much dependent on patient choice. It is then important that when two different forms of treatment are being evaluated the case-mix in each group is shown to be of equal distribution. The principle is the same as that for employing age and sex-matched controls; stratification by prognosis can be used in a similar manner. In a comparison of simple mastectomy and subcutaneous mastectomy in the NTPBCS we showed that there is no difference in overall survival between the two treatments and that this holds true when both groups of patients are stratified according to the NPI.[342–343]

b. Pathological prognostic factors play an extremely important role in the evaluation of screening programs for breast cancer, by helping to identify differences in the biology of screening-detected cancers compared with those presenting in symptomatic practice. In the prevalent round of mammographic screening there is a relative increase in the number of small carcinomas which are likely to be node negative, low histological grade and of a more favorable tumor type (e.g. tubular, tubular-mixed).[2,18–19,21,344] Patients with these cancers are therefore frequently located in the good prognostic group and usually, with an NPI value of < 3, in the excellent prognostic subgroup (EPG) (Fig. 18.16, Table 18.7). There is a marked shift of cases towards the more favorable end of the prognostic range in comparison with patients who present through the symptomatic clinics, with more than three times as many tumors in the EPG, and a very small percentage of cases in the PPG. Such data have obvious implications for selection of appropriate therapy, which is discussed in Chapter 22.

Within breast screening pathological prognostic factors have an important role in the *quality assurance* aspects of a program; apart from achieving a minimum cancer detection rate individual screening centers should monitor their performance in the detection of the favorable prognostic cases described above. Indeed, in the NHSBSP radiologists are set a small invasive cancer target: initially, with a tumor size of less than 10 mm, this was 15 per 10 000 women screened; currently it is required that 50% of invasive cancers measure less than 15 mm.[16,345] Although the ultimate success of a screening program depends on the demonstration of a significant reduction in mortality, pathological prognostic factors can be used as surrogates in some circumstances. For example, comparison of the NPI in cancers detected in the prevalent and incident rounds with those arising as interval cancers can be used to assess whether screening at the current interval of 3 years is the correct frequency.

STRATIFICATION OF PATIENTS FOR THERAPY

It is clear from the data presented earlier in this chapter that it is now feasible to place women with breast cancer into separate prognostic groups. It follows logically from this that the therapy used for patients in the GPG, who have an 80% chance of surviving 15 years (little difference from that of an age-matched population without breast cancer), should be different from that for those in the PPG of whom only 40% will be alive after 3 years and less than 15% at 15 years, a survival comparable with that of advanced breast cancer (stage 3 or tumors > 5 cm in diameter clinically). In Nottingham we have used the NPI as the basis for the selection of appropriate therapy for individual patients since 1990. These therapeutic decisions are made at a weekly prospective meeting in which the clinical and pathological data for

Table 18.7 Distribution of 134 invasive cancers detected in the prevalent round of mammographic screening in the Nottingham Breast Screening Service. Comparison is made with the distribution of 1629 cancers from an unscreened population

NPI Group	n	Screened (%)	Unscreened (%)
(EPG	59	44	13)
GPG	102	76	29
MPG	27	20	54
PPG	5	4	17

each patient are reviewed. The details of specific local and systemic therapy are discussed in Chapter 22 which should be read in conjunction with this account of prognostic factors.

SELECTION OF PATIENTS FOR SPECIFIC THERAPIES

Predictive prognostic indices such as the NPI place individuals in groups which can require further stratification should there be a choice of appropriate additional treatment, for example between adjuvant hormone and chemotherapy. Estrogen receptor is now widely used to identify those individuals who are likely to benefit from adjuvant or primary endocrine therapy. Predictors of response to chemotherapeutic regimens are more elusive.

There is evidence that response to chemotherapy can be predicted in patients with breast cancer through measurement of the proliferative activity of the tumor. It is widely accepted that tumors with a very high proliferative rate such as acute leukemias, high grade lymphomas and germ cell tumors can respond dramatically to chemotherapy schedules. Similar, although less dramatic, behavior has been reported in breast cancer. A relationship has been shown between S-phase fraction (SPF) and tumor response in patients with stage II–IIIa disease.[266] Tumors with a low SPF (< 5%) had a response rate of 46%. Those with an intermediate SPF (5–10%) had a response rate of 84% and of those with a high SPF (> 10%) all responded. There was considerable overlap between the groups but these results are encouraging and supportive data has emerged from thymidine labeling (TLI) studies on patients receiving adjuvant chemotherapy. Long-term follow-up has shown that patients with a high TLI had delayed recurrence in contrast to patients with a low tumor TLI in whom no benefit was observed.

More recently, specific molecular changes such as c-erbB-2 gene amplification and p53 gene mutation have been found to confer resistance to chemotherapy. The mechanisms are not clearly understood but these observations are likely to herald an era of investigation of specific therapeutic markers.[346]

CONCLUSIONS

In this chapter we have approached the subject of prognosis in breast cancer very much from the perspective of the routine diagnostic histopathology service with the objective of indicating which prognostic factors are of most value in determining appropriate therapy for individual patients. The Nottingham Prognostic Index, based on careful histopathological evaluation of tumor size, histological grade and lymph node stage, is a powerful and reproducible method of assessing prognosis and is the only integrated index which has been confirmed in prospective studies.[4,330] In the future more objective methods for estimating tumor differentiation and invasiveness may become available, but currently other techniques including molecular markers do not achieve significance in multivariate analysis when compared with histological grade. We will continue to assess the new markers and technologies, but it is likely that a molecular classification of breast cancer will only become commonplace when treatment strategies are based on specific genetic or biological events, comparable with the current use of hormone receptor assays to assess the suitability of a patient for hormone treatment.

The NPI fully satisfies the criteria suggested by McGuire and Clark[324] and endorsed by Hawkins.[323] In his recent review of prognostic factors in breast cancer Clark[5] stated that both the NPI and the Nottingham Index for patients with metastatic disease treated by endocrine therapy[347] 'provide an excellent basis for the evaluation of newer factors that have been more recently proposed'. The time has never been better for histopathologists to demonstrate the importance of their contribution to the management of patients with breast cancer. If we do not provide prognostic information to our clinical colleagues then others, including commercial laboratories, will fill the void.

REFERENCES

1. Nyström L, Rutqvist LE, Wall S et al. Breast cancer screening with mammography; overview of Swedish randomised trials. Lancet 1993; 341: 973–978.

2. Ellis IO, Galea MH, Locker A et al. Early experience in breast cancer screening: Emphasis on development of protocols for triple assessment. Breast 1993; 2: 148–153.

3. Clark GM. Integrating prognostic factors. Br Cancer Res Treat 1992; 22: 187–191.

4. Galea MH, Blamey RW, Elston CW et al. The Nottingham Prognostic Index in primary breast cancer. Br Cancer Res Treat 1992; 22: 207–219.

5. Clark GM. Do we really need prognostic factors for breast cancer? Br Cancer Res Treat 1994; 30: 117–126.

6. Pathology Reporting in Breast Screening Pathology. 2nd ed. NHSBSP Publications, no 3, 1995.

7. Cutler SJ, Black MM, Mork T et al. Further observations on prognostic factors in cancer of the female breast. Cancer 1969; 24: 653–657.

8. Carter GL, Allen C, Henson DE. Relation of tumour size, lymph node status, and survival in 24 740 breast cancer cases. Cancer 1989; 63: 181–187.

9. Elston CW, Gresham GA, Rao GS et al. The Cancer Research Campaign (Kings/Cambridge) trial for early breast cancer — pathological aspects. Br J Cancer 1982; 45: 655–669.

10. Fisher ER, Sass R, Fisher B et al. Pathologic findings from the National Surgical Adjuvant Project for breast cancer (protocol no 4). Discrimination for tenth year treatment failure. Cancer 1984; 53: 712–723.

11. Neville AM, Bettelheim R, Gelber RD et al. Predicting treatment responsiveness and prognosis in node-negative breast cancer. J Clin Oncol 1992; 10: 696–705.

12. Gallager HS, Martin JE. An orientation to the concept of minimal carcinoma. Cancer 1971; 28: 1505–1507.

13. Beahrs OH, Shapiro S, Smart C et al. Summary report of the Working Group to review the National Cancer Institute-American Cancer Society Breast Cancer Demonstration Detection Projects. J Nat Cancer Inst 1979; 62: 641–709.

14. Hartman WH. Minimal breast cancer: an update. Cancer 1984; 53: 681–684.

15. Bedwani R, Vana J, Rosner D et al. Management and survival of female patients with 'minimal' breast cancer: as observed in the long-term and short-term surveys of the American College of Surgeons. Cancer 1981; 47: 2769–2778.

16. Royal College of Radiologists. Quality Assurance Guidelines for Radiologists. NHSBSP Publications. 1990.

17. Rosen PP, Groshen S. Factors influencing survival and prognosis in early breast carcinoma (T1N0M0-T1N1M0). Assessment of 644 patients with median follow up of 19 years. Surg Clin North Am 1990; 70: 937–962.

18. Gibbs NM. Comparative study of the histopathology of breast cancer in a screened and unscreened population investigated by mammography. Histopathol 1985; 9: 1307–1318.

19. Tabar L, Duffy SW, Krusemo UB. Detection method, tumour size and node metastases in breast cancers diagnosed during a trial of breast cancer screening. Eur J Cancer Clin Oncol 1987; 23: 959–962.

20. Frisell J, Eklund G, Hellström L, Somell A. Analysis of interval breast carcinomas in a randomized screening trial in Stockholm. Br Cancer Res Treat 1987; 17: 219–225.

21. Anderson TJ, Lamb J, Donnan P et al. Comparative pathology of breast cancer in a randomised trial of screening. Br J Cancer 1991; 64: 108–113.

22. Sloane JP. National Coordinating Group for Breast Screening Pathology. Consistency of histopathological reporting of breast lesions detected by screening: findings of the UK National External Quality Assessment (EQA) Scheme. Eur J Cancer 1994; 30A: 1414–1419.

23. Fisher ER, Gregorio RM, Fisher B. The pathology of invasive breast cancer. A syllabus derived from findings of the National Surgical Adjuvant Breast Cancer Project (protocol no 4). Cancer 1975; 36: 144–156.

24. Azzopardi JG. Problems in breast pathology. London: W B Saunders, 1979.

25. Page DL, Anderson TJ, Sakamoto G. Infiltrating carcinoma: major histological types. In: Page DL, Anderson TJ, eds. Diagnostic histopathology of the breast. London: WB Saunders, 1987; 193–235.

26. Tavassoli FA. Infiltrating carcinomas, common and familiar special types. In: Tavassoli FA, ed. Pathology of the breast. Norwalk: Appleton and Lange, 1992; 293–347.

27. Ellis IO, Elston CW. Tumors of the breast. In: Fletcher CDM, ed. Diagnostic Histopathology of tumours. London, Edinburgh: Churchill Livingstone, 1995; 635–689.

28. Patey DH, Scarff RW. The position of histology in the prognosis of carcinoma of the breast. Lancet 1928; 1: 801–804.

29. Bloom HJG, Richardson WW. Histological grading and prognosis in breast cancer. A study of 1409 cases of which 359 have been followed for 15 years. Br J Cancer 1957; 11: 359–377.

30. Elston CW, Ellis IO. Pathological prognostic factors in breast cancer. I. The value of histological grade in breast cancer: experience from a large study with long-term follow-up. Histopathol 1991; 19: 403–410.

31. Black MM, Opler SR, Speer FD. Survival in breast cancer cases in relation to structure of the primary tumor and regional lymph nodes. Surg Gynecol Obstet 1955; 100: 543–551.

32. Dalton LW, Page DL, Dupont WD. Histological grading of breast carcinoma: a reproducibility study. Cancer 1994; 73: 2765–2770.

33. Frierson HF, Wolber RA, Berean KW et al. Interobserver reproducibility of the Nottingham modification of the Bloom and Richardson histological grading scheme for infiltrating ductal carcinoma. Am J Clin Pathol 1995; 105: 195–198.

34. Robbins P, Pinder S, deKlerk N et al. Histological grading of breast carcinomas. A study of interobserver agreement. Hum Pathol 1995; 26: 873–879.

35. Commission European. European Guidelines for Quality Assurance in Mammography Screening. 2nd ed. de Wolf CJM, Perry NM, eds. Luxembourg: Office for Official Publications of the European Communities, 1996.

36. Connelly JL, Fechner RE, Kempson RL et al. Recommendations for the reporting of breast carcinoma. Hum Pathol 1996; 27: 220–224.

37. Pereira H, Pinder SE, Sibbering DM et al. Pathological prognostic factors in breast cancer. IV: Should you be a typer or a grader? A comparative study of two histological prognostic features in operable breast carcinoma. Histopathol 1995; 27: 219–226.

38. Haagensen CD, ed. Diseases of the breast. Philadelphia: Saunders, 1986.

39. Harris JR, Hellman S, Henderson IC, Kinne DW. Breast diseases. 2nd ed. Philadelphia: Lippincott, 1991.

40. Barr LC, Baum M. Time to abandon TNM staging of breast cancer? Lancet 1992; 339: 915–917.

41. Ferguson DJ, Meier P, Karrison T et al. Staging of breast cancer and survival rates: an assessment based on 50 years of experience with radical mastectomy. J Am Med Assoc 1982; 248: 1337–1341.

42. Veronesi U, Galimberti V, Zurrida S et al. Prognostic significance of number and level of axillary node metastases in breast cancer. Breast 1993; 2: 224–228.

43. Nemoto T, Vana J, Bedwani RN. Management and survival of female breast cancer: results of a national survey by the American College of Surgeons. Cancer 1980; 45: 2917–2924.

44. Handley RF. Observations and thoughts on carcinoma of the breast. Proc R Soc Med 1972; 65: 437–444.

45. Blamey RW, Davies CJ, Elston CW et al. Prognostic factors in breast cancer: the formation of a prognostic index. Clin Oncol 1979; 5: 227–236.

46. Haybittle JL, Blamey RW, Elston CW et al. A prognostic index in primary breast cancer. Br J Cancer 1982; 45: 361–366.

47. Todd JH, Dowle C, Williams MR et al. Confirmation of a prognostic index in primary breast cancer. Br J Cancer 1987; 56: 489–492.

48. Locker AP, Ellis IO, Morgan DAL et al. Factors influencing local recurrence after excision and radiotherapy for primary breast cancer. Br J Surg 1989; 76: 890–894.

49. Steele RJC, Forrest APM, Gibson T. The efficacy of lower axillary sampling in obtaining lymph node status in breast cancer: a controlled randomized trial. Br J Surg 1985; 72: 368–369.

50. O'Dwyer PJ. Editorial. Axillary dissection in primary breast cancer; the benefits of node clearance warrant reappraisal. Br Med J 1992; 302: 360–361.

51. Cabanes PA, Salmon RJ, Vilcoq JR et al. Value of axillary dissection in addition to lumpectomy and radiotherapy in early breast cancer. Lancet 1992; 339: 1245–1248.

52. Du Toit RS, Locker AP, Ellis IO et al. Evaluation of the prognostic value of triple node biopsy in early breast cancer. Br J Surg 1990; 77: 163–167.

53. Mambo NC, Gallager HS. Carcinoma of the breast. The prognostic significance of extranodal extension of axillary disease. Cancer 1977; 39: 2280–2285.

54. Cascinelli N, Greco M, Bufalino R et al. Prognosis of breast cancer with axillary node metastases after surgical treatment only. Eur J Cancer Clin Oncol 1987; 23: 795–799.

55. Fisher ER, Gregorio RM, Redmond C et al. Pathologic findings from the National Surgical Adjuvant Breast Project (protocol no 4). III. The significance of extranodal extension of axillary metastases. Am J Clin Pathol 1976; 65: 439–444.

56. Hartveit F. Paranodal tumour in breast cancer: extranodal extension versus vascular spread. J Pathol 1984; 144: 253–256.

57. Huvos AG, Hutter RVP, Berg JW. Significance of axillary macrometastases and micrometastases in mammary cancer. Ann Surg 1971; 173: 44–46.

58. Fisher ER, Palekar A, Rockette H et al. Pathologic findings from the National Surgical Adjuvant Breast Project (protocol no 4). V. Significance of axillary nodal micro and macro metastases. Cancer 1978a; 42: 2032–2038.

59. Rosen PP, Beattie EJ, Saigo PE et al. Occult axillary lymph node metastases from breast cancers with intramammary lymphatic tumor emboli. Am J Surg Pathol 1982; 6: 639–641.

60. Wells CA, Heryet A, Brochier J et al. The immunohistochemical detection of axillary micrometastases in breast cancer. Br J Cancer 1984; 50: 193–197.

61. Sedmak DD, Meineke TA, Knechtges DS, Anderson J. Prognostic significance of cytokeratin-positive breast cancer metastases. Mod Pathol 1989; 2: 16–20.

62. Springall RJ, Rytina ERC, Millis RR. Incidence and significance of micrometastases in axillary lymph nodes detected by immunohistochemical techniques. J Pathol 1990; 160: 174A.

63. International Breast Cancer Study Group. Prognostic importance of occult axillary lymph node micrometastases from breast cancers. Lancet 1990; 335: 1565–1568.

64. Hainsworth PJ, Tjandra JJ, Stillwell RG et al. Detection and significance of occult metastases in node-negative breast cancer. Br J Surg 1993; 80: 459–463.

65. Fisher ER, Palekar AS, Gregorio RM et al. Pathologic findings from the National Surgical Adjuvant Project for breast cancers (protocol no 4). IV. Significance of tumour necrosis. Hum Pathol 1978b; 9: 523–530.

66. Galea MH, Athanassiou E, Bell J et al. Occult regional lymph node metastases from breast carcinoma: immunohistological detection with antibodies CAM 5.2 and NCRC-11. J Pathol 1991; 165: 221–227.

67. Nasser IA, Lee AKC, Bosari S et al. Occult axillary lymph node metastates in 'node-negative' breast carcinoma. Hum Pathol 1993; 24: 950–957.

68. de Mascarel I, Bonichon F, Coindre JM, Trojani M. Prognostic significance of breast cancer axillary lymph node micrometastases assessed by two special techniques: re-evaluation with longer follow-up. Br J Cancer 1992; 66: 523–527.

69. Trojani M, de Mascarel I, Coindre JM, Bonichon F. Micrometastases to axillary lymph nodes from invasive lobular carcinoma of breast: detection by immunohistochemistry and prognostic significance. Br J Cancer 1987; 56: 838–839.

70. McGuckin MA, Cummings MC, Walsh MD et al. Occult axillary node metastases in breast cancer: their detection and prognostic significance. Br J Cancer 1996; 73: 88–95.

71. Hartveit F, Lilleng PK. Breast cancer: two micrometastatic variants in the axilla that differ in prognosis. Histopathol 1996; 28: 241–246.

72. Hartveit F, Samsonen G, Tangen M, Halvorsen JF. Routine histological investigation of the axillary nodes in breast cancer. Clin Oncol 1982; 8: 121–126.

73. Rosen PP. The pathology of invasive breast carcinoma. In: Harris JR, Hellman S, Henderson IC, Kinne DW, eds. Breast diseases. 2nd ed. Philadelphia: Lippincott, 1991; 245–296.

74. Groote AD, Oosterhuis JW, Molenaar WM et al. Methods in laboratory investigation. Radiographic imaging of lymph nodes in lymph node dissection specimens. Lab Invest 1985; 52: 326–329.

75. Durkin K, Haagensen CD. An improved technique for the study of lymph nodes in surgical specimens. Ann Surg 1980; 191: 419–429.

76. Morrow M, Evans J, Rosen PP, Kinne DW. Does clearing of axillary lymph nodes contribute to accurate staging of breast carcinoma? Cancer 1984; 53: 1329–1332.

77. Lee AKC, De Lellis RA, Silverman ML et al. Lymphatic and blood vessel invasion in breast carcinoma; a useful prognostic indicator? Hum Pathol 1986a; 17: 984–987.

78. Sears HF, Janus C, Levy W et al. Breast cancer without axillary metastases. Are there subpopulations? Cancer 1982; 50: 1820–1827.

79. Dawson PJ, Ferguson DJ, Karrison T. The pathologic findings of breast cancer in patients surviving 25 years after radical mastectomy. Cancer 1982; 50: 2131–2138.

80. Roses DF, Bell DA, Fotte TJ et al. Pathologic predictors of recurrence in stage 1 (T1NOMO and T2NOMO) breast cancer. Am J Clin Pathol 1982; 78: 817–820.

81. Bettelheim R, Penman HG, Thornton-Jones H et al. Prognostic significance of peritumoral vascular invasion in breast cancer. Br J Cancer 1984a; 50: 771–777.

82. Nime FA, Rosen PP, Thaler HT et al. Prognostic significance of tumour emboli in intramammary lymphatics in patients with mammary carcinoma. Am J Surg Pathol 1977; 1: 25–30.

83. Nealon TF, Nkongho A, Grossi CE et al. Treatment of early cancer of the breast (T1NOMO and T2NOMO) on the basis of histologic characteristics. Surgery 1981; 89: 279–289.

84. Rosen PP. Tumor emboli in intramammary lymphatics in breast carcinoma: Pathological criteria for diagnosis and clinical significance. Pathol Annu 1983; 18: 215–232.

85. Dawson PJ, Karrison T, Ferguson DJ. Histologic features associated with long-term survival in breast cancer. Hum Pathol 1986; 17: 1015–1021.

86. Pinder S, Ellis IO, O'Rourke S et al. Pathological prognostic factors in breast cancer. III. Vascular invasion: relationship with recurrence and survival in a large series with long-term follow-up. Histopathol 1994; 24: 41–47.

87. Örbo A, Stalsberg H, Kunde D. Topographic criteria in the diagnosis of tumor emboli in intramammary lymphatics. Cancer 1990; 66: 972–977.

88. Lee AKC, De Lellis RA, Wolfe HJ. Intramammary lymphatic invasion in breast carcinomas. Evaluation using ABH isoantigens as endothelial markers. Am J Surg Pathol 1986b; 10: 589–594.

89. Bettelheim R, Mitchell D, Gusterson BA. Immunocytochemistry in the identification of vascular invasion in breast cancer. J Clin Pathol 1984b; 37: 364–366.

90. Martin SA, Perez-Reyes N, Mendelsohn G. Angioinvasion in breast carcinoma; an immunohistochemical study of factor VIII-related antigen. Cancer 1987; 59: 1918–1922.

91. Ordonez NG, Brooks T, Thompson S et al. Use of Ulex europeus agglutinin I in the identification of lymphatic and blood vessel invasion in previously stained microscopic slides. Am J Surg Pathol 1987; 11: 543–550.

92. Saigo PE, Rosen PP. The application of immunohistochemical stains to identify endothelial-lined channels in mammary carcinoma. Cancer 1987; 59: 51–54.

93. Gilchrist KW, Gould VE, Hirschl S et al. Interobserver variation in the identification of breast carcinoma in intramammary lymphatics. Hum Pathol 1982; 13: 170–172.

94. Davis BW, Gelber R, Goldhirsh A et al. Prognostic significance of peritumoral vessel invasion in clinical trials of adjuvant therapy for breast cancer with axillary node metastases. Hum Pathol 1985; 16: 1212–1218.

95. Rosen PP, Saigo PE, Brown DW et al. Predictors of recurrence in stage 1 (T1NOMO) breast carcinoma. Ann Surg 1981; 193: 15–25.

96. Kemperman H, Borger J, Hart A et al. Prognostic factors for survival after breast conserving therapy for Stage I and II breast cancer; the role of local recurrence. Eur J Cancer 1995; 31A: 690–698.

97. O'Rourke S, Galea MH, Euhus D et al. An audit of local recurrence after simple mastectomy. Br J Surg 1994; 81: 386–389.

98. Page DL, Anderson TJ, Connolly JL, Schnitt SJ. Miscellaneous features of carcinoma. In: Page DL, Anderson TJ, eds. Diagnostic histopathology of the breast. Edinburgh: Churchill Livingstone, 1987; 269–299.

99. Carter D, Elkins RC, Pipkin RD et al. Relationship of necrosis and tumour border to lymph node metastases and 10 year survival in carcinoma of the breast. Am J Surg Pathol 1978; 2: 39–46.

100. Gilchrist KW, Gray R, Fowble B et al. Tumor necrosis is a prognostic predictor for early recurrence and death in lymph node-positive breast cancer: a 10 year follow-up study of 728 Eastern Cooperative Oncology Group Patients. J Clin Oncol 1993; 11: 1929–1935.

101. Parham DM, Hagen N, Brown RA. Morphometric analysis of breast carcinoma: association with survival. J Clin Pathol 1988; 41: 173–177.

102. Parham DM, Hagen N, Brown RA. Simplified method of grading primary carcinomas of the breast. J Clin Pathol 1992; 45: 517–520.

103. Elston CW, Ellis IO. Method for grading breast cancer (letter). J Clin Pathol 1993; 46: 189–190.

104. World Health Organization. International histological classification of tumours. Histologic types of breast tumours. Geneva: World Health Organization, 1981.

105. Linell F, Ljungberg O, Andersson I. Breast carcinoma. Aspects of early stages, progression and related problems. Acta Pathol Microbiol Scand 1980; 272: 1–233.

106. Linell F, Rank F. Comments on histologic classifications with reference to histogenesis and prognosis. Universitetsförlaget Dialogos, Lund. 1989.

107. Silverberg SG, Chitale AR. Assessment of the significance of the proportion of intraductal and infiltrating tumor growth in ductal carcinoma of the breast. Cancer 1973; 32: 830–837.

108. Matsukuma A, Enjoji M, Toyoshima S. Ductal carcinoma of the breast. An analysis of the proportion of intraductal and invasive components. Pathol Res Prac 1991; 187: 62–67.

109. Ellis IO, Galea M, Broughton N et al. Pathological prognostic factors in breast cancer. II. Histological type. Relationship with survival in a large study with long-term follow-up. Histopathol 1992; 20: 479–489.

110. Van Dongen JA, Fentiman IS, Harris JR et al. In situ breast cancer: the EORTC consensus meeting. Lancet 1989; ii: 25–27.

111. Schnitt SJ, Connelly JL, Harris JR et al. Pathologic predictors of early local recurrence in stage I and stage II breast cancer treated by primary radiation therapy. Cancer 1984; 53: 1049–1057.

112. Fourquet A, Campana F, Zafrani B et al. Prognostic factors of breast recurrence in the conservative management of early breast cancer: a 25 year follow-up. Int J Rad Oncol Biol Physiol 1989; 17: 719–725.

113. Holland R, Connelly JL, Gelman R et al. The presence of an extensive intraduct component following a limited excision correlates with prominent residual disease in the remainder of the breast. J Clin Oncol 1990; 8: 113–118.

114. Jacquemier J, Kurtz JM, Amalric R et al. An assessment of extensive intraductal component as a risk factor for local recurrence after breast-conserving therapy. Br J Cancer 1990; 61: 873–876.

115. Gage I, Schnitt SJ, Nixon AJ et al. Pathologic margin involvement and the risk of recurrence in patients treated with breast-conserving therapy. Cancer 1996; 78: 1921–1928.

116. Leroux R. Reaction giganto cellulaire du stroma dans un epithelioma mammaire. Bull Cancer (Paris) 1931; 20: 692–697.

117. Factor SM, Biempica L, Ratner I et al. Carcinoma of the breast with multinucleated reactive stromal giant cells. Virchows Arch (A) Pathol Anat 1977; 374: 1–12.

118. Agnantis NT, Rosen PP. Mammary carcinoma with osteoclast-like giant cells: a study of eight cases with follow-up data. Am J Clin Pathol 1979; 72: 383–389.

119. Holland R, van Haelst UJGM. Mammary carcinoma with osteoclast-like giant cells. Cancer 1984; 53: 1963–1973.

120. Bertrand G, George P, Bertrand AF. Carcinome mammaire à stroma-reaction giganto-cellulaire premier cas masculin. Ann Pathol 1986; 6: 144–147.

121. Sugano I, Nagao K, Kondo Y et al. Cytologic and ultrastructural studies of a rare breast carcinoma with osteoclast-like giant cells. Cancer 1983; 52: 74–78.

122. Saout L, Leduc M, Suy-Beng PT, Meignie P. Présentation d'un nouveau cas de carcinome mammaire cribriforme associé à une réaction histocytaire giganto-cellulaire. Arch Anat Cytol Pathol 1985; 33: 58–61.

123. Tavassoli FA, Norris HJ. Breast carcinoma with osteoclastlike giant cells. Arch Pathol Lab Med 1986; 110: 636–639.

124. Reale D, Guarino M, Bianchini E et al. Infiltrating lobular carcinoma of the breast, alveolar variant, with stromal reactive osteoclast-like giant cells. Description of a case. Pathologica 1993; 85: 525–532.

125. Shivas AA, Douglas JG. The prognostic significance of elastosis in breast carcinoma. J Roy Coll Surg Edinb 1972; 17: 315–320.

126. Mitchell RE, Mitchell RM, Shugg D, Wyld C. The prognosis of breast cancer based on histological assessment. Aust NZ J Surg 1979; 49: 305–312.

127. Glaubitz LC, Bowen JH, Cox EB. Elastosis in human breast cancer. Correlation with sex steroid receptors and comparison with clinical outcome. Arch Pathol Lab Med 1984; 108: 27–30.

128. Anastassiades OT, Bouropoulou V, Kontogeorgos G. Duct elastosis in infiltrating carcinoma of the breast. Pathol Res Pract 1979; 165: 411–421.

129. Humeniuk V, Forrest APM, Hawkins RA, Prescott R. Elastosis and primary breast cancer. Cancer 1983; 52: 1448–1452.

130. Reyes MG, Bazile DB, Tosch T, Rubenstone AI. Periductal elastic tissue of breast cancer. Arch Pathol Lab Med 1982; 106: 610–614.

131. Millis RR. Correlation of hormone receptors with pathological features in human breast cancer. Cancer 1980; 42: 2869–2871.

132. Masters JRW, Sangster K, Hawkins RA, Shivas AA. Elastosis and oestrogen receptors in human breast cancer. Br J Cancer 1976; 33: 342–343.

133. Underwood JCE. A morphometric analysis of human breast carcinoma. Br J Cancer 1972; 26: 234–237.

134. Sistrunk WE, MacCarty WC. Life expectancy following radical amputation for carcinoma of the breast — a clinical and pathological study of 218 cases. Ann Surg 1922; 75: 61–69.

135. Hueper WC. The clinical significance and application of histologic grading of cancers. Ann Surg 1932; 95: 321–326.

136. Hamlin IME. Possible host resistance in carcinoma of the breast: a histological study. Br J Cancer 1968; 22: 383–401.

137. Alderson MR, Hamlin I, Staunton MD. The relative significance of prognostic factors in breast carcinoma. Br J Cancer 1971; 25: 646–656.

138. Giani C, Pianchera A, Breccia M et al. Relationship between progesterone receptor and productive fibrosis as an index of tumour differentiation in breast cancer. Tumori 1988; 74: 287–293.

139. Giani C, Campani D, De Negri F et al. Relationship between progesterone receptor, axillary node status and productive fibrosis in ductal infiltrating carcinoma of the breast. Appl Pathol 1989; 7: 225–232.

140. Parker MG. Nuclear hormone receptors. London: Academic Press, 1991.

141. Beatson JT. Treatment of inoperable cases of carcinoma of the mamma; suggestions for new method of treatment with illustrative cases. Lancet 1896; ii: 104–107.

142. Huggins C, Burgenstal BM. Inhibition of human mammary and prostatic cancer by adrenalectomy. Cancer Res 1952; 12: 134–141.

143. Pearson OH, Ray BS, Harrold CC et al. Hypophysectomy in the treatment of advanced cancer. JAMA 1956; 161: 17–21.

144. Dresser R. The effect of ovarian irradiation on the bone metastases of cancer of the breast. Am J Radiol 1936; 35: 384.

145. Sheth SP, Allegra JC. The comprehensive management of benign and malignant diseases. In: Bland KI, Copeland EM, eds. Vol 44. Philadelphia: WB Saunders, 1991.

146. Haddow A, Watkinson JM, Paterson E et al. Influence of synthetic oestrogens upon advanced malignant disease. Br Med J 1944; 2: 393–398.

147. Jensen EV, Jacobson HI. Buyers guide to the mechanism of oestrogen action. Recent Prog Horm Res 1962; 18: 387.

148. NIH consensus development conference on steroid receptors in breast cancer. Cancer 1980; 46: 2759–2963.

149. Greene GL, Nolan C, Engler JP et al. Monoclonal antibodies to human estrogen receptor. Proc Natl Acad Sci USA 1980; 77: 5115–5119.

150. Jensen EV, Greene GL, De Sombre ER. The estrogen-receptor immunoassay in the prognosis and treatment of breast cancer. Lab Manager 1986; 24: 25–42.

151. King WJ, Greene GL. Monoclonal antibodies localize oestrogen receptor in nuclei of target cells. Nature. 1984; 307: 745–747.

152. McCarty KSJ, Miller LS, Cox EB, Konrath J, McCarty KSS. Estrogen receptor analyses: Correlation of biochemical and immunohistochemical methods using monoclonal antireceptor antibodies. Arch Pathol Lab Med 1985; 109: 716–721.

153. Pertschuk LP, Eisenberg KB, Carter AC, Feldman JG. Immunohistologic localization of estrogen receptors in breast cancer with monoclonal antibodies. Cancer 1985; 55: 513–518.

154. Gaskell DJ, Hawkins RA, Tesdale AL et al. The differing predictive values of oestrogen receptor assays for large breast cancers. Postgrad Med J 1992; 68: 900–903.

155. McClelland RA, Berger U, Miller LS, Powles TJ, Coombes RC. Immunocytochemical assay for oestrogen receptor in patients with breast cancer. Relationship to biochemical assay and to outcome of therapy. J Clin Oncol 1986; 4: 1171–1176.

156. Seymour L, Meyer K, Esser J et al. Estimation of ER and PR by immunocytochemistry in breast cancer. Comparison with radioligand binding methods. Am J Clin Pathol 1990; 94: S35–40.

157. Anderson J, Orntoft T, Poulson SH. Semiquantitative oestrogen receptor assay in formalin-fixed paraffin sections of human breast cancer tissue using monoclonal antibodies. Br J Cancer 1986; 53: 691–694.

158. De Rosa CM, Ozello L, Greene GL, Habif DV. Immunostaining of oestrogen receptor in paraffin sections of breast carcinoma using monoclonal antibody D753P: Effects of fixation. Am J Surg Pathol 1987; 11: 943–950.

159. Jackson P, Teasdale J, Cowen PN. Development and validation of a sensitive immunohistochemical oestrogen receptor assay for use on archival breast tissue. Histochem 1990; 92: 149–152.

160. Paterson DA, Reid CP, Anderson TJ, Hawkins RA. Assessment of oestrogen receptor content of breast carcinoma by immunohistochemical techniques on fixed and frozen tissue and by chemical ligand binding assay. J Clin Pathol 1990; 43: 46–51.

161. Snead DJR, Bell JA, Dixon AR et al. Methodology of immunohistochemical detection of oestrogen receptor in human breast carcinoma in formalin fixed paraffin embedded tissue: a comparison with frozen section morphology. Histopathol 1993; 23: 233–238.

162. Goulding H, Pinder S, Cannon P et al. A new method for the assessment of oestrogen receptor status on routine formalin-fixed tissue samples. Hum Pathol 1995; 26: 291–294.

163. Robertson JFR, Bates K, Pearson D et al. Comparison of two oestrogen receptor assays in the prediction of the clinical course of patients with advanced breast cancer. Br J Cancer 1992; 65: 727–730.

164. Hawkins RA, Sangster K, Tesdale A et al. The cytochemical detection of oestrogen receptors in fine needle aspirates of breast cancer: correlation with biochemical assay and prediction of response to endocrine therapy. Br J Cancer 1988; 58: 77–80.

165. Cowen PN, Teasdale J, Jackson P, Reid BJ. Oestrogen receptor in breast cancer: prognostic studies using a new immunohistochemical assay. Histopathol 1990; 17: 319–325.

166. Jackson DP, Payne J, Bell S et al. Extraction of DNA from exfoliative cytology specimens and its suitability for analysis and the polymerase chain reaction. Cytopathol 1990; 1: 87–96.

167. Poulson HS, Jensen J, Hermansen C. Human breast cancer: Heterogeneity of estrogen binding sites. Cancer 1981; 43: 1791.

168. Chiu KY. Use of microwave for rapid immunoperoxidase staining of paraffin sections. Med Lab Sci 1987; 44: 3–5.

169. Shi SR, Key ME, Kalra KL. Antigen retrieval in formalin-fixed, paraffin embedded tissues: An enhancement method for immunohistochemical staining based on microwave oven heating of tissue sections. J Histochem Cytochem 1991; 39: 741–748.

170. Cuevas EC, Bateman AC, Wilkins BS et al. Microwave antigen retrieval in immunocytochemistry: A study of 80 antibodies. J Clin Pathol 1994; 47: 448–452.

171. King WJ, Greene GL. Monoclonal antibodies localize oestrogen receptor in nuclei of target cells. Nature 1984; 307: 745–747.

172. Barnes DM, Millis RR. Oestrogen receptors: the history, the relevance and the methods of evaluation. In: Kirkham N, Lemoine NR, eds. Progress in Pathology vol 2. Edinburgh: Churchill Livingstone, 1995: 89–114.

173. Williams MR, Todd JH, Ellis IO et al. Oestrogen receptors in primary and advanced breast cancer: An eight year review of 704 cases. Br J Cancer 1987; 55: 67–73.

174. Nicholson RI. Why ER level may not reflect endocrine responsiveness in breast cancer. Rev End Rel Cancer 1992; 40: 252–258.

175. Walker KJ, Price-Thomas JM, Candlish W et al. Influence of the antioestrogen tamoxifen on normal breast tissue. Br J Cancer 1991; 64: 764–768.

176. McGuire WL, Chambers GC, Fuqua SA. Abnormal estrogen receptor in clinical breast cancer. J Steroid Biochem Mol Biol 1992; 43: 243–247.

177. Ceriani R, Thompson K, Peterson JA. Surface differentiation antigens of human mammary epithelial cells carried on the human milk fat globule. Proc Natl Acad Sci (USA) 1977; 74: 582–586.

178. Burchell J, Taylor-Papadimitriou J. Antibodies to human milk fat globule molecules. Cancer Invest 1989; 7: 53–61.

179. Taylor-Papadimitriou J, D'Souza B, Burchell J et al. The role of tumor-associated antigens in the biology and immunotherapy of breast cancer. Ann NY Acad Sci 1993; 698: 31–47.

180. Heyderman E, Steele K, Ormerod MG. A new antigen on the epithelial membrane: Its immunoperoxidase

localisation in normal and neoplastic tissues. J Clin Pathol 1979; 32: 35–39.

181. Gendler SJ, Lancaster CA, Taylor-Papadimitriou J et al. Molecular cloning and expression of human tumor-associated polymorphic epithelial mucin. J Biol Chem 1990; 265: 15286–15293.

182. Hilkens J, Vos HL, Wesseling J et al. Is episialin/MUC1 involved in breast cancer progression? Cancer Lett 1995; 90: 27–33.

183. Price MR, Edwards S, Owainati A et al. Multiple epitopes on a human breast carcinoma associated antigen. Int J Cancer 1985; 36: 567–574.

184. Devine PL, McKenzie IFC. Mucins: structure, function, and association with malignancy. Bioessays 1992; 14: 619–625.

185. Lalani EN, Berdichevsky A, Straus H et al. Development of a mouse model system for the study of immunological responses to the human polymorphic epithelial mucin. J Pathol 1990; 161.

186. Ho SB, Kim YS. Carbohydrate antigens on cancer-associated mucin-like molecules. Semin Cancer Biol 1991; 2: 389–400.

187. Ho SB, Niehans GA, Lyftogt C et al. Heterogeneity of mucin gene expression in normal and neoplastic tissues. Cancer Res 1993; 53: 641–651.

188. Hilkens J, Buijs F, Hilgers J. Monoclonal antibodies against human milk fat globule membranes detecting differentiation antigens of the mammary gland and its tumours. Int J Cancer 1984; 34: 197–206.

189. Salomon DS, Brandt R, Ciardiello F, Normanno N. Epidermal growth factor-related peptides and their receptors in human malignancies. Crit Rev Oncol Hematol 1995; 19: 183–232.

190. Normanno N, Ciardiello F, Brandt R, Salomon DS. Epidermal growth factor-related peptides in the pathogenesis of human breast cancer. Br Cancer Res Treat 1994; 29: 11–27.

191. Fantl WJ, Johnson DE, Williams LT. Signalling by receptor tyrosine kinases. Annu Rev Biochem 1993; 62: 453–481.

192. Rajkumar T, Gullick WJ. The type I growth factor receptors in human breast cancer. Br Cancer Res Treat 1994; 29: 3–9.

193. Tonelli QJ, Sorof S. Epidermal growth factor requirement for development of cultured mammary gland. Nature 1980; 285: 250–252.

194. Taylor-Papadimitriou J, Shearer M, Stopker MGP. Growth requirements of human mammary epithelial cells in culture. Int J Cancer 1977; 20: 903–908.

195. Fitzpatrick SL, Lachance MP, Schultz GS. Characterisation of epidermal growth factor receptor and action on human breast cancer cells in culture. Cancer Res 1984; 44: 3442–3447.

196. Carpenter G, Cohen S. Epidermal growth factor. Ann Rev Biochem 1979; 48: 198–216.

197. Gullick WJ. The role of the epidermal growth factor receptor and the c-erbB-2 protein in breast cancer. Int J Cancer Suppl 1990; 5: 55–61.

198. Gullick WJ. Growth factors and oncogenes in breast cancer. Prog Growth Factor Res 1990; 2: 1–13.

199. Chrysogelos SA, Dickson RB. EGF receptor expression, regulation, and function in breast cancer. Br Cancer Res Treat 1994; 29: 29–40.

200. Carpenter G. Receptors for epidermal growth factor receptor and other polypeptide mitogens. Ann Rev Biochem 1987; 56: 881–914.

201. Coussens L, Yang-Feng TL, Liao YC et al. Tyrosine kinase receptor with extensive homology to EGF receptor shares chromosomal location with neu oncogene. Science 1985; 230: 1132–1139.

202. Ozanne B, Shum A, Richards CS et al. Evidence for an increase of EGF receptors in epidermoid malignancies. Cancer cells: growth factors and transformation. Cold Spring Harbour Laboratory. 1985; 41–48.

203. Harris AL. What is the biological, prognostic, and therapeutic role of the EGF receptor in human breast cancer? Br Cancer Res Treat 1994; 29: 1–2.

204. Fox SB, Smith K, Hollyer J, Greenall M, Hastrich D, Harris AL. The epidermal growth factor receptor as a prognostic marker: results of 370 patients and review of 3009 patients. Br Cancer Res Treat 1994; 29: 41–49.

205. Sharma AK, Horgan K, McClelland RA et al. A dual immunocytochemical assay for oestrogen and epidermal growth factor receptors in tumour cell lines. Histochem J 1994; 26: 306–310.

206. Sainsbury JRC, Farndon JR, Needham GK, Malcolm AJ, Harris AL. Epidermal growth factor receptor status as a predictor of early recurrence and of death from breast cancer. Lancet 1987; i: 1398–1402.

207. Lewis S, Locker A, Todd JH et al. Expression of epidermal growth factor receptor in breast carcinoma. J Clin Pathol 1990; 43: 385–389.

208. Grimaux M, Romain S, Remvikos Y, Martin PM, Magdelenat H. Prognostic value of epidermal growth factor receptor in node-positive breast cancer. Br Cancer Res Treat 1989; 14: 77–90.

209. Khazaie K, Schirrmacher V, Lichtner RB. EGF receptor in neoplasia and metastasis. Cancer Metastasis Rev 1993; 12: 255–274.

210. Marquardt H, Hunkapiller MW, Hood LE, Todaro GJ. Rat transforming growth factor type 1: structure and relationship to epidermal growth factor. Science 1984; 223: 1079–1082.

211. Todaro GJ, Fryling C, Delarco JE. Transforming growth factors produced by certain tumour cell lines: polypeptides that interact with epidermal growth factor receptors. Proc Natl Acad Sci USA 1980; 77: 5258–5261.

212. Roberts AB, Frolick CA, Anzano MA, Sporn MB. Transforming growth factors from neoplastic and non-neoplastic tissues. Fed Proc 1983; 42: 2621–2625.

213. Bates SE, Davidson NE, Valverius EM et al. Expression of transforming growth factor alpha and its messenger ribonucleic acid in human breast cancer: Its regulation by estrogen and its possible functional significance. Mol Endocrinol 1988; 2: 543–555.

214. Partridge M, Green MR, Langdon JD, Feldmann M. Production of TGF-α and TGF-β by cultured keratinocytes, skin and oral squamous cell carcinomas — potential autocrine regulation of normal and malignant epithelial cell proliferation. Br J Cancer 1989; 60: 542–548.

215. Cheifitz S, Weatherbee JA, Tsang ML et al. The transforming growth factor β system, a complex pattern of cross-reactive ligands and receptors. Cell 1987; 45: 409.

216. Silberstein GB, Daniel CW. Reversible inhibition of mammary gland growth by transforming growth factor-β. Science 1987; 237: 291–293.

217. Knabbe C, Lippman ME, Wakefield LM et al.

Evidence that transforming growth factor-β is a hormonally related negative growth factor in human breast cells. Cell 1987; 48: 417–428.

218. Shippley GD, Pittlekow MR, Willie JJ et al. Reversible inhibition of normal prokeratinocyte proliferation by type B transforming growth factor inhibitor in serum free medium. Cancer Res 1986; 46: 2068.

219. Yamamoto T, Ikawa S, Akiyama T et al. Similarity of protein encoded by the human c-erbB-2 gene to epidermal growth factor receptor. Nature 1986; 319: 230–234.

220. Weinberger C, Thompson CC, Ong ES et al. The c-erb-A gene encodes a thyroid hormone receptor. Nature 1986; 324: 641–646.

221. Maguire HC, Greene MI. The neu (c-erbB-2) oncogene. Semin Oncol 1989; 16: 148–155.

222. Hudziak RM, Lewis GD, Winget M, Fendly BM, Shepard HM, Ullrich A. p185HER2 monoclonal antibody has antiproliferative effects in vitro and sensitized human breast tumour cells to tumour necrosis factor. Mol Cell Biol 1989; 9: 1165–1172.

223. Venter DJ, Kumar S, Tuzi NL, Gullick WJ. Overexpression of the c-erbB-2 oncoprotein in human breast carcinomas: Immunohistochemical assessment correlates with gene amplification. Lancet 1987; ii: 69–71.

224. van de Vijver MJ, Peterse JL, Mooi MJ et al. Neu protein overexpression in breast cancer: association with comedo type ductal carcinoma in situ and limited prognostic value in stage II breast cancer. N Eng J Med 1988; 319: 1239–1245.

225. Lammie GA, Barnes DM, Millis RR, Gullick WJ. An immunohistochemical study of the presence of c-erbB-2 protein in Paget's disease of the nipple. Histopathol 1989; 15: 505–514.

226. Barnes DM. Editorial: Breast cancer and a proto-oncogene. Br Med J 1989; 299: 1061.

227. Lovekin C, Ellis IO, Locker A et al. c-erbB-2 oncoprotein expression in primary and advanced breast cancer. Br J Cancer 1990; 63: 439–443.

228. Slamon DJ, Godolphin W, Jones LA et al. Studies of the HER-2/neu proto-oncogene in human breast and ovarian cancer. Science 1989; 244: 707–712.

229. Wright C, Angus B, Nicholson S et al. Expression of c-erbB-2 oncoprotein: A prognostic marker in human breast cancer. Cancer Res 1989; 49: 2087–2091.

230. Barnes DM, Lammie GA, Millis RR et al. An immunohistochemical evaluation of c-erbB-2 expression in human breast carcinoma. Br J Cancer 1988; 58: 448–452.

231. Drebin JA, Link VC, Weinberg RA, Greene MI. Inhibition of tumour growth by a monoclonal antibody reactive with an oncogene encoded tumour antigen. Proc Natl Acad Sci USA 1986; 83: 9129–9133.

232. Kadowaki T, Kasuga M, Tobe K et al. A 190 000 Mw glycoprotein phosphorylated on tyrosine residues in Epidermal Growth Factor stimulated KB cells is the product of the c-erbB-2 gene. Biochem Biophys Res Com 1987; 144: 699–704.

233. Kokai Y, Myers J, Wada T et al. Synergistic interaction of p185c neu and the EFG receptor leads to transformation of rodent fibroblasts. Cell 1989; 58: 287–292.

234. De Potter CR. The neu-oncogene: more than a prognostic indicator? Hum Pathol 1994; 25: 1264–1268.

235. De Potter CR, Schelfhout AM. The neu-protein and breast cancer. Virchows Arch (A) Pathol Anat 1995; 426: 107–115.

236. Carraway KL, Sliwkowski MX, Akita R et al. The erbB3 gene product is a receptor for heregulin. J Biol Chem 1994; 269: 14303–14306.

237. Sliwkowski MX, Schaefer G, Akita RW et al. Coexpression of erbB2 and erbB3 proteins reconstitutes a high affinity receptor for heregulin. J Biol Chem 1994; 269: 14661–14665.

238. Plowman GD, Green JM, Culouscou JM, Carlton GW, Rothwell VM, Buckley S. Heregulin induces tyrosine phosphorylation of HER4/p180erbB4. Nature 1993; 366: 473–475.

239. Carraway KL, Cantley LC. A neu acquaintance for erbB3 and erbB4: a role for receptor heterodimerization in growth signaling. Cell 1994; 78: 5–8.

240. Travis A, Bell JA, Wencyk P et al. C-erbB-3 in human breast carcinoma: expression and relation to prognosis and established prognostic indicators. Br J Cancer 1996; 74: 229–233.

241. Rajkumar T, Gooden CS, Lemoine NR et al. Expression of the c-erbB-3 protein in gastrointestinal tract tumours determined by monoclonal antibody RTJ1 [published erratum appears in J Pathol 1993 Oct; 171: 154]. J Pathol 1993; 170: 271–278.

242. Quinn CM, Ostrowski JL, Lane SA et al. c-erbB-3 protein expression in human breast cancer: comparison with other tumour variables and survival. Histopathol 1994; 25: 247–252.

243. Alimandi M, Romano A, Curia MC et al. Cooperative signaling of ErbB3 and ErbB2 in neoplastic transformation and human mammary carcinomas. Oncogene 1995; 10: 1813–1821.

244. Slamon DJ, de Kerion JB, Verma IM, Cline MJ. Expression of cellular oncogenes in human malignancies. Science 1984; 224: 256–262.

245. Nishimura S, Sekiya T. Human cancer and cellular oncogenes. Biochem J 1987; 243: 313–327.

246. Lemoine NR. Molecular biology of breast cancer. Ann Oncol 1994; 4: 31–37.

247. Ozbun MA, Butel JS. Tumor suppressor p53 mutations and breast cancer: a critical analysis. Adv Cancer Res 1995; 66: 71–141.

248. Elledge RM, Allred DC. The p53 tumor suppressor gene in breast cancer. Br Cancer Res Treat 1994; 32: 39–47.

249. Eeles RA, Bartkova J, Lane DP, Bartek J. The role of TP53 in breast cancer development. Cancer Surv 1993; 18: 57–75.

250. Biggs PJ, Warren W, Venitt S, Stratton MR. Does a genotoxic carcinogen contribute to human breast cancer? The value of mutational spectra in unravelling the aetiology of cancer. Mutagenesis 1993; 8: 275–283.

251. Gelmann EP, Lippman ME. Understanding the role of oncogenes in human breast cancer. In: Sluyser M, ed. Growth factors and oncogenes in breast cancer. VCH Publishers. Weinheim, Germany, 1987.

252. Weinberg RA. The action of oncogenes in the cytoplasm and nucleus. Science 1985; 230: 770–774.

253. Walker RA, Wilkinson N. p21 ras protein expression in benign and malignant human breast. J Pathol 1988; 156: 147–153

254. Agnantis NJ, Petraki C, Markoulatos P, Spandidos DA.

Immunohistochemical study of the ras oncogene expression in human breast lesions. Anti Cancer Res 1986; 6: 1157–1160.

255. Honran Hand P, Thor A, Wunderlich D et al. Monoclonal antibodies of predefined specificity detect activated ras gene expression in human mammary and colon carcinomas. Proc Natl Acad Sci USA 1984; 81: 5227–5231.

256. Ohuchi N, Thor A, Page DL et al. Expression of the 21000 molecular weight ras protein in a spectrum of benign and malignant human mammary tissues. Cancer Res 1986; 46: 2511–2519.

257. Candlish W, Kerr IB, Simpson HW. Immunocytochemical detection and significance of p21 ras family oncogene product in benign and malignant breast disease. J Pathol 1986; 150: 163–167.

258. Ghosh AK, Moore M, Harris M. Immunohistochemical detection of ras oncogene p21 product in benign and malignant mammary tissue in man. J Clin Path 1986; 39: 428–434.

259. Yee LD, Kacinski BM, Carter D. Oncogene structure, function and expression in breast cancer. Semin Diagn Pathol 1989; 6: 110–125.

260. Walker RA, Senior PV, Jones JL et al. An immunohistochemical and in situ hybridization study of c-myc and c-erbB-2 expression in primary human breast carcinomas. J Pathol 1989; 158: 97–105.

261. Escot C, Theillet C, Lidereau R et al. Genetic alterations of the c-myc protooncogene (MYC) in human primary breast carcinomas. Proc Natl Acad Sci USA 1986; 83: 4834–4838.

262. Locker AP, Dowle CS, Ellis IO et al. C-myc oncogene product expression and prognosis in operable breast cancer. Br J Cancer 1989; 60: 669–672.

263. Meyer JS, Friedman E, McCrate MM et al. Prediction of early course of breast carcinoma by thymidine labeling. Cancer 1983; 51: 1879–1886.

264. Tubiana M, Pejovic MJ, Renaud A et al. Kinetic parameters and the course of the disease in breast cancer. Cancer 1981; 47: 937–943.

265. Bonadonna G, Valagussa P, Tancini G et al. Current status of Milan adjuvant chemotherapy trials for node-positive and node-negative breast cancer. NCI Monograph 1986; 1: 45–49.

266. Remvikos Y, Beuzebocp P, Zajdela A. Correlation of proliferative activity of breast cancer with response to cytotoxic chemotherapy. J Nat Cancer Inst 1989; 81: 1383–1387.

267. Wright NA, Hall PA. Cell proliferation in pathology. J Pathol 1993; 170: 327–330.

268. Wright NA. Cell proliferation in health and disease. In: Anthony PP, MacSween RNM, eds. Recent Advances in Histopathology. Edinburgh: Churchill Livingstone, 1984; 17–34.

269. Uyterlinde AM, Schipper NW, Baak JPA. Comparison of extent of disease and morphometric and DNA flow cytometric prognostic factors in invasive ductal breast cancer. J Clin Pathol 1987; 40: 1432–1436.

270. Gerdes J, Schwab V, Lemke H, Stein H. Production of a mouse monoclonal antibody reactive with a human nuclear antigen associated with cell proliferation. Int J Cancer 1983; 31: 13–20.

271. Gerdes J, Lelle RJ, Pickartz H et al. Growth fractions in breast cancers determined in situ with monoclonal antibody Ki-67. J Clin Pathol 1986; 39: 977–980.

272. Barnard NJ, Hall PA, Lemoine NR, Kadar N. Proliferative index in breast carcinoma determined in situ by Ki67 immunostaining and its relationship to clinical and pathological variables. J Pathol 1987; 152: 287–295.

273. Bouzubar N, Walker KJ, Griffiths K et al. Ki67 immunostaining in primary breast cancer; pathological and clinical associations. Br J Cancer 1989; 59: 943–947.

274. Pinder SE, Wencyk P, Sibbering DM et al. Assessment of the new proliferation marker MIBI in breast carcinoma using image analysis: Associations with other prognostic factors and survival. Br J Cancer 1995; 71: 146–149.

275. Ogata K, Kurki P, Celis JE et al. Monoclonal antibodies to a nuclear protein (PCNA/Cyclin) associated with DNA replication. Exp Cell Res 1987; 168: 476–486.

276. Prelich G, Tan CK, Kostura M et al. Functional identity of proliferating cell nuclear antigen and a DNA polymerase-d. 1987; 326: 515–517.

277. Garcia RL, Coltrera MD, Gown AM. Analysis of proliferative grade using anti-PCNA/Cyclin monoclonal antibodies in fixed embedded tissues. Am J Pathol 1989; 134: 733–739.

278. Schneider J, Bak M, Efferth T et al. P-Glycoprotein expression in treated and untreated human breast cancer. Br J Cancer 1989; 60: 815–818.

279. Porter-Jordan K, Lippman ME. Overview of the biologic markers of breast cancer. Hematol Oncol Clin North Am 1994; 8: 73–100.

280. Rochefort H. Oestrogens, proteases and breast cancer. From cell lines to clinical applications. Eur J Cancer 1994; 10: 1583–1586.

281. Gion M, Mione R, Dittadi R et al. Relationship between cathepsin D and other pathological and biological parameters in 1752 patients with primary breast cancer. Eur J Cancer 1995; 5: 671–677.

282. Eng Tan P, Benz CC, Dollbaum C et al. Prognostic value of Cathepsin D expression in breast cancer: immunohistochemical assessment and correlation with radiometric assay. Ann Oncol 1994; 5: 329–336.

283. Castiglioni T, Merino MJ, Elsner B et al. Immunohistochemical analysis of cathepsins D, B, and L in human breast cancer. Hum Pathol 1994; 25: 857–862.

284. Roger P, Montcourrier P, Maudelonde T et al. Cathepsin D immunostaining in paraffin-embedded breast cancer cells and macrophages: correlation with cytosolic assay. Hum Pathol 1994; 25: 863–871.

285. O'Donoghue AE, Poller DN, Bell JA et al. Cathepsin D in primary breast carcinoma: adverse prognosis is associated with expression of cathepsin D in stromal cells. Br Cancer Res Treat 1995; 33: 137–145.

286. Joensuu H, Toikkanen S, Isola J. Stromal cell cathepsin D expression and long-term survival in breast cancer. Br J Cancer 1995; 71: 155–159.

287. Morrow CS, Cowan KH. Mechanisms and clinical significance of multidrug resistance. Oncol 1988; 2: 55–64.

288. Charpin C, Vielh P, Duffaud F et al. Quantitative immunocytochemical assays of P-glycoprotein in breast carcinomas: correlation to messenger RNA expression and to immunohistochemical prognostic indicators. J Natl Cancer Inst 1994; 86: 1539–1545.

289. De La Torre M, Larsson R, Nygren P et al. Expression of the multidrug-resistance gene product in untreated human breast cancer and its relationship to prognostic markers. Acta Oncol 1994; 33: 773–777.

290. Pesce CM. Defining and interpreting diseases through morphometry. Lab Investigation 1987; 56: 568–575.

291. Baak JPA, Oort J. A manual of morphometry in diagnostic pathology. Berlin: Springer, 1983.

292. Aziz DC, Barathur RB. Quantitation and morphometric analysis of tumors by image analysis. J Cell Biochem Suppl 1994; 19: 120–125.

293. Brugal G. Analysis of microscopic preparations. In: Jasmin G, Proschek L, eds. Methods and achievements in experimental pathology, vol 11. Basel: Karger, 1984; 1–33.

294. Hedley DW, Friedlander MI, Taylor IW et al. Method for analysis of cellular DNA content of paraffin embedded pathological material using flow cytometry. J Histochem Cytochem 1983; 31: 1333.

295. Hedley DW, Friedlander ML, Taylor IW. Application of DNA flow cytometry to paraffin embedded archival material for the study of aneuploidy and its clinical significance. Cytometry 1985; 6: 327–333.

296. Hedley DW. Flow cytometry using paraffin embedded tissue: five years on. Cytometry 1989; 10: 229–241.

297. Auer G, Eriksson E, Azavedo E et al. Prognostic significance of nuclear DNA content in mammary adenocarcinoma in humans. Cancer Res 1984; 44: 394–396.

298. Walker RA, Camplejohn RS. DNA flow cytometry of human breast carcinomas and its relationship to transferrin and epidermal growth factor receptors. J Pathol 1986; 150: 37–42.

299. Locker AP, Dilks B, Gilmour A et al. Aspiration cytology diagnosis of breast lesions by nuclear DNA content. Br J Surg 1990; 77: A707.

300. Gasparini G, Harris AL. Clinical importance of the determination of tumour angiogenesis in breast carcinoma: much more than a new prognostic tool. J Clin Oncol 1995; 13: 765–782.

301. Folkman J, Cole P, Zimmerman S. Tumor behaviour in isolated perfused organs: in vitro growth and metastasis of biopsy material in rabbit thyroid and canine intestinal segment. Ann Surg 1966; 164: 491–502.

302. Folkman J. Tumor angiogenesis: Therapeutic implications. New Eng J Med 1971; 285: 1182–1186.

303. Folkman J. What is the evidence that tumors are angiogenesis dependent? J Natl Cancer Inst 1990; 82: 4–6.

304. Liotta L, Kleinerman J, Saidel G. Quantitative relationships of intravascular tumor cells, tumor vessels and pulmonary metastasis following tumor implantation. New Eng J Med 1974; 299: 1330–1334.

305. Liotta LA, Kleinerman J, Saidel GM. The significance of hematogenous tumor cell clumps in the metastatic process. Cancer Res 1976; 36: 889–894.

306. Nagy JA, Brown LF, Senger DR et al. Pathogenesis of tumour stroma generation: a critical role for leaky blood vessels and fibrin deposition. Biochem Biophys Acta 1989; 948: 305–326.

307. Fidler IJ, Ellis LM. The implications of angiogenesis for the biology and therapy of cancer metastasis. Cell 1994; 79: 185–188.

308. Weidner N, Carroll RP, Flax J et al. Tumor angiogenesis correlates with metastasis in invasive prostatic cancer. Am J Pathol 1993; 143: 401–409.

309. Macchiarini P, Fontanini G, Hardin MJ et al. Relation of neovascularisation to metastasis of non-small-cell lung cancer. Lancet 1992; 340: 145–146.

310. Weidner N, Semple JP, Welch WR, Folkman J. Tumour angiogenesis and metastasis — correlation in invasive breast carcinoma. New Eng J Med 1991; 324: 1–8.

311. Weidner N, Folkman J, Pozza F et al. Tumour angiogenesis: a new significant and independent prognostic indicator in early stage breast cancer. J Natl Cancer Inst 1992; 84: 1875–1887.

312. Toi M, Kashitani J, Tominaga T. Tumour angiogenesis is an independent prognostic indicator in primary breast carcinoma. Int J Cancer 1993; 55: 371–374.

313. Horak ER, Leek R, Klenk N et al. Angiogenesis, assessed by platelet/endothelial cell adhesion molecule antibodies, as an indicator of node metastases and survival in breast cancer. Lancet 1992; 340: 1120–1124.

314. Bosari S, Lee AK, De Lellis RA et al. Microvessel quantitation and prognosis in invasive breast carcinoma. Hum Pathol 1992; 23: 755–761.

315. Folkman J. Editorial. Angiogenesis and breast cancer. J Clin Oncol 1994; 12: 441–443.

316. Hall NR, Fish DE, Hunt N et al. Is the relationship between angiogenesis and metastasis in breast cancer real? Surg Oncol 1992; 1: 223–229.

317. Cohen P, Guidi A, Harris J, Schnitt S. Microvessel density and local recurrence in patients with early stage breast cancer treated by wide excision alone (WEA) (abstr). Mod Pathol 1994; 7: 14A.

318. Sightler HE, Borrowsky AD, Dupont WD et al. Evaluation of tumour angiogenesis as a prognostic marker in breast cancer (abstr). Mod Pathol 1994; 7: 22A.

319. Van Hoef MEHM, Knox WF, Dhesi SS. Assessment of tumour vascularity as a prognostic factor in lymph node negative invasive breast cancer. Eur J Cancer 1993; 29A: 1141–1145.

320. Goulding H, Rashid NFNA, Robertson JFR et al. Assessment of angiogenesis in breast cancer. An important factor in prognosis? Hum Pathol 1995; 26: 1196–1200.

321. Costello P, McCann A, Carney DN et al. Prognostic significance of microvessel density in lymph node negative breast carcinoma. Hum Pathol 1995; 26: 1181–1184.

322. Page DL, Jensen RA. Editorial. Angiogenesis in human breast carcinoma: what is the question? Hum Pathol 1995; 26: 1173–1174.

323. Hawkins RA. Prognostic factors: seeking a shaft of light or getting lost in the woods? — a personal view from Sherwood Forest. Breast 1993; 2: 125–129.

324. McGuire WL, Clark GM. Prognostic factors and treatment decisions in axillary node-negative breast cancer. New Eng J Med 1992; 326: 1756–1761.

325. Greenhough RB. Varying degrees of malignancy in cancer of the breast. J Cancer Res 1925; 9: 452–463.

326. Bloom HJG. Prognosis in carcinoma of the breast. Br J Cancer 1950a; 4: 259–288.

327. Bloom HJG. Further studies on prognosis of breast carcinoma. Br J Cancer 1950b; 4: 347–367.

328. Henson DE, Ries L, Freedman LS, Carriaga M. Relationship among outcome stage of disease and

histologic grade for 22 616 cases of breast cancer. Br Cancer Res Treat 1991; 22: 207–219.

329. Chevallier B, Mosseri V, Dauce JP et al. A prognostic score in histological node negative breast cancer. Br J Cancer 1990; 61: 436–440.

330. Brown JM, Benson EA, Jones M. Confirmation of a long-term prognostic index in breast cancer. Breast 1993; 2: 144–147.

330a. Balslev I, Axelsson CK, Zedeler K et al. The Nottingham Prognostic Index applied to 9,149 patients from the studies of the Danish Breast Cancer Cooperative Group (DBCG). Br Cancer Res Treat 1994; 32: 281–290.

331. Miller WR, Ellis IO, Sainsbury JRC, Dixon JM. Prognostic factors. ABC of breast diseases. Br J Med 1994; 309: 1573–1576.

332. O'Reilly SM, Barnes DM, Camplejohn RS et al. The relationship between C-erbB-2 expression, S-phase fraction and prognosis in breast cancer. Br J Cancer 1991; 63: 444–446.

333. Ellis IO, Bell J, Todd J et al. Evaluation of immunoreactivity with monoclonal antibody NCRC-11 in breast carcinoma. Br J Cancer 1987; 56: 295–299.

334. Morris ES, Elston CW, Bell JA et al. An evaluation of the cell cycle-associated monoclonal antibody Ki-S1 as a prognostic factor in primary invasive adenocarcinoma of the breast. J Pathol 1995; 176: 55–62.

335. Dowle CS, Owainati A, Robins A et al. The prognostic significance of the DNA content of human breast cancer. Br J Surg 1987; 74: 133–136.

336. Poller DN, Hutchings CE, Galea M et al. p53 protein expression in human breast cancer: relationship to expression of epidermal growth factor, C-erbB-2 protein overexpression, and oestrogen receptor. Br J Cancer 1992; 66: 583–588.

337. Fenlon S, Ellis IO, Bell J et al. *Helix pomatia* and *Ulex europeus* lectin binding in human breast carcinoma. J Pathol 1987; 152: 169–176.

338. Breast Cancer Trialists Collaborative Group. Systemic treatment of early breast cancer by hormonal, cytotoxic or immunotherapy. Lancet 1992; 339: 1–15.

339. Poller DN, Silverstein MJ, Galea M et al. Ductal carcinoma in situ of the breast. A proposal for a new simplified histological classification. Association between cellular proliferation and c-erbB-2 protein expression. Mod Pathol 1994; 7: 257–262.

340. Cardiff RD. Cellular and molecular aspects of neoplastic progression in the mammary gland. Eur J Cancer Clin Oncol 1988; 24: 15–20.

341. Poller DN, Ellis IO. Oncogenes and tumor morphology prediction. Mod Pathol 1993; 6: 376–377.

342. Hinton CP, Doyle PJ, Blamey RW et al. Subcutaneous mastectomy for primary operable breast carcinoma. Br J Surg 1984; 71: 469–472.

343. Cheung KL, Blamey RW. Subcutaneous mastectomy for primary breast cancer or ductal carcinoma in situ. Eur J Surg Oncol 1997; 23: 343–347.

344. Rajakariar R, Walker RA. Pathological and biological features of mammographically detected invasive breast carcinomas. Br J Cancer 1995; 71: 150–154.

345. Royal College of Radiologists. Quality Assurance Guidelines for Radiologists. Revised January 1997. NHSBSP Publications no 15. 1997.

346. Epstein R. Editorial. Treating breast cancer before surgery. Br Med J 1996; 313: 1345–1346.

347. Williams MR, Todd JH, Nicholson RI et al. Survival patterns in hormone treated advanced breast cancer. Br J Surg 1986; 73: 752–755.

Miscellaneous malignant tumors

GENERAL INTRODUCTION

The most common malignant lesions of the breast are those of epithelial origin and malignancy of the mesenchymal tissues is rare. However histopathological specimens from breast stromal elements, including malignancies derived from adipose tissue, fibroblasts, myofibroblasts, neural tissue and vascular structures may be seen. More commonly lymphomas may arise in or infiltrate the breast and secondary malignancies may be deposited in this site.

SARCOMAS

INTRODUCTION

True mammary sarcomas are said to have been described first by Chelius in 1828[1] and comprise less than 1% of malignancies of the breast. We believe that these lesions should be classified histogenetically and phyllodes tumors with sarcomatous elements should be identified separately (see Ch. 9); indeed rhabdomyosarcomatous and chondrosarcomatous elements are commoner as a component of phyllodes tumors than in a pure form in the breast although an extensive search for the epithelial elements of these tumors may be required to establish the correct diagnosis. Metaplastic carcinomas may also mimic mammary sarcomas but positive immunoreactivity with anti-cytokeratin antibodies in the former will distinguish these entities (see also Ch. 15).

Previously the term 'stromal sarcoma' of the breast[2] was widely used to imply breast sarcomas other than malignant phyllodes tumor and lymphoma. We believe that this term is rather loosely defined and unhelpful and many such tumors reported prior to the widespread use of immunohistochemistry may actually have been metaplastic carcinomas. Stromal sarcomas are not now recognized as true entities and will not be discussed further here. Carcinoma with sarcomatoid metaplasia and granular cell myoblastoma have also been included in the category of 'mammary sarcomas' by some authors;[1] the inclusion of a variety of tumor types such as these makes interpretation of results from past studies difficult. The true incidence of breast sarcomas is therefore unclear. It is believed, however, that malignant fibrous histiocytoma (MFH) and fibrosarcoma are the most frequently seen breast sarcomas after angiosarcoma[3] with rhabdomyosarcoma and liposarcoma reported more often than leiomyosarcoma.

PROGNOSIS

Because of the variety of tumors previously included in the category of breast sarcoma it is difficult to provide a reliable prediction of their behavior, but these neoplasms rarely metastasize to the axillary lymph nodes[1] and generally spread through the blood stream with secondary deposits in the lungs. The prognosis of these tumors may also be predicted by the degree of differentiation using morphological criteria including mitotic count, the presence or absence of necrosis, nuclear pleomorphism and cellularity.[4] Tumor necrosis has been reported to be the best predictor of survival and recurrence free interval in patients with soft tissue sarcomas[5] and in the presence of this feature, or of a focally infiltrating edge, an otherwise low grade lesion should be reclassified to an intermediate category. The same features which are associated with poor prognosis in soft tissue sarcomas elsewhere can be used to predict aggressive behavior of lesions in the breast, including high histological grade, mitotic count and infiltrating margins.[4–6] The significance of tumor size in predicting the behavior of primary breast sarcomas is less clear. Whilst some authors have suggested that tumor size is of prognostic significance,[1,7–8] and in particular that those

smaller than 5 cm have a better prognosis than larger lesions[1], other series have not found tumor size to be of such importance.[5,9]

ANGIOSARCOMA

Introduction

Angiosarcomas are the most common of the pure sarcomas occurring in the breast and may arise de novo or following irradiation therapy.[10–12] The development of vascular sarcomas of the extremities after radiation treatments has long been recognized[13] although there has been debate over the histogenetic origin of these lesions.[14] Angiosarcoma of the breast occurring after wide local excision and radiotherapy has been described more recently and may occur relatively soon after initial treatment[15] with important implications for patients having conservation therapy.[16]

Clinical features

Angiosarcoma occurs predominantly during the third and fourth decades, with a mean of 35[17] to 40 years.[18] These tumors are extremely rare in men and occur almost predominantly in women as a painless mass which may fluctuate in size or show pulsatility with a bruit. More rarely diffuse enlargement of the breast is found with no discrete lump palpable. The overlying skin may show blue, red or violaceous discoloration.

Macroscopic appearances

Tumors range in size from 1 to 14 cm with a mean of 5 cm in extent[18] and often have poorly defined margins. The lesions are often soft and friable with hemorrhagic, blood-filled spaces or foci of necrosis seen on the cut surface which may produce a honeycombed or cystic appearance.

Microscopic appearances

The microscopic appearances of angiosarcomas are extremely variable and this may cause considerable diagnostic difficulties. Indeed on review between 37%[17] and 50%[18] of angiosarcomas of the breast have been found to have been misdiagnosed originally as benign lesions such as hemangiomas, lymphangiomas or hematomas. The histological patterns of angiosarcomas of the breast have been classified into three grades reflecting the prognosis of these tumors[19-20] and most diagnostic difficulty is encountered with grade 1 lesions. Adequate sampling of these

neoplasms is vital as an admixture of patterns may be seen and grade 3 foci may be surrounded by areas of grade 1 morphology.

Up to 40% of breast angiosarcomas are of histological grade 1.[20] These lesions are composed of well-formed anastomozing vascular channels which infiltrate the adjacent breast stroma

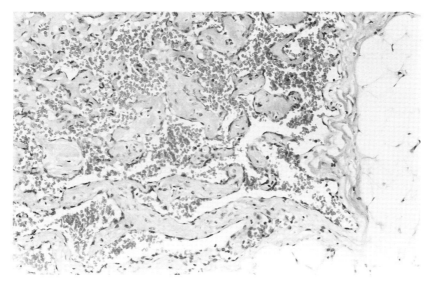

Fig. 19.1A Grade 1 angiosarcoma of breast. The lesion is well circumscribed, and an area of sclerosis is visible at the top left. Reproduced by kind permission of Dr Cecily Quinn. Haematoxylin–eosin × 125.

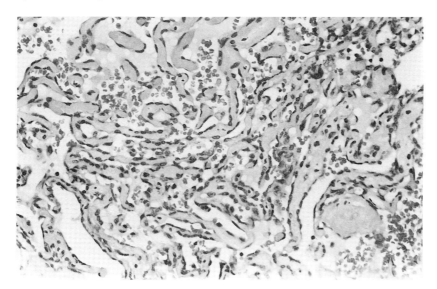

Fig. 19.1B Grade 1 angiosarcoma of breast. Higher magnification of another part of the tumour shown in Figure 19.1A. The tumour is composed of anastamozing vascular channels lined by flattened endothelial cells. Reproduced by kind permission of Dr Cecily Quinn. Haematoxylin–eosin × 125.

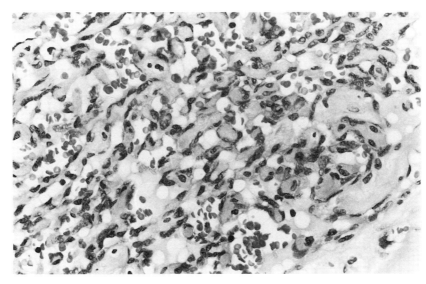

Fig. 19.1C   Grade 1 angiosarcoma of breast. Although this field is from a rather more compact area than that shown in Figure 19.1B, there is no endothelial tufting and nuclei appear regular. No mitoses are seen. Haematoxylin–eosin × 400.

(Fig. 19.1A and B). The tumor cells are flat with minimal endothelial tufting and papillary proliferations, although the nuclei may be hyperchromatic (Fig. 19.1B and C). Nucleoli are occasionally prominent but few mitoses are seen.

Grade 2 lesions are seen less frequently than grade 1 and grade 3 tumors and comprise about 20% of cases of breast angiosarcoma.[20] The appearances are essentially similar to grade 1 angiosarcomas but with endothelial tufting, focal papillary formations and nuclear pleomorphism (Fig. 19.2A and B). Mitoses may be more prominent. A spindle cell and solid pattern is not a major component of grade 2 lesions.

Approximately 40% of breast angiosarcomas are of histological grade 3.[20] In these tumors overtly sarcomatous areas are identified with only occasional well-defined vascular spaces. Hemorrhage and 'blood lakes' may be seen. The tumor may have a spindle, solid or papillary architecture (Fig. 19.3A–C). Nuclear pleomorphism may be marked and mitoses are frequent. Necrosis is a useful diagnostic feature and is only present in grade 3 tumors (Fig. 19.4).

Differential diagnosis

As noted above angiosarcomas may be misdiag-nosed as benign lesions due to the relatively bland nature of the neoplastic endothelial cells. The vascular channels in hemangiomas may rarely be anastomozing but they are not as infiltrative and tend to grow around ducts and lobules, whilst angiosarcomas invade breast parenchymal structures. In venous hemangiomas muscular elements may be identified within the walls of some vessels; this is not seen in angiosarcomas. In addition the size of the lesion may itself be helpful; hemangiomas rarely reach a size of 2 cm, whilst angiosarcomas are usually larger than this (see Ch. 11).

Pseudoangiomatous hyperplasia may present as a breast mass in premenopausal women.[21] This lesion is composed of anastomozing slit-like spaces which are lined by 'endothelial-like' cells and may involve intralobular stroma (Fig. 19.5A and B). Although the cells lining the spaces are not true endothelial cells and are believed to be myofibroblastic in origin this lesion may cause significant difficulties in interpretation and on occasions has been misdiagnosed as low grade angiosarcoma.[22] Pseudoangiomatous hyperplasia does not however infiltrate fat and occurs within dense collagenous stroma. Immunohistochemical assessment with vascular markers such as CD31 and CD34 may also prove useful in differentiating these entities; as described, the spindle cells in

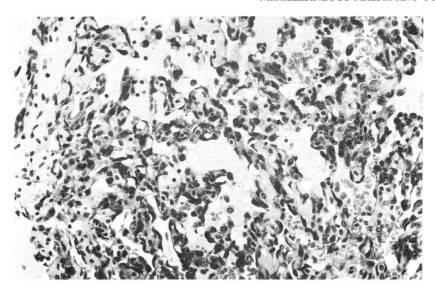

Fig. 19.2A   Grade 2 angiosarcoma of breast. The tumor is composed of irregular vascular channels; even at this magnification endothelial tufting is apparent. Hematoxylin–eosin × 125.

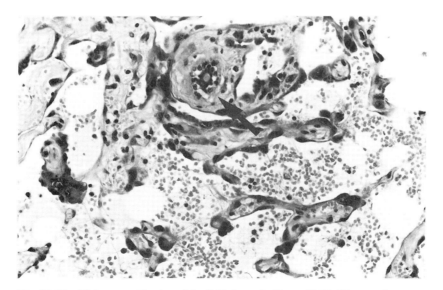

Fig. 19.2B   Higher magnification of the field shown in Figure 19.2A. The vascular channels surround a small breast duct (arrowhead). The endothelial cells are more prominent than in a grade 1 lesion, with some nuclear pleomorphism. Compare with Figure 19.1B. Hematoxylin–eosin × 400.

pseudoangiomatous hyperplasia are not truly endothelial and show no immunoreactivity with these antibodies.

At the other end of the spectrum grade 3 angiosarcomas may be mimicked by metaplastic breast carcinomas (see Ch. 15, Fig. 15.39A–D)[23–24] and should also be distinguished from other breast sarcomas. Although *Ulex europaeus* lectin and factor VIII-related antigen staining is not consistent in angiosarcomas,[25] immunohistochemical assessment with the vascular markers CD31 and CD34 is helpful (Fig. 19.6).[26–27] It should, how-

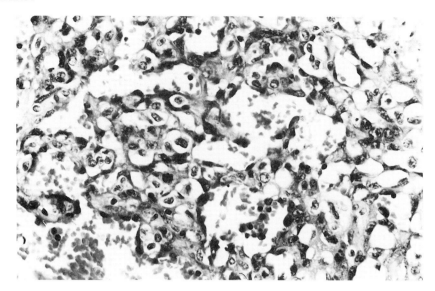

Fig. 19.3A Grade 3 angiosarcoma of breast. The vascular spaces are ill defined and endothelial cells show marked nuclear pleomorphism. Hematoxylin–eosin × 400.

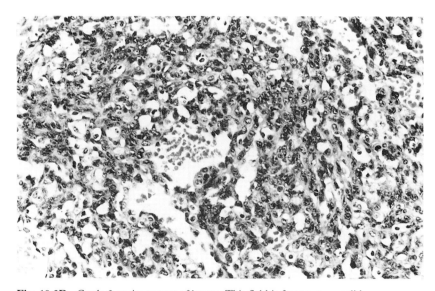

Fig. 19.3B Grade 3 angiosarcoma of breast. This field is from a more solid area of the tumor showing in Figure 19.3A; a 'blood lake' is seen at the center left. Hematoxylin–eosin × 185.

ever be noted that CD31 positivity has been described in occasional carcinomas[27] and CD34 immunoreactivity is seen in dermatofibrosarcoma protruberans as well as other vascular tumors.[27–28] A panel of epithelial markers is also required to exclude metaplastic carcinoma since expression may be inconsistent (see also Ch. 15).[23] A search

for Weibel-Palade bodies by electron microscopy may also be useful.

Prognosis

In the past angiosarcoma of the breast has been regarded as an aggressive tumor and many reports

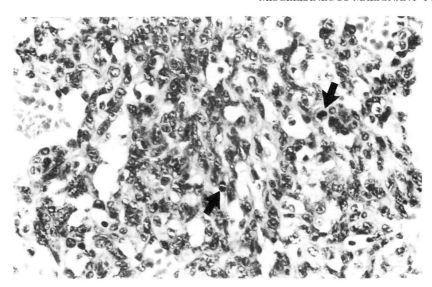

Fig. 19.3C   Higher magnification of the field shown in Figure 19.3B. Note the spindle cell structure, with marked nuclear pleomorphism and mitotic figures (arrowheads). Hematoxylin–eosin × 400.

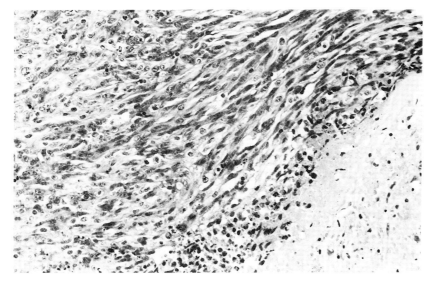

Fig. 19.4   Grade 3 angiosarcoma of breast. The lesion has a dominantly spindle cell pattern, with an area of necrosis. From a local recurrence of the tumor shown in Figure 19.3A 6 months after mastectomy. Hematoxylin–eosin × 185.

have recorded a poor prognosis.[17] Despite this, long-term survivors have been noted[29,30] and it is now clear that the prognosis is related to the histological appearances of the lesions. Grade 1 tumors have a relatively good prognosis with an 81% 10-year predicted survival but grade 3 angiosarcomas have a poor survival with only 14% of patients alive after 10 years.[20] Some authors have also reported that tumor size is of prognostic importance.[30–31] Metastases are most often seen in the lungs, liver, skin, bone and brain but involvement of the contralateral breast is also common.

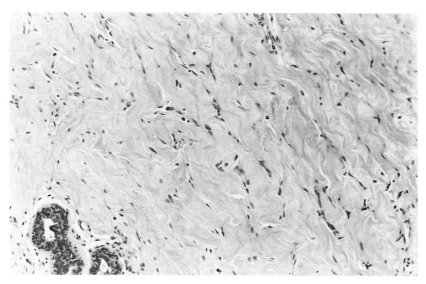

Fig. 19.5A Pseudoangiomatous hyperplasia. Normal breast ducts are seen at the lower left, with cleft-like spaces in the adjacent stroma. Hematoxylin–eosin × 125.

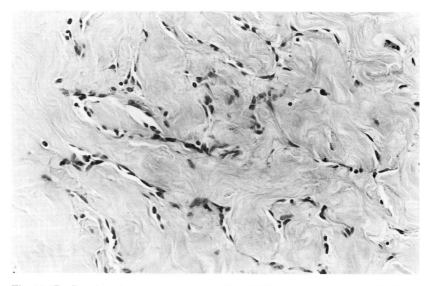

Fig. 19.5B Pseudoangiomatous hyperplasia. The cleft-like spaces appear to be lined by endothelial cells and resemble thin walled blood vessels. Immunostaining for the vascular markers CD 31 and CD 34 was, however, negative. From the same case as that shown in Figure 19.5A. Hematoxylin–eosin × 185.

LYMPHANGIOSARCOMA (POSTMASTECTOMY ANGIOSARCOMA)

Introduction

The first six cases of vascular sarcoma arising in association with chronic lymphedema postmas-tectomy were described by Stewart and Treves in 1948,[32] hence the eponymous name Stewart–Treves syndrome. In addition to chronic lymph-edema, which is recognized as a predisposing factor, a possible relationship to radiotherapy has been suggested but not definitely established. It is

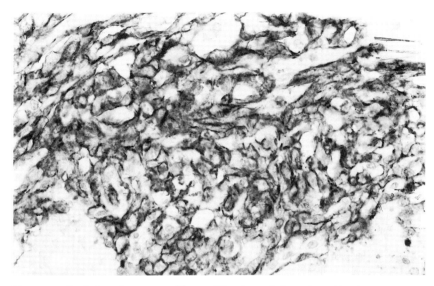

Fig. 19.6 Grade 3 angiosarcoma of breast. The diagnosis is confirmed by the demonstration of positive expression with the endothelial marker CD 31. Immunostaining for CD 31 × 400.

now widely accepted that these lesions are of vascular origin and not foci of recurrent mammary carcinoma.[33] It remains controversial, however, whether they arise from neoplastic blood vessels or lymphatic channels[14,34–35] or show differentiation towards both endothelial types. Because of this uncertainty it is best to avoid the designations lymphangiosarcoma or hemangiosarcoma and use the general term angiosarcoma for these postmastectomy vascular sarcomas.

Macroscopic and microscopic appearances

Most of the angiosarcomas of edematous extremities associated with previous breast cancer present at least 10 years after mastectomy as apparent bruising and swelling or mass or blistering lesions on the ipsilateral arm.[36] Microscopically the features are essentially similar to mammary angiosarcomas, as described above. Typically the tumors are variable in appearance, with well-developed capillary-like vessels lined by hyperchromatic endothelial cells and poorly differentiated areas within the same lesion. Although some of the spaces contain clear or faintly eosinophilic fluid, others bear erythrocytes. Elsewhere dilated lymphatic channels may be seen as evidence of the associated chronic lymphedema.

The differential diagnosis of these angiosarcomas includes recurrent carcinoma. This can be distinguished by reactivity of the neoplastic endothelial cells to Factor VIII related antigen, *Ulex europaeus* I,[35] CD31 and CD34 and no immunoreactivity with epithelial markers. As with mammary angiosarcoma, Weibel-Palade bodies may be seen ultrastructurally.[35]

Prognosis

The prognosis of patients with postmastectomy angiosarcomas is extremely poor and only early detection and extensive surgery appears to provide any opportunity for control.[36] Despite this the 5-year survival remains at about 5%.[37]

FIBROSARCOMA AND MALIGNANT FIBROUS HISTIOCYTOMA (MFH)

Introduction

Malignant fibrous histiocytoma (MFH) is reported by some authors to be the most frequent primary breast sarcoma after angiosarcoma.[3,6] Pitts et al, for example, reported that all 20 of the 'pure' sarcomas of the breast in their series were of MFH type, although, interestingly, two cases showed epithelial antigen immunoreactivity.[38] The wide variation in the proportion of types of breast sarcoma in the literature would support the view of some authorities that the designation MFH covers a heterogeneous group of malignant tumors,[39] many of which can, and should be, grouped according to histogenetic origin.

Macroscopic appearances

The macroscopic appearances of fibrosarcoma and MFH of the breast do not differ significantly. Tumors generally range from 1 to 14.5 cm in size.[40] The margins of the tumors are variable; some have clearly defined edges, others have

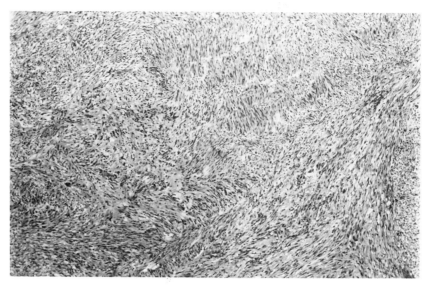

Fig. 19.7A Fibrosarcoma — malignant fibrous histiocytoma of breast. The tumor is composed of interlacing bands of spindle cells arranged in a typical 'herringbone' pattern. Hematoxylin–eosin × 125.

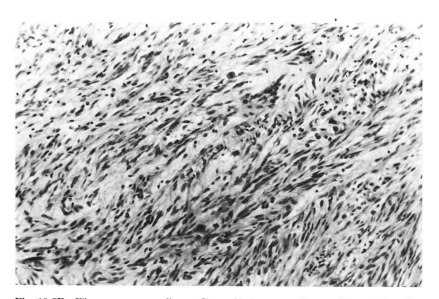

Fig. 19.7B Fibrosarcoma — malignant fibrous histiocytoma of breast. The spindle cells have elongated nuclei and there is little nuclear pleomorphism. From the same case as Figure 19.7A. Hematoxylin–eosin × 185.

irregular margins and some are apparently formed of multiple nodules. The cut surface is often firm and rubbery with a white/gray or pink/tan color although more rarely the mass may have a mucoid appearance. Focal calcifications may be identified macroscopically. Low grade lesions often have a whorled cut surface. Necrosis and hemorrhage are only seen in high grade tumors.

Microscopic appearances

As elsewhere in the soft tissues, breast fibrosarcomas are cellular tumors formed of spindle cells often arranged in a herringbone pattern (Fig. 19.7A).[41] In most cases little pleomorphism is seen, the neoplastic cells being of monomorphic appearance with tapering rather than oval nuclei. Mitoses are variable in number (Figs 19.7B, 19.8).

Five variants of MFH have been reported: pleomorphic, myxoid, angiomatoid, giant cell and inflammatory, but it is no longer widely believed that these tumors derive from histiocytic cells. For a fuller description of the histological features of these variants, soft tissue tumor texts are recommended.[41–42] However, as noted above, the pleomorphic subtype of MFH (which, from literature review, is probably the form most commonly diag-

nosed in the breast) is not believed to be a specific entity but a variety of neoplasms with morphologically similar appearances. The shared features of these tumors include marked pleomorphism with multinucleated cells and a storiform architectural pattern with chronic inflammatory cells and foamy macrophages often seen in the background.[41]

Differential diagnosis

Although typical leaf-like processes and epithelial lined clefts may be relatively sparse in a malignant phyllodes tumor with extensive stromal overgrowth their presence excludes fibrosarcoma as a diagnosis. Multiple sections and thorough sampling may, however, be required before the epithelial elements of a phyllodes tumors are found (see also Ch. 9). The differential diagnosis of fibrosarcoma in the breast also includes monophasic metaplastic carcinoma. Diligent search for more overtly epithelial elements in the latter may be helpful, but immunohistochemical examination with a variety of epithelial markers is invaluable; cytokeratin immunopositivity is seen in metaplastic carcinomas but not in true stromal lesions (see Ch. 15).

Fibromatosis may bear a close resemblance to

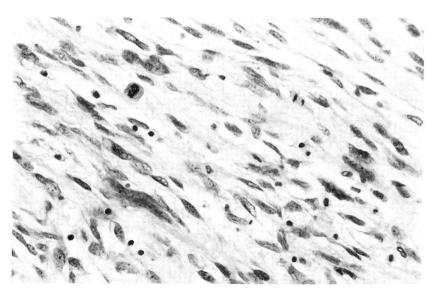

Fig. 19.8 Fibrosarcoma — malignant fibrous histiocytoma of breast. In this example there is marked nuclear pleomorphism and mitoses are present. Hematoxylin–eosin × 400.

low grade fibrosarcoma[43–44] and attention should be paid to the cellularity of the lesion, the architectural pattern with a herringbone or storiform distribution of malignant cells, a higher mitotic count and the presence of hyperchromasia in the latter. In nodular fasciitis mitotic figures are often prominent but are not abnormal, in comparison with fibrosarcoma when atypical mitoses may be identified. In addition the background pattern of nodular fasciitis includes a myxoid stroma with scattered chronic inflammatory cells which may be a helpful distinguishing feature.

Dermatofibrosarcoma protruberans (DFSP) is a low grade infiltrative cutaneous and subcutaneous lesion which may recur locally but rarely metastasizes. These tumors occur very rarely in the breast[45–46] and should be distinguished from fibrosarcomas and fibromatoses because of their very different clinical behavior. The expression of CD 34 in DFSP can be an invaluable aid in diagnosis.[28]

High grade lesions must be distinguished from other pleomorphic sarcomas if the designation MFH is to retain any significance. Immunohistochemistry is required and electron microscopy may be needed to identify the histogenetic origin of the lesion. Whilst pleomorphic rhabdomyosarcoma, liposarcoma and leiomyosarcoma most commonly produce such histological appearances, other tumors may, more rarely, be of pleomorphic morphology.[41]

Prognosis

Jones et al grouped tumors which had been coded as either fibrosarcoma or MFH in the Armed Forces Institute of Pathology (AFIP) files into histological grade according to the predominant histological pattern, the number of mitoses and the degree of nuclear atypia.[40] None of the group of patients with low grade fibrosarcoma died of tumor within a mean follow-up of 8 years and none had developed distant metastases.[40] The prognosis of patients with MFH of the breast is, however, more difficult to predict from literature review because of the problems with classification of these tumors. The 64%[38] to 69%[40] survival of patients with high grade fibrosarcoma/MFH reported by both Pitts et al[38] and Jones et al[40]

contrasts with the report of few patients surviving more than 2 years.[6] Further series of cases based on strictly defined diagnostic criteria are required before the behavior of these high grade sarcomas of the breast is clear.

LIPOSARCOMA

Introduction

Liposarcoma of the breast is distinctly uncommon. It may arise directly from adipose tissue within the breast or as a component of a malignant phyllodes tumor.[47–48] This latter form is more usual and pure liposarcoma arising de novo is very rare. Mammary liposarcoma generally presents with a slowly enlarging, sometimes painful breast mass in a patient between 26 to 76 years of age.[49] A single case report of liposarcoma of the breast occurring after radiotherapy for breast carcinoma has been published.[50]

Macroscopic and microscopic appearances

These tumors are often large at the time of presentation and measure on average 8 cm in diameter; they may, however, be up to 19 cm in size.[49] Although many appear well circumscribed macroscopically, liposarcomas of the breast are often lobulated or have infiltrative edges. The cut surfaces show the same features as soft tissue liposarcomas in other sites with a gelatinous, myxoid appearance or a more solid fleshy pattern, depending on histological sub-type.

The microscopic appearances of liposarcomas in the breast are essentially the same as those arising in other soft tissues.[41–42] In most reports of liposarcoma of the breast the subtype of tumor has not been clearly defined but the majority appear to be of the pleomorphic variety. These are composed of neoplastic cells of widely varying sizes and shapes with giant cell forms and abundant mitotic figures. Myxoid and well-differentiated forms of liposarcoma of the breast have however, very rarely, been described. The former sub-type shows the classical 'chicken wire' capillary pattern in a myxoid matrix with lipoblasts of varying maturity. The well-differentiated sub-type resembles a lipoma but with lipoblasts present, often adjacent to fibrous septae; in this form a lymphoid or plasma cell infiltrate may be prominent. Austin et al found that none of their 13 cases of pure liposarcoma (unassociated with phyllodes tumor) was of pure round-cell form;[49] this type of liposarcoma thus appears to be extremely rare.

Differential diagnosis

Vacuolated cells may occur in a variety of lesions and lipoblasts must be distinguished from cells containing mucin, glycogen or foreign material. Thus the differential diagnosis includes signet ring carcinomas either of primary or secondary origin as well as other metastatic deposits. Granulomatous inflammation and fat necrosis may mimic these malignant tumors and in the breast a foreign body type reaction to leaked silicone may resemble liposarcoma. Histochemistry and immunohistochemistry may be useful; mucin stains are negative in liposarcoma, as is immunoreactivity with cytokeratin and macrophage markers but positive immunostaining with S100 antibody is seen. At one end of the spectrum liposarcomas should be differentiated from benign lipomas by the careful search for lipoblasts and at the other end should be distinguished from other pleomorphic sarcomas. In the breast, liposarcomas most commonly arise in association with a phyllodes tumor and careful search for epithelial elements forming clefts should be undertaken.

Prognosis

The rarity of liposarcomas of the breast makes prediction of prognosis difficult, particularly when published data is contradictory. Although an aggressive behavior has been suggested, especially when associated with pregnancy, a lower rate of metastases and a better prognosis than other breast sarcomas has also been reported.[6,8] In particular, well-differentiated or well-circumscribed lesions and tumors arising in the male breast appear to have a better prognosis.[49] However, whilst breast liposarcomas overall appear to have a relatively low recurrence rate, those tumors which recur do so rapidly, often within one year of diagnosis.[49] A pleomorphic sub-type or the presence of an infiltrating edge are associated with

increased risk of recurrence[49] and if these features are seen a more guarded prognosis should be given.

OSTEOSARCOMA

Introduction

Pure osteogenic sarcoma is extremely rare and many of the reported cases probably represent osteosarcomatous elements within metaplastic carcinomas. Similar changes can also be seen within phyllodes tumors and a previous history of a fibroadenoma or phyllodes tumor is given in many of the published reports. In some cases a history of previous irradiation may be obtained; osteogenic sarcoma is the commonest histological type of radiation-induced sarcoma.[51-52] Osteosarcoma of the breast usually occurs in older patients and presents as a slowly enlarging mass which may be mistaken clinically for a calcified fibroadenoma.[53]

Macroscopic and microscopic appearances

The lesion is generally well circumscribed, may be lobulated and often has a gritty cut surface. Foci which are overtly calcified or bony may be seen and central necrosis can sometimes be identified.[54] The microscopical appearances are variable but neoplastic osteoid and bone are seen in a background of spindle cells in which abundant mitoses are often present (Fig. 19.9A and B). Admixed foci of osteoclastic giant cells and neoplastic cartilage may be identified. Some tumors may, however, have a deceptively benign structure with osteoid seams sandwiched between layers of plump spindle cells.

Differential diagnosis

Primary osteosarcomas should be differentiated from metaplastic carcinoma with osteosarcomatous elements (see Ch. 15) and from those lesions arising in phyllodes tumors (see Ch. 9). A useful point of distinction lies in the fact that in pure osteosarcoma the *whole* lesion shows the same pattern throughout, whilst in the other two entities the osteogenic structure is *focal*. Once they

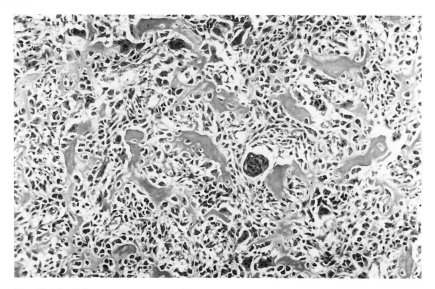

Fig. 19.9A   Primary osteosarcoma of breast. The whole of the tumor mass is composed of neoplastic osteoid and no epithelial elements were identified. Reproduced with permission from Dr F Bonnar. Hematoxylin–eosin × 125.

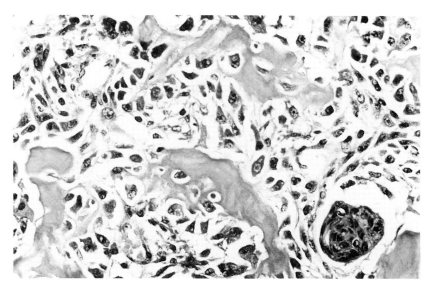

Fig. 19.9B   Primary osteosarcoma of breast. Higher magnification of field shown in Figure 19.9A. Hematoxylin–eosin × 400.

have been excluded, in the majority of cases the diagnosis is not difficult. Rarely however osteosarcomas of the breast may mimic benign lesions such as osseous metaplasia; two of 35 cases reviewed at the AFIP were originally reported as 'benign change' or myositis ossificans due to their bland nature.[55] On review these two tumors were well circumscribed, but were composed of spindle cells which were mitotically active and infiltrating adjacent tissue. Both patients subsequently developed metastatic deposits.

Prognosis

Despite the bland appearance of some tumors, osteosarcomas of the breast behave in an aggressive fashion with local recurrence within weeks or months and distant metastases within 2 years of diagnosis.[55] Dissemination is characteristically to the lungs.

LEIOMYOSARCOMA

Introduction

This is one of the rarest primary breast sarcomas with less than 20 cases reported in the literature. It seems most likely that these lesions arise from pluripotent mesenchymal cells rather than vascular walls[56] and many, although not all, appear to have developed in the area of the nipple or areola.[57–58] In common with other breast sarcomas, leiomyosarcoma has been recorded as part of a malignant phyllodes tumor.[47] Leiomyosarcoma appears to be most common in women in their sixth decade. The tumor has frequently been present for some time prior to excision suggesting a slow rate of growth.

Macroscopic and microscopic appearances

Macroscopically these lesions are well circumscribed masses measuring between 1.5 cm and 9.0 cm in size[59] with a predominantly gray-white cut surface. Areas of hemorrhage may be present.

Microscopically leiomyosarcomas of the breast resemble malignant smooth muscle tumors arising elsewhere in soft tissues; neoplastic smooth muscle bundles are arranged in a whorled pattern. Tumor cells are spindle-shaped with oval and blunt-ended nuclei (Fig. 19.10A and B) and may surround entrapped breast ducts. Moderate atypia with varying numbers of multinucleated giant cells have been reported in almost all cases of breast leiomyosarcoma.[57] Necrosis may be seen. A focal 'rounded cell appearance' has been reported[59] and an epithelioid variant has also been described in the breast.[60]

Nielsen has proposed that smooth muscle tumors of the breast with more than two mitotic figures per 10 high power fields should be classified as malignant.[61] Other authors have suggested a category of 'indeterminate prognosis' for tumors with 1–3 mitoses per HPF.[62] However, based on literature review of the 10 cases of breast leiomyosarcoma reported up to 1988 Arista-Nasr found no association between either mitotic count or tumor size and aggressiveness.[57] Although these tumors are generally thought to have a better prognosis than other breast sarcomas[63] they may behave insidiously with recurrence or death many years after initial diagnosis.[57,61] We believe that further series with long-term follow-up are required before definitive statements with regard

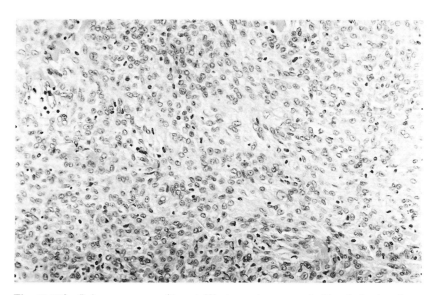

Fig. 19.10A   Leiomyosarcoma of breast. The tumor is composed of interlacing bundles of plump spindle cells. Hematoxylin–eosin × 185.

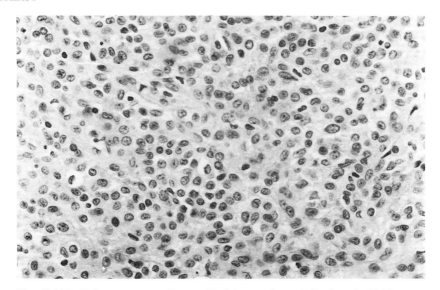

Fig. 19.10B   Leiomyosarcoma of breast. Nuclei are oval or spindle shaped with blunt ends and there is moderate pleomorphism. From the same case as that shown in Figure 19.10A. Hematoxylin–eosin × 400.

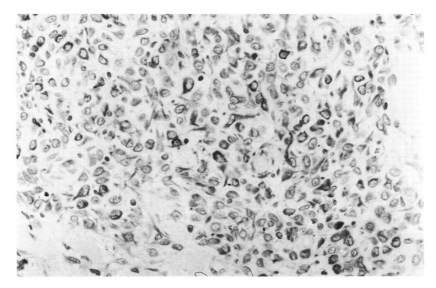

Fig. 19.10C   Leiomyosarcoma of breast. Focal positive cytoplasmic immunoreactivity for desmin is demonstrated. Immunostaining for desmin × 400.

to prognosis of patients with breast leiomyosarcoma can be made, but it is evident that relapse of disease may occur very many years after diagnosis. Thus if mitoses are present, particularly if prominent, it may be prudent to give a more guarded prognosis.

Differential diagnosis

Leiomyosarcomas should be distinguished from benign smooth muscle tumors which show no mitotic figures or necrosis. Other spindle cell lesions may cause diagnostic difficulties; the herringbone pattern and tapering nuclei of a fibrosarcoma are not seen in a leiomyosarcoma which is composed of interwoven fasicles of tumor cells with oval nuclei. Smooth muscle actin (SMA) and desmin immunoreactivity in leiomyosarcomas may be helpful in diagnosis (Fig. 19.10C); the latter is however seen in only about 70% of malignant smooth muscle tumors.[41] Conversely, epithelial membrane antigen (EMA), S100, and cytokeratin positivity may also be present in leiomyosarcomas,[57] the latter marker particularly in frozen section material.[64]

RHABDOMYOSARCOMA

Secondary rhabdomyosarcoma either presenting as a breast mass or developing during disease dissemination is a well recognized phenomenon and may be seen in young females.[65–67] Primary alveolar and embryonal tumors may also arise in the breast of young women or girls[68–71] but, in common with other breast sarcomas, rhabdomyosarcoma occurs more commonly as a component of a metaplastic carcinoma[72] or phyllodes tumor than in a pure form.

Primary pleomorphic rhabdomyosarcomas are highly cellular and composed of spindle to round cells with rhabdomyoblasts scattered throughout the tumor (Fig. 19.11A and B). The rhabdomyoblasts are large and bizarre and cross-striations are found with difficulty. Mitoses are frequent. These lesions should be distinguished from other pleomorphic sarcomas and in this respect immunohistochemical expression of muscle markers is helpful (Fig. 19.11C). Electron microscopy may be required to establish the correct diagnosis in some tumors.

An insufficient number of cases of breast rhabdomyosarcoma have been reported for the prognosis to be clear. Four cases of primary rhabdomyosarcoma in the AFIP files[55] (although one was largely within the pectoralis muscle and may not truly have been of mammary origin) were all in women over 40 years of age and all were aggressive. Two of the four patients had metastatic disease within a year of presentation.

CHONDROSARCOMA

Pure mammary chondrosarcoma is extremely rare[73] and chondromatous areas are more commonly seen within metaplastic carcinomas.[74–75] Macroscopically chondrosarcomas of the breast are well-defined lobulated masses. The seven

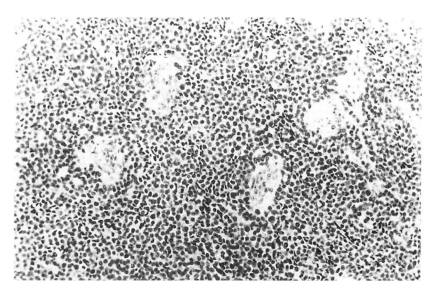

Fig. 19.11A   Rhabdomyosarcoma of breast, solid type. Note the closely packed cellular structure and focal fibrous septae. From a 23-year-old female who presented with a rapidly enlarging breast lump. Hematoxylin–eosin × 125.

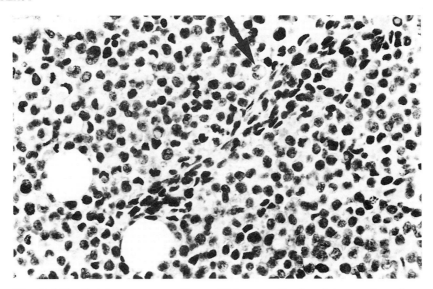

Fig. 19.11B   Rhabdomyosarcoma of breast. Higher magnification of the case shown in Figure 19.11A. The tumor cells are large with bizarre nuclei having ill-defined borders, and occasional rhabdomyoblasts are seen (arrowhead). Hematoxylin–eosin × 400.

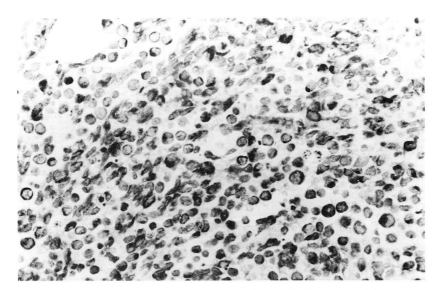

Fig. 19.11C   Rhabdomyosarcoma of breast. Extensive positive immunoreactivity for desmin is evident in the tumor cell cytoplasm. Immunostaining for desmin × 400.

cases reported at the AFIP showed a variety of appearances; some were cellular tumors formed of round or spindle cells with nodules of cartilage whilst others had a cellular periphery surrounding a chondroid and myxoid matrix.[55] The mesenchymal cells in metaplastic carcinoma retain cytokeratin immunoreactivity[76] and this may be useful in definitive diagnosis of these lesions.

OTHER RARE SARCOMAS

Some series of breast sarcomas include brief mention of lesions diagnosed as, for example, clear cell sarcoma, alveolar soft part sarcoma, neurogenic sarcoma, malignant schwannoma, neurofibrosarcoma and synovial sarcoma;[6,55,73,77] insufficient detail has been given to evaluate many of these reports. Hemangiopericytomas have also been described very rarely.[78] The Surveillance, Epidemiology and End Results (SEER) data, examining the possibility of an association between breast implants and breast sarcomas, intriguingly have reported that second to hemangiosarcoma, endometrial stromal sarcoma was the most common breast sarcoma from 1973–1990;[79] one can only assume that this code was used for 'stromal sarcoma (not otherwise specified)' rather than implying a true origin from the endometrium. These authors also recorded cases of malignant granular cell tumor, chondrosarcoma and malignant hemangioendothelioma as well as fibroxanthoma of the breast.

MALIGNANT LYMPHOMA

Primary non-Hodgkin's lymphoma of breast

Introduction

Primary breast lymphoma is uncommon, amounting to less than 0.5% of malignant breast tumors in women.[80] The disease is even rarer in men.[81] Histological specimens from secondary lymphomas are also uncommon; although patients with disseminated lymphoma may develop breast masses, these are not usually biopsied. It is, however, well recognized that Burkitt's lymphoma often involves the breast extensively in women who are pregnant or lactating[82] and a similar pattern of primary breast lymphoma of Burkitt's type is recognized.[80,83] These patients are also often young, puerperal or pregnant and may have bilateral disease. The second type of primary breast lymphoma, which is more common in the Western world and comprises over 80% of cases, is seen in older women with unilateral disease.[80,83]

The most common mode of presentation is with a breast lump indistinguishable from primary carcinoma, which is frequently the clinical diagnosis; however some lesions are now identified mammographically.[84] The 'B' symptoms of lymphoma including night sweats and fever are rare. The well defined nature of the lesions may suggest a diagnosis of fibroadenoma in younger patients.

There has been an increase in reports of primary lymphoma probably due to improved awareness of the entity and increased use of immunohistochemistry as a diagnostic aid. Criteria for the diagnosis of primary breast lymphoma have been described[80] and include (a) that adequate pathological material should be available for review, (b) that the breast should be the site of the primary or major manifestation of the disease clinically and (c) that there is no prior documentation of preceding similar histological type of lymphoma. In addition it has been suggested that a close association between breast tissue and the infiltrating lymphoma should be identified.[85]

Macroscopic appearances

Macroscopically the lesions are usually well-circumscribed, firm grayish-white to tan masses sometimes with a pearly cut surface and measuring between 1 and 7 cm[81] although larger tumors have been recorded up to 19 cm in size.[83] Overtly hemorrhagic foci may be present.

Microscopic appearances

Despite their well defined macroscopical appearance, primary breast lymphomas are diffusely infiltrative histologically and surround breast parenchymal structures (Fig. 19.12A). Malignant lymphoid cells may infiltrate into mammary ductules and lobules and expand those structures producing so-called lymphoepithelial lesions (Fig. 19.12B).[86] Vascular involvement is also common in both primary and secondary lymphomas of the breast with infiltration and separation of the layers of the walls of vessels.[87] Other histological features vary according to the histological subtype of breast lymphoma.

The relative rarity of the disease, the different histological classifications and the variation in immunohistochemical techniques in the literature makes accurate assessment of the incidence of histological types and behavior of primary breast lymphoma difficult. Nevertheless it is clear that the greatest number of cases are of a B cell lineage. Most secondary lymphomas involving the breast are also of B cell type and T cell lymphomas of the breast are rare.[87–89]

The neoplastic cells show a wide variety of mor-

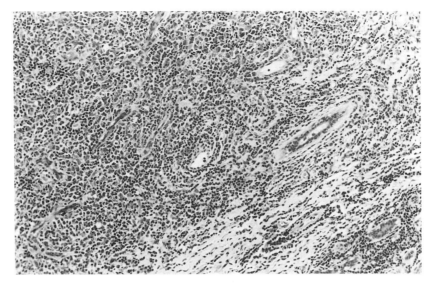

Fig. 19.12A   Primary breast lymphoma. There is a diffuse infiltrate of lymphoma cells around ductal structures. Hematoxylin–eosin × 125.

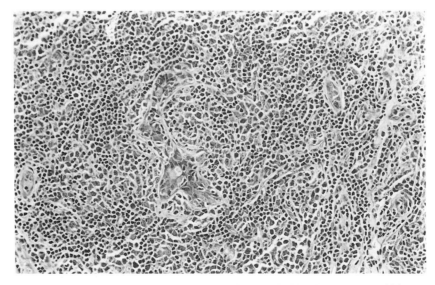

Fig. 19.12B   Primary breast lymphoma. In this field lymphoid cells are present within a duct, forming a lymphoepithelial lesion. From the same case as that shown in Figure 19.12A. Hematoxylin–eosin × 185.

phological appearances with low, intermediate and high grade breast disease, as seen elsewhere. The majority of mammary lymphomas are of high grade B cell type (Fig. 19.13A) and are described as being of centroblastic,[81,90–91] centroblastic/poly-morphous,[92] diffuse large cell[83,87] or diffuse large cell non-cleaved[80] morphology depending on the

favored classification system. The tumor cells have the same appearance as in other sites; centroblasts are large cells with scanty basophilic cytoplasm. Several nucleoli are prominent within a round or oval nucleus and are often situated close to the nuclear membrane. Scattered immunoblasts may also be seen with a single large nucleolus which is

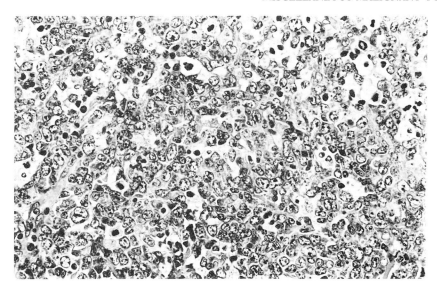

Fig. 19.13A   Primary breast lymphoma, diffuse large B cell type. The tumor cells resemble centroblasts. Hematoxylin–eosin × 400.

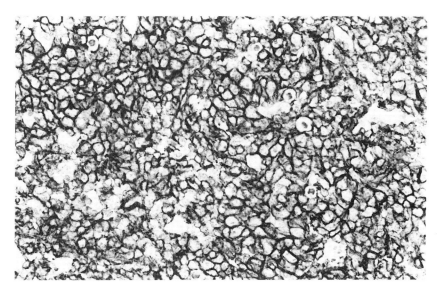

Fig. 19.13B   Primary breast lymphoma. The tumor cells show positive expression for the B cell marker, CD 20. From the same case as that shown in Figure 19.13A. Immunostaining for CD 20 × 400.

often centrally placed in a pale nucleus. Mitoses are usually frequent. Centrocytic-centroblastic lymphoma both follicular and/or diffuse[84,86,90] and lymphoplasmacytoid lymphoma of the breast have also been reported. This latter form of disease appears to be less frequently seen than in other extranodal sites.[81,86]

The preponderance of B cell tumors would suggest an origin for many of these lesions in mucosa associated lymphoid tissue (MALT). Some authors have reported lymphoepithelial lesions in association with breast lymphoma, particularly at the periphery of the mass.[84,87,91] Others have not, however, found features of MALT in breast lymphomas;[83,92] for example Bobrow et al showed that the lymphoid cells which were infiltrating acini were morphologically different from the tumor cell population and had a T cell immunophenotype.[92] In many cases of breast lymphoma lymphoid cells are seen infiltrating acini and ducts and we would recommend that their morphology and immunoreactivity should be carefully examined to determine whether these are true lymphoepithelial lesions.

Other features to support the diagnosis of a MALT origin have been noted such as plasma cell differentiation of lymphoma cells,[91] the presence of Dutcher bodies and reactive germinal centers with follicular colonization.[84] The reported association with lymphocytic lobulitis would also support the suggestion that some breast lymphomas are of MALT origin.[93]

Differential diagnosis

Primary breast lymphoma must be distinguished from breast carcinoma; invasive lobular carcinoma in particular may be mistaken for lymphoma histologically, due to the discohesive 'single file' growth and targetoid pattern of both lesions. As noted above, the neoplastic cells in a lymphomatous infiltrate may infiltrate the ductular and acinar epithelium, expanding these structures and pushing the epithelium into the lumen mimicking lobular neoplasia.[86] In both FNAC and tissue sections medullary carcinoma may also enter the differential diagnosis.[83,91]

On frozen section the diagnosis of breast lymphoma may be a particular problem. Cohen and Brooks reported that eight cases of lymphoma in their series of 35 cases were misdiagnosed on frozen section; three had been called carcinoma, one severe chronic inflammation, one granulocytic sarcoma and three pseudolymphoma.[87] It may not be possible to reach a definitive diagnosis on frozen section and in difficult cases we would advise deferring until paraffin sections and even immunohistochemical assessment has been performed.

Immunohistochemical examination is mandatory in primary breast lymphomas both to enable correct diagnosis and accurate immunophenotyping (Fig. 19.13B) and we would agree with Bobrow et al who suggest that, as a minimum,

markers against CD45, CD45RO, CD3, CD20 and an epithelial marker be employed.[92] In addition PGP9.5 positivity can be seen in small cell carcinomas which may very rarely metastasize to the breast. In FNAC samples containing abundant discohesive cells with little cytoplasm the diagnosis may lie between lymphoma and carcinoma; in these cases repeat FNAC or biopsy may be required to provide further material for immunohistochemical assessment. It may not be possible on FNAC specimens to employ all the immunohistochemical markers which are desired, but cytokeratin and CD45 immunostaining can be assessed and a definitive diagnosis of lymphoma rather than carcinoma can be made. Needle core biopsy or diagnostic biopsy can then be obtained for further evaluation of grade and type of lymphoma.

It should be noted that estrogen receptor positivity cannot be used to differentiate lymphoma from carcinoma definitively. Although estrogen receptor positivity has not been reported, to the best of our knowledge, in lymphomas by an immunohistochemical technique,[88] occasional breast lymphomas have shown estrogen and progesterone receptor positivity by dextran coated charcoal assay[80,92] and indeed have responded to tamoxifen therapy.[94]

The name 'pseudolymphoma' has been used to include lesions composed of a mixed cell population with reactive follicles and germinal centers.[95–96] It has been suggested that this is a benign disease process[97] possibly associated with injury[96,98] or underlying immunological abnormality.[95] We do not advise the use of this term which is unhelpful and misleading. With the advent of immunohistochemistry and molecular techniques the classification of 'pseudolymphoma' has been used less widely, but it remains true that malignant lymphoma must be distinguished from reactive and benign lymphoid infiltrates of the breast. Expression of both B and T cell markers and lack of light chain restriction will confirm the polyclonal nature of these lesions. Benign intramammary lymph nodes and inflammatory conditions may also be mistaken for lymphoma in FNAC specimens but in these samples recognition of the polymorphic nature of the lymphoid cell should enable correct diagnosis.

Prognosis

Primary breast lymphomas have a proclivity for metastasizing to other MALT sites including the contralateral breast; in a literature review carried out by Hugh et al recurrences were found in the other breast in 16 of 73 cases.[80] Other common sites of recurrence include lymph nodes, the chest or abdominal wall, central nervous system, lungs, spleen, bone, kidneys, ovary and gastro-intestinal tract. Rapid dissemination of disease to ovaries and the central nervous system is also seen in the younger patients with Burkitt's type lymphoma. It is widely agreed that these latter women have a poor prognosis with a median survival of only about 10 months.[80]

However, with the exception of the Burkitt's type breast lymphoma, the variation in the patterns of lymphoma reported makes prediction of prognosis in an individual patient difficult; from analysis of combined series, an overall 5-year survival of 48% is seen.[86] In individual units, however, 5-year survivals as high as 74%[86] and even 85%[90] have been reported. It is clear that, as with disease elsewhere, behavior is related to the stage, type and grade of disease[81,86,90,99–100] and overall the prognosis appears to be essentially similar to localized lymphoma in other sites.[101] In conclusion, whilst some groups have suggested that primary breast lymphoma spreads more rapidly than those at other extranodal tissue[81] we believe that this depends on the histological features and stage of disease.

Hodgkin's disease

Convincing cases of primary Hodgkin's disease of the breast are exceedingly uncommon and usually of nodular sclerosing type.[90,102] For example, although Meis et al reported six cases of Hodgkin's disease of the breast, lymph nodes (some with adjacent breast tissue) were involved in five of these patients.[103] It seems probable that intramammary nodes were the initial site of the disease rather than breast parenchyma. Secondary Hodgkin's lymphoma of the breast is also seen infrequently.

PLASMACYTOMA

Primary breast involvement in multiple myeloma

is rare and the majority of mammary extra-medullary plasmacytomas occur in the course of known systemic disease (although this may only be recognized in retrospect).[104] The breast has also been reported as a site of relapse of myeloma.[105] However, if the presence of disseminated disease is not recognized, biopsy may be performed and sheets of lymphoplasmacytoid or neoplastic plasma cells are seen histologically. These are usually relatively uniform although atypical and binucleate forms may be seen and the 'clockface nucleus' of normal plasma cells may not be prominent. Plasmablastic forms may also be seen.[106] There is little stromal response to the tumor but an associated mixed inflammatory response may be noted. The most significant differential diagnosis is infiltrating lobular carcinoma; the absence of intracellular mucin and associated in situ carcinoma may be helpful, but positive immunoreactivity for immunoglobulins, light chain restriction and the absence of cytokeratin expression is more helpful in the diagnosis of plasmacytoma/myeloma.

LEUKEMIA

There are many reports of leukemia occurring in patients who have had treatment, either radiotherapy or chemotherapy or both, for breast carcinoma (see Ch. 20) but clinical presentation as a breast mass is much less common. Bilateral or multiple leukemic deposits may be seen in association with acute lymphoblastic leukemia (ALL)[107] or chronic lymphocytic leukemia (CLL)[108] and as with myeloma, the breast may be the presenting site of deposits of leukemia which herald the relapse of disease.[109] If hematological malignancy is considered clinically FNAC may be helpful;[110] further histochemical and immunohistochemical examination can be performed and the necessity for diagnostic excision avoided.

Acute myeloblastic leukemia (AML) may present as a soft tissue mass and chloromas (granulocytic sarcomas)[111–112] of the breast have been reported, although rarely. These may occur at initial presentation or during the course of known AML and are usually unilateral well-defined masses. Patients with deposits but no evidence of systemic disease usually develop AML within 2 years. If resected the tumor mass is typically of green color, hence the term 'chloroma', although the color fades in contact with air. Histologically a diffuse infiltrate of granulocytic precursor cells with granular cytoplasm and irregular nuclei is seen. The presence of eosinophils may be helpful in aiding the diagnosis of granulocytic sarcoma. These lesions of AML within the breast may mimic infiltrating lobular carcinoma and also lymphoma[111] and we recommend a high index of suspicion along with immunohistochemical and histochemical examination to identify the myeloid origin of the neoplastic cells.

METASTASES WITHIN THE BREAST

Introduction

Metastases occur frequently within the breast at a late stage in patients with known disseminated malignancy. Conversely it is unusual for a patient to present with a breast mass which is subsequently found to be a secondary deposit from an occult primary tumor in another organ. Perhaps surprisingly, metastases within the breast are usually solitary and present as well circumscribed painless lumps, often in the upper outer quadrant.

Multiple well defined nodules[113] or more rarely a diffuse infiltrate by metastatic tumor may be seen, mimicking so-called 'inflammatory' carcinoma.

Macroscopic and microscopic appearances

Metastatic deposits in the breast are very rarely excised but are usually well-defined masses, sometimes with associated satellite nodules. A multitude of malignancies have been reported to metastasize to the breast but melanoma (Fig. 19.14A and B), lymphoma/leukemia and lung carcinoma are the most frequently seen.[114] Neuroendocrine tumors including oat cell carcinomas and carcinoids may also disseminate to the breast.[67,115]

Tumors of epithelial origin from which metastatic deposits may be seen include ovarian carcinoma which shows a predilection for metastasizing to the breast.[116] Primary breast adenocarcinoma may also metastasize to the opposite breast and should be considered in a patient who has had previous breast carcinoma, although most contralateral lesions are, in fact, second primary tumors. Reports of metastatic deposits within the breast from gastrointestinal,[117–118] renal,[119] thyroid,[120] cervical[113] and in men, prostatic carcinoma have also been recorded.

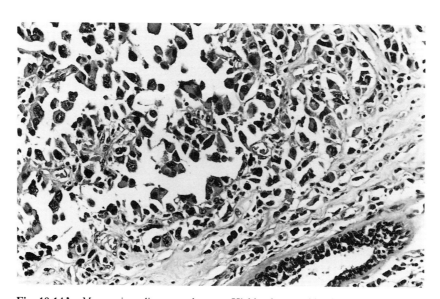

Fig. 19.14A Metastatic malignant melanoma. Highly pleomorphic discohesive tumor cells infiltrate the breast tissue. A normal duct is seen at the lower right of the field. Hematoxylin–eosin × 185.

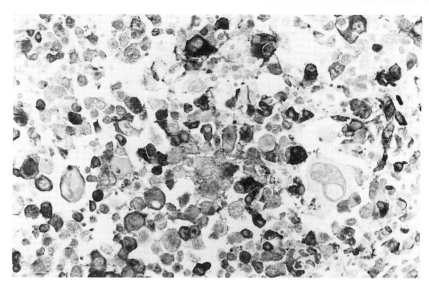

Fig. 19.14B Metastatic malignant melanoma. The diagnosis is confirmed by the demonstration of focal positive cytoplasmic expression with the HMB 45 antibody. Immunostaining for HMB 45 × 400.

The majority of breast malignancies in children are metastatic lesions;[66,69] rhabdomyosarcomas, particularly of alveolar type, are well recognized as metastasizing to the breast in childhood.[65,71,115] Metastatic neuroblastoma may also be seen.[70]

Differential diagnosis

A full clinical history is mandatory if misdiagnosis of metastatic deposits within the breast is to be avoided. If the overall histological features are not typical of a breast carcinoma the absence of associated in situ carcinoma and the presence of abundant intravascular deposits of tumor throughout the breast may be helpful features to suggest the correct diagnosis of a metastatic deposit.[67] In cases where it is difficult to determine whether a tumor has originated in the breast or elsewhere tumor markers may help to suggest the probable site of origin. This is particularly useful if it provides appropriate treatment options for the clinicians. We perform immunohistochemical examination with a panel of antibodies including cytokeratins 7 and 20, CEA, CEA/NCA, epithelial membrane antigen, Ca 19.9 and Ca 125 with the addition of estrogen receptor, alpha-B-crystallin, alpha-feto protein, prostate specific antigen, prostatic acid phosphatase and thyroglobulin, where appropriate, in selected cases.[121-122] Nevertheless in our experience the prognosis of patients with metastatic disease in the breast is almost uniformly poor.

REFERENCES

1. Gutman H, Pollock RE, Ross MI et al. Sarcoma of the breast: implications for extent of therapy. The MD Anderson experience. Surg 1994; 116: 505–509.
2. Berg JW, DeCosse JJ, Fracchia AA, Farrow J. Stromal sarcomas of the breast. A unified approach to connective tissue sarcomas other than Cystosarcoma Phyllodes. Cancer 1962; 15: 418–424.
3. Callery CD, Rosen PP, Kinne DW. Sarcoma of the breast. A study of 32 patients with reappraisal of classification and therapy. Ann Surg 1985; 201: 527–532.
4. Costa J, Wesley RA, Glatstein E et al. The grading of soft tissue sarcomas. Results of a clinicopathologic correlation in a series of 163 cases. Cancer 1984; 53: 530–541.
5. Barnes L, Pietruszka M. Sarcomas of the breast: A clinico-pathologic analysis of ten cases. Cancer 1977; 40: 1577–1585.
6. Pollard SG, Marks PV, Temple LN, Thompson HH. Breast sarcoma. A clinicopathologic review of 25 cases. Cancer 1990; 66: 941–944.
7. Norris HJ, Taylor HB. Sarcoma and related

mesenchymal tumours of the breast. Cancer 1968;
18: 1233–1243.

8. Ciatto S, Bonardi R, Cataliotti L, Cardona G.
Sarcomas of the breast: a multicenter series of 70 cases.
Neoplasma 1992; 39: 375–379.

9. Salvadori B, Greco M, Galluzzo D et al. Surgery for
malignant mesenchymal tumors of the breast: A series
of 31 cases. Tumori 1982; 68: 325–329.

10. Moskaluk CA, Merino MJ, Danforth DN, Medeiros
LJ. Low-grade angiosarcoma of the skin of the breast: a
complication of lumpectomy and radiation therapy for
breast carcinoma. Hum Pathol 1992; 23: 710–714.

11. Givens SS, Ellerbroek NA, Butler JJ et al. Angiosarcoma
arising in an irradiated breast. A case report and review
of the literature. Cancer 1989; 64: 2214–2216.

12. Del Mastro L, Garrone O, Guenzi M et al.
Angiosarcoma of the residual breast after conservative
surgery and radiotherapy for primary carcinoma. Ann
Oncol 1994; 5: 163–165.

13. Tomita K, Yokogawa A, Oda Y, Terahata S.
Lymphangiosarcoma in postmastectomy lymphedema
(Stewart-Treves syndrome): ultrastructural and
immunohistologic characteristics. J Surg Oncol 1988;
38: 275–282.

14. Capo V, Ozzello L, Fenoglio CM et al. Angiosarcomas
arising in edematous extremities: immunostaining for
factor VIII-related antigen and ultrastructural features.
Hum Pathol 1985; 16: 144–150.

15. Fineberg S, Rosen PP. Cutaneous angiosarcoma and
atypical vascular lesions of the skin and breast after
radiation therapy for breast carcinoma. Am J Clin
Pathol 1994; 102: 757–763.

16. Roukema JA, Leenen LP, Kuizinga MC, Maat B.
Angiosarcoma of the irradiated breast: a new problem
after breast conserving therapy? Neth J Surg 1991;
43: 114–116.

17. Chen KTK, Kirkegaard DD, Bocian JJ. Angiosarcoma
of the breast. Cancer 1980; 46: 368–371.

18. Rainwater LM, Martin J Jr, Gaffey TA, van Heerden
JA. Angiosarcoma of the breast. Arch Surg 1986;
121: 669–672.

19. Donnell RM, Rosen PP, Lieberman PH et al.
Angiosarcoma and other vascular tumours of the
breast: Pathologic analysis as a guide to prognosis. Am
J Surg Pathol 1981; 5: 629–642.

20. Rosen PP, Kimmel M, Ernsberger D. Mammary
angiosarcoma. The prognostic significance of tumor
differentiation. Cancer 1988; 62: 2145–2151.

21. Vuitch MF, Rosen PP, Erlandson RA.
Pseudoangiomatous hyperplasia of mammary stroma.
Hum Pathol 1986; 17: 185–191.

22. Ibrahim RE, Sciotto CG, Weidner N.
Pseudoangiomatous hyperplasia of mammary stroma.
Some observations regarding its clinicopathologic
spectrum. Cancer 1989; 63: 1154–1160.

23. Banerjee SS, Eyden BP, Wells S et al.
Pseudoangiosarcomatous carcinoma: a
clinicopathological study of seven cases. Histopathol
1992; 21: 13–23.

24. Hashimoto K, Matsumoto M, Eto H et al.
Differentiation of metastatic breast carcinoma from
Stewart-Treves angiosarcoma. Use of anti-keratin and
anti-desmosome monoclonal antibodies and factor
VIII-related antibodies. Arch Dermatol 1985;
121: 742–746.

25. Walker RA. Ulex europeus I–peroxidase as a marker of
vascular endothelium: its application in routine
histopathology. J Pathol 1985; 146: 123–127.

26. Ohsawa M, Naka N, Tomita Y et al. Use of
immunohistochemical procedures in diagnosing
angiosarcoma. Evaluation of 98 cases. Cancer 1995;
75: 2867–2874.

27. Miettinen M, Lindenmayer AE, Chaubal A.
Endothelial cell markers CD31, CD34, and BNH9
antibody to H- and Y-antigens — evaluation of their
specificity and sensitivity in the diagnosis of vascular
tumors and comparison with von Willebrand factor.
Mod Pathol 1994; 7: 82–90.

28. Aiba S, Tabata N, Ishii H, Ootani H, Tagami H.
Dermatofibrosarcoma protuberans is a unique
fibrohistiocytic tumour expressing CD34. Br J
Dermatol 1992; 127: 79–84.

29. Rosner D. Angiosarcoma of the breast: long-term
survival following adjuvant chemotherapy. J Surg Oncol
1988; 39: 90–95.

30. Hunter TB, Martin PC, Dietzen CD, Tyler LT.
Angiosarcoma of the breast. Two case reports and a
review of the literature. Cancer 1985; 56: 2099–2106.

31. Maddox JC, Evans HL. Angiosarcoma of skin and soft
tissue: A study of 44 cases. Cancer 1981;
48: 1907–1921.

32. Stewart FW, Treves N. Lymphangiosarcoma in
postmastectomy lymphedema: A report of six cases in
elephantiasis chirurgica. Cancer 1948; 1: 64–81.

33. Kanitakis J, Bendelac A, Marchand C et al. Stewart-
Treves syndrome: An histogenetic (ultrastructural and
immunohistological) study. J Cutan Pathol 1986;
13: 30–39.

34. Marsch WC. The Stewart-Treves syndrome: A
hemangiosarcoma in chronic lymphedema.
Ultrastructural analysis at various stages of clinical
development. Hautarzt 1987; 38: 82–87.

35. Kindblom LG, Stenman G, Angervall L.
Morphological and cytogenetic studies of angiosarcoma
in Stewart-Treves syndrome. Virchows Archiv (A)
Pathol Anat Histopathol 1991; 419: 439–445.

36. Stewart NJ, Pritchard DJ, Nascimento AG, Kang YK.
Lymphangiosarcoma following mastectomy. Clin
Orthop 1995; 320: 135–141.

37. Clements WDB, Kirk SJ, Spence RAJ. A rare late
complication of breast cancer treatment. Br J Clin
Pract 1993; 47: 219–220.

38. Pitts WC, Rojas VA, Gaffey MJ et al. Carcinomas with
metaplasia and sarcomas of the breast. Am J Clin
Pathol 1991; 95: 623–632.

39. Fletcher CD. Pleomorphic malignant fibrous
histiocytoma: fact or fiction? A critical reappraisal based
on 159 tumors diagnosed as pleomorphic sarcoma. Am
J Surg Pathol 1992; 16: 213–228.

40. Jones MW, Norris HJ, Wargotz ES, Weiss SW.
Fibrosarcoma-malignant fibrous histiocytoma of the
breast. A clinicopathological study of 32 cases. Am J
Surg Pathol 1992; 16: 667–674.

41. Fletcher CDM. Soft tissue tumors. In: Fletcher
CDM, ed. Diagnostic histopathology of tumors.
Edinburgh: Churchill Livingstone, 1995;
vol 2; 1043–1096.

42. Enzinger FM, Weiss SW, eds. Soft tissue tumours. 3rd
ed. St Louis: Mosby, 1995.

43. Payan HM, England DM. Fibrosarcoma mimicking

breast fibromatosis. Am J Med Genet Suppl 1987; 3: 257–262.

44. Wargotz ES, Norris HJ, Austin RM, Enzinger FM. Fibromatosis of the breast. A clinical and pathological study of 28 cases. Am J Surg Pathol 1987; 11: 38–45.

45. De Wilde R, Hesseling M, Holzgreve W, Raas P. Traumatically-induced dermatofibrosarcoma protuberans of the breast. Zentralbl Gynakol 1988; 110: 633–635.

46. Perry DA, Schultz LR, Dehner LP. Giant cell fibroblastoma with dermatofibrosarcoma protuberans-like transformation. J Cutan Pathol 1993; 20: 451–454.

47. Isimbaldi G, Sironi M, Declich P et al. A case of malignant phyllodes tumor with muscular and fatty differentiations. Tumori 1992; 78: 351–352.

48. Powell CM, Rosen PP. Adipose differentiation in cystosarcoma phyllodes. A study of 14 cases. Am J Surg Pathol 1994; 18: 720–727.

49. Austin RM, Dupree WB. Liposarcoma of the breast: a clinicopathologic study of 20 cases. Hum Pathol 1986; 17: 906–913.

50. Arbabi L, Warhol MJ. Pleomorphic liposarcoma following radiotherapy for breast carcinoma. Cancer 1982; 49: 878–880.

51. Brady MS, Gaynor JJ, Brennan MF. Radiation-associated sarcoma of bone and soft tissue. Arch Surg 1992; 127: 1379–1385.

52. Wiklund TA, Blomqvist CP, Raty J et al. Postirradiation sarcoma. Analysis of a nationwide cancer registry material. Cancer 1991; 68: 524–531.

53. Bianchi S, Malatantis G, Cardona G, Zampi G. Osteogenic sarcoma of the breast. A case report. Tumori 1992; 78: 43–46.

54. Going JJ, Lumsden AB, Anderson TJ. A classical osteogenic sarcoma of the breast: histology, immunohistochemistry and ultrastructure. Histopathol 1986; 10: 631–641.

55. Tavassoli FA. Mesenchymal lesions. In: Pathology of the breast. Norwalk: Appleton and Lange, 1992; 517–563.

56. Yamashina M. Primary leiomyosarcoma in the breast. Jpn J Clin Oncol 1987; 17: 71–77.

57. Arista-Nasr J, Gonzalez-Gomez I, Angeles-Angeles A et al. Primary recurrent leiomyosarcoma of the breast. Case report with ultrastructural and immunohistochemical study and review of the literature. Am J Clin Pathol 1989; 92: 500–505.

58. Lonsdale RN, Widdison A. Leiomyosarcoma of the nipple. Histopathol 1992; 20: 537–539.

59. Waterworth PD, Gompertz RH, Hennessy C et al. Primary leiomyosarcoma of the breast. Br J Surg 1992; 79: 169–170.

60. Wei CH, Wan CY, Chen A, Tseng HH. Epithelioid leiomyosarcoma of the breast: report of a case. J Formos Med Assoc 1993; 92: 379–381.

61. Nielsen BB. Leiomyosarcoma of the breast with late dissemination. Virchows Arch (A) Pathol Anat 1984; 403: 241–245.

62. Boscaino A, Ferrara G, Orabona P et al. Smooth muscle tumors of the breast: clinicopathologic features of two cases. Tumori 1994; 80: 241–245.

63. Alessi E, Sala F. Leiomyosarcoma in ectopic areola. Am J Dermatopathol 1992; 14: 165–169.

64. Brown DC, Theaker JM, Banks PM et al. Cytokeratin expression in smooth muscle and smooth muscle tumours. Histopathol 1987; 11: 477–486.

65. Beattie M, Kingston JE, Norton AJ, Malpas JS.

66. Nasopharyngeal rhabdomyosarcoma presenting as a breast mass. Pediatr Hematol Oncol 1990; 7: 259–263.

66. Pettinato G, Manivel JC, Kelly DR et al. Lesions of the breast in children exclusive of typical fibroadenoma and gynecomastia. A clinicopathologic study of 113 cases. Pathol Annu 1989; 2: 296–328.

67. Vergier B, Trojani M, de Mascarel I et al. Metastases to the breast: differential diagnosis from primary breast carcinoma. J Surg Oncol 1991; 48: 112–116.

68. Torres V, Ferrer R. Cytology of fine needle aspiration biopsy of primary breast rhabdomyosarcoma in an adolescent girl. Acta Cytol 1985; 29: 430–434.

69. Rogers DA, Lobe TE, Rao BN et al. Breast malignancy in children. J Pediatr Surg 1994; 29: 48–51.

70. Boothroyd A, Carty H. Breast masses in childhood and adolescence. A presentation of 17 cases and a review of the literature. Pediatr Radiol 1994; 24: 81–84.

71. Sugar J, Sapi Z. Alveolar rhabdomyosarcoma — a case report. Arch Geschwulstforsch 1988; 58: 445–448.

72. Carstens HB, Cooke JL. Mammary carcinosarcoma presenting as rhabdomyosarcoma: an ultrastructural and immunocytochemical study. Ultrastruct Pathol 1990; 14: 537–544.

73. Thilagavathi G, Subramanian S, Samuel AV et al. Primary chondrosarcoma of the breast. J Indian Med Assoc 1992; 90: 16–17.

74. Lamovec J, Kloboves-Prevodnik V. Teleangiectatic sarcomatoid carcinoma of the breast. Tumori 1992; 78: 283–286.

75. Silverman JF, Geisinger KR, Frable WJ. Fine-needle aspiration cytology of mesenchymal tumors of the breast. Diagn Cytopathol 1988; 4: 50–58.

76. Santeusanio G, Pascal RR, Bisceglia M, Costantino AM, Bosman C. Metaplastic breast carcinoma with epithelial phenotype of pseudosarcomatous components. Arch Pathol Lab Med 1988; 112: 82–85.

77. Meunier B, Leveque J, Le Prise E et al. Three cases of sarcoma occurring after radiation therapy of breast cancers. Eur J Obstet Gynecol Reprod Biol 1994; 57: 33–36.

78. Arias SJ Jr, Rosen PP. Hemangiopericytoma of the breast. Mod Pathol 1988; 1: 98–103.

79. Engel A, Lamm SH, Lai SH. Human breast sarcoma and human breast implantation: a time trend analysis based on SEER data (1973–1990). J Clin Epidemiol 1995; 48: 539–544.

80. Hugh JC, Jackson FI, Hanson J, Poppema S. Primary breast lymphoma. An immunohistologic study of 20 new cases. Cancer 1990; 66: 2602–2611.

81. Giardini R, Piccolo C, Rilke F. Primary non-Hodgkin's lymphomas of the female breast. Cancer 1992; 69: 725–735.

82. Wright DH. Histogenesis of Burkitt's lymphoma: a B-cell tumour of mucosa-associated lymphoid tissue. IARC Sci Publ 1985; 60: 37–45.

83. Jeon HJ, Akagi T, Hoshida Y et al. Primary non-Hodgkin malignant lymphoma of the breast. An immunohistochemical study of seven patients and literature review of 152 patients with breast lymphoma in Japan. Cancer 1992; 70: 2451–2459.

84. Mattia AR, Ferry JA, Harris NL. Breast lymphoma. A B-cell spectrum including the low grade B-cell lymphoma of mucosa associated lymphoid tissue. Am J Surg Pathol 1993; 17: 574–587.

85. Wiseman C, Liao KT. Primary lymphoma of the breast. Cancer 1972; 29: 1705–1712.

86. Brustein S, Filippa DA, Kimmel M et al. Malignant lymphoma of the breast. A study of 53 patients. Ann Surg 1987; 205: 144–150.

87. Cohen PL, Brooks JJ. Lymphomas of the breast. A clinicopathologic and immunohistochemical study of primary and secondary cases. Cancer 1991; 67: 1359–1369.

88. Ariad S, Lewis D, Cohen R, Bezwoda WR. Breast lymphoma. A clinical and pathological review and 10-year treatment results. S Afr Med J 1995; 85: 85–89.

89. Kosaka M, Tsuchihashi N, Takishita M et al. Primary adult T-cell lymphoma of the breast. Acta Haematol 1992; 87: 202–205.

90. Dixon JM, Lumsden AB, Krajewski A et al. Primary lymphoma of the breast. Br J Surg 1987; 74: 214–216.

91. Lamovec J, Jancar J. Primary malignant lymphoma of the breast. Lymphoma of the mucosa-associated lymphoid tissue. Cancer 1987; 60: 3033–3041.

92. Bobrow LG, Richards MA, Happerfield LC et al. Breast lymphomas: a clinicopathologic review. Hum Pathol 1993; 24: 274–278.

93. Aozasa K, Ohsawa M, Saeki K et al. Malignant lymphoma of the breast. Immunologic type and association with lymphocytic mastopathy. Am J Clin Pathol 1992; 97: 699–704.

94. Millis RR, Bobrow LG, Rubens RD, Isaacson PG. Histiocytic lymphoma of breast responds to tamoxifen. Br J Cancer 1988; 58: 808–809.

95. Jeffery KM, Pantazis CG, Wei JP. Pseudolymphoma of the breast associated with Graves' thyrotoxicosis. Breast Disease 1994; 7: 169–173.

96. Lin JJ, Farha GJ, Taylor RJ. Pseudolymphoma of the breast. I. In a study of 8654 consecutive tylectomies and mastectomies. Cancer 1980; 45: 973–978.

97. Chang DW, Weiss PR. Pseudolymphoma of the breast. Plast Reconstr Surg 1995; 95: 145–147.

98. Maldonado ME, Sierra RD. Pseudolymphoma of the breast: Case report and literature review. Mil Med 1994; 159: 469–471.

99. Grande M. Breast involvement in malignant blood diseases. A report of four cases and review of the literature. Recenti Prog Med 1990; 81: 474–478.

100. Nielsen VT, Vetner M. Malignant lymphoma of the breast. A review of the literature and seven Danish cases. Ugeskrift for Laeger 1981; 143: 661–664.

101. Smith MR, Brustein S, Straus DJ. Localized non-Hodgkin's lymphoma of the breast. Cancer 1987; 59: 351–354.

102. Raju GC, Jankey N, Delpech K. Localized primary extranodal Hodgkin's disease (Hodgkin's lymphoma) of the breast. J R Soc Med 1987; 80: 247–249.

103. Meis JM, Butler JJ, Osborne BM. Hodgkin's disease involving the breast and chest wall. Cancer 1986; 57: 1859–1865.

104. Ben-Yehuda A, Steiner-Saltz D, Libson E, Polliack A. Plasmacytoma of the breast. Unusual initial presentation of myeloma: report of two cases and review of the literature. Blut 1989; 58: 169–170.

105. Ross JS, King TM, Spector JI et al. Plasmacytoma of the breast. An unusual case of recurrent myeloma. Arch Intern Med 1987; 147: 1838–1840.

106. Jarczok K, Rozek-Lesiak K, Kubinska E. Breast and subcutaneous plasmoblastic infiltrations in the course of plasmoblastoma. Folia Haematol Int Mag Klin Morphol Blutforsch 1987; 114: 234–237.

107. Jain AK, Gupta RC, Bhardwaj B, Leelani N. Acute lymphoblastic leukaemia presenting as breast mass. J Assoc Physicians India 1992; 40: 335–336.

108. Gogoi PK, Stewart ID, Keane PF et al. Chronic lymphocytic leukaemia presenting with bilateral breast involvement. Clin Lab Haematol 1989; 11: 57–60.

109. Sagar TG, Maitreyan V, Majhi U, Shanta V. Breast involvement in acute lymphoblastic leukaemia. J Assoc Physicians India 1989; 37: 718–719.

110. Miura H, Konaka C, Kawate N et al. Fine-needle aspiration cytology of metastatic breast tumor originating from leukemia. Diagn Cytopathol 1992; 8: 605–608.

111. Chua ET. A case of granulocytic sarcoma of the breast and review of the literature. Singapore Med J 1989; 30: 311–312.

112. Pettinato G, De Chiara A, Insabato L, De Renzo A. Fine needle aspiration biopsy of a granulocytic sarcoma (chloroma) of the breast. Acta Cytol 1988; 32: 67–71.

113. Kumar L, Tanwar RK, Karak PK, Shukla NK. Breast metastasis from primary cervical cancer. Asia Oceania J Obstet Gynaecol 1994; 20: 345–348.

114. Nunez DA, Sutherland CG, Sood RK. Breast metastasis from a pharyngeal carcinoma. J Laryngol Otol 1989; 103: 227–228.

115. Sneige N, Zachariah S, Fanning TV et al. Fine-needle aspiration cytology of metastatic neoplasms in the breast. Am J Clin Pathol 1989; 92: 27–35.

116. Yamasaki H, Saw D, Zdanowitz J, Faltz LL. Ovarian carcinoma metastasis to the breast: case report and review of the literature. Am J Surg Pathol 1993; 17: 193–197.

117. Cavazzini G, Colpani F, Cantore M et al. Breast metastasis from gastric signet ring cell carcinoma, mimicking inflammatory carcinoma. A case report. Tumori 1993; 79: 450–453.

118. Alexander HR, Turnbull AD, Rosen PP. Isolated breast metastasis from gastrointestinal carcinomas: report of two cases. J Surg Oncol 1989; 42: 264–266.

119. Monticelli J, Machiavello JC, Birtwisle-Peyrottes I et al. Breast metastasis revealing cancer of the kidney. Apropos of a new case and review of the literature. J Chir 1994; 131: 160–161.

120. Ordonez NG, Katz RL, Luna MA, Samaan NA. Medullary thyroid carcinoma metastatic to breast diagnosed by fine-needle aspiration biopsy. Diagn Cytopathol 1988; 4: 254–257.

121. Ellis IO, Hitchcock A. Tumour marker immunoreactivity in adenocarcinoma. J Clin Path 1988; 41: 1064–1067.

122. Pinder SE, Balsitis M, Ellis IO et al. The expression of alpha B-crystallin in epithelial tumours: a useful tumour marker? J Pathol 1994; 174: 209–215.

Effects of treatment

INTRODUCTION

An increased proportion of patients now have breast conserving therapy rather than mastectomy for first line surgical treatment of breast carcinoma. This is frequently followed by radiotherapy to the breast. Both pre- and postoperative chemotherapy may also be utilized in different treatment regimens of patients with primary breast cancer. Fine needle aspiration cytology (FNAC) specimens or biopsies of clinical or mammographic abnormalities in the residual breast may thus show changes due to irradiation or systemic therapies which may mimic residual, recurrent or second malignancies. It is therefore vital that adequate clinical information is given about previous treatments when any specimen is sent to the laboratory.

Second malignancies, both mammary and non-mammary in origin are also seen in patients treated for breast cancer and these must be considered when new clinical or radiological lesions are identified. In addition systemic treatments for breast cancer may produce changes in distant tissues. Hormone therapies in particular have well recognized effects on endometrium.

RADIOTHERAPY

EFFECTS ON NON-NEOPLASTIC BREAST TISSUE

Many of the features of radiotherapy alter with time and the histological changes seen depend somewhat on the duration between irradiation treatment and examination. In essence many of the appearances are similar to those described in other tissues. Irradiated breast skin, for example, shows identical changes to that from other sites.[1] Fat necrosis, which can mimic recurrent carcinoma both clinically and mammographically, may also be seen (Fig. 20.1).[2–3]

Within the breast parenchyma both the stromal component and the epithelium may show radiation changes. Stromal fibrosis with reactive 'radiation fibroblasts', as seen elsewhere in the body, can be identified (Fig. 20.2A and B). The nuclei of these fibroblasts may be variable in size and

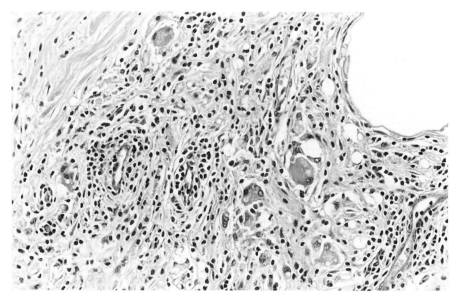

Fig. 20.1 Irradiation associated fat necrosis. The lesion consists of a mixture of foamy macrophages, giant cells and lymphocytes with prominent blood vessels. Hyalinized connective tissue is seen at the top left. The biopsy was taken from a residual palpable mass which developed at the previous tumor site after local excision and postoperative irradiation. Hematoxylin–eosin × 185.

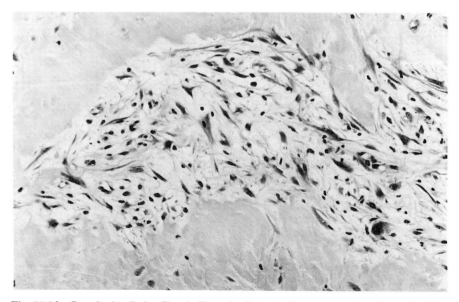

Fig. 20.2A Reactive irradiation fibrosis. Dense hyalinized collagen surrounds a focus of cellular loose connective tissue in which plump fibroblasts are clearly visible. Hematoxylin–eosin × 185.

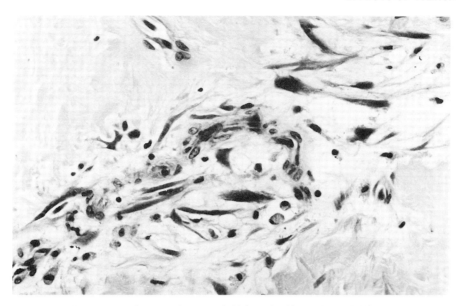

Fig. 20.2B   Higher magnification of another field from the biopsy shown in Figure 20.2A. The fibroblast nuclei are greatly enlarged and hyperchromatic. In some the nuclear outlines are indistinct. From a residual nodule at the site of a previous excision biopsy for carcinoma, one month post irradiation. FNAC had revealed cells suspicious of malignancy. Hematoxylin–eosin × 400.

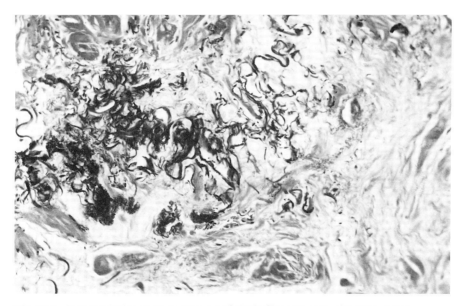

Fig. 20.3   Post-irradiation elastosis. Tangles of elastic fibers are seen with rather dense hyalinized collagen. This biopsy was taken several months after irradiation therapy. Hematoxylin–eosin × 125.

hyperchromatic or hypochromatic with 'smudged' outlines;[4] nucleoli may also be visible. The fibrosis may be extensive and a severe reaction is a particular complication of radiotherapy in patients with underlying connective tissue diseases.[5–6] Elastosis is also seen in association with radiotherapy (Fig. 20.3) but this is a non-specific feature which may be present in benign breast conditions and

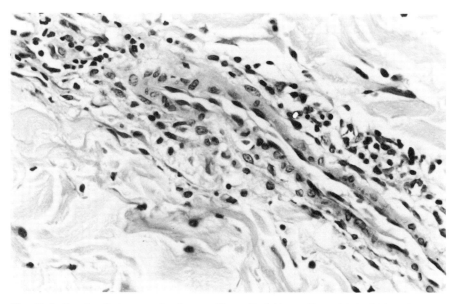

Fig. 20.4   Post-irradiation vascular damage. The wall of this small arteriole is thickened and the endothelial nuclei enlarged and hyperchromatic. Note the perivascular lymphocytic infiltrate. Hematoxylin–eosin × 400.

after surgery alone and is thus of little diagnostic help.

Vascular changes, as seen in other tissues subject to irradiation, can be identified (Fig. 20.4) and include fibroblastic thickening of the intima and fragmentation of the elastic lamina of vessel walls. Endothelial cell changes, including the development of large hyperchromatic nuclei, are thought to be relatively specific for irradiation.[4]

The most characteristic radiation changes, however, involve the terminal duct lobular units where atypical epithelial cells are present within the surrounding lobular stroma which is usually hyalinized and sclerotic (Fig. 20.5A and B).[4,7] The epithelial changes are seen in all irradiated patients but show considerable variation in severity, apparently unrelated to radiation dose.[7] Nuclei are hyperchromatic and enlarged, but nucleoli are inconspicuous and chromatin is homogeneous without the 'clumping' seen in malignancy. The cytoplasm of the cells is often vacuolated. Myoepithelial cells are reported to be unaffected by radiotherapy.[4]

The epithelial atypia described may mimic residual or recurrent carcinoma. However, although the epithelial cells are plump and may appear to fill the terminal duct lobular units, the latter are not significantly distended and a lack of stratification and mitotic activity may be helpful in determining that the features are due to irradiation. Neither the monotony of the regular cells of lobular carcinoma in situ nor the pleomorphism, conspicuous nucleoli, mitoses and loss of polarity of ductal carcinoma in situ (DCIS) within lobules ('cancerization of lobules') is present. Although epithelial atypia may be seen in larger ducts, as reported with chemotherapy, this is always accompanied by the more characteristic changes in the terminal duct lobular unit. Necrosis is not usually identified.

The epithelial features associated with radiotherapy may also be seen in foci of sclerosing adenosis thus making histological interpretation more difficult. The overall architectural pattern on low power examination is then not that of carcinomatous infiltration, but remains lobulocentric and this is a useful discriminatory feature. To diagnose residual or recurrent carcinoma in these circumstances may be a particular problem in frozen section material and a definite diagnosis may not be possible on such preparations. In general frozen section requests should be discouraged when small foci of recurrent carcinomas are suspected in patients who have had radiotherapy.

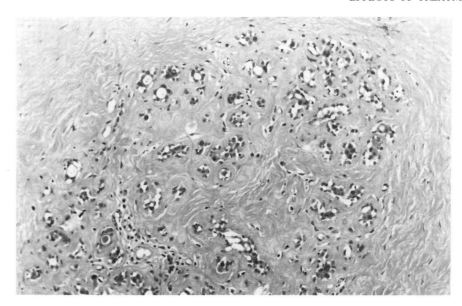

Fig. 20.5A Post-irradiation lobular sclerosis. The rounded outline of the lobule is still apparent, but there is marked intralobular fibrosis with hyalinization. Hematoxylin–eosin × 125.

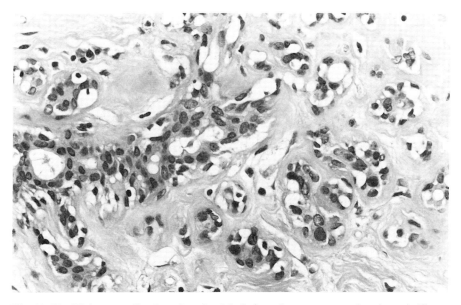

Fig. 20.5B Higher magnification of another lobule from the same case as that shown in Figure 20.5A. The epithelial nuclei show moderate nuclear pleomorphism. Cytoplasmic vacuolation is also conspicuous. Hematoxylin–eosin × 400.

It is worth noting however that recurrent breast carcinomas are usually similar in appearance to the original tumor and review of the previous reports and histological slides may be invaluable.

The lack of the architectural assistance gained from histological examination of an excision biopsy specimen may make the assessment of needle core and cytological preparations from the irradiated breast very difficult (Fig. 20.5C). It has been reported that the cytological features in particular

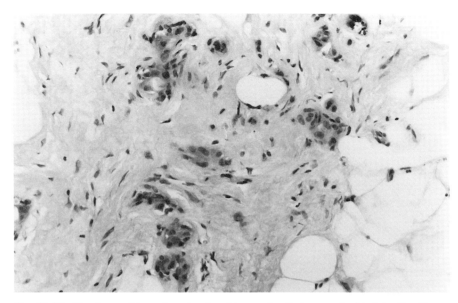

Fig. 20.5C Needle core biopsy from irradiated breast. Small clusters of epithelial cells with no apparent myoepithelial layer or lobular structure are present within a dense fibrous stroma. These appearances were interpreted by the pathologist who reported the biopsy as strongly suspicious of malignancy. From the same case as that shown in Figure 20.5A and B; no evidence of recurrent tumor was identified. Hematoxylin–eosin × 185.

may be indistinguishable from malignancy.[8] With experience, however, FNAC can be a useful technique and a sensitivity of 86% and a specificity of 98% has been obtained for lesions from irradiated breasts.[9] Caution is, however, required in the interpretation of cytological atypia in FNAC from irradiated tissues and the cellularity of the sample is more useful diagnostically;[9] paucicellular samples are uncommon from foci of recurrent or residual malignancy, but are usual from the non-neoplastic irradiated breast. If scanty highly atypical cells are seen in a smear it may be necessary to issue a C4 (suspicious) rather than a C5 (malignant) report.

EFFECTS ON RESIDUAL CARCINOMA

The tissue changes present in residual breast carcinoma cells after radiotherapy are essentially similar in nature to those seen in non-neoplastic breast tissue. Cytoplasmic vacuolation may be identified and carcinoma cell nuclei may show marked pleomorphism with the presence of bizarre forms;[10] extensive tumor necrosis may be encountered (Fig. 20.6). As described above the fibrosis of the stroma may lead to difficulties in distinguishing small foci of carcinoma cells which have become entrapped (Fig. 20.7) from radiation changes in sclerosing adenosis and non-neoplastic conditions. In these circumstances immunohistochemistry with epithelial markers and smooth muscle actin may be invaluable; the epithelial nature of the cells can be confirmed, but smooth muscle actin immunoreactivity will be seen surrounding entrapped benign tubules.

EFFECTS ON OTHER TISSUES

The development of second malignancies in patients who have had radiotherapy is well recognized and includes both bone and soft tissue sarcomas.[11–12] Lymphangiosarcoma is associated with lymphedema following radical breast surgery and irradiation (Stewart–Treves syndrome) but is rare[13–14] (see Ch. 19). Angiosarcoma may follow radiotherapy for breast carcinomas but is also very uncommon[15–16] (see Ch. 19).

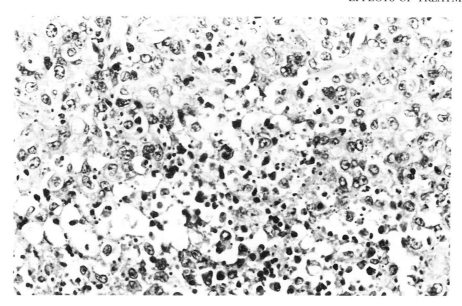

Fig. 20.6   Post-irradiation tumor necrosis. Few apparently viable tumor cells are seen and there is marked karyorhexis and karyolysis with bizarre nuclear forms. Hematoxylin–eosin × 400.

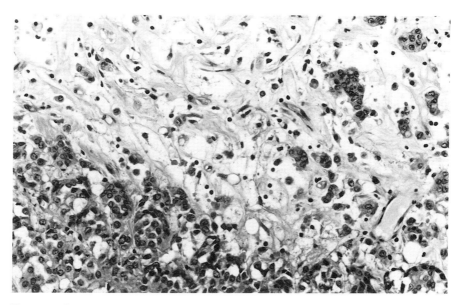

Fig. 20.7   Post-irradiation tumor fibrosis. Relatively well preserved tumor is present at the lower left of the field, whilst groups of residual carcinoma cells are seen within cellular fibrous tissue to the right. Hematoxylin–eosin × 185.

CHEMOTHERAPY

EFFECTS ON NON-NEOPLASTIC BREAST TISSUE

Chemotherapy in the residual non-neoplastic breast causes changes similar to those in the irra-diated organ. Atrophy of epithelial structures is seen in lobules with a variable degree of intra-lobular fibrosis[17] (Fig. 20.8A). Indeed lobular atrophy occurs in up to 65% of cases and is seen in both pre- and postmenopausal women.[18] Bland fibrous obliteration of acini may occur and fibrous

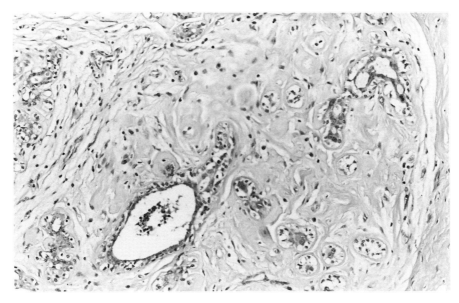

Fig. 20.8A Post-chemotherapy lobular sclerosis. The terminal duct is dilated and there is a marked reduction in the number of lobular acini, with extensive intralobular fibrosis. From a patient who had received neoadjuvant cytotoxic therapy for a locally advanced breast carcinoma. Hematoxylin–eosin × 125.

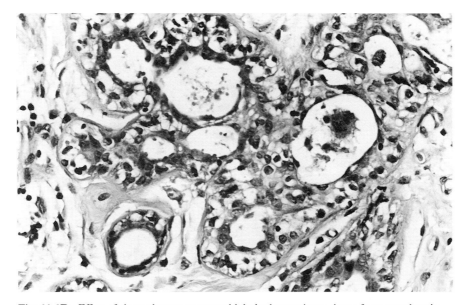

Fig. 20.8B Effect of chemotherapy on normal lobular breast tissue. Apart from cytoplasmic vacuolation myoepithelial cells are relatively well preserved compared with secretory epithelial cells. From the same case as that shown in Figure 20.8A. Hematoxylin–eosin × 400.

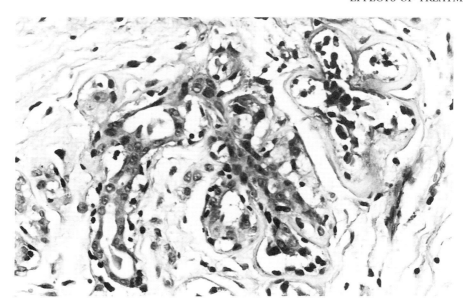

Fig. 20.8C   Effect of chemotherapy on normal lobular breast tissue. In this lobule there is moderate nuclear atypia and some hyperchromatic nuclei are present. From the same case as that shown in Figure 20.8A. Hematoxylin–eosin × 400.

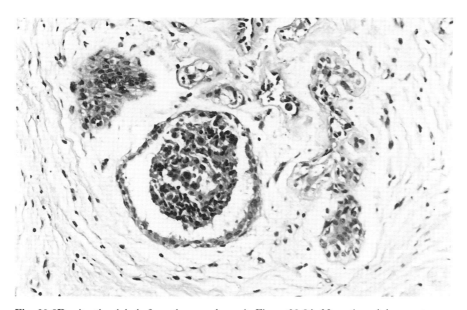

Fig. 20.8D   Another lobule from the case shown in Figure 20.8A. Necrotic and degenerate epithelial cells are seen within the lumen of the duct. Hematoxylin–eosin × 185.

or fatty involution of the stroma elsewhere in the breast may be identified, possibly related to suppression of ovarian function. Complete replacement of the parenchyma by adipose tissue has been noted in over 40% of cases.[17] An increase in elastic tissue is also common and a lymphoid infiltrate, often around ducts, is seen in over one-quarter of cases. As with radiotherapy, myoepithelial cells are rarely affected (Fig. 20.8B).

Epithelial atypia is present in the lobules in

approximately 30% to 50% of cases but, unlike irradiation change, is equally common in ducts where this feature may be seen in 40–50% of specimens.[17–18] Epithelial cells may be enlarged with prominent nuclei, small nucleoli, thick nuclear membranes and pale vacuolated cytoplasm, essentially similar to the features of irradiation in breast tissue (Fig. 20.8C). The nuclear membrane remains well-defined and hyperchromasia is less prominent than in residual or recurrent carcinoma cells. Uncommonly, necrosis and consequent calcification may occur within the duct lumen and can thus produce a suspicious mammographic appearance necessitating FNAC or biopsy (Fig. 20.8D).

EFFECTS ON RESIDUAL CARCINOMA

Residual carcinomatous foci may show similar histopathological changes as a result of chemotherapy to those described following irradiation. These features may be degenerative and transient.[19] It has been reported, however, that malignant cells can be mistaken for histiocytes with increased quantities of vacuolated eosinophilic cytoplasm and eccentric, sometimes hyperchromatic, vesicular nuclei.[17] Vacuolization of the cytoplasm is seen in approximately 60% of cases and may also be seen in metastatic deposits within lymph nodes.[18] Other authors have reported vacuolization of the tumor cell nuclei in approximately 40% of cases.[20] Chromatin clumping and prominent nucleoli may be seen and multinucleated forms identified. The typical desmoplastic stroma is not invariably present; instead connective tissue may be dense and hyalinized. Significant difficulties in diagnosis can occur when small foci of residual or recurrent carcinoma are admixed with genuine histiocytes and foreign body type giant cells adjacent to the site of a previous biopsy.

Although some authors have reported that carcinoma cells retain an overtly malignant appearance after chemotherapy[19] we believe that in difficult cases immunohistochemical profiles may be invaluable; carcinoma cells retain cytokeratin and epithelial membrane antigen (EMA) expression post chemotherapy despite the alteration in morphological appearance.[17] It is of interest to note that infiltrating lobular carcinomas are said not to show the cytological effects of chemotherapy seen in other types of breast carcinoma.[21]

Although primary chemotherapy rarely causes difficulties in diagnosis, with the exception of the distinction of small foci of residual disease as noted above, this treatment has been suggested to alter the histological grade of tumors. This has obvious consequences for the use of this variable in predicting prognosis. The claim is difficult to assess; nuclear changes including pleomorphism are produced by chemotherapy and thus this component of histological grade may be affected. The initial diagnosis of breast carcinoma has often been made on cytological material and thus histological examination of tissue pre- and post-chemotherapy cannot be compared. A proportion of cases may show complete remission with treatment, leaving only those cases resistant to therapy. Cytomegaly, nuclear enlargement and pleomorphism with hyperchromasia and multinucleation were reported by Frierson and Fechner in cases of breast cancer after induction chemotherapy, but there was little change in histological grade. In this small series one tumor showed a difference and was of higher grade in the mastectomy specimen due to a higher mitotic count.[22] We have ourselves found little difference in the histological features, including grade, of breast carcinomas before, during and after a course of chemotherapy although others have suggested that the changes in morphology associated with chemotherapy preclude accurate cytological or histological assessment of grade.[19]

EFFECTS ON OTHER ORGANS

Systemic chemotherapy has been implicated in the development of second malignancies and patients who have received alkylating agents in particular may develop leukemia.[23] The relative risk is thought to be less than 5 fold and peaks before 10 years.[24] Most commonly second malignancies develop in the contralateral breast[25] but other sites include rectum, skin, bone,[26] colon and female genital tract.[25,27] These new malignancies may develop in patients with primary breast cancer who have not received systemic treatment, particularly in young patients,[28] and it is difficult to ascribe the development of second tumors purely to previous treatments for primary breast cancer. Eleven percent of breast cancer patients will develop a second primary tumor outside the breast (at a mean of approximately 7 years)[27] and it is important to consider the possibility of a new primary tumor, as well as metastatic cancer, in biopsy material from any site from patients who have had breast carcinoma. Although approximately 30% of patients die directly as a consequence of their breast cancer[27,29] a greater number (50%) are reported to die as a result of a second primary, non-mammary, malignancy thought to be metastatic in origin.[27]

HORMONE THERAPY

INTRODUCTION

The effects of hormone treatment on residual or recurrent carcinoma and on adjacent non-neoplastic breast tissue have received little attention; most studies have been from earlier decades and often larger doses of steroid hormones were given than would now be used. The changes reported in both non-neoplastic breast and residual carcinoma are similar.

EFFECTS ON NON-NEOPLASTIC BREAST TISSUE

In 1953 Huseby and Thomas performed a study on 36 postmenopausal women receiving estrogens for advanced breast cancer.[30] They reported epithelial changes, particularly in medium and small ducts, including the presence of abundant basophilic cytoplasm in the cells which were frequently large and columnar. Prominent nucleoli were seen in enlarged nuclei. These authors suggested that hormone treatment induced 'extension of the duct system' with changes in the periductal stroma which was less dense and more basophilic than previously. Lobules were more abundant in number. Lymphocytes and plasma cells were seen in the intralobular stroma. Lobular epithelial cells also appeared to be 'stimulated' and in some cases secretory vacuoles were seen. An increase in interlobular fibrous stroma was noted.

EFFECTS ON RESIDUAL CARCINOMA

Few studies have been published on the effects of hormone therapies on residual carcinoma cells. Godwin and Escher in 1941 reported that fibrosis and cytoplasmic vacuolation were seen in the breast tumors of patients treated with steroid hormones and noted that in some cases the features mimicked irradiation changes.[31] Emerson et al[32] described 'loosening' of the stroma surrounding the tumor cells often with an associated lymphoid and plasma cell infiltrate. Tumor cells underwent degenerative change and developed swollen, pale, vacuolated cytoplasm with pyknotic or karyolytic nuclei. Subsequent fibrosis occurred with 'elastic deposition' and finally formation of dense acellular scar tissue.[33]

EFFECTS ON OTHER ORGANS

Tamoxifen has an estrogenic effect on vaginal epithelium[34] and a stimulatory effect on the endometrium particularly if given in high doses. An association with endometrial polyps, hyperplasia, atypia and adenocarcinoma has been reported.[35–37] In a recent series 21% of asymptomatic postmenopausal breast cancer patients on tamoxifen treatment had endometrial lesions; 12% had 'simple' endometrial hyperplasia, 3% complex hyperplasia, 4% endometrial polyps and 2% had endometrial carcinoma.[38] In other series up to 35–39% of postmenopausal women on tamoxifen have developed pathological changes in the endometrium compared with 10–20% of control patients.[39–40] It therefore appears likely that in postmenopausal women tamoxifen acts as an estrogen agonist on the endometrium. A tendency for the incidence of endometrial pathology to increase with length of duration of tamoxifen therapy has also been reported; 31% of patients receiving tamoxifen for more than 4 years were found to have an endometrial pathology compared with 21% and 13% of women who had taken the drug for less than 2 years or 2 to 4 years respectively, although this did not reach statistical significance.[38]

One of the most common histological findings is the presence of endometrial polyps,[35] particularly in postmenopausal women;[41] these may have an unusual histological appearance with decidualization of the stroma.[42] Cohen et al found a decidual reaction in all 11 asymptomatic patients in their series who had received tamoxifen and progestogens for 3 months or longer;[43] one patient who had received treatment for only one month had atrophic endometrium on biopsy. Thus a combination of tamoxifen and progestogens for a length of time appears to result in decidualization of the endometrial stroma which may be seen in histological specimens.

Up to 16% of patients have developed atypical hyperplasia of the endometrium in some series[39] and there is now convincing evidence that tamoxifen treatment in patients with breast cancer is associated with an increased incidence of endometrial malignancy.[44–48] Accurate assessment of the degree of risk is difficult but in several series the relative risk of endometrial carcinoma has been reported to be doubled;[47] in a large case control study, for example, a relative risk of 2.3 was reported by Van Leuween et al.[46] Some studies have recorded an even greater relative risk of up to 6.4[45] although in others no increase in endometrial carcinoma has been found.[49–51]

Women receiving tamoxifen who acquire endometrial carcinomas may develop these more rapidly than a control population; some authors have suggested that these tumors are more often of high grade and a poor prognosis.[52] Conversely in a large multicenter study of 89 patients treated with tamoxifen who had developed endometrial cancer a high frequency of superficial and well differentiated tumors was found.[53] In other series the histopathological features of endometrial carcinomas of women on tamoxifen have not been significantly different from those in control patients.[47,54] Other authors have reported a higher than expected incidence of unusual histological forms of uterine tumors, including increased numbers of clear cell carcinomas, leiomyosarcomas of epithelioid and myxoid appearance and mixed Mullerian tumors in breast cancer patients receiving tamoxifen.[37,53,55–56]

It has been suggested that tamoxifen acts as a growth promoter of underlying endometrial disease[53] and it seems likely that both length of duration of treatment and the presence of pre-existing endometrial abnormalities may influence the incidence of endometrial pathology in breast cancer patients. In view of the increasing evidence of an association between duration of tamoxifen treatment and development of non-mammary carcinomas the National Cancer Institute in the USA has suggested that adjuvant tamoxifen therapy is not warranted for more than 5 years.[57–58]

Elsewhere in the female genital tract an increase in pathology has been reported in association with tamoxifen treatment; adenomyosis has been noted in up to 57% of postmenopausal women[59] and ovarian cysts are also common[60] in women receiving this therapy. Some authors have suggested that the incidence of ovarian tumors is higher in women receiving tamoxifen.[61]

SURGERY

Fibrous scarring after surgery and radiotherapy is seen in about one-quarter of women[62] and may mimic residual or recurrent carcinoma clinically and mammographically. Biopsy may be required to exclude malignancy although some authors suggest that fine needle aspiration cytology is cost effective and reliable in distinguishing scar tissue from carcinomatous foci within scar lesions.[63] As with radiotherapy, FNAC samples from residual carcinomatous foci are usually cellular with overtly malignant cells compared with smears from areas of fibrous scarring which are almost acellular, usually with a predominance of macrophages. Mammographic calcifications may be identified in patients who have had wide local excision of a primary breast carcinoma with subsequent radiotherapy. A high index of suspicion should be retained for new calcifications in the post-irradiated breast which are more often associated with residual or recurrent carcinoma than non-neoplastic irradiation changes.[64]

REFERENCES

1. Fajardo LF. Pathology of radiation injury. New York: Masson Publishing, 1982.
2. Clarke D, Curtis JL, Martinez A et al. Fat necrosis of the breast simulating recurrent carcinoma after primary radiotherapy in the management of early stage breast carcinoma. Cancer 1983; 52: 442–445.
3. Rostom AY, el-Sayed ME. Fat necrosis of the breast: an unusual complication of lumpectomy and radiotherapy in breast cancer. Clin Radiol 1987; 38: 31.
4. Girling AC, Hanby AM, Millis RR. Radiation and other pathological changes in breast tissue after conservation treatment for carcinoma. J Clin Pathol 1990; 43: 152–156.
5. Robertson JM, Clarke DH, Pevzner MM, Matter RC. Breast conservation therapy. Severe breast fibrosis after radiation therapy in patients with collagen vascular disease. Cancer 1991; 68: 502–508.
6. Fleck R, McNeese MD, Ellerbroek NA et al. Consequences of breast irradiation in patients with pre-existing collagen vascular disease. Int J Radiat Oncol Biol Phys 1989; 17: 829–833.
7. Schnitt SJ, Connolly JL, Harris JR, Cohen RB. Radiation-induced changes in the breast. Hum Pathol 1984; 15: 545–550.
8. Bondeson L. Aspiration cytology of radiation-induced changes of normal breast epithelium. Acta Cytol 1987; 31: 309–310.
9. Filomena CA, Jordan AG, Ehya H. Needle aspiration cytology of the irradiated breast. Diagn Cytopathol 1992; 8: 327–332.
10. Haagensen CD. Radiotherapy only for breast carcinoma. In: Haagensen CD, ed. Diseases of the breast. Philadelphia: WB Saunders, 1986; 954–975.
11. Amendola BE, Amendola MA, McClatchey KD, Miller C Jr. Radiation-associated sarcoma: a review of 23 patients with postradiation sarcoma over a 50-year period. Am J Clin Oncol 1989; 12: 411–415.
12. Taghian A, de Vathaire F, Terrier P et al. Long-term risk of sarcoma following radiation treatment for breast cancer. Int J Radiat Oncol Biol Phys 1991; 21: 361–367.
13. Clements WDB, Kirk SJ, Spence RAJ. A rare late complication of breast cancer treatment. Br J Clin Pract 1993; 47: 219–220.
14. Kiricuta IC, Dammrich J. Lymphangiosarcoma of arm after chronic lymphedema: a rare long-term complication after radical mastectomy in breast cancer patients. Case report and overview. Strahlenther Onkol 1993; 169: 291–295.
15. Wijnmaalen A, van Ooijen B, van Geel BN et al. Angiosarcoma of the breast following lumpectomy, axillary lymph node dissection, and radiotherapy for primary breast cancer: three case reports and a review of the literature. Int J Radiat Oncol Biol Phys 1993; 26: 135–139.
16. Taat CW, van Toor BS, Slors JF et al. Dermal angiosarcoma of the breast: a complication of primary radiotherapy? Eur J Surg Oncol 1992; 18: 391–395.
17. Kennedy S, Merino MJ, Swain SM, Lippman ME. The effects of hormonal and chemotherapy on tumoral and nonneoplastic breast tissue. Hum Pathol 1990; 21: 192–198.
18. Aktepe K, Kapucuoglu N, Pak I. The effects of chemotherapy on breast cancer tissue in locally advanced breast cancer. Histopathol 1996; 29: 63–67.
19. Rasbridge SA, Gillett CE, Seymour AM et al. The effects of chemotherapy on morphology, cellular proliferation, apoptosis and oncoprotein expression in primary breast carcinoma. Br J Cancer 1994; 70: 335–341.
20. Morrow M, Braverman A, Thelmo W et al. Multimodal therapy for locally advanced breast cancer. Arch Surg 1986; 121: 1291–1296.
21. Brifford M, Spyratos F et al. Sequential cytopunctures during preoperative chemotherapy for primary breast carcinoma. Cytomorphologic changes, initial tumor ploidy, and tumor regression. Cancer 1989; 63: 631–637.
22. Frierson HF, Fechner RE. Histologic grade of locally advanced infiltrating ductal carcinoma after treatment with induction chemotherapy. Am J Clin Pathol 1994; 102: 154–157.
23. Geller RB, Boone LB, Karp JE et al. Secondary acute myelocytic leukemia after adjuvant therapy for early-stage breast carcinoma. A new complication of cyclophosphamide, methotrexate, and 5-fluorouracil therapy. Cancer 1989; 64: 629–634.
24. Forbes JF. Long-term effects of adjuvant chemotherapy in breast cancer. Acta Oncol 1992; 31: 243–250.
25. La Francis IE, Cooper RB. Second primary malignancies associated with primary female breast cancer: a review of the Danbury Hospital experience. Conn Med 1992; 56: 411–414.
26. Doherty MA, Rodger A, Langlands AO, Kerr GR. Multiple primary tumours in patients treated with radiotherapy for breast cancer. Radiother Oncol 1993; 26: 125–131.
27. Mamounas EP, Perez-Mesa C, Penetrante RB, Driscoll DL, Blumenson LE, Tsangaris TN. Patterns of occurrence of second primary non-mammary malignancies in breast cancer patients: results from 1382 consecutive autopsies. Surg Oncol 1993; 2: 175–185.
28. Lee CG, McCormick B, Mazumdar M et al. Infiltrating breast carcinoma in patients age 30 years and younger: long term outcome for life, relapse, and second primary tumors. Int J Radiat Oncol Biol Phys 1992; 23: 969–975.
29. Parham DM, Robertson AJ, Guthrie W, Swanson Beck J. How fatal is breast cancer? A prospective study of breast carcinoma deaths in Tayside. Br J Cancer 1993; 67: 1086–1089.
30. Huseby RA, Thomas LB. Histological and histochemical alterations in the normal breast tissues of patients with advanced breast cancer being treated with estrogenic hormones. Cancer 1953; 7: 54–74.
31. Godwin JT, Escher G. Hormone treated primary operable breast carcinoma. A pathological study of 33 cases. Cancer 1951; 4: 136–140.
32. Emerson WJ, Kennedy BJ, Graham JN, Nathanson IT. Pathology of primary and recurrent carcinoma of the human breast after administration of steroid hormones. Cancer 1953; 6: 641–679.
33. Emerson WJ, Kennedy BJ, Taft EB. Correlation of histological alterations in breast cancer with response to hormone therapy. Cancer 1960; 13: 1047–1052.
34. Lahti E, Vuopala S, Kauppila A et al. Maturation of vaginal and endometrial epithelium in postmenopausal breast cancer patients receiving long-term tamoxifen. Gynecol Oncol 1994; 55: 410–414.

35. Lahti E, Blanco G, Kauppila A et al. Endometrial changes in postmenopausal breast cancer patients receiving tamoxifen. Obstet Gynecol 1993; 81: 660–664.

36. Uziely B, Lewin A, Brufman G et al. The effect of tamoxifen on the endometrium. Br Cancer Res Treat 1993; 26: 101–105.

37. Seoud MA, Johnson J, Weed JC Jr. Gynecologic tumors in tamoxifen-treated women with breast cancer. Obstet Gynecol 1993; 82: 165–169.

38. Cohen I, Altaras MM, Shapira J et al. Time-dependent effect of Tamoxifen therapy on endometrial pathology in asymptomatic postmenopausal breast cancer patients. Int J Gynecol Pathol 1996; 15: 152–157.

39. Kedar RP, Bourne TH, Powles TJ et al. Effects of tamoxifen on uterus and ovaries of postmenopausal women in a randomised breast cancer prevention trial. Lancet 1994; 343: 1318–1321.

40. Cohen I, Rosen DJ, Shapira J et al. Endometrial changes with tamoxifen: comparison between tamoxifen-treated and nontreated asymptomatic, postmenopausal breast cancer patients. Gynecol Oncol 1994; 52: 185–190.

41. McGonigle KF, Lantry SA, Odom Maryon TL et al. Histopathologic effects of tamoxifen on the uterine epithelium of breast cancer patients: Analysis by menopausal status. Cancer Letters 1996; 101: 59–66.

42. Corley D, Rowe J, Curtis MT et al. Postmenopausal bleeding from unusual endometrial polyps in women on chronic tamoxifen therapy. Obstet Gynecol 1992; 79: 111–116.

43. Cohen I, Figer A, Altaras MM et al. Common endometrial decidual reaction in postmenopausal breast cancer patients treated with tamoxifen and progestogens. Int J Gynecol Pathol 1996; 15: 17–22.

44. Robinson DC, Bloss JD, Schiano MA. A retrospective study of tamoxifen and endometrial cancer in breast cancer patients. Gynecol Oncol 1995; 59: 186–190.

45. Fornander T, Rutqvist LE, Cedermark B et al. Adjuvant tamoxifen in early breast cancer: occurrence of new primary cancers. Lancet 1989; 1: 117–120.

46. van Leeuwen FE, Benraadt J, Coebergh JW et al. Risk of endometrial cancer after tamoxifen treatment of breast cancer. Lancet 1994; 343: 448–452.

47. Fisher B, Costantino JP, Redmond CK et al. Endometrial cancer in tamoxifen-treated breast cancer patients: findings from the National Surgical Adjuvant Breast and Bowel Project (NSABP) B–14. J Natl Cancer Inst 1994; 86: 527–537.

48. Sasco AJ, Chaplain G, Amoros E, Saez S. Endometrial cancer following breast cancer: Effect of tamoxifen and castration by radiotherapy. Epidemiol 1996; 7: 9–13.

49. Neven P, de Muylder X, Van Belle Y et al. Tamoxifen and the uterus and endometrium. Lancet 1989; 1: 375–376.

50. 'Nolvadex' Adjuvant Trial Organisation. Controlled trial of tamoxifen as a single adjuvant agent in the management of early breast cancer. Br J Cancer 1988; 57: 608–611.

51. Ribeiro G, Swindell R. The Christie hospital adjuvant tamoxifen trial — status at 10 years. Br J Cancer 1988; 57: 601–603.

52. Magriples U, Naftolin F, Schwartz PE, Carcangiu ML. High-grade endometrial carcinoma in tamoxifen-treated breast cancer patients. J Clin Oncol 1993; 11: 485–490.

53. Mignotte H, Rodier JF, Lesur A et al. Endometrial carcinoma associated with adjuvant tamoxifen therapy for breast cancer: a French multi-centre analysis of 89 cases. Breast 1995; 4: 200–202.

54. Barakat RR, Wong G, Curtin JP et al. Tamoxifen use in breast cancer patients who subsequently develop corpus cancer is not associated with a higher incidence of adverse histologic features. Gynecol Oncol 1994; 55: 164–168.

55. Silva EG, Tornos CS, Follen-Mitchell M. Malignant neoplasms of the uterine corpus in patients treated for breast carcinoma: the effects of tamoxifen. Int J Gynecol Pathol 1994; 13: 248–258.

56. Sasco AJ, Raffi F, Satge D et al. Endometrial mullerian carcinosarcoma after cessation of tamoxifen therapy for breast cancer. Int J Gynecol Obstet 1995; 48: 307–310.

57. National Cancer Institute. Clinical announcement: adjuvant therapy of breast cancer — tamoxifen update. Cancer Net 1995.

58. Bulbrook RD. Long term adjuvant therapy for primary breast cancer. More than five years of tamoxifen is no longer justified. Br Med J 1996; 312: 389–390.

59. Cohen I, Beyth Y, Tepper R et al. Adenomyosis in postmenopausal breast cancer patients treated with tamoxifen: A new entity? Gynecol Oncol 1995; 58: 86–91.

60. Shushan A, Peretz T, Uziely B et al. Ovarian cysts in premenopausal and postmenopausal tamoxifen-treated women with breast cancer. Am J Obstet Gynecol 1996; 174: 141–144.

61. Cohen I, Beyth Y, Tepper R et al. Ovarian tumors in postmenopausal breast cancer patients treated with tamoxifen. Gynecol Oncol 1996; 60: 54–58.

62. Dershaw DD, Shank B, Reisinger S. Mammographic findings after breast cancer treatment with local excision and definitive irradiation. Radiol 1987; 164: 455–461.

63. Malberger E, Edoute Y, Toledano O, Sapir D. Fine-needle aspiration and cytologic findings of surgical scar lesions in women with breast cancer. Cancer 1992; 69: 148–152.

64. Solin LJ, Fowble BL, Troupin RH, Goodman RL. Biopsy results of new calcifications in the postirradiated breast. Cancer 1989; 63: 1956–1961.

Male breast disease

GENERAL INTRODUCTION

In Chapter 1 we pointed out that the breasts are modified apocrine sweat glands, which during childhood consist in both females and males of an insignificant nipple-areolar complex and an associated rudimentary branching duct system. Whilst the female breast undergoes major changes during puberty the male breast is non-functioning and retains its vestigial prepubertal structure in adulthood. Male breast is therefore composed of a small nipple areolar complex together with relatively few underlying ducts. These ducts correspond in general structure to the lactiferous ducts of the female breast, but are much shorter; they are lined by the characteristic bilayer of secretory and myoepithelial cells. The ducts are surrounded by dense connective tissue and small amounts of adipose tissue. Lobular structures do not normally develop in the male breast, even in men exposed to endogenous or exogenous hormonal stimulation. However, lobular structures have been described in gynecomastia[1-6] and in this situation some authors have ascribed their presence to estrogen therapy.[7-8] Furthermore, pathological lesions traditionally associated with an origin in lobules such as fibroadenoma, fibroadenomatoid hyperplasia, phyllodes tumor and lobular carcinoma in situ have all been recorded in males, albeit rather rarely.[4-5,9-12] Developmental abnormalities such as accessory nipples and breast tissue do occur in males, but are extremely uncommon.

Male breast lesions occur much less frequently than female breast disease. The two most common conditions are gynecomastia and carcinoma, but most entities which occur in the female breast, apart of course from lactational lesions, have been reported in males, on an anecdotal basis.

GYNECOMASTIA

INTRODUCTION

This term is derived from the Greek (gynos = woman, mastos = breast) and refers to the clinical finding of breast development more in keeping with the female than the male phenotype. It is a relatively common condition, but accurate estimates of the overall frequency are very difficult to obtain because of case selection bias — many men with breast enlargement simply do not consult a doctor. Even in autopsy studies, the reported frequency varies from 3 to 55%.[2,13–14] It has been estimated that the overall frequency in older men is about 30%.[15] Gynecomastia may occur at almost any age, but is most frequent during puberty and in men over 50 years. Transient neonatal breast enlargement is often seen in infants, but the nodules usually regress spontaneously over a few weeks and this physiological change hardly justifies use of the term gynecomastia. Prepubertal gynecomastia is rare, and in the majority of cases the cause is unknown.[16]

CLINICAL FEATURES

A mild degree of breast enlargement is encountered with surprising frequency in pubertal boys, typically between the ages of 12 and 16 years; Bannayan and Hajdu[1] give the frequency as 60–70% (although this appears to have been a selected series). It is usually bilateral and consists of an ill defined diffuse thickening which may be tender. One breast may be larger than the other. This type of gynecomastia is almost always transient and usually regresses within a year or two of onset. Occasionally the enlargement persists into adulthood but surgical intervention is rarely required.[17]

In adulthood breast hypertrophy occurs most frequently over the age of 50. It may appear to be unilateral on presentation, but in most cases bilateral masses eventually become apparent. There is usually a palpable mass beneath the areola, measuring from 2 to 5 cm in diameter. This may be soft or firm, well defined or diffuse and is not infrequently tender. The differential diagnosis is carcinoma of the breast, and in cases where the lesion is unilateral biopsy may be necessary to establish the correct diagnosis. This can be achieved using fine needle aspiration cytology or needle core biopsy (see Ch. 2).

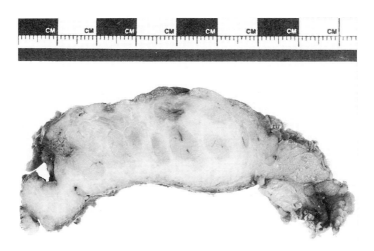

Fig. 21.1 Gynecomastia. This is the diffuse form in which there is an admixture of connective tissue stroma and adipose tissue.

MACROSCOPIC APPEARANCES

The gross appearances are rather non specific. In the more common diffuse form there is an ill defined greyish-white mass which merges with adjacent adipose tissue (Fig. 21.1). In more discrete forms there is a well defined circumscribed mass, which appears separate from the surrounding tissues.

MICROSCOPIC APPEARANCES

The histological appearances are variable, depending on the relative proportions of epithelial and stromal tissue. Two main patterns are seen, the so-called florid type in which there is an abundance of ductular structures and the fibrous type in which a rather acellular stroma dominates. It has been suggested that these patterns represent

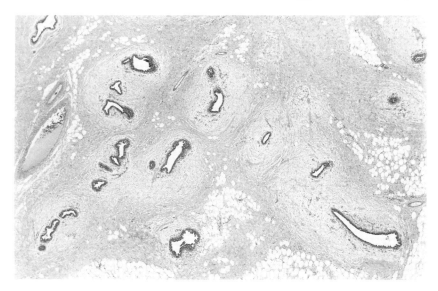

Fig. 21.2A   Gynecomastia, florid type. There is a proliferation of ducts and stroma intermingled with adipose tissue. Hematoxylin–eosin × 23.

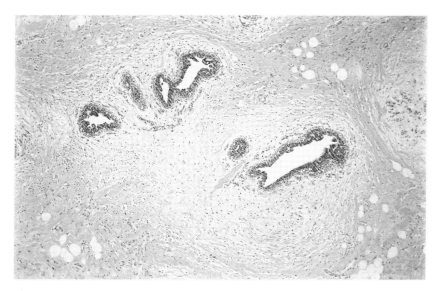

Fig. 21.2B   At this magnification the loose, cellular periductal connective tissue can be distinguished from the less cellular stroma in the background. Same case as Figure 21.2A. Hematoxylin–eosin × 57.

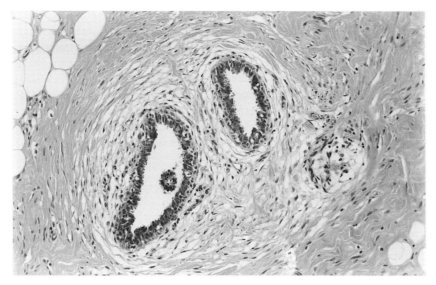

Fig. 21.2C   Higher magnification of another area from the same case as Figure 21.2A and B, to show the characteristic periductal stroma and ductal epithelial bilayer. Hematoxylin–eosin × 125.

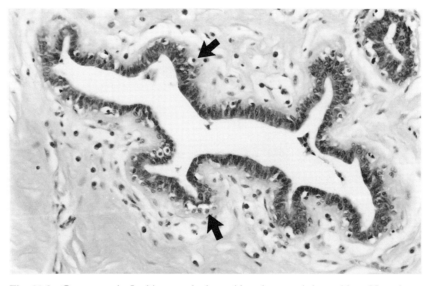

Fig. 21.3   Gynecomastia. In this example the periductal stroma is less evident. Note the outer layer of myoepithelial cells with clear cytoplasm (arrowheads). Hematoxylin–eosin × 185.

two ends of a temporal spectrum, with progression from the florid to the fibrous type as the lesion develops, even in those cases in which estrogen therapy is implicated,[1,18–19] and this view has become widely accepted.[20] However, following a study of over 100 cases of gynecomastia

Pages and Ramos[21] have refuted this claim, finding no correlation between morphological pattern and age of the patient or duration of the lesion, although the florid pattern was more frequently associated with estrogen therapy.

The florid type of gynecomastia is characterized by an increased number of irregularly branching ducts which are surrounded by a loose, cellular, periductal stromal connective tissue element (Fig. 21.2A, B and C). In routine hematoxylin and eosin sections the latter usually has a bluish tinge due to the presence of acidic mucosubstances. A variable amount of adipose tissue is present. The ducts are normally lined by the characteristic bilayer of epithelial and myoepithelial cells (Figs 21.2C, 21.3) but proliferation of the epithelial cells is common. This is usually of mild degree with small focal tufts (Fig. 21.4A and B) but in some cases appears florid, with distinct papillary projections (Fig. 21.5) which occasionally exhibit squamous metaplasia.[22] Florid epithelial hyperplasia may mimic the appearances of micropapillary ductal carcinoma in situ, but the papillary projections lack the bulbous nature of

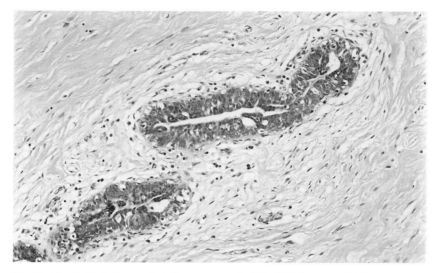

Fig. 21.4A   Epithelial hyperplasia in gynecomastia. This field shows a mild degree. Hematoxylin–eosin × 125.

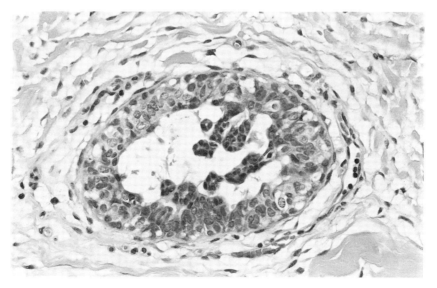

Fig. 21.4B   Another duct from the case shown in Figure 21.4A. Focal epithelial tufts are present. Hematoxylin–eosin × 400.

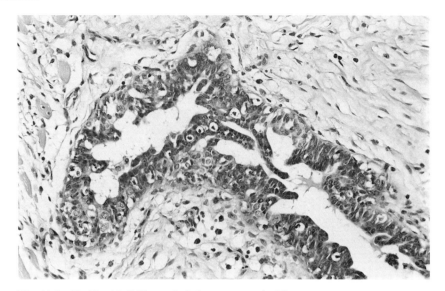

Fig. 21.5   Florid epithelial hyperplasia in gynecomastia. There are numerous micropapillary projections, but these appearances should not be mistaken for ductal carcinoma in situ. The epithelial proliferation lacks the appropriate monotony for such a diagnosis and the papillary tufts are composed of both epithelial and myoepithelial cells. Hematoxylin–eosin × 185.

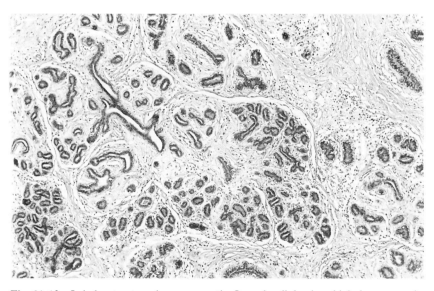

Fig. 21.6A   Lobular structures in gynecomastia. Several well developed lobules are seen in this field. Elsewhere the characteristic features of the florid type of gynecomastia were seen. Hematoxylin–eosin × 57.

the latter.[20] Atypical ductal hyperplasia is extremely rare, but examples are illustrated by Andersen and Gram[2] and Tavassoli.[6]

As noted earlier lobules are not normally found in the male breast, but have been described in gynecomastia (Figs 21.6A and B, 21.7). Estimates of the frequency vary widely, from less than 0.1%[1] in a large clinical series to 7% in an autopsy series.[7] They are said to be more common in the fibrous type than the florid type[20] but we

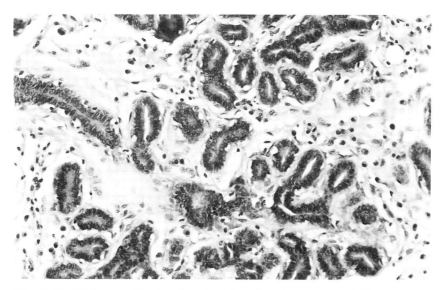

Fig. 21.6B   Higher magnification of another lobule from the case shown in Figure 21.6A. Hematoxylin–eosin × 185.

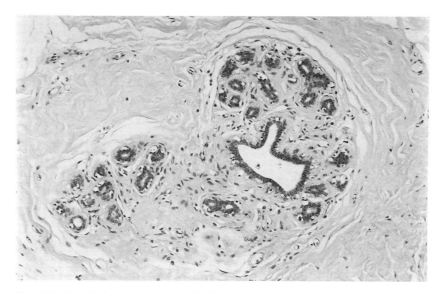

Fig. 21.7   Lobule from an example of the fibrous type of gynecomastia. Note the intralobular fibrosis. Hematoxylin–eosin × 125.

have seen lobular structures more often in the latter.

In the fibrous type of gynecomastia there are fewer ductal structures, and these are set in a sparsely cellular hyalinized stroma (Fig. 21.8A and B). Epithelial proliferation is usually less marked than in the florid type. Not surprisingly, in a minority of cases a mixed or intermediate morphological pattern may be seen, with features of both main types. In addition, other changes such as apocrine metaplasia[13,20] and fibrocystic change[23] have been described.

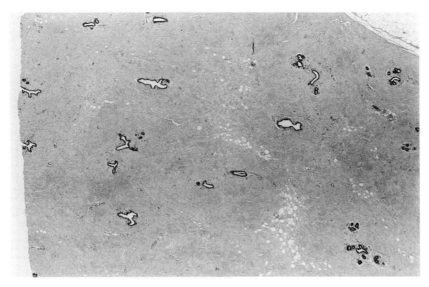

Fig. 21.8A   Gynecomastia, fibrous type. Widely dispersed ducts are separated by a dense fibrous stroma. Hematoxylin–eosin × 23.

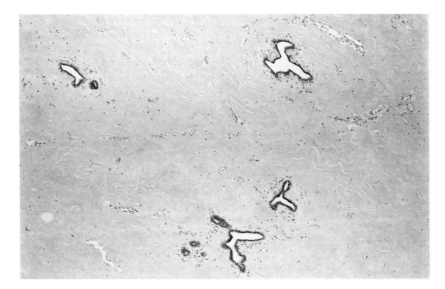

Fig. 21.8B   Higher magnification of field shown in Figure 21.8A. The stroma appears hyalinized and is relatively acellular. Hematoxylin–eosin × 57.

PATHOGENESIS

Gynecomastia is generally thought to represent a mammary response to estrogens, either due to excessive end organ sensitivity or because of absolute or relative hyperestrogenism. A large number of causal agents and diseases have been described in association with gynecomastia; these may be grouped under the general heading shown in Table 21.1. They are discussed in more detail elsewhere.[6,16]

In the relatively common pubertal and senescent gynecomastia no specific hormonal abnormality is found and this is, of course, also true for idiopathic gynecomastia.

Both estrogen and androgen therapy can cause

Table 21.1 Causal agents and diseases associated with gynecomastia

Endogenous hormonal imbalance
Puberty
Senescence

Exogenous hormonal therapy
Drugs
Neoplasms
Gonadal dysfunction
Systemic diseases
Idiopathic

gynecomastia. Clinically the most frequent example is stilbestrol therapy for prostatic carcinoma. The list of other drugs which have been implicated in the etiology of gynecomastia exceeds 50[6,16] and includes antihypertensive agents, cytotoxic agents, diuretics, narcotics and antidepressants. Drug-related gynecomastia is said to be more frequently unilateral than hormonally induced lesions.[1] It presents at variable times during therapy and usually regresses once the causative agent is discontinued.

Gynecomastia has been recorded with a number of hormone-producing benign and malignant neoplasms including Leydig cell tumors and germ cell tumors of testis, functional adrenal tumors, pituitary tumors and hepatoma.[6,20]

Gynecomastia is frequently associated with gonadal dysfunction, and is seen particularly in Klinefelter's syndrome (XXY).[15-16] Although Klinefelter's syndrome is also an uncommon risk factor for male breast cancer there appears to be no etiological connection with gynecomastia.

Finally, a wide range of systemic diseases are known on occasion to be associated with gynecomastia. These include cirrhosis of the liver, chronic renal failure, chronic lung disease and prolonged malnutrition.

DIFFERENTIAL DIAGNOSIS

Since the majority of male breast lesions present as a unilateral or bilateral mass the differential diagnosis covers the whole diagnostic spectrum. Preoperative fine needle aspiration cytology (FNAC) or needle core histology are useful in distinguishing benign from malignant lesions. For example, if gynecomastia is the most likely diagnosis on clinical grounds, a benign FNAC may obviate the need for excision biopsy.

Should excision biopsy prove necessary there are few serious diagnostic pitfalls. Simple obesity causing breast enlargement can be distinguished easily from gynecomastia by the abundant adipose tissue and absence of proliferation of ducts and stroma. Differentiation from the rare fibroadenoma and phyllodes tumor is discussed in the next section.

Differentiation of gynecomastia from invasive carcinoma is relatively straightforward. Although ductular structures may be small and compressed in the fibrous type, mimicking an infiltrative pattern, the presence of a bilayer of epithelial cells precludes a diagnosis of malignancy. The finding of florid ductular epithelial proliferation may pose more difficult problems in differentiation from ductal carcinoma in situ. Andersen and Gram[2,13] found atypical ductal hyperplasia (ADH) in 6.5% of cases of surgically resected gynecomastia and 7% in an autopsy series. They concluded that the clinical significance of ADH should not be overestimated. We agree with this cautious approach; in our experience DCIS is exceedingly rare in gynecomastia and should only be diagnosed when the morphological features are unequivocal.

PROGNOSIS AND MANAGEMENT

Gynecomastia is a benign, relatively common and often reversible enlargement of the male breast. Whilst its presence may cause embarrassment and psychological problems, treatment should still be relatively conservative. For example, patients with the transient gynecomastia of puberty may well require reassurance and counseling, but surgical intervention is rarely indicated. Similarly, if an underlying cause can be identified treatment of that condition may induce regression of the gynecomastia. Formal treatment of gynecomastia should be considered in idiopathic cases, when the underlying cause is not reversible, or where the condition is persistent or symptomatic.[16]

Medical treatment, which is in general effective, is based on drugs such as dihydrotestosterone, danazol and tamoxifen. They should probably only be used in selected cases, and benefits need to be balanced against side-effects.

Surgical excision is mainly indicated in the older age group, particularly when the lesion is unilateral and there is a clinical suspicion of carcinoma.

FIBROADENOMA AND RELATED LESIONS

Biphasic lesions such as fibroadenoma and phyllodes tumor are extremely rare in the male breast, and have usually been reported solely on an anecdotal basis. Indeed Page and colleagues[20] stated categorically that true fibroadenoma had not been documented in the male breast. He pointed out that gynecomastia may bear a superficial resemblance to fibroadenoma, and Tavassoli[6] has noted that in some reports in the older literature the terms were often used synonymously. The main reason given for the rarity of fibroadenoma in the male breast is the absence in the normal breast of lobular structures referred to previously.

The most convincing cases in the literature are from recent reports. Nielsen[5] has described a single case in a 69-year-old male who had been on long term digoxin therapy and spironolactone for 4 years. He developed bilateral gynecomastia and on histological examination definite lobular struc-tures were observed. Throughout both breasts there were multiple firm nodules which had the histological structure of fibroadenomas. Because many of these were confluent Nielsen used the term 'fibroadenomatoid hyperplasia' to describe the lesion, following the terminology suggested by Symmers.[24] Since the breast enlargement did not commence until the spironolactone therapy began he suggested that the drug was the most likely causative agent. Tavassoli[6] has recorded a further seven examples of male fibroadenoma taken from the files of the Armed Forces Institute of Pathology, four of which had been reported separately.[12] The age range was 19–79 years, and four were over 50. The ethnic origin of three patients was Japanese. One patient was receiving hormone therapy for carcinoma of the prostate, and another had been on antihypertensive agents for several years; in both cases there was a background of gynecomastia with lobule formation. We have encountered a single case of fibroadenoma in the male breast (Fig. 21.9A and B). The patient was aged 23 years and no predisposing factors were identified. He presented with unilateral breast enlargement.

Phyllodes tumor has been observed rather more frequently than fibroadenoma in the male, but the total number of cases in the literature is

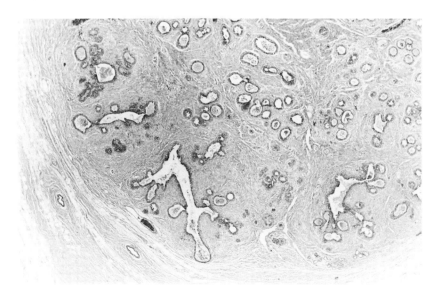

Fig. 21.9A Fibroadenoma. The lesion measures 1.5 cm in diameter and is sharply circumscribed. The changes of gynecomastia were present in the adjacent breast tissue, forming an overall mass 8 cm in maximum diameter. Hematoxylin–eosin × 23.

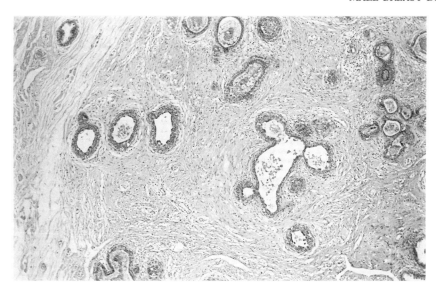

Fig. 21.9B   Higher magnification of lesion shown in Figure 21.9A. The pattern is predominantly pericanalicular, with focal dilatation of ductal structures. Hematoxylin–eosin × 57.

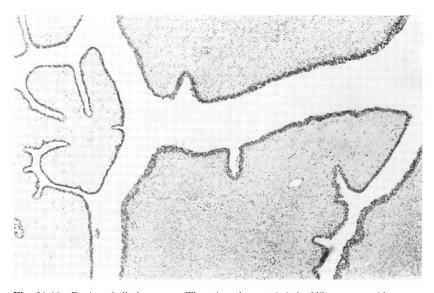

Fig. 21.10   Benign phyllodes tumor. There is a characteristic leaf-like pattern with cellular stroma. Elsewhere in the lesion the appearances resembled a cellular fibroadenoma. Hematoxylin–eosin × 50. (Reproduced from Histopathology with permission from Dr D Hilton and Professor R N M MacSween (ed).)

still less than 12.[4,6,11–12,25] The age range is 15–74 years, with most patients in the older age group. In the majority of cases there is associated gyneco-mastia, often with lobule formation. All the lesions showed appearances indistinguishable from phyllodes tumor in the female, although in

the case reported by Hilton and colleagues[11] in a 15-year-old boy there was a mixed pattern, some areas resembling a cellular fibroadenoma and others showing the leaf-like structure of a benign phyllodes tumor (Fig. 21.10). One of the two cases reported by Tavassoli[6] appears to have behaved as a malignant tumor, with multiple recurrences; no other malignant cases have been recorded.

As noted above these biphasic lesions must be distinguished morphologically from gynecomastia. Their relative circumscription and organized structure are features in favor of fibroadenoma and phyllodes tumor.

CARCINOMA OF THE MALE BREAST

INTRODUCTION

Male breast carcinoma (MBC) is uncommon. Tavassoli[6] quoted figures from the American Cancer Society indicating that 1000 new cases are diagnosed annually in the United States, with approximately 300 deaths each year, whilst Ribiero[26] gave a mortality figure for the United Kingdom of approximately 90 per year. It has long been the received wisdom that males account for approximately 1% of all breast carcinomas[6,26–27] although higher figures have been quoted, including 2.4% by Norris and Taylor.[28] The data on which these figures are based should be interpreted with caution as they are often derived from retrospective analysis of cases from tertiary referral centers. In fact, modern studies show that male breast cancer is even rarer than previously assumed, probably of the order of 0.5 to 0.8%.[29–32] In a comprehensive retrospective study in Nottingham for the 20 years 1974–1994 only 43 cases of male breast cancer were identified;[33] during the same period over 6000 females presented as new cases.

It has also become generally accepted that MBC affects an older population, presents late and is frequently fatal,[27] although the morphological characteristics of the tumors are little different from those seen in women.

CLINICAL FEATURES

Male breast cancer may occur at any age from childhood to extreme old age; the reported range is 12 years to 96 years, with a mean of 60–65 years.[6,26–27,30–31,33–38] This mean age at presenta-

tion is approximately 10 years later in males than in females.[26,34]

The great majority of patients (over 80%) present with a unilateral palpable breast lump, which is not surprising in view of the small size of the male breast.[26–27,33] In a minority (less than 10%) the presenting sign is a nipple abnormality, usually a sero-sanguinous discharge and, rarely, eczema due to Paget's disease. Breast pain is an uncommon symptom. Synchronous bilateral disease appears to be extremely rare; a figure of 1.4% is cited by Borgen et al[34] but this may reflect selection bias (bilateral cancers are more likely to be reported than unilateral cancers, unless the study is genuinely community based). The average time from the onset of symptoms to clinical presentation appears to be shortening. Borgen et al[34] noted that prior to 1950 the average delay was 18 months, whilst in their own series this had reduced to 18 weeks. Our own experience is in keeping with the latter figure, with an average duration of 6 months (range 1 week–3 years).[33]

MACROSCOPIC APPEARANCES

Not surprisingly the majority of male breast carcinomas are situated in the subareolar region. There is little difference in gross features from tumors in the female. Invasive carcinomas usually form a hard, irregular stellate mass, often with associated yellow streaks indicating an in situ component. They vary in size from under 1 cm to over 5 cm, with a mean of 2–2.5 cm. Because of the small size of the breast, larger tumors tend to invade into skin and underlying pectoral muscle. There may be associated indrawing of the nipple and, rarely, Paget's disease of the nipple is present. Pure in situ carcinoma is uncommon. The lesion is less obvious grossly than invasive carcinoma, with an ill defined area of thickening in which yellow streaks may be visible.

MICROSCOPIC APPEARANCES

In published series the vast majority of invasive carcinomas have been shown to be of no special type (ductal NST); figures quoted range from

Table 21.2 Histological tumor type in male breast carcinoma

Type	Series						
	Norris and Taylor 1969[28]	Visfeldt and Scheike 1973[8]	Heller et al 1978[39]	Cutuli et al 1991[40]	Borgen et al 1992[34]	Gough et al 1993[27]	Willsher et al 1996[38]
Pure DCIS	8 (7%)	0	4 (4%)	15 (3.7%)	16 (14%)	3 (2.5%)	2 (5%)
Ductal NST	84 (74%)	157 (88%)	68 (70%)	356 (88%)	87 (82%)[c]	116 (94%)[e]	37 (86%)
Infiltrating lobular	0	0	0	0	0	1	0
Medullary	0	4	0	0	} 2	0	0
Tubular/Cribriform	1[a]	5	1	0		0	0
Mucinous	1	5	1	0	0	1	0
Tubular mixed	0	0	0	0	0	0	1
NST/Special type	0	0	0	0	0	0	3
Papillary	9	5	4[d]	9	0	2	0
Miscellaneous	10	3[b]	19[f]	24	1	1	0
Total	113	179	97	404	106	124	43

[a]Termed 'well-differentiated'.
[b]Paget's disease of nipple not otherwise specified.
[c]Includes 51 cases of ductal NST + DCIS.
[d]Intracystic.
[e]Includes four cases of Paget's disease and one ductal NST + DCIS.
[f]Not reviewed.

75% to 97%[8,20,27–28,34,38–40] (Table 21.2) with the majority at the upper end of that range. Morphologically these tumors have the same characteristics as seen in the female, with an infiltrative structure of sheets and trabeculae of tumor cells set within a connective tissue stroma. All other morphological types which are found in the female also occur in males, but are uncommon. Infiltrating lobular carcinoma is particularly rare, perhaps related to the lack of normal lobules in the male breast and in several large series no cases were identified (Table 21.2). In 1982 Schwartz[41] noted that eight previous cases of small cell carcinoma of the male breast had been reported in the literature and included one of his own; he considered these to be examples of infiltrating lobular carcinoma. Perhaps the first unequivocal case, with associated lobular carcinoma in situ (LCIS), was reported by Sanchez and colleagues[9] in a man with Klinefelter's syndrome. Since then only three further cases have been reported, two as single case reports[10,42] and one as part of a large series;[27] all three patients were genetically normal. Medullary and special type carcinomas (tubular, invasive cribriform, mucinous) are also rare (Table 21.2).[43] We encountered no medullary or pure special type cases in our own series[38] although there was one tubular mixed carcinoma and the three mixed ductal NST/special type cases had a mucinous element (Fig. 21.11A and B). Argyrophilia has

been reported in a relatively high proportion of cases (21%) in a series of 134 male breast carcinomas.[44] There was ultrastructural evidence of dense core granulation and positive immunostaining for chromogranin was found in 60% of cases. However, no correlation with prognosis was established and the relevance of the diagnosis of argyrophilic carcinoma must therefore remain in doubt. Other, rare histological types which have been described include apocrine, adenoid cystic and secretory carcinoma.[45–50]

Formal histological grading has been carried out in only a limited number of studies (Table 21.3). No consistent pattern is seen, but the number of cases studied is relatively small and the results should be interpreted with caution since

Table 21.3 Histological grade in male breast carcinoma

Series	Grade %			
	1	2	3	No. in study
Visfeld and Scheike, 1973[8]	29	54	17	150
Lundy et al, 1986[51]	2	7	6	15
Hultborn, Friberg and Hultborn, 1987[30–31]	19	49	32	143
Gough et al, 1993[27,a]	2	10	81[b]	124
Rogers, Day and Fox, 1993[52]	14	62	24	21
Cutuli et al, 1995[36]	20	58	22	223
Payne et al, 1995[54]	12	28	60	30
Willsher et al, 1996[38]	2	27	70	41

[a]7% ungraded.
[b]Grades 3 and 4 — method not specified.

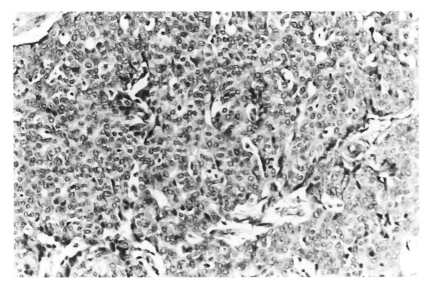

Fig. 21.11A   Invasive carcinoma of mixed ductal NST and mucinous type. This field shows the NST pattern. Hematoxylin–eosin × 125.

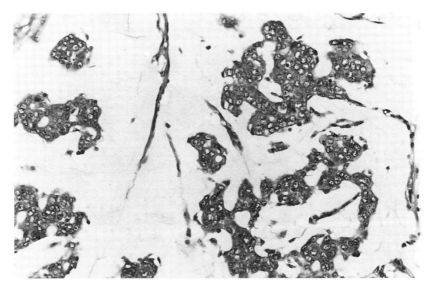

Fig. 21.11B   In this field from the same tumor as that shown in Figure 21.11A, islands and trabeculae are seen within a fibrillary mucinous 'lake'. Hematoxylin–eosin × 125.

the methods used have varied or, in some cases, have not been specified. In the largest study to date Visfeldt and Scheike[8] found that 29% of infiltrating ductal carcinomas were grade 1, whilst only 17% were grade 3. A similar relatively low percentage of high grade tumors has been obtained by several other groups.[30–31,40,51–52] In complete contrast a number of studies recently have shown a much higher proportion of poorly differentiated tumors with very few low grade carcinomas.[27,38,53–54] It is difficult to explain this marked discrepancy in view of the close similarity between the studies in the percentage of ductal NST carcinomas. Our figure of 70% grade 3 carcinomas is considerably higher than that reported for female breast carcinoma; in the large

Nottingham Tenovus Primary Breast Carcinoma Study 47% of cases were grade 3.[55]

In common with females pure ductal carcinoma in situ (DCIS) is observed in the male, although the reported frequency varies markedly, from 2.5% to 14% (Table 21.2). This almost certainly reflects differences in selection of cases between different series; in the majority of studies the frequency is between 3 and 8%. Cutuli and colleagues[35,56] state that in their study DCIS occurs at an earlier average age than invasive carcinoma (mean of 55 years compared with 63 years). All the usual morphological subtypes of DCIS are found although Cutuli et al[56] noted that a papillary pattern, either intraductal or intracystic, predominated. According to Tavassoli[6] over 50 cases of Paget's disease of the nipple have been recorded in males. Diagnostic problems may be encountered with the distinction from malignant melanoma, and, as in the female,[57] immunostaining with antibodies to cytokeratins are useful in confirming the correct diagnosis.[58] It appears that in the majority of cases there is an underlying invasive carcinoma as well as DCIS[27,30–31,39,58–59] and the prognosis is correspondingly poor.

PATHOGENESIS

The precise etiology of male breast cancer is unknown and for the great majority of cases no underlying predisposing factors can be identified. However, a number of potential risk factors have been identified and these are discussed briefly below.

Hyperestrogenism has been implicated theoretically by some authors[60] but the actual evidence is rather scanty and imprecise.[27] There is certainly no convincing data to suggest that exogenous estrogen, given for examples as therapy in prostatic carcinoma, is a predisposing factor. Klinefelter's syndrome is, however, a definite risk factor;[61–63] it has been estimated that the risk for development of breast cancer is increased 20-fold compared with normal males.[64]

The data concerning gynecomastia as a risk factor for male breast carcinoma are conflicting. As stated previously, gynecomastia is a relatively common phenomenon, and yet Crichlow,[65] in a review of 625 cases of MBC in the literature, found an association between the two in only 17 (3%). In contrast, Scheike and Visfeldt[64] in a study based on the Danish Cancer Registry, were able to establish the presence of histologically confirmed gynecomastia in 21 out of 187 cases of MBC (11%). They concluded that gynecomastia may be a premalignant state. More recently Rose[60] found a reported range of 2.7 up to 27%, but in many of the studies the diagnosis of gynecomastia was made on clinical grounds only, and the significance of the findings must be in doubt. At the present time it would appear that these associations are not sufficiently strong to implicate gynecomastia as a precursor lesion in male breast cancer.[61,63]

Although familial factors have not in general been regarded as contributory in male breast cancer there is increasing evidence of their importance in a minority of cases. In Crichlow's[65] review there were 10 cases of breast cancer in female blood relatives of 79 patients with MBC, but none were first degree and he felt that the data were of doubtful significance. Several anecdotal examples of an association in first degree male relatives were cited in the report by Schwartz et al[66] of MBC in father and son. In 1986 Kozak and colleagues[67] reported MBC in an uncle and nephew, and found 12 other cases in related males. In addition, there was a family history of breast cancer in first or second degree female relatives in 60% of the cases. More recently Borgen and colleagues,[34] reporting on 104 patients from two centers, one in New York and one in New Orleans, USA, found that 14% of their cases of MBC had a first degree and 9% had a second degree relative with breast cancer. These figures seem rather high, as does the rather non-specific report from Gough et al[27] that approximately 25% of 124 patients with MBC gave a family history of breast cancer. These latter two reports should be treated with some caution as case selection bias is almost certainly a factor in the associations recorded.

Prior radiation exposure has also been recorded on an anecdotal basis as a risk factor. Crichlow[65] found five cases in the literature, the carcinoma usually developing many years after the radiation therapy. By 1989 Eldar and colleagues,[68] reporting a case of encysted papillary carcinoma which occurred 30 years after radiation for keloid scars, could only find a total of 10 other reported cases. They concluded that although there are too few cases of MBC associated with prior irradiation to draw firm conclusions the risk is probably similar to that reported in females.

DIFFERENTIAL DIAGNOSIS

The main clinical differential diagnosis is clearly gynecomastia, and this has been discussed previously (p. 478). Little difficulty should be experienced at a histological level in distinguishing MBC from gynecomastia or the rarer fibro-adenoma and phyllodes tumor.

In cases in which there is no doubt that the lesion in the breast is malignant the possibility of a metastasis should always be considered. The most frequent metastatic tumors in the male breast are prostate, lung, kidney and malignant lymphoma. Metastatic prostatic carcinoma may cause the greatest diagnostic difficulty, as the cribriform and glandular pattern may mimic a breast primary. In most cases this problem can be resolved by the use of immunostaining for specific prostatic markers (prostate specific antigen — PSA; prostate specific acid phosphatase — PSAP). Similarly, malignant lymphoma and leukemic infiltrates can be distinguished from poorly differentiated carcinoma with differential immunostaining for lymphoid and epithelial markers.

PROGNOSIS AND MANAGEMENT

Mortality

It has long been the received wisdom that male breast cancer has a worse prognosis than breast cancer in females;[28,69–71] much of the data are reviewed by Tavassoli.[6] Erlichman et al[70] found an actuarial 5-year disease-free survival of 45%, whilst the overall 5- and 10-year survival rates in the series from Spence et al[71] were 38 and 17% respectively; similar figures (46 and 29%) were obtained by Scheike.[69] A number of reasons have been proposed for the apparent differences in survival, including the later age of onset and more advanced stage at presentation in males. However, as we have noted before, many of the published studies of MBC are based on relatively small numbers of cases, often from tertiary referral centers (with the attendant likelihood of case selection bias), and no attempts were made to match series of male and female breast cancer for age, stage and other known prognostic factors. There is increasing evidence that when such factors are taken into account breast cancer in males carries a very similar prognosis to female breast cancer although reported survival rates vary considerably.[33–34,37–38,61,72] Heller et al[39] compared 5- and 10-year survival rates in 97 males with an earlier experience in females reported by the same group.[73] No difference was found at 5 years, but at 10 years the overall survival rate was only 40% in the men compared with 62% in the women. Interestingly, the difference in survival was limited to patients with stage 2 node positive disease. In their recent joint study from New Orleans and New York Borgen and colleagues[34] found that the overall 5-year survival for their series of 104 patients with MBC of 85%, was not significantly different from that reported for females undergoing mastectomy in the National Surgical Adjuvant Breast Project (NSABP) B-06 trial of 76%.[74] Ten-year data were not supplied. Guinee and colleagues[37] have carried out an even wider collaborative evaluation of prognosis in MBC involving 335 patients from 11 different centers throughout the world. Survival rates at 10 years were 84% for patients with histologically negative lymph nodes, 44% for those with 1 to 3 positive nodes and 14% for the group with 4 or more positive nodes. Using historical published data for females they concluded that there is no difference in prognosis between males and females with breast cancer when compared on the basis of histological lymph node involvement.

In Nottingham we have taken a rather different approach.[33] For each of the 41 male patients with invasive breast carcinoma three female patients were matched for age, pathological tumor size, histological grade and histological lymph node stage. The groups were also matched for date of diagnosis in order to allow for any potential impact of changing therapy over the 20 years period on which the study was based. We found a closely similar actuarial outcome between males and females in terms of both disease-free interval and overall survival when matched in this way.

In summary, the majority of modern studies indicate that there is no intrinsic difference in overall survival between males and females with breast cancer when known prognostic factors are taken into consideration. Previously perceived differences may be due to the inclusion of more patients of advanced stage and poorer histological grade in MBC series.

Prognostic factors

The traditional pathological prognostic factors (see Ch. 18) have a similar validity in male breast cancer to female breast cancer, with certain reservations referred to below.

Pathological tumor size has been confirmed in a substantial number of studies to provide independent prognostic information.[27,30–31,34,37–38,75] As expected, the larger the tumor the worse the prognosis.

Histological type in MBC, however, does not provide useful discriminatory information. This is due to the fact that the great majority of cases of MBC are of ductal NST type, with very few special type cases of more favorable prognosis (Table 21.2). Indeed, so few cases with special type features, such as tubular carcinoma, have been reported that their prognostic significance in MBC is impossible to assess.

In contrast histological grade has been shown to be a useful prognostic factor in a number of studies, despite considerable variation in the proportion of grades from series to series.[8,27,30–31,38,53–54] As expected prognosis is poorer in the higher histological grades, although in the study of Gough et al[27] this effect was only seen for disease-free interval. In distinction from the studies above Cunha et al[75] could find no significant association between histological grade and prognosis, but the number of cases studied, 44, was small and the method used, that of Bloom and Richardson,[76] known to be suboptimal.

Not surprisingly the most powerful traditional factor is lymph node stage, assessed histologically,[27,30–31,34,37–39] and the effect is closely similar to that in females. For most studies the long term survival for patients with histologically negative nodes is in excess of 75% whilst progressive node involvement reduces survival to less than 20% for four or more nodes involved.

Biological prognostic factors known to have some prognostic significance in female breast cancer have also been studied in male breast cancer. Both estrogen receptor protein (ER) and progesterone receptor protein (PR) have been identified in a high proportion of MBC, using the dextran coated charcoal method (DCC), enzyme-linked immunoabsorbent assay (ELISA) and immunostaining (ERICA).[26,33–34,38,52–54,77–78] Most studies have reported that ER is expressed in at least 80% of MBC and PR in up to 75% of cases, considerably in excess of the figures for female breast cancer. To date no entirely convincing explanation has been advanced for this difference. It may be related to the relative lack of exposure to endogenous estrogens or the older age group for MBC. There is little evidence that hormone receptor status has utility as a prognostic factor in MBC[34,38,52–53] although ER status is being used increasingly to select patients for hormone therapy such as tamoxifen.[34,79]

In contrast with female breast cancer there have been very few studies of proliferative activity in MBC to date, probably because until very recently the best antibody, Ki-67, which detects a nuclear antigen expressed in proliferating cells, was only effective on frozen sections.[80–81] The new monoclonal antibody, MIB-1, which was raised against recombinant parts of the Ki-67 antigen, has the considerable advantage that it can be used on paraffin sections from formalin fixed material following heat enhanced antigen retrieved (usually by microwave).[82] Using the median value for the percentage of cells exhibiting positive nuclear staining, 23.5, Pich and colleagues[53] found a significant correlation with overall survival, in a series comprising only 27 patients. Interestingly they found no significant correlation between MIB-1 expression and histological grade, although the latter correlated with survival. In the only other study to date Willsher and colleagues[38] obtained slightly different results, possibly because they used positivity or negativity of expression for the cut-off point, rather than the median value. There was a significant correlation with histological grade, but only a trend towards significance with overall survival. Such differences are almost certainly due to the small number of cases examined in each series. Further studies are clearly required.

Expression of epithelial mucin antigens (EMA) has been shown to provide prognostic information in female breast cancer.[83–84] Using the same antibody, NCRC-II, we obtained a very similar staining pattern in MBC to that in females,[38] with an overall positive expression of 78%. Unfortunately, there were insufficient cases to carry out subgroup analysis for survival studies. Similar results were obtained by Lundy and colleagues[51] using the antibody DF 3 which has its epitope on the same Mucin 1 molecule as NCRC-II.

There have been relatively few studies of the expression of c-erbB-2 in MBC. Three have shown relatively high levels of positive staining of over 40%.[38,54,85] Our own figure of 45% is considerably higher than that obtained in our series of female breast cancer,[86] probably because of the large number of high grade tumors in the males. In one series,[87] rather surprisingly, no c-erbB-2 expression was found in 21 cases of MBC and further studies are required to evaluate this discrepancy. None of the studies has shown c-erbB-2 to be a significant prognostic factor in MBC.

It is difficult to assess the role of growth factors in MBC. In one study of 21 cases, 76% showed positive Epidermal Growth Factor Expression (EGFR)[77] whilst a much lower figure, 20%, was obtained in our own series of 41 patients.[38] We found no correlation with prognosis, but without providing survival data and ignoring the fact that over 80% of their cases were ER positive, Fox et al[77] speculated that the high percentage of cases expressing EGFR in their study might explain the poor prognosis of MBC.

To date two studies have evaluated the tumor supressor gene p53 in MBC. Both obtained just over 50% positivity,[38,54] a slightly higher figure than that found in females.[88] In our study there was a non-significant trend towards an association with survival,[38] but more data are required to evaluate the clinical relevance of this association.

In summary, the traditional pathological prognostic factors for female breast cancer, such as tumor size, histological grade and lymph node stage, have similar validity in MBC. With the exception of ER status which may prove useful in stratification of patients for hormonal therapy, there is insufficient available data to make a judgment on the value of biological markers of prognosis, although assessment of both proliferative activity using MIB-1 and expression of the tumor suppressor gene p53 show some promise.

Management

In many centers the management of male breast cancer is very similar to that in females,[26–27,33–34] although protocols may vary slightly. Primary surgery is usually some form of mastectomy, with a trend towards a simple rather than a radical operative technique. Conservation surgery is less of an option in MBC than in females because of the small size of the breast, and the acknowledged importance of obtaining complete local excision. Postoperative radiotherapy to skin flaps and axilla is usually given for patients with axillary node involvement. Primary radiotherapy is the preferred option for patients with locally advanced tumors.

Although in some centers tamoxifen has been given to all stage 2 and 3 patients[26] there is an increasing tendency, as in females, to base systemic therapy on hormone receptor expression, reserving adjuvant hormone therapy for patients whose tumors are ER positive.[34] The role of adjuvant and secondary cytotoxic therapy is less certain as so few studies have been carried out. However, it is likely that protocols will, in future, follow those for female breast cancer.[34] We have suggested that, since the biological behavior of MBC is closely similar to female breast cancer, prognostic factors such as those which form the Nottingham Prognostic Index should be used to select patients for appropriate therapy.[33,38]

MISCELLANEOUS LESIONS

It will be appreciated from the previous sections that, apart from gynecomastia, male breast disease is relatively uncommon. Nevertheless the spectrum of lesions which occurs in the female is generally recapitulated in the male, albeit as rare examples presented in anecdotal case reports. They can be considered broadly in two groups, epithelial and mesenchymal.

EPITHELIAL

Because the male breast normally lacks lobules fibrocystic change is exceedingly rare. McClure and colleagues[23] reported the case of a 28-year-old male in whom unilateral gynecomastia was associated with lobule formation and fibrocystic change. The latter displayed apocrine metaplasia and florid epithelial hyperplasia of usual type including papillary structures. Banik and Hale[89] described a case of fibrocystic change in an even younger male (21 years) with no evidence of associated gynecomastia. Apocrine change and florid epithelial hyperplasia of papillary pattern were dominant features and the cystic collections had an apparent lobular morphology.

Sclerosing adenosis has been reported as an incidental finding at autopsy in a 41-year-old male who died from small cell carcinoma of bronchus.[90] The lesion was associated with lobular structures and the authors speculated that ectopic hormone production by the bronchial primary may have been a predisposing factor.

Waldo and colleagues[91] described an example of adenoma of the nipple in an 83-year-old male who had received diethylstilbestrol therapy over 10 years for prostatic carcinoma. From a review of the literature they concluded that this was the seventh such case reported in males at that time. The authors speculated that in their case the nipple lesion may have been induced by the hormone therapy. Benign ductal papillomas are also known to occur in the male breast. The lesion reported by Sara and Gotfried was found in a 71-year-old male who had received phenothiazine therapy for 10 years.[92]

Several cases of mammary duct ectasia with periductal mastitis have been reported in the male.[93–94] The patients have been over 45 years in age and all presented with a tender breast mass. Histologically the appearances were identical to those seen in the female, with markedly dilated ducts containing foamy macrophages and periductal inflammation and fibrosis.

MESENCHYMAL

Mesenchymal tumors are particularly uncommon in males. The most frequent is a benign spindle cell tumor designated as a myofibroblastoma by Wargotz and colleagues.[95] They searched the files of the Armed Forces Institute of Pathology for all mesenchymal lesions of the breast. From a total of 230 cases they found 16 with the same morphological features, 11 of which had occurred in males. Since then other series have shown a female predominance[96–97] and it is probable that they occur with equal frequency in men and women. The tumors are nodular in outline and well demarcated from the surrounding breast tissue. They rarely exceed 3 cm in maximum diameter although Ali and colleagues[98] have reported giant myofibroblastoma in a male of over 80 which measured 10 cm. Microscopically they are composed of bundles and sheets of plump, bipolar spindle cells arranged in fascicular clusters separated by broad bands of collagen, which is often hyalinized. In the majority of cases the spindle cells are regular in appearance and mitoses are rare. On ultrastructural examination Wargotz et al[95] considered that the majority of spindle cells were myofibroblastic in origin and this has also been shown by Ali et al.[98] Most studies have found positive immunostaining for desmin and/or smooth muscle actin[95–97,99] and the general consensus has been that myofibroblastoma is the correct designation for these lesions. Hamele-Bena et al[97] have gone a step further and suggested that myofibroblastoma and pseudoangiomatous stromal hyperplasia (PASH) represent, respectively, localized and diffuse benign tumors of myofibroblastic origin. However, Begin[100] in a single case report has drawn slightly different conclusions. He considered the majority of cells to be fibroblastic on ultrastructural examination, with a minority of smooth muscle cells and no myofibroblasts. Desmin and muscle-specific actin immunostaining was present in approximately 50 and 20% of the cell population respectively. On this basis Begin[100] has suggested that the designation of myogenic stromal tumor is more appropriate. We have seen two examples of this entity in our consultation practice, one in a female and one in a male (Fig. 21.12A–D). In all cases recorded to

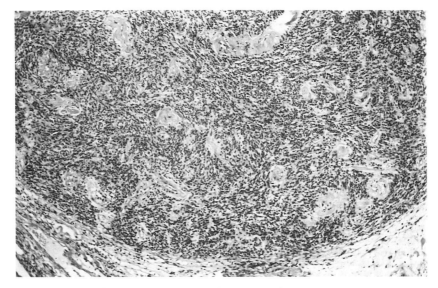

Fig. 21.12A   Myofibroblastoma. The lesion has a well defined, nodular outline, with a fasciculated structure. From an 84-year-old man who presented with a painless swelling in one breast. (Reproduced with permission from Dr Jane Armes.) Hematoxylin–eosin × 57.

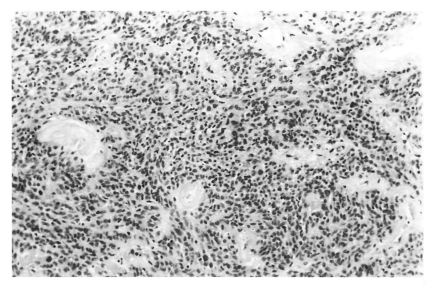

Fig. 21.12B   In this field there are bundles of plump spindle cells with intervening collagen bands. Same case as Figure 21.12A. Hematoxylin–eosin × 100.

date excision has been curative with no recurrences or metastases.

Other benign mesenchymal lesions recorded in the male breast have included nerve sheath tumors,[101–102] hemangiomas,[6,103] hemangiopericytoma[104] and adenomyoepithelioma.[105]

Malignant mesenchymal tumors appear to be extremely rare in the male breast. Anecdotally, leiomyosarcoma,[106] angiosarcoma,[107] malignant phyllodes tumor[6] and an unusual giant cell tumor of uncertain histogenesis have been reported.[108]

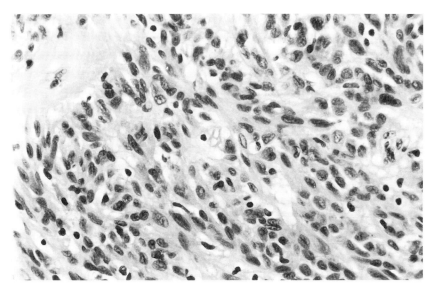

Fig. 21.12C Fasciculated groups of bipolar spindle cells are seen, with little nuclear pleomorphism. Same case as Figure 21.12A. Hematoxylin–eosin × 400.

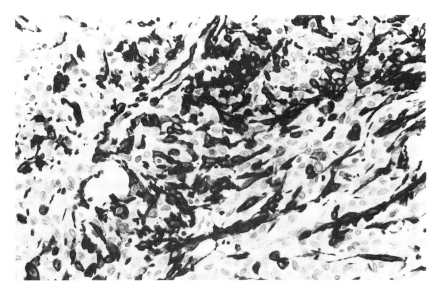

Fig. 21.12D Positive immunoreactivity for smooth muscle actin is demonstrated in approximately 50% of the spindle cells in this field. Same case as Figure 21.12A. Immunostaining for anti-smooth muscle actin × 400.

REFERENCES

1. Bannayan GA, Hajdu SI. Gynecomastia: clinicopathologic study of 351 cases. Am J Clin Pathol 1972; 57: 431–437.
2. Anderson JA, Gram JB. Gynecomasty. Histological aspects in a surgical material. Acta Path Microbiol Immunol Scand (A) 1982a; 90: 185–190.
3. Haibach H, Rosenholtz MJ. Prepubertal gynecomastia with lobules and acini: a case report and review of the literature. Am J Clin Pathol 1983; 80: 252–255.
4. Nielsen VT, Andreasen C. Phyllodes tumour of the male breast. Histopathol 1987; 11: 761–765.

5. Nielsen BB. Fibroadenomatoid hyperplasia of the male breast. Am J Surg Pathol 1990; 14: 774–777.

6. Tavassoli FA. Male breast lesions. In: Tavassoli FA, ed. Pathology of the breast. Norwalk: Appleton and Lange, 1992; 637–659.

7. Schwartz IS, Wilens SL. The formation of acinar tissue in gynecomastia. Am J Pathol 1963; 43: 797–807.

8. Visfeldt J, Scheike O. Male breast cancer. I. Histologic typing and grading of 187 Danish cases. Cancer 1973; 32: 985–990.

9. Sanchez AG, Villanueva AG, Redondo C. Lobular carcinoma of the breast in a patient with Klinefelters syndrome. A case with bilateral, synchronous histologically different breast tumors. Cancer 1986; 57: 1181–1183.

10. Nance KVA, Reddick RL. In situ and infiltrating lobular carcinoma of the male breast. Hum Pathol 1989; 20: 1220–1222.

11. Hilton DA, Jameson JS, Furness PN. A cellular fibroadenoma resembling a benign phyllodes tumour in a young male with gynaecomastia. Histopathol 1991; 18: 476–477.

12. Ansah-Boateng Y, Tavassoli FA. Fibroadenoma and cystosarcoma phyllodes of the male breast. Mod Pathol 1992; 5: 114–116.

13. Anderson JA, Gram JB. Male breast at autopsy. Acta Path Microbiol Immunol Scand (A) 1982b; 90: 191–197.

14. Sandison AT. An autopsy study of the adult human breast. In: Natl Cancer Inst. Monograph No 8. Washington DC: US Govt Printing Office, 1962; 77–80.

15. Carlson HE. Gynecomastia. New Eng J Med 1980; 303: 795–799.

16. Eberlein TJ. Gynecomastia. In: Harris JR, Hellman S, Henderson IC, Kinne DW, eds. Breast diseases. Philadelphia: Lippincott, 1991; 46–50.

17. Haagensen CD. Abnormalities of breast growth, secretion and lactation of physiological origin. In: Haagensen CD, ed. Diseases of the breast. 3rd ed. Philadelphia: Saunders, 1986; 56–74.

18. Williams MJ. Gynecomastia. Its incidence, recognition and host characterization in 447 autopsy cases. Am J Med 1963; 34: 103–112.

19. Nicolis GL, Modlinger RS, Gabrilove JL. A study of the histopathology of human gynecomastia. J Clin Endocrinol 1971; 32: 173–178.

20. Page DL, Anderson TJ, Johnson RL. The male breast and gynaecomastia. In: Page DL, Anderson TJ, eds. Diagnostic histopathology of the breast. Edinburgh: Churchill Livingstone, 1987; 30–42.

21. Pages A, Ramos R. Contribution à l'étude des gynécomasties. A propos de 112 cas. Ann Pathol 1984; 4: 137–142.

22. Gottfried MR. Extensive squamous metaplasia in gynecomastia. Arch Pathol Lab Med 1986; 110: 971–973.

23. McClure J, Bannerjee SS, Sandilands DGD. Female type cystic hyperplasia in a male breast. Pstgrad Med J 1985; 61: 441–443.

24. Symmers WSC. The Breasts. In: Symmers WSC, ed. Systemic pathology. 3rd ed. Vol 4. Edinburgh: Churchill Livingstone, 1978; 1759–1861.

25. Bartoli C, Zurrida SM, Clemente C. Phyllodes tumor in a male patient with bilateral gynecomastia induced by oestrogen therapy for prostatic carcinoma. Eur J Surg Oncol 1991; 17: 215–217.

26. Ribiero G. Male breast carcinoma — a review of 301 cases from the Christie Hospital and Holt Radium Institute, Manchester. Br J Cancer 1985; 51: 115–119.

27. Gough DB, Donohue JH, Evans MM et al. A 50-year experience of male breast cancer: is outcome changing? Surg Oncol 1993; 2: 325–333.

28. Norris HJ, Taylor HB. Carcinoma of the male breast. Cancer 1969; 23: 1428–1435.

29. Gardner MJ, Winter PD, Taylor CP, Acheson ED. Atlas of cancer mortality in England and Wales 1968–1978. Chichester: Wiley, 1983.

30. Hultborn R, Friberg S, Hultborn KA. Male breast carcinoma. I. A study of the total material reported to the Swedish Cancer Registry 1958–1967 with respect to clinical and histopathologic parameters. Acta Oncol 1987a; 26: 241–256.

31. Hultborn R, Friberg S, Hultborn KA et al. Male breast carcinoma. II. A study of the total material reported to the Swedish Cancer Registry 1958–1967 with respect to treatment, prognostic factors and survival. Acta Oncol 1987b; 26: 327–341.

32. Boring CC, Squires TS, Tong T. Cancer statistics, 1991. CA 1991; 41: 19–36.

33. Willsher PC, Leach IH, Ellis IO et al. Male breast cancer: a comparison of outcome with breast cancer in females. Am J Surg 1997a; 173: 185–188.

34. Borgen PI, Wong GY, Vlamis V et al. Current management of male breast cancer. A review of 104 cases. Ann Surg 1992; 215: 451–457.

35. Cutuli BF, Lacroze M, Dilhuydy JM et al. Cancer du sein chez l'homme: fréquence et types des cancers associés, antéreurs, synchrones et métachrones. Bull Cancer 1992a; 79: 689–696.

36. Cutuli B, Lacroze M, Dilhuydy JM et al. Male breast cancer: results of the treatments and prognostic factors in 397 cases. Eur J Cancer 1995; 31A: 1960–1964.

37. Guinee VF, Olssen H, Moller T et al. The prognosis of breast cancer in males. Cancer 1993; 71: 154–161.

38. Willsher PC, Leach IH, Ellis IO et al. Male breast cancer: pathological and multiple immunohistochemical features. The Breast 1997b; submitted for publication.

39. Heller KS, Rosen PP, Schottenfeld D et al. Male breast cancer: a clinicopathologic study of 97 cases. Ann Surg 1978; 188: 60–65.

40. Cutuli BF, Florentz P, Lacroze M et al. Cancer du sein chez l'homme. Étude rétrospective multicentrique: analyse de 444 cas. Bull Cancer 1991; 78: 503.

41. Schwartz IS. Small cell breast carcinoma in men. Hum Pathol 1982; 13: 185.

42. Michaels BM, Nunn CR, Roses DF. Lobular carcinoma of the male breast. Surgery 1994; 115: 402–405.

43. Taxy JB. Tubular carcinoma of the male breast. Report of a case. Cancer 1975; 36: 462–465.

44. Scopsi L, Androla S, Saccozzi R et al. Argyrophilic carcinoma of the male breast. A neuroendocrine tumor containing predominantly chromogranin B (Secretogranin I). Am J Surg Pathol 1991; 15: 1063–1071.

45. Miliauskas JR, Leong AS-Y. Adenoid cystic carcinoma in a juvenile male breast. Pathol 1991; 23: 298–301.

46. Bryant J. Male breast cancer: a case of apocrine

carcinoma with psammoma bodies. Hum Pathol 1981; 12: 751–753.

47. Hartman AW, Magrish P. Carcinoma of the breast in children: case report: six year old boy with adenocarcinoma. Ann Surg 1955; 141: 792–797.

48. Karl SR, Ballantine TVN, Zaino R. Juvenile secretory carcinoma of the breast. J Pediatr Surg 1985; 20: 368–371.

49. Krausz T, Jenkins D, Grontoft O et al. Secretory carcinoma of the breast in adults: emphasis on late recurrence and metastasis. Histopathol 1989; 14: 25–36.

50. Roth JA, Discafani C, O'Malley M. Secretory breast carcinoma in a man. Am J Surg Pathol 1988; 12: 150–154.

51. Lundy J, Mishriki Y, Viola MV et al. A comparison of tumor-related antigens in male and female breast cancer. Br Cancer Res Treat 1986; 7: 91–96.

52. Rogers S, Day CA, Fox SB. Expression of Cathepsin D and estrogen receptor in male breast carcinoma. Hum Pathol 1993; 24: 148–151.

53. Pich A, Margaria E, Chiusa L. Proliferative activity is a significant prognostic factor in male breast carcinoma. Am J Pathol 1994; 145: 481–489.

54. Payne S, Bruce DM, Heys SD et al. Prognostic parameters in male breast cancer. J Pathol 1995; 175 (Suppl): 143A.

55. Elston CW, Ellis IO. Pathological prognostic factors in breast cancer. I. The value of histological grade in breast cancer: experience from a large study with long-term follow-up. Histopathol 1991; 19: 403–410.

56. Cutuli BF, Florentz P, Lacroze M et al. Cancer du sein chez l'homme: étude de 15 cas de carcinome canulaire in situ (CCIS) pur. Bull Cancer 1992b; 79: 1045–1053.

57. Hitchcock A, Topham S, Bell J et al. Routine diagnosis of mammary Paget's disease. A modern approach. Am J Surg Pathol 1992; 16: 58–61.

58. Stretch JR, Denton KJ, Millard PR, Horak E. Paget's disease of the male breast clinically and histopathologically mimicking melanoma. Histopathol 1991; 19: 470–472.

59. Serour F, Birkenfeld S, Amsterdam E et al. Paget's disease of the male breast. Cancer 1988; 62: 601–605.

60. Rose DP. Endocrine epidemiology of male breast cancer (Review). Anticancer Res 1988; 8: 845–850.

61. Van Geel AN, Van Slooten EA, Mavrunac M et al. A retrospective study of male breast cancer in Holland. Br J Surg 1985; 72: 724–727.

62. Evans DB, Crichlow RW. Carcinoma of the male breast and Klinefelters syndrome: is there an association? CA Cancer J Clin 1987; 37: 246–251.

63. Sasco AJ, Lowenfels AB, Pasker-De Jong P. Epidemiology of male breast cancer. A meta-analysis of published case-control studies and discussion of selected aetiological factors. Int J Cancer 1993; 53: 538–549.

64. Scheike O, Visfeldt J. Male breast cancer. 4. Gynecomastia in patients with breast cancer. Acta Path Microbiol Scand Sect (A) 1973; 81: 359–365.

65. Crichlow RW. Carcinoma of the male breast. Surg Gynec Obstet 1972; 134: 1011–1019.

66. Schwartz RM, Newell RB, Hauch JF, Fairweather WH. A study of familial male breast carcinoma and a second report. Cancer 1980; 46: 2697–2701.

67. Kozak FK, Hall JG, Baird PA. Familial breast cancer in males. A case report and review of the literature. Cancer 1986; 58: 2736–2739.

68. Eldar S, Nash E, Abrahamson J. Radiation carcinogenesis in the male breast. Eur J Surg Oncol 1989; 15: 274–278.

69. Scheike O. Male breast cancer. Acta Path Microbiol Scand Sect (A) 1975; Suppl 251: 1–35.

70. Erlichman C, Murphy KC, Elkahim T. Male breast cancer: a 13 year review of 89 patients. J Clin Oncol 1984; 2: 903–909.

71. Spence RAJ, Mackenzie G, Anderson JR et al. Long-term survival following cancer of the male breast in Northern Ireland. Cancer 1985; 55: 648–652.

72. Vercoutere AL, O'Connell TX. Carcinoma of the male breast. An update. Arch Surg 1984; 119: 1301–1304.

73. Schottenfeld D, Nash AG, Robbins GF et al. Ten year results of the treatment of primary operable breast carcinoma. Cancer 1976; 38: 1001–1007.

74. Fisher B, Redmond C, Poisson R et al. Eight year results of a randomized clinical trial comparing total mastectomy and lumpectomy with or without irradiation in the treatment of breast cancer. New Eng J Med 1989; 320: 822–828.

75. Cunha F, André S, Soares J. Morphology of male breast carcinoma in the evaluation of prognosis. Path Res Pract 1990; 186: 745–750.

76. Bloom HJG, Richardson WW. Histological grading and prognosis in breast cancer. A study of 1409 cases of which 359 have been followed for 15 years. Br J Cancer 1957; 11: 359–377.

77. Fox S, Rogers S, Day C, Underwood JCE. Oestrogen receptor and epidermal growth factor receptor expression in male breast carcinoma. J Pathol 1992; 166: 13–18.

78. Kardas I, Seitz G, Limon J et al. Retrospective analysis of prognostic significance of the estrogen-inducible pS2 gene in male breast carcinoma. Cancer 1993; 72: 1652–1656.

79. Kinne DW, Hakes TB. Special therapeutic problems: male breast cancer. In: Harris JR, Hellman S, Henderson IC, Kinne DW, eds. Breast diseases. Philadelphia: Lippincott, 1991; 782–790.

80. Gerdes J, Schwab V, Lemke H, Stein H. Production of a mouse monoclonal antibody reactive with a human nuclear antigen associated with cell proliferation. Int J Cancer 1983; 31: 13–20.

81. Gerdes J, Lemke H, Baisch H et al. Cell cycle analysis of a cell proliferation associated human nuclear antigen defined by the monoclonal antibody Ki 67. J Immunol 1984; 133: 1710–1715.

82. Cattoretti G, Becker MH, Key G et al. Monoclonal antibodies against recombinant parts of the Ki 67 antigen (MIB 1 and MIB 3) detect proliferating cells in microwave-processed formalin-fixed paraffin sections. J Pathol 1992; 168: 357–363.

83. Ellis IO, Hinton C, MacNay J et al. Immunocytochemical staining of breast carcinoma with the monoclonal antibody NCRC-II: a new prognostic indicator. Br Med J 1985; 290: 881–883.

84. Ellis IO, Bell J, Todd J et al. Evaluation of immunoreactivity with monoclonal antibody NCRC-II in breast carcinoma. Br J Cancer 1987; 56: 295–299.

85. Blin N, Kardas I, Welter C et al. Expression of the

c-erbB-2 protooncogene in male breast cancer: lack of prognostic significance. Oncol 1993; 50: 408–411.

86. Lovekin C, Ellis IO, Locker A et al. C-erbB-2 oncoprotein in primary and advanced breast cancer. Br J Cancer 1991; 63: 439–443.

87. Fox SB, Day CA, Rogers S. Lack of c-erbB-2 oncoprotein expression in male breast carcinoma. J Clin Pathol 1991; 44: 960–961.

88. Poller DN, Hutchings CE, Galea M et al. p53 protein expression in human breast cancer: a relationship to expression of epidermal growth factor, C-erbB-2 protein overexpression, and oestrogen receptor. Br J Cancer 1992; 66: 583–588.

89. Banik S, Hale R. Fibrocystic change in the male breast. Histopathol 1988; 12: 214–216.

90. Bigotti G, Kasznica J. Sclerosing adenosis in the breast of a man with pulmonary oat cell carcinoma. Hum Pathol 1986; 17: 861–863.

91. Waldo ED, Sidhu GS, Hu AW. Florid papillomatosis of male nipple after diethylstilboestrol therapy. Arch Pathol 1975; 99: 364–366.

92. Sara AS, Gottfried MR. Benign papilloma of the male breast following chronic phenothiazine therapy. Am J Clin Pathol 1987; 87: 649–650.

93. Tedeschi LG, McCarthy PE. Involutional mammary duct ectasia and periductal mastitis in a male. Hum Pathol 1974; 5: 232–236.

94. Mansel RE, Morgan WP. Duct ectasia in the male. Br J Surg 1979; 66: 660–662.

95. Wargotz ES, Weiss SW, Norris HJ. Myofibroblastoma of the breast. Sixteen cases of a distinctive benign mesenchymal tumor. Am J Surg Pathol 1987; 11: 493–502.

96. Julien M, Trojani M, Coindre JM. Myofibroblastoma of the breast. Report of 8 cases. Ann Pathol 1994; 14: 143–147.

97. Hamele-Bena D, Cranor ML, Sciotto C et al. Uncommon presentation of mammary myofibroblastoma. Mod Pathol 1996; 9: 786–790.

98. Ali S, Teichberg S, DeRisi DC, Urmacher C. Giant myofibroblastoma of breast. Am J Surg Pathol 1994; 18: 1170–1176.

99. Lee AH, Sworn MJ, Theaker JM, Fletcher CDM. Myofibroblastoma of the breast: An immunohistochemical study. Histopathol 1993; 22: 75–78.

100. Begin LR. Myogenic stromal tumor of the male breast (so-called myofibroblastoma). Ultrastruct Pathol 1991; 15: 613–622.

101. Lipper S, Willson CF, Copeland KC. Pseudogynecomastia due to neurofibromatosis — a light microscopic and ultrastructural study. Hum Pathol 1981; 12: 755–759.

102. Martinez-Onsurbe P, Fuentes-Vaamonde E, Gonzalez-Estecha A et al. A neurilemmoma of the breast in a man. A case report. Acta Cytol 1992; 36: 511–513.

103. Shousha S, Theodorou NA, Bull TB. Cavernous haemangioma of breast in a man with contralateral gynaecomastia and a family history of breast carcinoma. Histopathol 1988; 13: 221–223.

104. Jimenez-Ayala M, Diez-Nau MD, Larrad A. Haemangiopericytoma in a male breast. Report of a case with cytologic, histologic and immunochemical studies. Acta Cytol 1991; 35: 234–238.

105. Tamura G, Monma N, Suzuki Y et al. Adenomyoepithelioma (myoepithelioma) of the breast in a male. Hum Pathol 1993; 24: 678–681.

106. Hernandez FJ. Leiomyosarcoma of male breast originating in the nipple. Am J Surg Pathol 1978; 2: 299–304.

107. Rainwater LM, Martin JK, Gaffey TA et al. Angiosarcoma of the breast. Arch Surg 1986; 121: 669–672.

108. Lucas JG, Sharma HM, O'Toole RV. Unusual giant cell tumor arising in a male breast. Hum Pathol 1981; 12: 840–844.

Clinical aspects of malignant breast lesions

INTRODUCTION

The diagnostic pathway for, and the management of, breast cancer have changed greatly over the past 20 years. Despite these changes the number of women dying of this disease has remained high; in the United Kingdom (UK) approximately 24 000 cases are diagnosed per annum and there are around 15 000 deaths. The results of trials of mammographic screening have shown that this measure can reduce mortality from breast cancer[1] and the implementation of population screening for women aged 50–64 in the UK should result in such a diminution.

As a sequitur to the worldwide trials of adjuvant systemic therapies, some women certainly gain a substantial lengthening of life from hormonal and cytotoxic treatments.[2] New agents of these classes have been introduced over the last few years, aimed at both more effective therapy and reduction of side effects.

Other measures introduced in the last decade have resulted in a better quality of life for women with breast cancer: rapid and accurate diagnosis; counseling for a better understanding by the patient of her disease and therapies; less radical therapies for primary breast cancer — including removal of the primary growth with breast conservation; the offer of informed choice in treatment, which in itself has been shown to reduce psychological morbidity; the recognition and treatment of such morbidity; better radiotherapeutic techniques with much less side effect from radiation; new hormonal and cytotoxic agents and methods of giving them; new agents to combat side effects of cytotoxic therapy; bone stabilizing agents, particularly useful in hypercalcemia; better pain relief.

The consequence of these changes is that breast cancer care now requires much greater expertise and experience in the disciplines involved: mammography from radiographers, mammographic reading by radiologists, new surgical techniques, counseling and oncological management, all backed by expert pathology. The concept of team working is now well established, both in diagnosis and treatment.

In the UK a recent report to the Chief Medical Officer[3] has recognized these changes and recommends that care is to be carried out by designated Breast Units, which will provide expertise from breast cancer specialists in each discipline; audit of agreed standards will be an important part of this process.

CARCINOMA OF THE BREAST

DIAGNOSIS

The majority of breast cancers still present with symptoms through the general practitioner (GP) but in the UK in the 50–64 age group many cancers are now found at screening. From 1980 in the Nottingham Breast Unit in women in this age group, 298 primary operable breast cancers — invasive and in situ — have been diagnosed at screening and 377 from GP referral.

Cancers detected at screening are, by definition, largely found as mammographic abnormalities. Although two-thirds of screen detected cancers are palpable, further imaging remains the initial investigation of such abnormalities, resulting in reclassification into 'no lesion present', 'probably benign lesion', 'indeterminate' and 'suspicious of cancer'. Those judged to have a definite lesion, are investigated by fine needle aspiration cytology (FNAC) or needle core biopsy; these may be guided by ultrasound or carried out by X-ray stereotaxis.

The most common symptoms in the GP referral clinic are lump and pain; nipple abnormalities are less common (discharge, indrawing or eczema) and other symptoms uncommon (Table 22.1). In the symptomatic clinic, clinical examination is the initial investigation and women in

Table 22.1 Symptoms of women referred to the Nottingham Breast Clinic in 1995 ($n = 4341$)

Main presenting symptom	n
Lump	2577
Pain	587
Nipple problems	293
Deformity	34
Inflammation	18
Other	189
Asymptomatic (usually for advice on family history)	643

whom there is no significant finding (many of those complaining of pain; those in whom the complaint of 'lump' is not confirmed; multiduct nipple discharge; inpulled nipple judged normal, etc) are reassured without further investigation.

When a significant lesion is found a tissue diagnosis is required (see Ch. 2) and imaging makes little further contribution to *diagnosis*. Further imaging is important in *management* — giving preoperative sizes of cancers or in meeting the criteria for the nonoperative management of benign lumps (see Ch. 13). The use of in-clinic diagnostic needling procedures has resulted in 92% of the last 100 cancers on our Unit being diagnosed preoperatively. Nipple eczema (Fig. 22.1) should be regarded as Paget's disease (see Ch. 14) until proved otherwise. A very small nipple biopsy to confirm the diagnosis is easily undertaken in the out-patient clinic with a sharp scalpel blade.

MANAGEMENT OF 'RISK'

Many epidemiological factors have been claimed for breast cancer, particularly hormonal. There is no hard evidence that the majority are anything but associations with other factors, rather than primary determinants of risk. Furthermore, the risk levels ascribed to most do not allow selection of a group for screening.[4] The exception is genetic risk. Once a family history has been established the degree of risk may be estimated by use of the Claus model;[5] this identifies women with as high as a 30% probability of developing breast cancer by the age of 50, in women with multiple relatives with breast or ovarian cancers.

The highest risk level that can be given from family history alone is a 40% lifetime risk. Since the genetic abnormality within the family has a

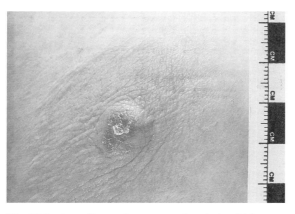

Fig. 22.1   A small area of eczema on the nipple which proved to be Paget's disease on biopsy.

50:50 chance of being passed to any individual, this level for the individual is not 40% but either 80% or the normal risk for any woman (around 8%). It is now clear that women with certain mutations of the BRCA1 and BRCA2 genes and probably other genes, carry such a risk.[6,7]

The other established predictor of risk is the finding of certain specific histological entities (Chs 5 and 6) in the breast on biopsy. These are presumably not primary risk factors in their own right but the morphological expression of somatic mutations increasing risk, sometimes dictated by the presence of germline mutations (Fig. 22.2).

Lines of management of women at risk include surgery, screening or medical therapies.

Removal of both breasts, albeit with reconstruction, is too radical an approach for most women to consider, unless they have the risk levels shown

by women with mutations of certain genes. With two (BRCA1[6] and BRCA2[7]) and perhaps three (AT) genes sequenced within the last year at the time of writing, mutational analysis will become increasingly available. This means that an 80% lifetime risk (and 60% chance of developing breast cancer before the age of 50) can be ascribed to some women. Under these circumstances surgeons would be willing to undertake prophylactic surgery.

Our choice is bilateral subcutaneous mastectomy,[8] preserving the skin over the breast together with the nipple and areola and inserting a silicone implant (Fig. 22.3). This is much the simplest, shortest and cheapest option and if prophylactic mastectomy and reconstruction is advised more often than at present, it is probably all that breast units can afford. It may result in a perfect appearance, but if unsuccessful in achieving a good result it does not prevent the subsequent use of more complicated procedures.

Population *screening* is not cost effective below the age of 50 since it achieves a non-significant 13% reduction in population mortality from breast cancer.[1] The possibility remains that screening a high risk group might be worthwhile: the reduction in younger women is only one-third of that in older women, but by selecting a population with three times the normal incidence, the net effect should be the same. We have established a 'Family History' clinic, at which women at risk

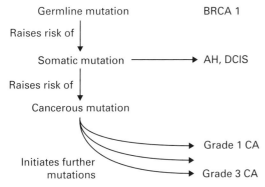

Fig. 22.2   A genetic cascade hypothesis for the etiology of breast cancer (AH: atypical hyperplasia; DCIS: ductal carcinoma in situ; CA: invasive carcinoma).

Germline mutation   BRCA 1

Raises risk of ↓

Somatic mutation ——————→ AH, DCIS

Raises risk of ↓

Cancerous mutation

Initiates further mutations ——————→ Grade 1 CA
——————→ Grade 3 CA

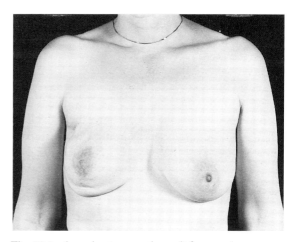

Fig. 22.3   A moderate cosmetic result from a subcutaneous mastectomy and insertion of silicone implant. The patient will appear normal dressed in a bra' and will not have to wear an external prosthesis.

(usually indicated by family history) and under the age of 50 are screened. Our early results[9] show that the women selected are indeed at high risk: 29 in situ and invasive cancers have arisen (diagnosed at screening or presenting in between screenings) in a total of 2559 women-years; the expected number in the normal age-matched population is 3. The prevalent screen of these high risk women detected nine cases per 1000 screens and the incident screen 3.3 per thousand: it is encouraging that these are comparable figures to the detection rates found in whole population screening of women aged 50–64 in the United Kingdom National Health Service Breast Screening Programme (NHSBSP). The result requires confirmation in a larger series of patients and outcome in the patients detected has to be shown to be better than that in symptomatic women of the same age, before it is established that screening of a high risk group of young women is successful.

It has been suggested that the long term application of the peripheral estrogen blocker, tamoxifen, may provide a *medical* means of prevention in high-risk women.[10] This is based on the observation that the number of contralateral breast cancers appearing in follow-up of women with breast cancer is lower in women who are on adjuvant tamoxifen; the figures from the Early Breast Cancer Trialists Collaborative Group[11] show 122 contralateral cancers in the tamoxifen treated and 184 women in the controls. Although this appears to provide evidence of a prevention effect there is another interpretation. Women with proven primary breast cancers may have complete response to tamoxifen therapy with apparent disappearance of the tumor for periods up to and beyond 10 years.[12] A number of contralateral breast cancers will have begun their growth but not yet reached the size necessary for detection; similarly on the receipt of tamoxifen some of these will not progress until the endocrine response wears off. This would result in apparent but not true prevention. The use of tamoxifen in prevention is being tested in an international clinical trial (IBIS).

DUCTAL CARCINOMA IN SITU (DCIS)

The finding of DCIS means that there is a high chance of the development of an invasive carcinoma within the tissue showing this change. The evidence on the exact risk level is slim (Ch. 14) but our estimate is that high grade DCIS has around a 75% chance within each subsequent 10-year period and low grade perhaps a 25% chance, both high enough to warrant intervention.

The work of Holland and his colleagues[13] has shown that ductal carcinoma in situ is often extensive but most importantly is unicentric; some lesions are small, especially among those discovered at screening.[14] Twenty percent of the cancers detected at screening are in situ, whereas only 5% of symptomatic cancers are in situ. This reflects the fact that DCIS is often impalpable, perhaps presenting as a lumpy area in the breast indistinguishable from the normal range.

Extensive DCIS requires mastectomy (simple or subcutaneous) but since DCIS is unicentric, those with the smaller lesions (under 4 cm in our practice) are offered treatment with breast conservation. In many centers this is carried out by wide local excision to clear margins with no measured margin extent required, followed by radiotherapy (RT) to the intact breast. Whether RT confers benefit after such surgery is the subject of several clinical trials.[15–16] In Nottingham we have ensured 10 mm clearance at the circumferential margins (Fig. 22.4) and have not given RT: although the series is small ($n = 48$) at a median follow-up of 5 years there are only three recurrences and only one of these is invasive.[17]

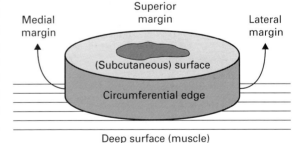

Fig. 22.4 The principle of wide local excision of a primary breast cancer. All tissue between skin and muscle is removed. The circumferential margin is closely examined by the pathologist and at this edge a depth of 1 cm of tumor free tissue is required all round.

THE MANAGEMENT OF PRIMARY INVASIVE CARCINOMA

Following treatment of the primary tumor the recurrences which may occur are classified as local (LR), regional (RR) and distant metastases (DM). Each differs in the factors which dictate whether they are likely to occur. Treatment of the primary tumor has to be directed at minimizing each of these; however, treatments carry side effects and a balance has to be struck for each between prophylactic effect and side effect.

Whether *distant metastatic spread* has occurred and will eventually become apparent and inevitably lead to death of the patient, is determined before diagnosis. When the cancer has metastasized by the time of diagnosis, even if it is successfully excised so that neither local nor regional recurrence occurs, the woman dies from distant metastatic spread. However even in symptomatically detected tumors 25% or more appear likely to be cured by local treatment (surgery ± radiotherapy). In cancers detected at breast cancer screening around 60% appear likely to be cured by removal of the primary tumor (Fig. 22.5).

Those that are not cured may obtain an advantage in survival terms from the application of adjuvant systemic therapies, hormonal or cytotoxic.[2] The overall effect is not large and appears to be an extension of life rather than a cure.[18] Cytotoxic therapy in all who receive it and hormonal therapy in premenopausal women have considerable side effects. Their use should be restricted to women who have distant metastases at diagnosis and who are therefore not cured by their local therapy; hence the importance of recognizing these women by prognostic discrimination.

Local recurrence depends upon whether there is local spread around the primary tumor in the breast tissue when this has been retained in breast conserving operations or in the dermal lymphatics around the tumor.

LR in the treated breast following breast conservation therapy by local excision plus radiotherapy can be very distressing, since at the least it means conversion to mastectomy and at the worst the recurrence is uncontrollable (Fig. 22.6).[19–20]

The incidence of local recurrence following mastectomy can be reduced by the application of radiotherapy (RT) to the skin flaps. However if all women are given RT, 75% do not suffer LR[21] and would be overtreated whilst 5–10% suffer regional recurrence even if given RT.[22]

LR occurs because of a combination of factors in the primary tumor and can be largely averted if women with these factors are given RT;[21] it is therefore important that they are recognized at the time of primary treatment (see below).

Regional recurrence (RR), enlarging lymph nodes invaded by breast cancer (usually axillary, occasionally supraclavicular or internal mammary), is unsurprisingly more common if the regional nodes are neither cleared surgically nor irradiated at the time of initial therapy. Without this prophy-

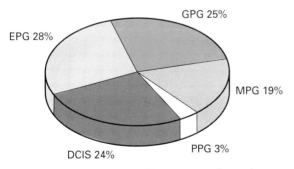

Fig. 22.5 The distribution of breast cancers detected at population screening, according to prognostic groups. A total of 75% are either carcinoma-in-situ or invasive cancers lying in the good and excellent prognostic groups, with a high chance of cure from their primary surgery. (DCIS: ductal carcinoma in situ; EPG: excellent prognostic group; GPG: good prognostic group; MPG: moderate prognostic group; PPG: poor prognostic group).

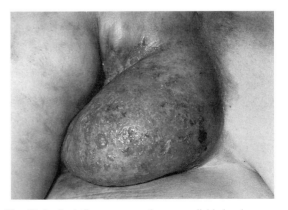

Fig. 22.6 An inflammatory and uncontrollable local recurrence following treatment with breast conservation.

laxis RR is by no means inevitable, occurring in only some 30%[22–23] and is in most cases controlled by surgery or radiotherapy applied at recognition of recurrence.[22–23] Thus a few more women die with uncontrolled axillary recurrence in those not receiving axillary nodal prophylaxis than in those undergoing clearance or RT[22] but this is offset by the morbidity from prophylactic treatments.[24] Ideally all uncontrolled recurrence should be prevented and all patients should have an undisturbed tumor free interval, even if distant metastatic spread later becomes apparent; hence the importance of recognizing factors which place women at high risk of RR and especially of uncontrolled RR, so that prophylactic therapy may be applied to them and not given to those at low risk (see below).

Treatment with breast conservation

In Nottingham the operation used for breast conservation is wide local excision. This does not mean a radical removal of the tumor, such as is carried out at quadrantectomy; the latter gives a bad cosmetic result in around one-quarter of the cases.[25] The technique used in Nottingham gives generally excellent cosmesis (Fig. 22.7).

At operation the subcutaneous and deep planes are dissected widely around the tumor and the surgeon removes a cylinder of tissue, taking all tissue between skin and muscle and aiming for a 15–20 mm palpable margin around the tumor; the apparent margin is checked with specimen X-ray (Fig. 22.8) and if the tumor appears nearer to one margin than the surgeon intended then re-excision of that edge of the cavity is carried out at the time. The specimen is orientated with stitches and the external surface of the specimen is inked before the pathologist cuts into it (see Ch. 2).

As a result of an audit of our first 250 cases,[19] women with tumors measured preoperatively as exceeding 30 mm in diameter are not now offered treatment with breast conservation. Postoperatively the margins are checked histologically and at least 5 mm clearance around the circumferential (Fig. 22.4) margin is required, otherwise the margin is reexcised to achieve that distance. The other important feature which correlated with subsequent LR was vascular invasion (VI)[19] (Ch. 18). If the pathologist reports that VI is present then the other factors associated with LR[19,26] are considered: these are young age (<50) and tumor size. The combination of VI, age <50 and a tumor greater than 20 mm carried a very high risk of LR in our initial series.[19] Women with this profile or with multiple margins involved with invasive carcinoma or DCIS are now advised that conversion to mastectomy is necessary: this means that 12% of cases originally offered breast conservation are converted to mastectomy;[27] the remainder proceed to radiotherapy to the intact breast.

This policy has resulted in a LR rate after breast conservation of only 2.2% at a median of 5 years follow-up.[27] Our previous recurrence rate

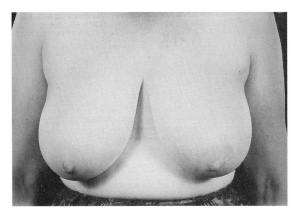

Fig. 22.7 Wide local excision of a breast cancer followed by intact breast irradiation generally gives a good cosmetic result: here is shown an excellent result.

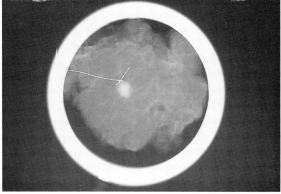

Fig. 22.8 Specimen X-ray of an impalpable invasive cancer removed with wide local excision.

in the unselected series[19] was 21% at the same time of follow-up. Since the new selection policy was introduced (1988) 12% have been excluded from breast conserving therapy by the histological criteria, 5% have suffered local recurrence and 3% required re-excision of margins before continuing with breast conserving treatment; these add up to 20%, close to the 21% recurrence in our unselected original series, which serves to confirm that the new policy has indeed identified most of those who would have suffered LR if treated with breast conservation. The policy relies heavily on careful histological assessment of the specimen.

Prophylaxis against local recurrence following mastectomy

In women choosing or advised to undergo simple mastectomy, without irradiation of the skin flaps, LR in our series of 966 patients was 23% at a median of 7 years follow-up.[21] This is comparable to LR in other series of mastectomies without flap irradiation.[22] In 50% of cases LR in the flaps is a single spot,[28] treated by excision. The appearance of multiple spots or of a widespread eczematous appearance caused by dermal lymphatic invasion, means that long term local control will be difficult.[21,28]

For the reasons given earlier we sought to identify a subgroup with a high enough incidence of LR to justify giving prophylactic radiotherapy; the features that predicted for LR in the flaps were histological grade 3, lymph node invasion and VI.[21] VI is thus a factor that is important in the genesis of LR both after mastectomy and wide local excision; it is of less importance in the prediction of DM and survival (Ch. 18).

The combination of all three factors predicted a subsequent LR rate after mastectomy of 44% and the presence of any two of over 30%.[21] The presence of two or more of these factors is used in Nottingham to select for prophylactic flap irradiation. Only 33% of those undergoing mastectomy are selected for flap irradiation and this includes 90% of those who would otherwise develop the more aggressive local recurrences (see above).[21]

Subcutaneous mastectomy, preserving the skin over the breast and the nipple and with the later placement of silicone implants, is offered to women who are advised not to have treatment with breast conservation because of the selection factors but wish for a better cosmetic result than given by simple mastectomy. Using both the Nottingham Prognostic Index (Ch. 18) and the presence of VI to stratify patients, we have been able to demonstrate that LR occurs with no greater frequency after subcutaneous mastectomy than after simple mastectomy.[8]

Prophylaxis against regional recurrence

Yet again analysis has been made for predictive factors. A combination of lymph node positivity at node sampling and of a grade 3 primary tumor identifies a group with a 53% chance of symptomatic RR by 10 years of follow-up.[23] A small randomized trial has shown that RR was markedly reduced in these patients by prophylactic RT;[23] it is now our standard policy to give RT to this group, regardless of whether the primary tumor is treated by breast conservation or simple or subcutaneous mastectomy.

Regional node sampling

Selection policies for prophylaxis against RR and LR (above) and for adjuvant systemic therapy (below) require knowledge as to whether axillary nodes are involved with carcinoma. As we do not carry out a full axillary clearance for prophylaxis, axillary sampling is necessary.

Nodal sampling of the axilla is carried out in all invasive cancers. The dissection is low in the axilla, working if possible below the intercostobrachial nerve (the lateral intercostal cutaneous branch of T2). This nerve crosses the axilla horizontally and since the plane of axillary dissection is vertical, the nerve or its small branches are damaged in a higher dissection, leading to long lasting discomfort of the medial side of the upper arm, sometimes extending to the hand.

A minimum of four nodes are identified separately and removed. Four node sampling has been shown to be as accurate as node clearance up to the axillary vein in the determination of nodal status.[29]

We prefer this procedure to a partial clearance

(dissection up to the axillary vein), since the side effects are worse if a combination of surgery and radiotherapy is used for prophylaxis. This is why our biopsy is confined to the low axilla and if indicated, axillary radiotherapy may then be used without serious side effect.

Sampling of an internal mammary node (usually the second interspace node) is carried out for invasive cancers in the inner half of the breast.[30] At mastectomy a node lying at the apex of the axilla, just lateral to the first rib and below the axilla vein, is sampled.

The staging of patients according to the node sampling is described in Chapter 18, together with the incorporation of the nodal stage into the Nottingham Prognostic Index (NPI).

Selection for adjuvant systemic therapy

The prediction of survival is determined by the NPI. Survival curves for women under 70 with operable (<5 cm diameter) primary breast cancer are shown in Chapter 18. From these it may be seen that, for example, a woman in the EPG has only a 10% chance of death from breast cancer by 15 years. Consideration of the prognosis must be taken into account when the decision is made concerning the need for adjuvant systemic therapy.

Our prescription of adjuvant systemic therapy is shown in Table 22.2. The NPI of the patient is noted. If the patient falls into the excellent (EPG) or good (GPG) prognostic groups, then their chance of suffering metastases and death from breast cancer by 15 years is low; if adjuvant

systemic therapy were to be prescribed in these groups, the great majority of women would be receiving it for no effect.

In addition to prognosis, factors predictive of response to therapy (Ch. 18) are important. Estrogen receptor (ER) status predicts for response to endocrine therapy in the advanced situation and the adjuvant effect of tamoxifen is much more powerful in ER positive tumors.[11] That there is any apparent adjuvant endocrine effect in ER negative tumours when assessed by the dextran coated charcoal method is likely to be due to falsely negative results brought about by leaving operative specimens too long at room temperature before snap freezing samples for assay.[31]

Estrogen receptor status is therefore taken into consideration for women in the moderate (MPG) and poor (PPG) prognostic groups. If the tumour is ER+ (ERICA H-score >50 out of a possible 300) (see Ch. 18), then women in these groups are advised to receive hormone therapy. Menopausal status does not enter into the decision to receive endocrine therapy since the effect appears similar[11] in pre- and postmenopausal groups; postmenopausal women are prescribed tamoxifen (which is a peripheral estrogen antagonist) and premenopausal women receive ovarian suppression by use of goserelin (Zoladex), an LH/RH agonist.

This leaves those women in the MPG and PPG who have tumors with an ERICA H-score <50. These women are candidates for adjuvant chemotherapy but the toxicity of this treatment must be taken into consideration; nausea, mucositis, alopecia and general malaise are all distressing and early menopause may be undesirable. This toxicity has to be weighed against the comparatively small gain in prognostic terms and the fact that some of the gain is due to ovarian suppression.

Women in the PPG will shortly present with metastatic spread; their outlook is similar to patients presenting with locally advanced disease.[32] They therefore require adjuvant therapy if possible and cytotoxic therapy should be given, unless they are judged unfit.

Women in the MPG have a 40% chance of having avoided symptoms of distant spread by 15 years. The natural survival of older women in this group has to be taken into account (Fig. 22.9) and

Table 22.2 The advice given in the Breast Unit for the prescription of adjuvant systemic therapy, according to the Nottingham Prognostic Index (NPI)

NPI	Predicted 15-year survival	Adjuvant systemic therapy advised
Good prognostic group	85%	Nil
Moderate prognostic group	40%	ER+: endocrine ER–: depending on age, fitness and tumor size CT sometimes advised
Poor prognostic group	12%	ER+: Endocrine ER–: CT if fit

ER: Estrogen receptor.
CT: Cytotoxic therapy.

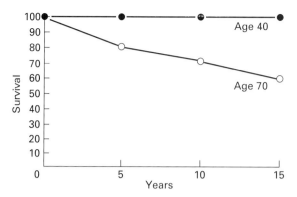

Fig. 22.9 Natural life expectancy of a woman of 40 years and a woman of 70 years.

for this reason as they approach 70 the gain from adjuvant therapy would be halved. Therefore cytotoxic therapy is reserved for the younger women in this group.

In many units only nodal status is taken into account in prescribing adjuvant therapy. It is noteworthy that the survival of women with a node negative, 2 cm grade 3 tumor is only 50% at 15 years; young women with such tumors in our Unit are advised to have adjuvant therapy. Conversely, a node positive 2 cm grade 1 tumor gives an 80% 15-year survival.

Multidisciplinary team management

Decisions on adjuvant irradiation and systemic therapies in the individual patients are made at a weekly meeting between the surgeons, clinical oncologist and pathologists of the Breast Unit. After this meeting the case management plan is explained to the patient by the surgeon or clinical oncologist. It is important that the breast care nurses attend the meeting, as they will have to counsel the patient and give a more detailed explanation of the treatment to be given. They will have come to know the patient from meeting them at diagnosis and at admission for surgery; their advice is therefore very helpful with regard to physical and psychological fitness for treatments such as cytotoxic therapy.

Treatment of elderly patients

The natural survival (Fig. 22.9) of the elderly woman must be considered when advising treat-

ment. In addition the older the patient the more likely her cancer is to be strongly estrogen receptor (ER) positive and primary treatment with hormonal agents is therefore an attractive proposition. Several clinical trials have compared initial hormone therapy with surgery[33–34] and have shown that although survival was not affected, the majority of women who started with hormone therapy eventually came to surgery. However considerable periods of control of the primary tumor, even over 10 years, can be achieved.[35]

A further trial[37] in Nottingham has shown that by selecting only women with tumors with high ER values (ERICA H score >100) for primary hormone therapy, those tumors that progress from the start are eliminated. Patients gaining a complete or partial response by 6 months of therapy are likely to go on to a good period of long term control. To commence only those with high ER positivity on hormone therapy and then to reassess at 6 months, operating on those with static disease, seems a reasonable policy.

Locally advanced breast cancer

Tumors of 5 cm diameter or more are termed 'locally advanced' in the Nottingham Breast Unit.

Two presentations may be recognized among tumors of this size. The cancer may present as a large lump, attached to and eventually ulcerating through the skin, often in elderly women who have known of the lump for some time. In contrast there may be sudden presentation of an edematous

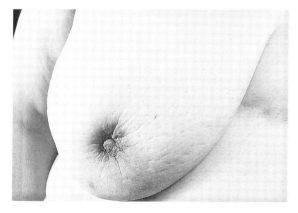

Fig. 22.10 A locally advanced primary tumor with peau d'orange and indrawing of the nipple.

breast, in which the skin shows peau d'orange and erythema (Fig. 22.10). In the latter case the tumor is aggressive and infiltrates the breast without forming a mass and these tumors often show no abnormality on mammography.

Although the overall prognosis is poor[32] some tumors with the former presentation are slow growing and may respond well to hormone therapy. Patients with the second presentation have a grave prognosis, with not only very poor survival but also a high risk of uncontrolled local and regional disease. Preoperative chemotherapy, radical surgery to breast and axilla and flap irradiation help to avert the local and regional problems.[36]

Breast cancer in pregnancy

Breast cancers occurring during pregnancy usually carry a poor outlook.[37] Those presenting in the second and third trimesters tend to be large and diffuse, which, as they lie in breasts which are very lumpy and difficult to examine, probably means they are diagnosed late. They are often poorly differentiated and ER negative. This is possibly because the ER positive, better differentiated tumors are controlled by the hormone changes of the pregnancy and do not therefore present clinically; the smaller, slower growing tumors may be concealed in the lumpy breast in pregnancy. Tumors of this kind require mastectomy rather than treatment with breast conservation. Any adjuvant treatment (systemic, local or regional) can be given after the pregnancy is over.

Breast cancer in males

One in 300 breast cancers arises in a male. This reflects the proportionate number of epithelial cells at risk. The differential diagnosis lies between gynecomastia (Ch. 21) and breast cancer but is usually clinically obvious.

Prognosis[38] and treatment are the same as for breast cancer in females although since there is little breast tissue, mastectomy must be the operation of choice for the primary tumor.

DISTANT METASTASES

Once a patient is diagnosed as having overt distant metastatic spread she is doomed to die from breast cancer. Treatments are therefore palliative but include systemic therapies, hormonal and cytotoxic, which can slow tumor growth or give temporary remissions.

The likelihood of gaining a remission or of dying very early from metastatic spread may be estimated using the Nottingham Metastatic Index.[39–40] The median survival overall is less than one year from the diagnosis of distant metastases, but around one in ten women will survive for more than 5 years.

A longer survival time is associated with a good response to hormone therapy[39–40] and this in turn is dependent upon the ER status of the tumor. Women with ER negative tumors are very unlikely to respond to hormone therapy.[41]

Diagnosis of metastatic spread

Imaging applied at the *time of treatment* of the primary tumor in an attempt to find occult metastases is worthless and costly. Even if a 'hot spot' is found on a bone scan, all that can be concluded is that distant spread has probably occurred. Only around 2–5% of scans are positive[42] whereas over 60% of patients with primary breast cancer can be shown to be likely to have metastatic spread using an index such as the NPI (Ch. 18).

The diagnosis of distant spread during *follow-up* comes from the investigation of symptoms and in this imaging is very important. Pain is initially investigated by bone radiographs (Fig. 22.11) and

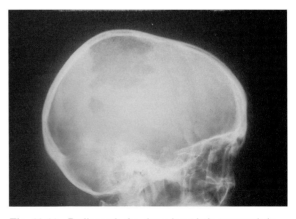

Fig. 22.11   Radiograph showing a large lytic metastasis in the skull vault.

if no abnormality is seen, by isotope bone scan and if necessary by magnetic resonance imaging (MRI). Breathlessness and cough may indicate lung metastases, investigated by chest radiographs and, possibly, computerized tomography (CT) scan. Liver ultrasound may be used to confirm the diagnosis when symptoms suggest spread to the liver. When metastases are large enough to give symptoms, serum tumor marker levels (CA 15.3 and CEA) are markedly raised in over 80% of patients[43] and this may be useful in making the diagnosis.

Management

Management of distant metastases has two aims, to slow the growth of the metastases by hormonal means or by cytotoxic therapy and to palliate.

Endocrine maneuvers may act by reducing circulating estradiol in premenopausal women by oophorectomy or ovarian suppression and in postmenopausal women by the use of aromatase inhibitors; by peripheral estrogen antagonists using tamoxifen; by other means using high dose progesterones or androgens.

Hormonal therapy is well tolerated and is the first systemic therapy to consider. In endocrine receptor positive tumors one-third to a half will show objective response to endocrine therapies[41] and once the metastases have relapsed, around half of the responders will gain a response to a second hormone therapy.[44]

Cytotoxic therapy is used as the initial treatment when a rapid response is required, such as when the patient is breathless, or when the tumor is hormone receptor negative. The response rate to the most commonly used combination regimen is 40–50% but the average response duration is shorter than is achieved by hormonal therapies.

The side effects are unpleasant and the more aggressive cytotoxic regimens can be life threatening.

The symptoms of metastatic spread require energetic palliation: anemia from bone marrow infiltration may require transfusion; radiotherapy is given for bone pain; orthopedic surgery is used to treat or avoid fractures; phosphonates to treat hypercalcemia and also to reduce bone pain and reduce the risk of fractures; pleural effusion (which may be due to lymphatic spread through the chest wall or to hematogenous lung metastases) requires drainage and pleurodesis; specialist pain relief, access to a palliative care unit and psychological and social service help are very important.

MALIGNANT MESENCHYMAL TUMORS

The experience of any unit of such tumors is small: in the past 15 years, in the Nottingham City Hospital Breast Unit we have diagnosed over 5000 breast cancers; we have seen only one phyllodes tumor (Ch. 9) which metastasized (and that was a patient seen at tertiary referral), two fibromatoses that occurred in underlying muscle rather than breast tissue and behaved in a locally aggressive fashion (Ch. 11), one angiosarcoma (Ch. 19) that metastasized and one that appears not to have done so.

Malignant (and potentially malignant) mesenchymal tumors must be treated by complete excision (wide local excision or mastectomy). Lymph node sampling is unnecessary since these tumors do not tend to spread regionally.

There is some evidence that radiotherapy may add to control of fibromatoses[45] as may the use of peripheral estrogen antagonists such as tamoxifen.[46]

REFERENCES

1. Nyström L, Rutqvist LE, Wall S et al. Breast cancer screening with mammography: overview of Swedish randomized trials. Lancet 1993; 341: 973–978.
2. Early Breast Cancer Trialists Collaborative Group. Systemic treatment of early breast cancer by hormonal, cytotoxic or immune therapy. Lancet 1992; 339: 71–85.
3. A Policy Framework for Commissioning Cancer Services. A Report by the Expert Advisory Group on Cancer to the Chief Medical Officers of England and Wales. Department of Health publication, April 1995.
4. Henderson IC. Risk factors for breast cancer development. Cancer (suppl) 1993; 31: 2127–2140.
5. Claus EB, Risch N, Thompson WD. Autosomal dominant inheritance of early onset breast cancer — implications for risk prediction. Cancer 1994; 73: 643–651.

6. Miki Y, Swensen J, Shattuck-Eidens D et al. A strong candidate for the breast and ovarian cancer susceptibility gene BRCA1. Science 1994; 266: 66–71.

7. Wooster R, Bignell G, Lancaster J et al. Identification of the breast cancer susceptibility gene BRCA2. Nature 1995; 378: 789–792.

8. Cheung KL, Blamey RW, Robertson JFR et al. Subcutaneous mastectomy for primary breast cancer or ductal carcinoma in situ. Eur J Surg 1997; 23: 343–347.

9. Kollias J, Sibbering DM, Holland PAM et al. Results of screening for women aged <50 with a family history of breast cancer (Abstr). Eur J Surg Oncol 1996; 22: 551.

10. Cuzick J. Chemoprevention of breast cancer with Tamoxifen. In: Hakama M, Beral V, Buiatti E, eds. Chemoprevention in cancer control. IARC Scientific Publications No 135, 1996; 95–106.

11. Early Breast Cancer Trialists Collaborative Group. Systemic treatment of early breast cancer by hormonal, cytotoxic or immune therapy. Oxford overview September 1995. Lancet 1997; in press.

12. Low SC, Dixon AR, Bell J et al. Tumour oestrogen receptor content allows selection of elderly patients with breast cancer for conservative Tamoxifen treatment. Br J Surg 1992; 79: 1314–1316.

13. Faverly DRG, Burgers L, Bult P, Holland R. Three dimensional imaging of mammary ductal carcinoma in situ: clinical implications. Semin Diagn Pathol 1994; 11: 193–198.

14. Evans AJ, Pinder SE, Ellis IO et al. Screening-detected and symptomatic ductal carcinoma in situ: mammographic features with pathologic correlation. Radiol 1994, 191: 237–240.

15. Fisher B, Costantino J, Redmond C et al. Lumpectomy compared with lumpectomy and radiation therapy for the treatment of intraductal breast cancer. N Eng J Med 1993; 328: 1581–1586.

16. Working Party of the Breast Cancer Trials Co-ordinating Subcommittee, United Kingdom Co-ordinating Committee on Cancer Research. Protocol of the UK randomized trial for the management of screen-detected ductal carcinoma in situ (DCIS) of the breast. UKCCCR 1989.

17. Sibbering DM, Blamey RW. The Nottingham Experience. In: Silverstein MJ, ed. Ductal carcinoma in situ. California: Williams and Wilkins, 1997; 367–377.

18. Blamey RW. Assessment of the predicted effects of adjuvant therapies in the individual. 5th Nottingham International Breast Cancer Conference, 1997.

19. Locker AP, Ellis IO, Morgan DAL et al. Factors influencing local recurrence after excision and radiotherapy for primary breast cancer. Br J Surg 1989; 76: 890–894.

20. Fisher ER, Sass R, Fisher B et al. Pathologic findings from the National surgical adjuvant breast project (Protocol 6): II. Relation of local breast recurrence to multicentricity. Cancer 1986; 57: 1717–1724.

21. O'Rourke JS, Galea MH, Morgan DA et al. Local recurrence after simple mastectomy. Br J Surg 1994; 81: 386–389.

22. Berstock DA, Houghton J, Haybittle J, Baum M. The role of radiotherapy following total mastectomy for patients with early breast cancer. World J Surg 1985; 9: 667–670.

23. Archer S, Morgan DAL, Sibbering DM et al. Regional recurrence in Stage I and Stage II breast cancer: selection of patients at high risk for radiotherapy. Eur J Surg Oncol, 1997; submitted for publication.

24. Kissin MW, Querci della Rovere G, Easton D, Westbury G. Risk of lymphoedema following the treatment of breast cancer. Br J Surg 1986; 73: 580–584.

25. Veronesi U, Volterrani F, Luini A et al. Quadrantectomy versus lumpectomy for small size breast cancer. Eur J Cancer 1990; 26: 671–673.

26. Vilcoq JR, Calle R, Stacey P, Ghossein NA. The outcome of treatment by tumorectomy and radiotherapy of patients with operable breast cancer. Int J Radiat Oncol Biol Phys 1981; 7: 1327–1332.

27. Sibbering DM, Galea MH, Morgan DAL et al. Safe selection criteria for breast conservation without radical excision in primary operable invasive breast cancer. Eur J Cancer 1995; 31: 2191–2195.

28. Blacklay PF, Campbell FC, Hinton CP et al. Patterns of flap recurrence following mastectomy. Br J Surg 1985; 72: 719–720.

29. Forrest APM, Everington D, McDonald CC et al. The Edinburgh randomized trial of axillary sampling or clearance after mastectomy. Br J Surg 1995; 82: 1504–1508.

30. Du Toit RS, Locker AP, Ellis IO et al. An evaluation of the prognostic value of triple node biopsy in early breast cancer. Br J Surg 1990; 77: 163–167.

31. Bishop HM. Oestrogen receptors in human breast cancer. MD Thesis, University of Nottingham 1982.

32. Willsher PC, Robertson JFR, Armitage N et al. Locally advanced breast cancer: long term results of a randomized trial comparing primary treatment with Tamoxifen or radiotherapy in post menopausal women. Eur J Surg Oncol 1996; 22: 34–37.

33. Bates T, Riley DL, Houghton J et al. Breast cancer in elderly women: a Cancer Research Campaign trial comparing treatment with Tamoxifen and optimal surgery with Tamoxifen alone. Br J Surg 1991; 78: 591–594.

34. Robertson JFR, Ellis IO, Elston CW, Blamey RW. Mastectomy or Tamoxifen as initial therapy for operable breast cancer in elderly patients: 5-year follow-up. Eur J Cancer 1992; 28: 908–910.

35. Willsher PC, Robertson JFR, Jackson L et al. Investigation of primary Tamoxifen therapy for elderly patients with operable breast cancer. The Breast 1997; 6: 150–154.

36. Willsher PC, Robertson JFR, Chan SY et al. Locally advanced breast cancer: early results of a randomized trial of multimodal therapy versus initial hormone therapy. Eur J Cancer 1997; 33: 45–49.

37. Guinee VF, Olsson H, Moller T et al. Effect of pregnancy on prognosis for young women with breast cancer. Lancet 1994; 343: 1587–1588.

38. Willsher PC, Leach IH, Ellis IO et al. A comparison of outcome of male breast cancer with breast cancer in women. Am J Surg 1997; 173: 185–188.

39. Williams MR, Todd JH, Nicholson RI et al. Survival patterns in hormone treated advanced breast cancer. Br J Surg 1986; 73: 752–755.

40. Roberston JRF, Nicholson RI, Dixon AR et al. Confirmation of a prognostic index for metastatic breast cancer. Br Cancer Res Treat 1992; 22: 221–227.

41. Robertson JFR, Bates K, Pearson D et al. Comparison of two oestrogen receptor assays in the prediction of the

clinical course of patients with advanced breast cancer. Br J Cancer 1992; 65: 727–730.

42. Bishop HM, Blamey RW, Morris AH et al. Bone scanning: its lack of value in the follow-up of patients with breast cancer. Br J Surg 1979; 66: 752–754.

43. Albuquerque K, Price MR, Badley RA et al. Pre-treatment serum levels of tumour markers in metastatic breast cancer: a prospective assessment of their role in predicting response to therapy and survival. Eur J Surg Oncol 1995; 21: 504–509.

44. Cheung KL, Willsher PC, Pinder SE et al. Predictors of response to secondline endocrine therapy for breast cancer. Br Cancer Res Treat 1997; 45: in press.

45. Kiel KD, Suit HD. Radiation therapy in the treatment of aggressive fibromatoses (Desmoid tumors) Cancer 1984; 54: 2051–2055.

46. Kinzbrunner B, Ritter S, Domingo J, Rosenthal CJ. Remission of rapidly growing desmoid tumors after Tamoxifen therapy. Cancer 1983; 52: 2201–2204.

Screening for breast cancer

INTRODUCTION

The ideal solution to the problem of mortality from breast cancer would be prevention; the effect of tamoxifen in primary prevention is under investigation, but at present no proven means of primary prevention exists. Adjuvant tamoxifen is known to reduce mortality in women with primary operable breast cancer,[1] but no study has yet looked at the effects of tamoxifen on population survival. At present screening is the only option of known value in improving population survival.

General principles of screening have been developed to predict whether screening for disease may be effective:

- The condition should be an important health problem.
- The natural history of the disease should be well understood.
- The disease must have a detectable preclinical phase.
- Early treatment should be more likely to lead to a favorable outcome.
- The screening tool must be specific, sensitive, safe, acceptable to the screened population and be widely available.
- There must be a mechanism for identifying and inviting the targeted population.
- Effective diagnostic and treatment facilities must be widely available.
- The screening test should be repeated at intervals determined by the natural history of the disease.
- The screening program must be cost effective in comparison with other health care measures.

This chapter will focus on the application of these principles to breast cancer screening. The first part of the chapter will deal with the natural history of breast cancer and evidence concerning which age groups to screen by which modality. The second, shorter part of the chapter is a more practical guide to the screening process.

EVIDENCE FOR SCREENING

EPIDEMIOLOGY

Breast cancer is the most common malignant tumor to affect women in Western industrialized countries and its incidence has gradually increased during the past 30 years. Breast cancer kills 15 000 women per annum in the United Kingdom and approaching 90% of these deaths occur in women over 50.[2] Breast cancer accounted for 19% of female cancer deaths and 5% of all female deaths in 1990. The Department of Health's Health of the Nation target for breast cancer is to reduce breast cancer deaths among women invited for screening by at least 25% by the year 2000.[2]

NATURAL HISTORY OF BREAST CANCER

A proportion of invasive breast cancer arises from ductal carcinoma in situ (DCIS), while some invasive tumors probably arise de novo. Invasive breast cancer usually grows in a predictable fashion. The incidence of spread to regional axillary and internal mammary lymph nodes (markers of metastatic spread) is related to the size of the invasive tumor at presentation.[3]

Very few invasive tumors less than 10 mm in size, even when they are of high histological grade, have metastasized to the regional lymph nodes and it has been suggested that at this early stage histological grade is prognostically less important[4] (see also Ch. 18). Such small breast cancers represent a subclinical phase of tumor development and are different in their characteristics from breast cancer which presents clinically, so-called symptomatic cancer, where tumor sizes are larger, lymph node involvement more frequent and tumor grade prognostically more important.[5–6]

It is possible that at least some breast cancers de-differentiate histologically over time (so-called 'phenotypic drift'), having an early, relatively indolent well-differentiated phase of development followed by de-differentiation and more rapid growth.[7] This is suggested by the grade profile of screen detected cancers compared with symptomatic cancer where screen detected cancers which are smaller are more likely to be well differentiated.[6,8–9] It has been suggested that the differing grade profiles of screen detected and symptomatic invasive cancers could be due to over-diagnosis by screening (detecting cancers that would never present clinically). In our view, histological de-differentiation is the more likely explanation of the different grade characteristics of screen detected and symptomatic invasive breast cancer.

DCIS is found much more frequently at mammographic screening than in symptomatic practice.[10–11] A proportion of these cases (especially those with low grade DCIS) may well represent over-diagnosis, that is, they would never develop a symptomatic breast cancer. However, screen detected DCIS is more likely to be high grade than symptomatic DCIS and, therefore, has a higher invasive potential.[12–14] The invasive tumors that develop from high grade DCIS are also more likely to be of high histological grade.[15] The detection of high grade DCIS before invasion has occurred may therefore be an important factor contributing to the mortality reduction achievable by screening.

EFFECTIVENESS OF BREAST SCREENING

If screening is to be effective it should detect breast cancers that have not metastasized and are therefore potentially curable, but which would eventually threaten the woman's life. As noted above the pathological prognostic factors for screen detected breast cancer are more favorable than in symptomatic cancer: they are smaller, more frequently node negative and of special histological type (tubular or tubular mixed);[16] they are less likely to be poorly differentiated, show high mitotic counts, tumor necrosis or be of ductal NST histological type. Screen detected cancers are also more often estrogen and progesterone receptor positive, with lower S phase fractions and lower expression of the oncogenes c-erbB-2 and p53.[6,8-9] The survival of women with screen detected cancers is also better than those with symptomatic cancer. These facts do not necessarily indicate a mortality reduction in the screened population. This is because of lead time bias, the occurrence of interval cancers and over-diagnosis.

Lead time bias

The lead time of a screening test is the interval between detecting the tumor at screening and the time the tumor would present clinically. Lead time bias occurs when a tumor is detected earlier by screening but the woman dies at the same time as if the tumor had presented clinically. In these circumstances the woman's tumor may well have better prognostic features than symptomatic tumors at diagnosis. Her survival from diagnosis will be longer than in symptomatic cases, but no prolongation of life will have been achieved. The quality of life in such a case may be diminished by the fact that the woman has knowledge of her breast cancer for a longer period of time.

Interval cancers

Interval cancers are cancers which present after a negative screen and before the next scheduled screening episode. It is possible that screening may be biased towards the detection of good prognosis tumors and that aggressive tumors might go undetected by screening and arise between screening episodes, presenting as interval cancers. If this is the case the prognostic profile and survival of screen detected cancers might be excellent but little mortality reduction would be achieved. The incidence and prognosis of interval cancers are therefore important in evaluating the success of a screening program.[17]

Over-diagnosis

Over-diagnosis occurs when screening detects tumors which would never threaten life. Over-diagnosis certainly occurs in mammographic screening especially in the prevalent (first) screening round. A proportion of low grade DCIS

(approximately 7% of prevalent round tumors) represents over-diagnosis as only about 30% will progress to invasive cancer within 10 years.[14,18] However, the number of invasive cancers in the control and screening arms of the Health Insurance Plan (HIP) mammographic screening trial after prolonged follow-up show the actual degree of over-diagnosis of invasive tumors to be small.[19]

Randomized controlled trials

Lead time bias, interval cancers and over-diagnosis mean that surrogate measures of outcome such as the prognostic profile and survival of screen detected cancers may not be effective in predicting the efficacy of screening. Randomized controlled trials are the only reliable way of assessing any mortality benefit from screening. If the breast cancer mortality of a group of women randomized to be screened is compared with an identical control group of women not offered screening then any mortality reduction achieved by screening can be measured over time. Lead time bias, interval cancers and over-diagnosis do not interfere with the outcomes of such trials. The first randomized controlled trial of mammographic screening was the HIP trial carried out in New York 30 years ago.[19] A number of similar trials have subsequently been carried out in Europe (The Swedish Two Counties,[4,7,20-21] Edinburgh,[22] Malmö,[11] Stockholm,[23] and Gothenburg[24] trials). The mortality reductions achieved and the 95% confidence intervals for the age ranges screened are shown in Figure 23.1.[25] Two of these trials, the Two Counties trial and the HIP trial, have shown statistically significant mortality reductions of 22% and 21% respectively. The other randomized controlled trials showed similar trends, but the mortality reductions have not so far reached statistical significance. Meta-analysis of the combined results suggest that a 22% reduction in mortality was achieved in the entire 40–74 year age range (relative risk 0.78, 95% confidence interval 0.70–0.87) in those invited for screening. In women aged 50–74 the mortality reduction achieved in these trials was 24% (RR 0.76, 95% confidence interval 0.67–0.87) (Fig. 23.1). The mortality reductions in the combined Swedish trials reached statistical significance in the 50–59

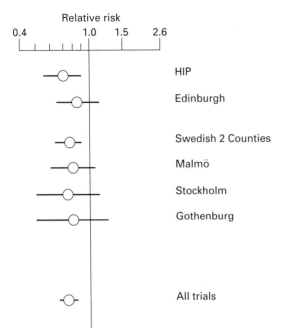

Relative risk

HIP

Edinburgh

Swedish 2 Counties

Malmö

Stockholm

Gothenburg

All trials

Fig. 23.1 The relative risk of breast cancer mortality in women aged 40–74 years invited for screening compared with those not invited is shown for each trial together with the 95% CI. The combined estimate is shown for all trials. (Reproduced from Wald et al. The Breast 1993; 2: 209–216 with kind permission.)

and 60–69 year age bands, providing convincing evidence of the efficacy of mammographic screening in women aged 50–69.[24] Significant mortality reductions were not observed in the 40–49 or 70–74 year age bands. The mortality reduction in those women who actually attended (age range 40–74) was 28%.[25] Other studies with either geographical controls (Guildford[26]) or those in women accepting screening (BCDDP,[27] Nijmegen,[28] Utrecht[29] and Florence[30]) all showed statistically significant mortality reductions, but case control studies are open to bias not present in randomized controlled trials.

SCREENING WOMEN UNDER 50 YEARS OF AGE

None of the six randomized controlled trials discussed above were specifically designed to assess the value of screening in women under 50 years of age. One trial designed to assess the value of screening women aged 40–49 (The Canadian trial[31]) did not show a significant mortality reduction (RR 1.36 95% confidence interval 0.84–2.21). However there were many defects in the design, implementation and quality in the Canadian trial and the validity of its results are in doubt. Women were examined physically before randomization and those with palpable tumors were not excluded from the study group resulting in a larger number of palpable tumors in the screening arm of the trial. Half of the mammograms performed in years 1–4 were judged to be of poor or unacceptable diagnostic quality, a matter over which external radiology quality assurance assessors resigned. At least one physician working in the trial refused to biopsy abnormalities unless they were palpable. A quarter of needle localization biopsies recommended were not performed and another quarter of women in the control group had mammography outside the trial. Furthermore the trial was not large enough to have sufficient statistical power to demonstrate any significant mortality reduction at the 15–20% level.[32]

The conclusion must be that the findings of the Canadian screening trial should be ignored when assessing the efficacy of screening by mammography in women aged 40–49. None of the other randomized controlled trials showed a significant mortality reduction in women aged 40–49. However a recent meta-analysis of the most recent data from the randomized controlled trials show a statistically significant mortality reduction in women aged 40–49 if the Canadian trial is excluded (RR 0.76, 95% CI 0.62–0.95).[33] Studies have shown that the prognostic factors of grade, lymph node stage and size are as valid in this age group as in older women suggesting that there is no *biological* reason why screening should not be effective.[34] There are, however, a number of other reasons why the achievement of a significant mortality reduction should be more difficult when screening women aged 40–49.

1. Breast cancer mortality and incidence is lower in younger women so that larger numbers are required to show a statistically significant benefit. The lower incidence of cancer in this age group will also lead to a lower specificity of recall.

2. Higher rates of DCIS in younger women and its slow progression to invasion means that

any mortality benefit gained from detecting DCIS will be delayed.[20] The mortality curves of women under 50 in the combined Swedish trials show a delayed mortality benefit beginning at 9 years. In one of the arms of the Swedish Two Counties trial this benefit appears to be increasing after 14 years.[21] With further follow-up this may become statistically significant. This possible late mortality benefit may be due to the bias towards the detection of DCIS when screening younger women.

3. Mammography is less sensitive in younger women because the relatively denser parenchyma obscures some subtle signs of cancers.[35] However, data from the Breast Cancer Detection Demonstration Project show that when women are screened by mammography combined with physical examination the proportion of tumors found by physical examination alone is low even in young women.[34] This is in marked contrast to the HIP study where many tumors in younger women were found by physical examination alone.[19] This difference is almost certainly due to the improved quality of mammography in more recent studies. Estimates of mammographic sensitivity at screening calculated from the Two Counties trial are 86%, 92% and 94% for women aged 40–49, 50–59 and 60–69 years of age respectively.[20]

4. Lower prevalence to incidence ratios and a shorter time to natural incidence of breast cancer after a negative screen in women under 50 suggests a shorter lead time for screening in this age group. The mean sojourn times calculated from data from the Two Counties trial for women aged 40–49 years, 50–59 years, 60–69 years and 70–74 years are 1.7, 3.3, 3.8 and 2.6 years respectively. This may be due to differences in tumor biology in women under 50. Tabar suggests that there is a larger proportion of poor prognosis grade 3 and medullary tumors in the younger age group. Estimates of tumor volume doubling times from the Two Counties trial are 178 days in women aged 40–49 and 255 days in women aged 50–74.[20] These data support the concept that the interval between screens should be shorter in younger women. The 'age trial' currently under way in the United Kingdom is the only trial in this age group to use annual mammography. As annual mammography may be required to screen

women under 50 effectively, the results of this trial are awaited with interest. (First reports are likely to be available after 2002.)

BREAST SELF EXAMINATION AND CLINICAL EXAMINATION

Although one of the screening trials to show a mortality benefit (the HIP trial[19]) used clinical examination, the other (the Two Counties trial[4]) did not. There is no evidence to show that when modern mammography is used clinical examination adds to any mortality benefit. No trial using clinical examination alone for screening has ever shown a significant reduction in breast cancer mortality. The specificity of clinical examination as a screening modality is also unacceptably low.[36]

A United Kingdom population screening trial using instruction in breast self examination as the screening method showed slightly better prognostic features in the study group, but this was not translated into a significant mortality reduction (RR 1.01, 95% CI 0.86–1.17).[37–38] Other trials of breast self examination have also failed to show a mortality benefit. However, it is reasonable to consider breast self examination as an adjunct to mammographic screening.

MAMMOGRAPHY AS A SCREENING TECHNIQUE

Mammography remains the most effective single method for detecting breast cancer in its preclinical phase. However, it has a number of disadvantages:

1. It is difficult to perform and interpret, requiring dedicated and expensive equipment and rigorous quality control measures to achieve adequate diagnostic images.

2. Mammography is uncomfortable, and a small proportion of women find the procedure unacceptably painful. Nevertheless, attendance rates for repeat screening examinations are excellent in women participating in the United Kingdom National Health Service Breast Screening Programme (NHSBSP). Re-attendance rates are

lower in older women entering a screening program.[39]

3. Mammography uses ionizing radiation and so is theoretically capable of inducing breast cancers as well as detecting them. Thorough reviews of radiation risks indicate that the carcinogenic effects of screening mammography are negligible.

Despite these points mammography is a sensitive screening tool and when followed by multidisciplinary assessment of screen detected abnormalities is highly specific in determining when surgical biopsy is required.

The sensitivity of screening mammography can be measured by comparing the numbers of interval cancers with the breast cancer incidence in a non-screened population. Such calculations show a 76% decrease in symptomatic breast cancer in the first year following a negative screen. This reduces to 41% and 21% in the second and third years after a negative screen.[17] Detection of interval cancers requires close cooperation between the screening center and local pathology departments and Cancer Registries. In the United Kingdom National Quality Assurance guidelines state that interval cancer numbers should be less than 1.2/1000 in the first 2 years after screening and less than 1.3/1000 in the third year. The prognosis of interval cancers is no worse than that of symptomatic cancer presenting in women of the same age, but is worse than that of screen detected cancer.[40] Review of the screening mammograms of interval cancers is a useful method of assessing the quality of screen reading. The proportion of screening films showing the cancer (false negatives) should be low. One recent series of interval cancers had a false negative rate of 22%.[40] Ideally this should be zero, but this false negative rate is lower than in most studies of interval cancers.

The specificity of mammography alone is shown by comparing the recall for assessment rate with the cancer detection rate. United Kingdom screening programs perform with an assessment rate of 10 times that of the cancer detection rate.[41] Multidisciplinary assessment improves this specificity greatly and this is indicated by the benign to malignant biopsy ratio. In the NHSBSP for the years 1990–1993 the prevalent round ratio was two cancers to one benign biopsy.[41]

SCREENING PRACTICE

BACKGROUND

The NHSBSP was set up following publication of the Forrest report.[42] The report recommended 3-yearly single view screening by mammography alone in women aged 50–64 years. It also recommended research to be carried out concerning the length of the screening interval and a comparison between a single and two views. The first centers began screening in 1987 and now over 90 centers provide a nation-wide service. At present The Netherlands, Sweden and Iceland also have established national programs; Norway, Germany and France are starting national projects and a European Union pilot scheme is also being undertaken in those member states which have not commenced screening on a national basis.

IDENTIFYING AND INVITING THE SCREENING POPULATION

Although many risk factors for breast cancer are known, only age and sex are strong enough to guide selection of the screening population. Women in the United Kingdom aged 50–64 are identified from Family Health Services Authorities (FHSA) which hold the computerized records of all patients registered with General Practitioners. After validation women are invited by letter to attend for screening. In inner cities where the population is more mobile, records can be quite inaccurate resulting in a decreased uptake. The average uptake for breast screening in the United Kingdom is just above 70%.[41] The lack of accurate population registers or problems of access can be a major obstacle to the establishment of effective screening programs in a number of countries.

INITIAL SCREEN AND SCREEN READING

Mammography

Mammographic screening should include two views of each breast. The mean recall rate and cancer detection rate of United Kingdom centers using two view mammography are 5.6% and

6.2/1000. These are significantly better than the equivalent rates of 6.6% and 5.6/1000 found in centers using single view mammography.[41] In the UKCCCR one view two view comparison trial, two view mammography detected 24% more cancers with a 15% lower recall rate, whilst the cost per cancer detected was similar.[43] Two view mammography at first screen was made mandatory in the NHSBSP from August 1995. The efficacy of one view compared to two view screening at subsequent screens has not yet been tested.

Film reading

The NHSBSP is funded for a single reading only. Double reading without consensus leads to increased sensitivity but decreased specificity. A recent study of double reading without consensus showed a 5% increase in cancer detection at the cost of a 1.8% increase in recall rate.[44] A similar study from Florence indicated a 4.6% increase in cancer detection with independent double reading.[45] A study using double reading with consensus showed a decrease in recall rate of 45% with a 9% increase in cancer detection.[46] Double reading appears to give only a modest increase in cancer detection and therefore may not be cost effective.

Recall

It is important that multidisciplinary assessment of screen detected abnormalities is carried out quickly and efficiently by the screening center.

Recall for assessment causes considerable anxiety, so it is important that the recall rate is kept as low as possible without compromizing sensitivity. Recall rates in the NHSBSP in 1990–1993 were 6.4% in the prevalent round and 3.0% at incident screens.[41] A list of mammographic abnormalities and their positive predictive value for malignancy following assessment is shown in Table 23.1.

ASSESSMENT

Assessment should be carried out by a multidisciplinary team including a radiologist, clinician, pathologist, radiographer and breast care nurse. Patients normally undergo further mammography and/or ultrasound and clinical examination is performed.

Fine needle aspiration cytology (FNAC) and/or needle core biopsy are carried out under image guidance if required. Needle core biopsy is particularly useful in the assessment of microcalcification. The estimate of risk of malignancy of a lesion is based on the combination of imaging and clinical findings. Patient management is based on the most suspicious of these findings. Lesions with a low risk of malignancy are returned to normal screening on the basis of benign FNAC or needle core biopsy results while lesions with a high risk of malignancy are removed irrespective of the FNAC/needle core biopsy results.[16] The aim of preoperative sampling in the latter case is to allow a preoperative diagnosis to be made in the patients with carcinomas so that therapeutic rather than

Table 23.1 Screen detected mammographic abnormalities; their positive predictive value for malignancy and management

Mammographic abnormality	Positive predictive value for malignancy following assessment	Management summary
Well-defined mass	0–5%	Not recalled unless new or growing; if recalled and solid, left in situ if FNAC/needle core biopsy is benign
Ill-defined mass	35%	Always recalled; if solid, are left in situ if two FNAC samples show benign cells or core biopsy indicates a fibroadenoma
Spiculate mass	90%	Are always removed whatever the FNAC/needle core biopsy result*
Architectural distortion	40%	Are always removed whatever the FNAC/needle core biopsy result*
Asymmetric density	<1%	Are not recalled unless new
Comedo calcification (rods/branching)	80%	Are always removed whatever the FNAC/needle core biopsy result*
Non-comedo suspicious calcification	30%	Are removed unless a needle core biopsy shows representative calcification in a benign lesion

*FNAC/Needle core result determines whether excision is *diagnostic* or *therapeutic*.

diagnostic surgery can be offered and informed counseling provided. A summary of the management of screen detected lesions is shown in Table 23.1. Preoperative diagnosis rates for malignancy of 90% for invasive carcinoma and 75% for DCIS can be achieved with judicious use of core biopsy and repeat procedures.[47] Needle core biopsy is also useful as a supplementary technique when equivocal (C3) FNAC results are obtained from masses thought to be benign on clinical and imaging grounds.

Patient management is best decided at a prospective pre-treatment multidisciplinary meeting where the pathological, imaging and clinical findings are discussed before the women are seen for their follow-up appointment.

SURGERY FOR SCREEN DETECTED ABNORMALITIES

Ideally diagnostic and therapeutic surgery should be carried out by the clinician who has also been involved in assessment and will have established a rapport with the patient. Approximately 50% of suspicious abnormalities requiring removal will be impalpable and need marker localization. Marker localization is best performed under ultrasound control, but stereotaxis is required for lesions not visible on ultrasound, such as calcifications. Close cooperation between the pathologist, radiologist and surgeon is needed to ensure that the correct lesion is excised. Immediate radiography of a compressed, orientated specimen is required for the surgeon in theatre to ensure that the lesion is removed in a diagnostic procedure and to obtain adequate margins of clearance in therapeutic wide local excisions (see Ch. 2). The NHSBSP standard requires that >80% of wire localization biopsies should have the wire within 10 mm of the lesion and that the abnormality should be removed at the first diagnostic operation in 95% of cases. More than 80% of diagnostic biopsies should weigh less than 20 grams.[48]

THE SCREENING INTERVAL

It is a basic tenet of screening that the screening interval (the time between screening examinations) should be less than the lead time provided by screening. Estimates of the sojourn time achieved by mammographic screening in the Two Counties trial in women aged 50–59 and 60–69 are 3.3 and 3.8 years respectively.[20] A sharp increase in interval cancers is observed in the third year after screening.[17] The 3-year screening interval of the NHSBSP may therefore be too long. As recommended in the Forrest report[42] a multicenter United Kingdom trial (the 'frequency trial') has taken place to assess the relative merits of annual compared with 3-yearly screening. Preliminary results suggest that the benefits of shortening the screening interval are likely to be marginal. All the other European screening programs have a shorter screening interval than the United Kingdom program.

COST EFFECTIVENESS OF MAMMOGRAPHIC SCREENING

The success of mammographic screening can be measured not only in terms of breast cancer mortality reduction, but also in cost effectiveness. A number of studies have been performed which indicate that 2-yearly screening is cost effective in women over the age of 50, but that screening women under 50 at this interval is not cost effective.[49–50] The reasons for lack of cost effectiveness in screening women under 50 include the lower incidence of breast cancer in this age group, the reduced sensitivity of mammography, the higher frequency of false positive screening results[51] and the need for annual screening.

SCREENING IN 'HIGH RISK' GROUPS

Many women are now aware of the increased risk of breast cancer associated with a family history of the disease in close relatives. This has led to a rise in the number of referrals for counseling and mammographic screening of women with a family history of breast cancer. Most units offer mammographic screening to women under 50 who have a first degree relative with breast cancer occurring at a young age. Screening should include counseling, an assessment of risk, instruction in breast self examination and be combined with physical examination. There have been no controlled trials to show a mortality benefit from family history screening and it is carried out on an empirical basis. As there are no proven therapeutic maneuvers to offer women with a family history of breast cancer except bilateral mastectomy, family history screening should only be offered to women presenting with anxiety concerning their family history risk. Raising anxiety in women by offering screening to women unaware of their increased risk is unjustified.

There is concern that offering mammographic screening to very young women with a strong family history may induce as many cancers as it finds. This has led to interest in non-mammographic methods of breast cancer screening. Research into the role of enhanced magnetic resonance mammography (MRM) in screening such women is being contemplated. At present the specificity and sensitivity of MRM in asymptomatic women is unknown. MRM screening of the breast would also be time consuming and expensive.

The other groups of women at 'high risk' who are offered regular mammographic screening are:

1. Women who have had a previous breast biopsy showing atypical ductal hyperplasia or lobular carcinoma in situ.
2. Women who have had breast conserving surgery for breast cancer.
3. Contralateral mammography for women who have had a mastectomy for breast cancer.

SUMMARY

Mammographic screening is of proven benefit in reducing breast cancer mortality in women aged 50 to 70 years. Screening women aged 40–49 is less effective than in older women. The value of screening women over the age of 70 has not been established. Breast self examination and clinical examination have never been shown to confer any breast cancer mortality benefit.

Breast screening is best carried out in dedicated screening units by properly trained staff. Assessment of screen detected abnormalities should be carried out by a multidisciplinary team who discuss case management at prospective meetings. Quality assurance guidelines should be established for breast screening programs and adhered to by participating units.

REFERENCES

1. Early Breast Cancer Trialists Collaborative Group. Systemic treatment of early breast cancer by hormonal, cytotoxic, or immune therapy. Lancet 1992; 339: 1–15.
2. Department of Health. The Health of the Nation, 1993.
3. Seidman JD, Schnaper LA, Aisner SC. Relationship of the size of the invasive component of the primary breast carcinoma to axillary lymph node metastasis. Cancer 1995; 75: 65–71.
4. Tabar L, Fagerberg G, Duffy SW et al. Update of the two-county program of mammographic screening for breast cancer. Rad Clin N Am 1992; 30: 187–210.
5. Elston CW, Ellis IO. Pathological prognostic factors in breast cancer. 1. The value of histological grade in breast cancer: experience from a large study with long term follow up. Histopathol 1991; 19: 403–410.
6. Rajakariar R, Walker RA. Pathological and biological features of mammographically detected invasive breast cancer. Br J Cancer 1995; 71: 150–154.
7. Tabar L, Fagerberg G, Day NE et al. Breast cancer treatment and natural history: new insights from results of screening. Lancet 1992; 339: 412–414.
8. Klemi PJ, Joensuu H, Toikkanen S et al. Aggressiveness of breast cancers found with and without screening. Br Med J 1992; 304: 467–469.
9. Cowan WK, Angus B, Henry J et al. Immunohistochemical and other features of breast carcinomas presenting clinically compared with those detected by cancer screening. Br J Cancer 1991; 64: 780–784.
10. Smart CR, Myers MH, Gloecker LA. Implications from SEER data on breast cancer management. Cancer 1978; 41: 787–789.
11. Andersson I, Aspergren K, Janzon L et al. Mammographic screening and mortality from breast cancer: the Malmo mammographic screening trial. Br Med J 1988; 297: 943–948.
12. Bellamy CO, McDonald C, Salter DM et al. Non invasive ductal carcinoma of the breast: the relevance of histologic categorization. Hum Pathol 1993; 24: 16–23.
13. Evans AJ, Pinder S, Ellis IO et al. Screening detected and symptomatic ductal carcinoma in situ: mammographic features with pathologic correlation. Radiol 1994; 191: 237–240.
14. Ketcham AS, Moffat FL. Vexed surgeons, perplexed patients and breast cancer which may not be cancer. Cancer 1990; 65: 387–393.
15. Lampejo OT, Barnes DM, Smith P, Millis RR. Evaluation of infiltrating ductal carcinomas with a DCIS

component: correlation of the histologic type of the in situ component with grade of the infiltrating component. Semin Diagn Pathol 1994; 11: 215–222.

16. Ellis IO, Galea MH, Locker A et al. Early experience in breast cancer screening: emphasis on development of protocols for triple assessment. Breast 1993; 2: 148–153.

17. Day N, McCann J, Camilleri-Ferrante C et al. Monitoring interval cancers in breast screening programmes: the East Anglian experience. J Med Screen 1995; 2: 180–185.

18. Page DL, Dupont WD, Rogers LW, Rados MS. Atypical hyperplastic lesions of the female breast. A long-term follow-up study. Cancer 1985; 55: 2698–2708.

19. Shapiro S, Venet W, Strax P, Venet L. Periodic screening for breast cancer: the Health Insurance Plan project and its sequelae, 1963–1986. Baltimore: Johns Hopkins University Press, 1988.

20. Tabar L, Fagerberg G, Chen HH et al. Screening for breast cancer in women aged under 50: mode of detection, incidence, fatality, and histology. J Med Screen 1995a; 2: 94–98.

21. Tabar L, Fagerberg G, Chen HH et al. Efficacy of breast cancer screening by age. New results from the Swedish Two-Counties Trial. Cancer 1995b; 75: 2507–2517.

22. Roberts MM, Alexander FE, Anderson TJ et al. Edinburgh trial of screening for breast cancer: mortality at 7 years. Lancet 1990; 335: 241–246.

23. Frisell J, Eklund G, Hellstrom L et al. Randomised study of mammography screening-preliminary report on mortality in the Stockholm Trial. Br Canc Res Treat 1991; 18: 49–56.

24. Nyström L, Rutqvist LE, Wall S et al. Breast cancer screening with mammography; overview of Swedish randomised trials. Lancet 1993; 341: 973–978.

25. Wald NJ, Chamberlain J, Hackshaw A. Consensus Statement. Report of the European Society for Mastology Breast Cancer Screening Evaluation Committee. Breast 1993; 2: 209–216.

26. UK trial of early detection of breast cancer. Breast cancer mortality after 10 years in the UK trial of early detection of breast cancer. Breast 1993; 2: 13–20.

27. Morrison AS, Brisson J, Khalid N. Breast cancer incidence and mortality in the breast cancer detection demonstration project. J Natl Cancer Inst 1988; 80: 1540–1547.

28. Verbeek ALM, Hendricks JHCL, Holland R et al. Mammographic screening and breast cancer mortality: age specific effects in the Nijmegen project, 1975–1982. Lancet 1985; i: 865–866.

29. Collette HJA, Rombach JJ, Day NE, De Waard F. Evaluation of screening for breast cancer in a non-randomised study (the DOM project) by means of a case-control method. Lancet 1984; i: 1224–1226.

30. Palli D, del Turco MR, Buiatti E. A case-control study of the efficacy of a non-randomised breast cancer screening programme in Florence. Int J Cancer 1986; 38: 501–504.

31. Miller AB, Baines CJ, To T, Wall C. Canadian National Breast Screening Study. 1. Breast cancer detection and death rates among women aged 40–49 years. Can Med Ass J 1992; 147: 1459–1476.

32. Kopans DB, Feig SA. The Canadian National Breast Screening Study: a critical review. Am J Roentgenol 1993; 161: 755–760.

33. Smart CR, Hendrick RE, Rutledge JH III, Smith RA.

34. Smart CR, Hartmann WH, Beahrs OH, Garfinkel L. Insights into breast cancer screening of younger women. Evidence from the 14 year follow up of the Breast Cancer Detection Demonstration Project. Cancer Suppl 1993; 72: 1449–1456.

35. Sibbering DM, Burrell HC, Evans AJ et al. Mammographic sensitivity in women under 50 presenting symptomatically with breast cancer. Breast 1995; 4: 127–129.

36. UK trial of early detection of breast cancer. Specificity of screening in the United Kingdom trial of early detection of breast cancer. Br Med J 1992; 304: 346–349.

37. Ellman R, Moss SM, Coleman D, Chamberlain J. Breast self examination programmes in the trial of early detection of breast cancer: ten year findings. Br J Cancer 1993; 68: 208–212.

38. Locker AP, Caseldine J, Mitchell AK et al. Results from a 7 year programme of breast self-examination in 89,010 women. Brit J Cancer 1989; 60: 401–405.

39. Scaf-Klomp W, Van Sonderen FLP, Stewart R et al. Compliance after 17 years of breast cancer screening. J Med Screen 1995; 2: 195–199.

40. Burrell HC, Sibbering DM, Wilson ARM et al. The mammographic features of interval cancers and prognosis compared with screen detected symptomatic breast cancers. Radiol 1996; 199: 811–817.

41. Moss SM, Michell M, Patnick J et al. Results from the NHS breast screening programme 1990–1993. J Med Screen 1995; 2: 186–190.

42. Forrest APM. Breast Cancer Screening. A report to the Health Ministers of England, Scotland and Northern Ireland. London: HMSO, 1986.

43. Wald NJ, Murphy P, Major P et al. UKCCCR multicentre randomised controlled trial of one and two view mammography in breast cancer screening. Br Med J 1995; 311: 1189–1193.

44. Anderson ED, Muir BB, Walsh JS, Kirkpatrick AE. The efficacy of double reading mammograms in breast screening. Clin Radiol 1994; 49: 248–251.

45. Ciatto S, del Turco MR, Morrone D et al. Independent double reading of screening mammograms. J Med Screen 1995; 2: 99–101.

46. Anttinen I, Pamilo M, Soiva M, Roiha M. Double reading of mammography screening films — one radiologist or two. Clin Radiol 1993; 48: 414–421.

47. Litherland JC, Evans AJ, Wilson ARM et al. The impact of core biopsy on pre-operative diagnosis rate of screen detected breast cancers. Clin Radiol 1996; 51: 562–565.

48. Quality assurance guidelines for surgeons in breast cancer screening. 2nd ed. NHSBSP Publications, April 1996.

49. Van Der Maas PJ, de Koning HJ, Van Ineveld BM et al. The cost effectiveness of breast cancer screening. Int J Cancer 1989; 43: 1055–1060.

50. de Koning HJ, Van Ineveld BM, Van Oortmarssen GJ et al. Breast cancer screening and cost effectiveness; policy alternatives, quality of life considerations and the possible impact of uncertain forces. Int J Cancer 1991; 49: 531–537.

51. Lidbrink E, Elfving J, Frisell J, Jonsson E. Neglected aspects of false positive findings of mammography in breast cancer screening: analysis of false positive cases from the Stockholm trial. Br Med J 1996; 312: 273–276.

Quality assurance in breast pathology

INTRODUCTION

As definitive diagnoses of breast cancer and related disorders are made almost exclusively by pathologists, the quality of pathology services is of crucial importance in ensuring that patients are managed appropriately. Furthermore, with an increasing number of treatment options, it is no longer sufficient for histopathologists simply to distinguish breast cancer from benign conditions and there is an increasing requirement for them to report consistently those pathological features of prognostic significance which help clinicians to make important management decisions, such as the extent of surgery and the use of adjuvant cytotoxic and hormonal therapy.

The introduction of mammographic screening for breast cancer has further increased the demands on pathologists. Improvements in the scope and quality of cytopathology services are required to reduce the number of unnecessary surgical operations as, combined with high quality imaging and clinical examination, fine needle aspiration cytology can improve confidence about benign diagnoses.[1] Screening has also had a major impact on histopathology at both the macroscopic and histological stages of the examination. The former has been affected mainly by the need for specimen radiography to localize and obtain accurate samples of impalpable radiographic abnormalities and the latter by the disproportionate number of early cancers and borderline lesions detected by screening. Ductal carcinoma in situ (DCIS), for example, accounts for about 5% of cancers in symptomatic women but for 15–20% in screened women.

In view of the increasing demands placed on

pathologists, quality assurance programs are becoming necessary to define and monitor standards of pathological examination and to correct deficiencies wherever they are identified. For the purposes of this chapter, histopathology and cytopathology will be treated separately although it is recognized that these two aspects of pathological examination are increasingly being undertaken by the same individuals.

The following account of quality assurance in breast pathology is largely concerned with defining standards and evaluating performance through external quality assessment. It should be remembered, however, that other factors are of vital importance in determining the quality of pathology services, particularly education, training, research, development and the provision of adequate material and human resources.

HISTOPATHOLOGY

MACROSCOPIC EXAMINATION

This is a crucial part of the examination of breast specimens for if the lesion responsible for symptoms or a radiological abnormality is not localized and sampled, the value of subsequent histological examination is negated. In the UK National Breast Screening Programme (NHSBSP), guidelines were therefore issued defining standards that are minimally acceptable in the gross examination of breast specimens[2] and much depends on pathologists monitoring and trying to improve their own standard of performance. It is, however, very difficult to monitor the quality of macroscopic examination by any external quality assessment procedure.

SPECIMEN RADIOGRAPHY

The necessity for specimen radiography has increased greatly since the introduction of mammographic screening as the technique is indispensable in detecting impalpable abnormalities. It has also been used to examine specimens from symptomatic women where it has been found that small carcinomas may occasionally be detected which would have gone unrecognized by conventional macroscopic examination.[3–4] In general, however, the use of the technique to examine breasts containing palpable abnormalities is not considered to be necessary. Neither is the technique thought to be suitable for assessing excision margins of impalpable lesions as it has been shown that the extent of DCIS as determined by histological examination is often significantly greater than that visualized by specimen radiography.[5]

For impalpable lesions, a radiograph of the intact specimen must first be made and, ideally, examined by the radiologist who reported the clinical mammogram to determine whether the lesion has been resected. A good working relationship between pathologist, surgeon and radiologist is essential to ensure that mammographic abnormalities are correctly identified and sampled. The specimen is then cut into slices and further radiographs taken. The slices should be thin enough to require no further trimming before they are embedded. The radiological abnormality is then sampled together with any other areas which appear suspicious on radiological or naked eye examination. The areas sampled can be marked on the specimen radiograph.

Although this method is regarded as an ideal way of localizing mammographic abnormalities, it is a two-stage procedure regarded as too time-consuming by some pathologists. A wide variety of one-stage procedures has thus been developed, usually employing some form of grid.

In one of these methods, biopsy specimens are securely mounted on pieces of perspex inlaid with a wire grid.[6] Using the grid coordinates, the mammographic abnormality is mapped to a particular area which is then sliced into. Any macroscopically detectable abnormality on the cut surface is sampled. If no abnormality is seen, the tissue overlying the appropriate grid squares is blocked in its entirety.

In another method,[7] the specimen is placed in a plastic petrie dish filled with paraffin wax and covered by a translucent and radiolucent plate containing numerous asymmetrically spaced holes 3–4 mm in diameter. A specimen radiograph is taken and a pin inserted through the hole nearest the mammographic abnormality, the tissue and into the underlying paraffin to which it is secured. The plate is removed and the tissue is sectioned.

A 1.5–2 cm area around the pin is separately processed.

In an even simpler method,[8] the radiologist, using the specimen radiograph as a guide, inserts a hypodermic needle into the tissue as close as possible to the center of the suspicious lesion. The specimen is then transported to the histopathology department where the pathologist slices the specimen along the plane of the needle and places it in fixative. After fixation, several blocks are taken adjacent to the needle shaft.

The advantage of these methods and their variants is that time and money are saved in avoiding a second specimen radiograph. There are, however, several disadvantages. The specimen may move on the grid or the localizing pin or needle may become dislodged. The pathologist is dependent on the surgeon or radiologist to undertake a procedure in a specified fashion in the operating theatre or radiology department. Sampling multiple abnormalities may be very difficult as the tissue loses its integrity when the first slice is cut. Finally, identifying lesions in thick specimens may be difficult given the two-dimensional nature of the radiograph.

The method adopted in a particular laboratory will clearly depend on local resources and preferences, but pathologists should be confident that they have characterized the mammographic abnormality histologically in at least 99% of cases.

EXCISION MARGINS

Given the increasing use of breast-conserving surgery, there is a perceived need for pathologists to determine adequacy of excision of carcinomas, particularly in local excision specimens. This is usually performed by coating the whole surface of the specimen with some marker material which will remain adherent to it during fixation, processing and section cutting. Commonly used materials are india ink, and colored gelatins and dyes such as Alcian blue. The specimen can then be sliced and blocks taken to include the excision margins nearest to the tumor borders. In some centers, the whole specimen is peeled like an orange so that the whole of the excision margin can be embedded (see also Ch. 2).

There is, however, a far from perfect correlation between the adequacy of excision as determined by the pathologist and the presence of residual carcinoma in the breast. Failure to find residual tumor in re-excision specimens removed because the pathologist reported the margins as involved may be due to destruction of residual tumor by the surgical procedure. Alternatively, there may be residual tumor in the specimen which is not detected because of sampling error. It is also possible that tumor may only reach the margin and not extend beyond it. The presence of residual tumor in the face of clear excision margins can easily be explained by sampling of inappropriate margins. Most breast carcinomas have irregular, ill-defined outlines and determining the one nearest the excision margin on macroscopic examination can be very difficult. Another problem is multicentric tumor. The incidence of multicentric breast cancer varies greatly in the literature, mainly according to how it is defined. In a review of 11 studies, Carter[9] found that the reported incidence of multifocality varied from 9 to 75% with a mean of 32%.

Clearly the pathologist's ability to predict the presence of residual tumor in the breast is somewhat limited and dependent on a number of factors including the extent of sampling, the degree of circumscription of the tumor and the distance from the margin. It is, however, generally accepted that pathologists should assess adequacy of excision, particularly in ductal carcinomas in situ and well-delineated, invasive tumors without metastatic disease where complete local excision is curative.

SAMPLING

It is very difficult to determine what is an acceptable level of sampling of breast specimens. The more extensive it is, the greater the likelihood will be that small carcinomas and risk lesions will be detected. The probability of finding such changes, however, has to be balanced against the cost of doing so.

With small biopsies, it is reasonable to expect the whole specimen to be blocked. With large specimens, however, this may involve an enormous amount of work, particularly for technical staff in cutting and staining sections from many blocks. This raises the important question of whether the role of the pathologist is merely to provide a diagnosis on a palpable or mammographic abnormality or to detect microscopic in situ and invasive carcinomas and atypical lesions associated with an increased risk of developing cancer.

Schnitt and Wang[10] investigated the problem of cost-effectiveness by reviewing 384 consecutive biopsies from symptomatic women in which gross examination revealed no abnormality. All tissue was submitted for histological examination and produced 3342 blocks. Carcinoma or atypical hyperplasia was detected in 26 cases (6.8%) comprising 12 of lobular carcinoma in situ (LCIS), four of atypical lobular hyperplasia (ALH), four of DCIS, three of atypical ductal hyperplasia (ADH) and three of invasive carcinoma. They calculated that if the first five blocks only had been taken from each case, then 1386 (41%) blocks would have been saved but six of the 26 malignant or borderline lesions would have been undetected. If sampling had been limited to 10 blocks per case, then 610 fewer blocks would have been taken, but all lesions would have been detected with the exception of a single case of LCIS. A very useful practical observation was that in all but one case the lesions were located in the fibrous part of the breast rather than the grossly fatty tissue. The authors suggested that a possible cost-effective method of sampling grossly benign biopsies is to submit a maximum of 10 blocks of fibrous breast tissue per case and only examine the remainder if carcinoma or atypical hyperplasia is found.

In a similar study of 157 biopsies from screened women,[11] it was found that 2183 blocks were required to sample the whole of each specimen (13 blocks per case). This resulted in the detection of carcinoma in 50 patients and atypical hyperplasia in 19. If sampling was restricted initially to areas containing radiological abnormalities and further tissue taken only if carcinoma or atypical hyperplasia was found, 38% fewer blocks would be required (leaving nine blocks per case) but one of the 50 cancers and four of the 19 atypical hyperplasias would have been missed. Although these studies do not allow any dogmatic state-ments to be made about the extent of sampling, they do give guidance to pathologists in planning a strategy for sampling breast biopsies within available resources. An important factor which needs to be taken into account is what action, if any, surgeons and other clinical staff will take when these lesions are discovered.

MICROSCOPIC EXAMINATION

Mammographic screening and larger numbers of treatment options have, in recent years, led to a requirement for increased standards of histopathological examination.

Although screening is primarily radiological, definitive diagnoses of cancer are almost invariably made by pathologists. Accurate diagnoses are essential not only to ensure appropriate patient management but also to monitor screening programs effectively. It is not sufficient merely to diagnose carcinomas and distinguish them from benign lesions and the reporting of features of prognostic significance is necessary (see p. 529). Furthermore, specimens generated by screening are significantly more difficult to interpret than those from symptomatic women due to the disproportionate number of borderline lesions. These lesions fall into two main categories; intraductal proliferations and infiltrative lesions which are benign or of low grade malignancy.

DCIS is now recognized to be a heterogeneous group of proliferations which vary according to cell type and growth pattern. Some forms, particularly those of low nuclear grade, may be difficult to distinguish from atypical ductal hyperplasia, and others from minimally invasive carcinomas. Classification of DCIS has traditionally been based on growth pattern, but has been undertaken with little enthusiasm given a generally perceived lack of clinical relevance. More recent studies, however, have provided evidence that cell type may be related to recurrence after local excision[12] and have consequently raised the question of the need for a reproducible and clinically relevant classification.

The main benign infiltrative lesion detected by screening is the radial scar which may bear a strong resemblance to low grade carcinoma, particularly of tubular type. Furthermore, recent work has shown that screen-detected radial scars may actually exhibit foci of malignant change.[13]

The significance of reporting prognostic features of invasive carcinomas is illustrated in Figure 24.1 which shows markedly different survival curves for patients who have been divided into three groups according to the Nottingham Prognostic Index.[14] This index is based on three pathological features, namely tumor size, histological grade and loco-regional lymph node involvement. The score for tumor size is obtained by multiplying its measurement in centimeters by 0.2. Grade is scored according to the method described by Elston and Ellis from 1–3.[15] Stage is based on a triple lymph node sampling technique; a score of 1 is given if all nodes are tumor free, 2 if tumor is present in the low axillary nodes only and 3 if tumor is present in the apical/axillary and internal

mammary nodes. Scores for each pathological feature are added together and the patient is assigned to the good prognosis group if it equals or is less than 3.4, the moderate group if it is equal to or less than 5.4 and the poor group if it exceeds 5.4 (see also Ch. 18).

Pathological features are useful not only to assign patients to appropriate management protocols (it would clearly be inappropriate, for example, for patients in group 1 to receive adjuvant chemotherapy), but also to monitor breast screening. Although the success of screening is ultimately measured by a reduction in the death rate of the screened population, statistically significant mortality data do not become available for many years after the onset of a program. Pathological features of prognostic significance can be used as a surrogate measure as the success of screening tends to be mirrored by more favorable pathological characteristics of the tumors detected. Pathological features, however, can only have the powerful prognostic significance illustrated in Figure 24.1 if they are reported consistently by all the pathologists providing the data.

In the quality assurance programme associated with the NHSBSP, the problem of reporting consistency was approached in three ways. First, a standard reporting form (Fig. 24.2) in pro-forma style was developed in consultation with all pathologists involved to ensure that the same data were provided from each patient using the same terminology. Secondly, the diagnostic criteria were defined and the use of the form described in an accompanying booklet 'Pathology Reporting in Breast Cancer Screening'.[2] Thirdly, a National External Quality Assessment scheme was set up to monitor reporting consistency, to identify where there are problems and investigate ways of tackling them.

EXTERNAL QUALITY ASSESSMENT

EQA schemes have been set up in many branches of histopathology in recent years. Most are of the 'consensus' variety where there is no prejudgment about the correct diagnosis which is generally accepted to be that made by the majority of participants unless there is clear evidence to the

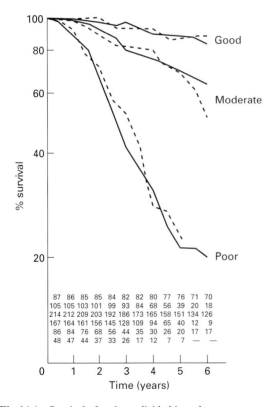

Fig 24.1 Survival of patients divided into three groups according to the Nottingham prognostic index. The continuous lines represent an original study of 387 patients and the discontinuous lines a subsequent prospective study of 320 patients. (Reproduced by kind permission of the British Journal of Cancer.)

BREAST SCREENING HISTOPATHOLOGY

Surname .... Forenames .... Date of Birth ....

Screening no .... Hospital no .... Report no ....

Side   ☐ Right   ☐ Left   Histological Calcification   ☐ Absent   ☐ Benign   ☐ Malignant

Specimen radiograph seen?   ☐ Yes   ☐ No   Mammographic abnormality present in specimen?   ☐ Yes   ☐ No   ☐ Unsure

Specimen type   ☐ Localisation biopsy   ☐ Open biopsy   ☐ Segmental excision   ☐ Mastectomy   ☐ Wide bore needle core

Specimen size (excluding mastectomies and needle core biopsies)   x   x   mm.

HISTOLOGICAL DIAGNOSIS   ☐ NORMAL   ☐ BENIGN   ☐ MALIGNANT

For BENIGN lesions please tick the lesions present

☐ Fibroadenoma   ☐ 'Fibrocystic change'

Papilloma   ☐ Single   ☐ Solitary cyst

☐ Multiple   ☐ Periductal mastitis/duct ectasia

☐ Complex sclerosing lesion/radial scar   ☐ Sclerosing adenosis

☐ Other (please specify) ....

EPITHELIAL PROLIFERATION

☐ Not present   ☐ Present with atypia ('ductal')

☐ Present without atypia   ☐ Present with atypia (lobular)

For MALIGNANT lesions please tick any of the following present

NON-INVASIVE

☐ Ductal   Subtype ....   ☐ Lobular   ☐ Paget's disease

MICROINVASION

☐ Not present   ☐ Possible   ☐ Present

INVASIVE

☐ 'Ductal' (not otherwise specified)   ☐ Tubular or cribriform carcinoma

☐ Medullary carcinoma   ☐ Mucoid carcinoma

☐ Lobular carcinoma

☐ Other primary carcinoma (please specify) ....

☐ Other malignant tumour (please specify) ....

MAXIMUM DIAMETER (invasive component) .... mm   (in-situ) .... mm

AXILLARY NODES   ☐ Not Present   Number positive ....   Total Number ....

OTHER NODES Site ....   ☐ Not Present   Number positive ....   Total Number ....

EXCISION   ☐ Reaches Margin   ☐ Does not reach margin (Distance .... mm)   ☐ Uncertain

GRADE   ☐ I   ☐ II   ☐ III   ☐ Not assessable

DISEASE EXTENT   ☐ Localised   ☐ Diffuse single quadrant   ☐ Multiquadrant   ☐ Not assessable

VASCULAR INVASION   ☐ Present   ☐ Not seen   COMMENTS/ADDITIONAL INFORMATION

SITE (Optional)

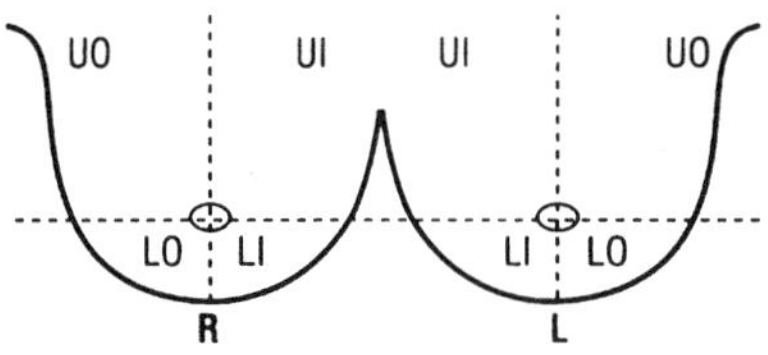

UO   UI   UI   UO

LO ⌖ LI   LI ⌖ LO

R   L

☐ Case for review?

PATHOLOGIST   DATE ....

Fig 24.2 Standard reporting form used for the UK National Breast Screening Programme and which was employed in an edited version for the EQA scheme described in the text. The form is presently undergoing modification mainly by replacing specimen size with weight, classifying DCIS according to nuclear grade and measuring invasive tumors according to the size of the invasive component or to the combined size of the invasive and in situ components if associated DCIS extends for more than 1 mm beyond the invasive disease.

contrary. This is in contrast to the so-called 'proficiency testing' schemes where the correct diagnoses are determined in advance by the organizers who thus function similarly to examiners conducting an examination. Although these schemes are effective at identifying sub-standard performance, they have little educational value as most participants will inevitably be of the required standard and there is little or no opportunity to discuss the slides.

Although 'consensus' schemes are also designed primarily to identify sub-standard performance, they have significant educational value by allowing participants regularly to compare and discuss their diagnoses with other participants. Furthermore, not every case needs to be suitable for assessing performance and some rare and difficult lesions can be included. Unsuitable cases are simply identified by an inadequate level of agreement by the participants.

Another advantage of 'consensus' schemes is that they allow valid studies of diagnostic consistency to be made as cases can be selected in a random manner within broad diagnostic categories.

The following account of EQA in breast histopathology is based mainly on the findings of the 'consensus' scheme set up in association with the NHSBSP.[16] This is a very large scheme and has allowed a number of conclusions to be drawn about the consistency with which pathologists report breast disease.

In this scheme, three sets of 12 slides are sent to each of 17 regional coordinators every 6 months. The coordinators then distribute them to as many consultant pathologists as possible within their regions over a period of about 6 months. At the time of writing, cases have been randomly selected in the following diagnostic categories: benign not otherwise specified, radial scar, atypical hyperplasia, in situ carcinoma and invasive carcinoma of varying size. Radial scar, atypical hyperplasia and in situ carcinoma were chosen because they were perceived as being particularly problematical in breast screening. Individual cases were not selected because they were thought to be particularly difficult or interesting examples, but were the first to be reported at any particular screening center after a specified date.

Participants report the sections using the standard reporting form shown in Figure 24.2, which is modified for the EQA scheme by excluding data which cannot be supplied by examining histological sections alone. The completed forms are sent to the UK National Cancer Screening Evaluation Unit where the responses are analyzed. The findings are presented to the participants in a number of different ways. Table 24.1 shows the results of one circulation in which 280 pathologists participated. The diagnoses have been divided into six major groups — benign, radial scar (including complex sclerosing lesion), atypical hyperplasia, in situ carcinoma, microinvasive carcinoma and invasive carcinoma. In the left-hand column are listed the slide numbers and in the right-hand column, the majority opinions. In eight cases, the majority of opinion was formed by more than 90% of all readings, whereas in the remaining four, it was formed by 43–81%. Not surprisingly, the

Table 24.1   Distributions of individual diagnoses on 12 slides

Slide No.	No. of responses	Benign n.o.s.*	Radial scar	Atypical hyperplasia	In situ carcinoma	Microinvasive carcinoma	Invasive carcinoma	Majority opinion
643	280	268	0	12	0	0	0	Benign
663	280	0	0	0	1	0	279	Invasive carcinoma
664	278	61	8	59	120	1	29	In situ carcinoma
665	280	0	0	0	1	0	279	Invasive carcinoma
666	279	2	47	27	17	3	183	Invasive carcinoma
667	280	2	3	15	226	22	12	In situ carcinoma
668	280	1	0	0	0	0	279	Invasive carcinoma
669	279	0	0	0	2	0	277	Invasive carcinoma
720	280	0	0	0	5	0	275	Invasive carcinoma
721	277	1	0	0	257	13	6	In situ carcinoma
723	278	2	11	0	4	0	261	Invasive carcinoma
1580	279	14	0	72	184	5	4	In situ carcinoma
Total	3350	351	69	185	817	44	1884	

*n.o.s.: not otherwise specified

majority diagnosis was in situ carcinoma in three of these four cases. In one of them (1580), the major problem was clearly in distinguishing in situ carcinoma from atypical hyperplasia whereas, in the other two (664 and 667), the alternative opinions were distributed more evenly among the other groups. Case 666 was highly unusual in that the majority opinion was of invasive carcinoma, but did not exceed 90%. This tumor was classified as of tubular type by most of the participants.

Table 24.2 shows the same diagnostic categories in the same circulation but this time the pathologists are listed in the left-hand column. It can be seen that each pathologist has a code number known only to themselves. No-one knows anyone else's code number and so the scheme is completely anonymous. Pathologists can read across the major categories and identify in the last column what is their overall level of agreement with the majority. Presenting data in this way has the major limitation of making no allowance for the clinical significance of any disagreement, but it nevertheless enables pathologists to compare regularly their diagnoses with those of others.

There is evidence that this leads to improvement in diagnostic consistency (see p. 536).

Table 24.3 summarizes the major findings of the scheme after the first six rounds. In the left-hand column are listed the majority diagnoses. The horizontal rows show what percentage of readings fell into the major categories for each majority diagnosis. Consequently, where the majority diagnosis was 'benign nos', this diagnosis was made in 88.6% of all readings. Had there been perfect agreement, the top left-hand box would have shown a figure of 100% as would every other box moving diagonally from the top left-hand corner of the table to the bottom right. It can be seen, in the 'benign nos' category, that a small percentage of diagnoses were of carcinoma. It is difficult to understand, on examining the histological sections, why these deviant diagnoses were made. Although it is possible that a small number of pathologists made serious mistakes of interpretation, it is also possible that they were due to clerical error.

The next line shows radial scar where the majority diagnosis was formed by 74.8% of all

Table 24.2   Individual diagnoses compared with majority diagnosis

Pathologist*	Benign nos	Radial scar	Atypical hyperplasia	In situ carcinoma	Microinvasive carcinoma	Invasive carcinoma	Agreement with majority
1	1	0	1	4	0	6	91%
2	1	0	1	3	0	7	91%
4	3	1	1	2	0	5	66%
5	3	1	1	2	0	5	66%
9	0	0	2	3	0	7	91%
10	1	1	0	3	0	7	91%
11	3	0	0	2	0	7	83%
12	1	1	0	3	0	7	83%

*The numbers are fictitious.

Table 24.3   Distribution of individual opinions for slides classified according to the majority opinion

Majority diagnosis	Benign nos	Radial scar	Atypical hyperplasia	In situ carcinoma (inc microinvasive)	Invasive carcinoma	No. of cases	Total readings
Benign nos	**88.6%**	3.6%	5.9%	1.1%	0.1%	17	4105
Radial scar	13.1%	**74.8%**	8.3%	0.9%	2.9%	10	2466
Atypical hyperplasia	37.4%	7.0%	**41.9%**	13.6%	0.1%	3	701
In situ carcinoma (inc microinvasive)	6.3%	0.5%	10.5%	**77.9%**	4.7%	21	5045
Invasive carcinoma	0.8%	3.3%	1.0%	2.6%	**92.1%**	21	5228
						72	17545

N.B.: In situ and microinvasive carcinoma are grouped together as the latter was never a majority diagnosis. Microinvasive carcinoma was defined, for the purposes of the UK screening programme, as a predominantly in situ carcinoma with one or more foci of invasion, none exceeding 1 mm in maximum dimension.
(Reproduced by permission of the European Journal of Cancer.)

readings. Only 2.9% were of invasive carcinoma. This is a surprising and encouraging finding as it had been anticipated that significant problems would be encountered in distinguishing radial scars from well-differentiated, low grade invasive carcinomas.

With atypical hyperplasia, however, the majority diagnosis was formed by only 41.9% of all readings. Nevertheless, most of the other diagnoses were of benign conditions and only 13.6% of in situ carcinoma. The majority diagnosis of in situ carcinoma was formed by 77.9% of all readings which was also a very encouraging finding and exceeded a national target set at the beginning of the screening program. In this category, 10.5% of diagnoses were of atypical hyperplasia. Where the majority diagnosis is DCIS or atypical hyperplasia, there is thus a 10–15% incidence of the other diagnosis. Only 4.7% of readings were of invasive carcinoma where in situ carcinoma was the majority diagnosis. Microinvasive carcinoma was never the majority diagnosis.

The low level of agreement in diagnosing atypical hyperplasia is not surprising and in keeping with findings in other reports.[17–18] Greater concordance was achieved in one study[19] although this was at the expense of a lower level of agreement on in situ carcinoma. Furthermore, this study exhibited several major differences from the UK scheme: (1) only six pathologists, chosen by the scheme organiser, participated; (2) the cases were selected by the organizer according to their histological appearance and the technical quality of the sections; (3) slides were covered with masking tape so that only lesions of interest were visible; (4) participants were provided with a written summary of diagnostic criteria and a set of teaching slides prior to the study. The first three of these different aspects would be inappropriate for an EQA scheme, whose aim is to determine diagnostic consistency with a minimum of artificiality. The last, however, is relevant. Although detailed diagnostic criteria for hyperplasia of usual type and ductal carcinoma in situ were laid down at the onset of the UK scheme, atypical hyperplasia was simply defined as a group of intermediate proliferations which did not fit easily into either of the other two categories. Detailed architectural and cytological criteria for diagnosing atypical ductal

hyperplasia have recently been published[20] and could form the basis of a more precise definition.

Not surprisingly, the majority diagnosis of invasive carcinoma was formed by a very high percentage of all readings but a small percentage of benign diagnoses were noted. A total of 3.3% of these were of radial scar, but 1.8% were benign n.o.s. or atypical hyperplasia for reasons which are not clear.

Although the majority diagnosis of ductal carcinoma in situ was composed of nearly 80% of readings overall, significant variations are encountered in the size of the majority from case to case. In those composed of cells of high nuclear grade, particularly with comedo necrosis, the majority diagnosis comprised over 90% of all readings and rarely less than 70%. In those composed of cells of low nuclear grade, the majority diagnosis may be formed by less than 40% of all readings and rarely more than 60%. Cases where opinion is significantly divided between DCIS and ADH are usually of this type. An EQA scheme of this type can thus help not only to determine the level of diagnostic agreement, but also to identify where problems of inconsistency occur.

Classifying DCIS was also examined. Using a classification entirely based on growth pattern resulted in Kappa values shown in Table 24.4. Kappa statistics are a way of measuring the level of agreement, taking into account that which would be expected by chance. A value of 1 indicates perfect agreement and 0 the level of agreement that would be expected by chance alone. Minus values indicate a level of disagreement greater than would be expected by chance. What is an acceptable value is determined by the nature and specificity of the diagnosis. A high value (in excess of 0.9) would be expected for diagnosing an ordinary invasive carcinoma, but lower values would be expected for the various borderline lesions or

Table 24.4 Kappa statistics after six circulations

	DCIS subtype (all participants)		
NOS	0.09	Solid	0.22
Comedo	0.44	Mixed	0.06
Cribriform	0.22	Other	0.11
Overall	0.23		

(Reproduced by permission of the European Journal of Cancer.)

for typing or grading tumors. A value of 0.7 is, however, generally regarded as acceptable. It can thus be seen from Table 24.4 that the level of consistency in classifying DCIS is unacceptably low and an improved system of classification is urgently required.

It is important to be able to determine the extent of DCIS as this is an important predictor of local recurrence not only in pure DCIS but also in association with invasive carcinomas. Wide ranges in size measurement are found for most cases of DCIS but histograms show that the measurements are often tightly grouped and that the wide ranges are due to a small number of outlying results (Fig. 24.3). There are, however, cases where there is a genuine lack of agreement on the size of DCIS (Fig. 24.4). In only eight out of 17 circulated cases were 80% of the size estimates within 3 mm of the median. In the remaining nine cases the measurements were more variable. Several reasons for size variation have been identified: (1) the lesion varies significantly in the different sections circulated to the participating pathologists; (2) the DCIS may merge with atypical ductal hyperplasia. In these circumstances, there is significant uncertainty about whether to include the atypical hyperplasia in the measurement. There is also significant uncertainty in determining where the DCIS stops and the atypical hyperplasia begins; (3) in some cases, DCIS presents as small, widely dispersed foci rather than as more compact masses of tumor; (4) the lesion may have different dimensions in different planes; (5) there is a tendency to round up or round down measurements, usually to the nearest 5 mm.

Although a high level of consistency is achieved in diagnosing radial scars, it has recently become apparent that they may contain foci of carcinoma or atypical hyperplasia with disproportionate frequency, particularly if detected by mammographic screening. In a recent study,[13] in situ or invasive carcinoma was found in as many as 43% of screen detected radial scars although this may represent an overestimate as the study contained a significant number of cases referred for second opinion because they presented diagnostic difficulty. A relationship was found between the presence of carcinoma and atypical hyperplasia and lesion size and patient age. Malignant change was

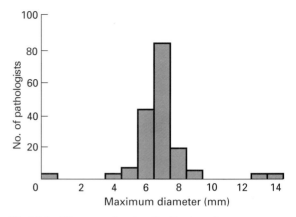

Fig 24.3 Histogram showing distribution of measurements of a case of DCIS made on 51 histological sections reported by 161 pathologists. The tumor was of similar size in all the circulated slides. The measurements are fairly tightly clustered, but there is a wide range due to a small number of outlying results. The explanation for these deviant measurements is not clear.

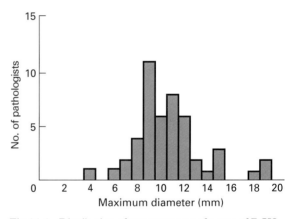

Fig 24.4 Distribution of measurements of a case of DCIS made on 51 histological sections. The lesion was of similar size in all circulated material but was irregular in outline and showed a very variable appearance, merging with areas of atypical hyperplasia. Only 51 pathologists attempted a measurement.

rarely encountered in lesions under 6 mm in size or in patients under 50 years of age. This probably explains the higher incidence of carcinoma in mammographically detected radial scars as smaller lesions are undetectable by radiography and, at least in the UK, screening is restricted to women who are at least 50 years of age. There is presently no evidence that women from whom uncomplicated scars are removed have a higher chance of developing cancer. None of the radial scars yet studied in the EQA scheme have shown foci of carcinoma or atypical hyperplasia.

Consistency of grading has been examined, with disappointing results. The grading procedure was very precisely defined before the onset of the scheme, even to the extent of measuring the high power fields in different microscopes in order to obtain accurate mitotic counts. The Kappa values for Grades 1, 2 and 3 for all participants were 0.36, 0.18 and 0.21 respectively. Somewhat higher values were obtained by 21 members of the UK National Coordinating Group for Breast Screening Pathology, but even these were unsatisfactory at 0.58, 0.40 and 0.38. The reasons for this lack of consistency in histological grading are not clear at the present time. It may be due to the inherent subjective nature of the method, although this now seems unlikely in view of several recent reports, all of which have demonstrated entirely satisfactory consistency with the Nottingham method.[21-23] It therefore seems much more likely that many of the participants did not actually consult the grading criteria. In a pilot study within the Trent region satisfactory Kappa values were obtained when 15–20 pathologists graded the same set of slides and followed the grading criteria strictly (Elston, 1995 — pers. comm.).

Surprisingly wide variations may be obtained in measuring invasive carcinomas. In most cases, however, measurements are tightly clustered and the wide ranges are due to a small number of outlying results (Fig. 24.5). As with DCIS, some cases do, however, show a large variation in tumor measurement as exemplified in Figure 24.6. Microscopically, this tumor exhibited a main mass surrounded by several small outlying foci of invasive carcinoma. It is important for clinicians and radiologists to remember that although tumors may appear to be well-circumscribed on clinical or radiological examination, they may be very poorly circumscribed microscopically and that reproducible measurements may consequently be very difficult to obtain in some cases. Figure 24.6 also shows the tendency for pathologists to round off measurements with peaks at 10 and 15 mm. In cancers with only one focus of tumor, over 90% of readings were within 3 mm of the median.

These findings indicate the kind of information that can be obtained from EQA schemes about

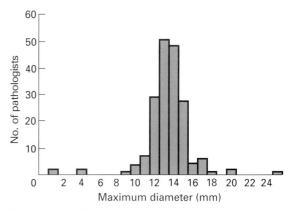

Fig 24.5 Distribution of measurements of an invasive carcinoma made on 51 histological sections by 203 pathologists. As in the case of DCIS illustrated in Figure 24.3, the results are tightly clustered with a few outlying results giving a broad range.

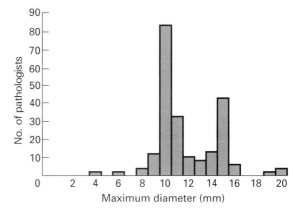

Fig 24.6 Distribution of measurements of an invasive carcinoma made by 107 pathologists on 51 circulated slides. The tumor was of similar overall size in all circulated material, but consisted of several separate foci.

pathologists' ability to report histological features consistently. They also point to possible methods of improving consistency. Such schemes can also be used to identify sub-standard performance although this has to be done on a consensus basis rather than on any preconception about what is the correct answer as in the so-called 'proficiency testing schemes' (see above, p. 531).

Care needs to be exercised in assessing substandard performance from consensus schemes. First of all, it is necessary to have an adequate number of participants in order for the consensus to have any validity. Secondly, it is inappropriate to assess performance on cases in which there is a significant level of disagreement. Thirdly, any diagnosis that deviates from the consensus should have clinical significance. Fourthly, there should be no evidence, e.g. from follow-up information, that the majority diagnosis is wrong. Finally, deviation from the majority diagnosis should occur persistently before any participant's performance is deemed sub-standard.

An important question is whether consensus schemes actually improve performance. Table 24.5 shows the overall Kappa values for new and old participants in each of six circulations of the UK Breast Pathology Scheme. The overall Kappa values appear rather low because they include the borderline cases. It can be seen in each of the circulations that the Kappa value is higher for experienced participants than participants who are taking part for the first time. Kappa values in each group, not surprisingly, change from one circulation to another as the cases vary in their level of difficulty. The differences between new participants and old participants cannot be explained by new participants with low scores leaving the scheme, i.e. failing to become old participants, as similar values are obtained if these are excluded. Consequently, this table provides evidence that participating in a scheme can itself improve diagnostic consistency.

Further evidence is obtained by comparing results with those obtained in a previous scheme funded by the Medical Research Council in the United Kingdom in association with a trial of early detection of breast cancer (TEDBC) in which Kappa values of 0.16, 0.67 and 0.76 were obtained for atypical hyperplasia, DCIS/microinvasive carcinoma and invasive carcinoma respectively.[17] All these values are lower than those achieved in the present UK national scheme where respective values of 0.25, 0.81 and 0.94 were obtained for 21 coordinators and 0.17, 0.70 and 0.83 for up to 250 non-coordinators. This achievement is all the more significant given that only nine pathologists participated in the TEDBC scheme and that the same slides were examined by all participants. It thus appears that efforts over several years from various quarters to improve diagnostic consistency in breast pathology in the UK have met with some success.

The scheme described above is, of necessity, artificial to some extent. Only one block per case was used and slides were unaccompanied by clinical details or information about macroscopic appearances. (This was felt not to be desirable given that the scheme was designed primarily to investigate the reporting of histological features.) Participants were obliged to report specific categories and there was no opportunity to express uncertainty. Furthermore, the sections were not cut and stained in the participants' own laboratories and may thus have exhibited appearances somewhat different from those to which they were accustomed. Finally, participants may not devote the same attention to EQA cases as to those which form part of their surgical workload. Nevertheless, this scheme and others like it have generated important information about consistency of reporting breast specimens.

Some of the problems that have been identified are predictable (e.g. diagnosing atypical hyperplasia) whereas others are not (e.g. measuring invasive carcinoma). Furthermore, it has been found that some conditions, e.g. radial scar, are diagnosed with much greater consistency than would have been anticipated.

Table 24.5 Overall Kappa statistics of new participants compared with old participants

Circulation	New participants		Old participants	
	No.	Kappa	No.	Kappa
1	185 (164)	0.53 (0.54)	15	0.58
2	64 (51)	0.52 (0.54)	144	0.59
3	29 (29)	0.65 (0.65)	187	0.74
4	33 (27)	0.69 (0.69)	212	0.72
5	15 (9)	0.61 (0.63)	230	0.69
6	11	0.55	240	0.57

Figures in brackets refer to new participants who persevered with the scheme, i.e. subsequently became old participants. (Reproduced by permission of the European Journal of Cancer.)

CYTOPATHOLOGY

Many of the approaches to quality assurance in breast cytopathology are the same as those in histopathology. They include issuing guidance on good working practice, standardizing terminology and diagnostic criteria and initiating slide exchange schemes to improve reporting consistency. Training and research are also indispensable in improving standards. In addition, performance can be monitored by relating findings to subsequent histological diagnoses which thus become a 'gold standard' reference in monitoring performance.[24]

Whereas guidance on practical procedures in histopathology largely concerns cut up and macroscopic examination, in cytopathology it relates mainly to obtaining and preparing high quality specimens. The former may fall within the province of cytopathologists themselves, unlike biopsy specimens which are the responsibility of the surgeon. The success of fine needle aspiration is directly related to the skill and experience of the operator. The number of staff involved should be restricted in order to ensure that they have adequate experience and trainees should be closely supervised. The aspirators may be clinicians or cytopathologists. The attendance of cytopathologists in breast clinics has the advantages of rapid, on the spot reporting and the opportunity to repeat the aspiration in the event of an unsatisfactory preparation, without recalling the patient to a subsequent outpatient clinic. Many cytopathologists, however, are unable to find the necessary time to spend in clinics in this way. Even greater skills are required to aspirate impalpable lesions which require localization by X-rays or ultrasound. These procedures are best carried out by radiologists who are specialists in breast imaging.

Guidance and training in the techniques for smearing aspirates and staining them is also vital. In breast screening programs, it is generally accepted that specimens which are unsatisfactory for whatever reason should not exceed 25% and in many centers it is much lower than this.

The decision about whether a patient requires a biopsy is based not only on the cytopathological data, but also on the findings of clinical examination and the imaging techniques employed. In order to be maximally effective, cytopathologists thus need to function as part of multidisciplinary teams.

As in histopathology, reporting consistency is best achieved by using a standard reporting form in which specimen type and localization procedure are given in addition to the cytological opinion. The last of these is usually divided into five categories:

1. unsatisfactory
2. benign
3. atypia, probably benign
4. suspicious of malignancy
5. definitely malignant.

Criteria for categorizing samples into these five major groups need to be stated clearly.

Investigating diagnostic consistency presents significantly greater problems in cytopathology than histopathology in view of the variations in staining technique and the uniqueness of cytological preparations. The inability to produce large numbers of identical preparations has two major drawbacks: (1) there is a reluctance to use slides for EQA purposes in view of their clinical importance; and (2) slide circulations take a very long time. Consensus and proficiency testing schemes have both been used in diagnostic cytopathology, particularly cervical cancer screening. In the latter, a coordinator usually visits a laboratory with a set of slides which, in the opinion of the scheme organizers, clearly fall into the major diagnostic categories. The slides are reported by pathologists and technical staff where appropriate and the reports are then assessed. If a participant's mark falls below a certain level, then the procedure is repeated. Further failures may necessitate participation in retraining schemes or, very rarely, in having to withdraw from cytological practice.

Consensus schemes are usually organized in small groups of pathologists or 'cells' around which the slides are circulated. Once they have been seen by all members of the cell, they can then be passed on to another one and recirculated. Analysis of reporting consistency can be undertaken at the end of the slide circulation. The general methods of analysis are similar to those employed for histopathology schemes although they are simpler as the number of features reported is much less.

The most effective and convenient method of monitoring a cytopathology service is to determine values for sensitivity and specificity in detecting carcinomas by relating cytological findings to subsequent histological diagnoses. It allows continuous monitoring of a cytopathology service, although it does not allow cytopathologists to compare their diagnoses with those of other pathologists in individual cases. A list of performance indices, together with how they are calculated, and acceptable values is shown in Table 24.6.

Table 24.6 Measures of performance in breast cytopathology[24]

Quality measure	Definition	Minimum acceptable value (palpable lesions)
Absolute sensitivity (C5)	The number of carcinomas diagnosed as such (C5) expressed as a percentage of the total number of carcinomas aspirated	>60%
Complete sensitivity	The number of carcinomas that were not definitely negative or inadequate on FNAC expressed as a percentage of the total number of carcinomas	>80%
Specificity	The number of correctly identified benign lesions (the number of C2 results minus the number of false negatives) expressed as a percentage of the total number of benign lesions aspirated	>60%
Positive predictive value	The number of correctly identified cancers (C5) expressed as a percentage of the total number of positive results	>95%
False negative rate*	The number of false negative results expressed as a percentage of the total number of carcinomas aspirated	<5%
False positive rate**	The number of false positive results expressed as a percentage of the total number of carcinomas aspirated	<1%
Inadequate rate	The number of inadequate specimens expressed as a percentage of the total number of cases aspirated	<25%

* A false negative case is defined as one which subsequently turns out (over the next 3 years) to be carcinoma having had a negative cytology result (this will by necessity include some cases where a different area from the lesion was aspirated but who turn up with interval cancer).

** A false positive case is defined as one which was given a C5 cytology result who turns out at open surgery to have a benign lesion (including atypical hyperplasia).

REFERENCES

1. Lamb J, Anderson TJ, Dixon MJ, Levack PA. Role of fine needle aspiration cytology in breast cancer screening. J Clin Pathol 1987; 40: 705.
2. Royal College of Pathologists Working Party. Pathology Reporting in Breast Cancer Screening. Screening Publications, 1990.
3. Bauermeister DE, Hall MH. Specimen radiography — a mandatory adjunct to mammography. Am J Clin Pathol 1973; 59: 782–789.
4. Rosen P, Snyder RE, Foote RW, Wallace T. Detection of occult carcinoma in the apparently benign breast biopsy through specimen radiography. Cancer 1970; 26: 944–952.
5. Holland R, Hendriks JHCL, Verbeek ALM, Mravunac M, Schuurmans Stekhoven JH. Extent, distribution, and mammographic/histological correlations of breast ductal carcinoma in situ. Lancet 1990; 335: 519–522.
6. Champ CS, Mason CH, Coghill SB, Robinson M. A perspex grid for localisation of non-palpable mammographic lesions in breast biopsies. Histopathol 1989; 14: 311–315.
7. Gauvin GP, Shortsleeve MJ, Ostheimer JT. A rapid technique for accurately localising microcalcifications in breast biopsy specimens. Am J Clin Pathol 1990; 93: 557–560.
8. Walker TM, Horton LWL, Menai Williams R. Impalpable breast lesions: marking of surgical specimens for pathology. Clin Radiol 1992; 45: 179–180.
9. Carter D. Margins of 'lumpectomy' for breast cancer. Hum Pathol 1986; 17: 330–332.
10. Schnitt SJ, Wang HH. Histologic sampling of grossly benign breast biopsies. How much is enough? Am J Surg Pathol 1989; 13: 505–512.
11. Schnitt SJ, Wang HH, Owings DV, Hann L. Sampling grossly benign breast biopsy specimens. Lancet 1989; ii: 1038.
12. Lagios MD. Duct carcinoma in situ. Pathology and treatment. Surg Clin N America 1990; 70: 853–871.
13. Sloane JP, Mayers MM. Carcinoma and atypical hyperplasia in radial scars and complex sclerosing lesions: importance of lesion size and patient age. Histopathol 1993; 23: 225–231.
14. Todd JH, Dowle C, Williams MR et al. Confirmation of a prognostic index in primary breast cancer. Br J Cancer 1987; 56: 489–492.
15. Elston CW, Ellis IO. Pathological prognostic factors in breast cancer. I. The value of histological grade in breast cancer: experience from a large study with long-term follow-up. Histopathol 1991; 19: 403–410.
16. Sloane JP and members of the National Coordinating Group for Breast Screening Pathology. Consistency of histopathological reporting of breast lesions detected by screening: findings of the UK National EQA Scheme. Eur J Cancer 1994; 30: 1414–1419.
17. Swanson Beck J and members of the Medical Research Council Breast Tumour Pathology Panel. Observer variability in reporting of breast lesions. J Clin Pathol 1985; 38: 1358–1365.
18. Rosai J. Borderline epithelial lesions of the breast. Am J Surg Pathol 1991; 15: 209–221.
19. Schnitt SJ, Connolly JL, Tavassoli FA et al. Interobserver reproducibility in the diagnosis of ductal proliferative breast lesions using standardised criteria. Am J Surg Pathol 1992; 16: 1133–1143.
20. Page DL, Rogers LW. Combined histologic and cytologic criteria for the diagnosis of mammary atypical ductal hyperplasia. Hum Pathol 1992; 23: 1095–1097.

21. Dalton LW, Page DL, Dupont WD. Histological grading of breast cancer: a reproducibility study. Cancer 1994; 73: 2765–2770.

22. Frierson HF Jr, Wolber RA, Berean KW et al. Interobserver reproducibility of the Nottingham modification of the Bloom and Richardson histologic grading scheme for infiltrating ductal carcinoma. Am J Clin Pathol 1995; 103: 195–198.

23. Robbins P, Pinder S, de Klerk N et al. Histological grading of breast carcinomas. A study of interobserver agreement. Hum Pathol 1995; 26: 873–879.

24. Cytology Sub-Group of the National Coordinating Committee for Breast Screening Pathology. Guidelines for Cytology Procedures and Reporting in Breast Cancer Screening. NHSBSP Publications, 1993.

Index